JOAQUIN O. UY, PH.D., M.D.

Radiology of Trauma

Textbook and Atlas

By H. Birzle, R. Bergleiter and E. H. Kuner

Translated by H. J. Kaufmann

1095 Figures

1978

W. B. Saunders Company Philadelphia · London · Toronto

Georg Thieme Publishers Stuttgart

AUTHORS:

Prof. Dr. HERMANN BIRZLE
Head of the Radiology Department at St.-Marien-Hospital Ludwigshafen/Rhein

Prof. Dr. RUDOLF BERGLEITER
Head of the Radiology Department at Katharinenhospital Stuttgart

Prof. Dr. EUGEN H. KUNER
Head of the Division of Trauma at Chirurgische Universitätsklinik Freiburg/Breisgau

TRANSLATOR:

Prof. Dr. HERBERT J. KAUFMANN
Hôpital des Enfants Malades,
149, Rue de Sevre, 75730 Paris

W. B. Saunders Company:
West Washington Square, Philadelphia, Pa. 19105

1 St. Anne's Rd., Eastbourne, East Sussex BN21 3UN, England

833 Oxford Street, Toronto, Ontario M8Z 5T9, Canada

English edition co-published 1978 by W. B. Saunders Company, Philadelphia, London, Toronto and Georg Thieme Verlag, Stuttgart

Radiology of Trauma

ISBN 0-7216-1703-4
LCCCN 76-20070

Last digit is the print number: 9 8 7 6 5 4 3 2 1

Translator's Foreword

Technological advances and mechanization in industry and homes as well as increased use of motor vehicles have brought us not only convenience in our present age but the threat of a multitude of traumatic injuries. The nature of injury may vary from youth to old age, but the risks are ever present. It is virtually unheard of for a person to grow up without requiring radiologic studies for obvious or suspected trauma at irregular intervals. The total of 102,500 deaths attributed to trauma among the population of the United States in 1975 is one measure of the magnitude of the problem. The cost to the national economy, estimated at 47.1 billion dollars, is another yardstick. The most tragic problem, besides the many deaths, is the huge number of 10.7 million disabling injuries. The accompanying Table shows these sad statistics; their inherent human drama and suffering can only be imagined.

Accidental Deaths and Injuries, 1975

	Number of Deaths	Number of Disabling Injuries	Cost
Motor Vehicle Accidents	46,000	1,800,000	$21.2 billion
(Pedestrians)	8,600		
Work Accidents	12,600	2,200,000	$16.0 billion
Home Accidents	25,500	400,000	$6.0 billion
Nonmotor Vehicle Public Accidents	22,500	2,800,000	$4.8 billion
Airplane Accidents	1,448	(Not available)	
Railroad Accidents	1,989	18,148	
TOTALS	102,500*	10,700,000**	$47.1 billion

* 4,100 counted in two categories
** 100,000 counted in two categories

(Figures supplied by National Safety Council estimates)

Against this background it is quite logical that in the United States there have been concentrated and successful efforts to develop traumatology into a specialty of its own within the last 15 years. Emergency room medicine within the hospital setting has taken a central place for the rapid and competent handling and care of all trauma patients, whereas in earlier days many would have been seen and treated in the private offices of the family physician or local surgeon. This development resulted in a continuously increasing need for qualified physicians especially trained and experienced in the diagnosis and management of trauma patients of all ages.

In the initial work-up of the injured patient, one of the key diagnostic tools is radiology. In order to offer the patient the best medical backup, the radiologist must evaluate the findings and the possible further usefulness of specialized radiologic techniques or investigations such as special views, fluoroscopy, tomography, neuroradiologic studies, angiographic procedures, nuclear medicine techniques, ultrasonography and CT scanning. It cannot be simply left to the emergency room physician, whether a specialist in traumatology or not, to review the x-ray films alone. This could be detrimental to the patient, who should have the timely benefit of competent radiologic consultation and not just the opinion of a radiologist on an x-ray report, ex post facto, dictated, typed and included in the case record, often many days later. In order to offer the patient an optimal radiologic work-up, immediate and repeated contacts are necessary with radiologists qualified to function in the many aspects of traumatology. Reality frequently dictates that radiologists in training – residents – cover the needs arising in the emergency room at all hours. This book attempts to provide for these and all radiologists the background information necessary for the optimal benefit of the trauma patient.

This book offers basic radiologic information to the radiologist responsible in these areas. Beyond this, however, it will be equally helpful to those primary physicians – the traumatologist, orthopedic surgeon, general surgeon, neurosurgeon and others – in whose hands the care of the injured patient truly lies.

November 1977

Herbert J. Kaufmann

Foreword

According to statistical data provided by the World Health Organization, annually 100,000 people die in traffic accidents, 1–1.5 million are severely injured and 3–4 million are slightly injured. Between 1953 and 1976, the number of traffic accidents increased from 473,000 to 1,417,000 (West German Federal Office of Statistics). Most accidents involving children occur in the street. Ninety per cent of the most serious injuries and 80 per cent of the fatalities involving children are traffic accidents (Rheinpfalz [daily newspaper] No. 215/77). It should be noted that traffic accidents comprise only 20 per cent of the total, about the same as for household accidents. The vast majority of accidents occur at the place of work, although a distinct decline has been recorded (1963: 2,618,544 – 1975: 1,760,713 [West German Federal Office of Statistics]). With the development of popular sports, the incidence of sports injuries has increased significantly. In 1967, 240,000 sport injuries were recorded. The most recent statistics, however, reveal that, alone in April 1974, 55,000 sport-related injuries were reported (West German Federal Office of Statistics). A significant decline in the total number of accidents is unlikely, rather, a further escalation in number should be anticipated. The conclusion, therefore, is that there will be a greater need for physicians well trained in traumatology in order to meet the challenge for more and better diagnostic radiologic services.

During the daily x-ray sessions with young residents in training, and from the many daily questions raised by clinical and surgical colleagues, it became evident that the knowledge necessary for proper diagnostic radiologic interpretation in traumatology can be acquired only slowly and in a setting where the person learning has an opportunity to profit from his or her own active participation.This refers not only to the ability to properly and reliably recognize traumatic changes on roentgenograms but also to the judgment to recognize indications for the further use of radiologic diagnostic measures when internal organs are involved. With this aim in mind, the younger residents working with me in the radiology department and various other departments of the Freiburg University Surgical Hospital have inspired me to write a book on traumatologic x-ray diagnosis. Georg Thieme Verlag was receptive to this idea.

By the nature of the topic, the effectiveness of such a book will rest on the strength of its illustrations. It was my intention not to show the most severe and unusual types of trauma but to present the basic x-ray symptoms and particularly x-rays that will cause the observer to collaborate actively while viewing them. The illustrations selected should give the beginner an opportunity to accumulate experience in viewing such material for which he would need a much longer time if he attempted to acquire this experience in daily practice.

I am thankful to many of my collaborators at this hospital for important cases presented here. The accumulation of documentary material and particularly clinical information has been greatly facilitated through the kind services of the secretaries of the Institute. I would like to thank our colleagues from the Surgical Clinic for letting us use clinical data.

I would like to express my gratitude to Dr. Kuner for his chapter Internal Fixation and Its Radiologic Evaluation.

I would also like to express my gratitude to Dr. Bergleiter for his chapter Neuroradiologic Diagnosis with Contrast Studies After Skull-Brain Trauma and Injuries to the Spine and the new Chapter Axial Computer Tomography in the Diagnosis of Skull-Brain Trauma.

Ludwigshafen, December 1977

Hermann Birzle

Contents

Introduction

The physician active in traumatologic-roentgenologic practice, whether in an office or a hospital, must be fully cognizant of the indications for x-ray examination in certain injuries and of the instances when special examinations are needed. He must know all the standard views and the most important special x-ray incidences and, in addition, he must be in a position to fully interpret them. This has as a prerequisite detailed knowledge of the respective normal x-ray appearances, of normal variations and of the distinction between the latter and true disease. The specialist in radiology, furthermore, must be fully familiar with the technical and equipment aspects of obtaining proper radiographs. Every physician involved in the use of ionizing radiation and the ancillary personnel working in an x-ray department must be fully trained in the performance of radiodiagnostic measures and must be equally aware of the potential genetic and somatic damage due to ionizing radiation (Graul and Stockhausen, 1968).

Normal Findings and Variations

The normal form, size and articulation of the bones and joints forming the skeletal system are known to the physician from his studies in anatomy. The comparative interpretation of these structures on an x-ray usually does not offer particular difficulties. The contours and the structure itself, as well as the density of the different individual skeletal parts, play an important role in traumatologic diagnosis. When there is doubt, a comparative roentgenogram of the corresponding uninjured region may offer full clarification. It is recommended, however, that the uninitiated first consult the specialized literature and not simply ask for unnecessary x-rays out of lack of knowledge. Variations and minor malformations of the skeletal system are often difficult to differentiate properly from traumatic alterations. This refers particularly to the many accessory bony elements and the sesamoid bones and also to other so-called possible sources of error, i. e., normal but sometimes impressive irregularities of bony contours and even structural irregularities. The main variants that are particularly relevant in the context of traumatologic radiologic diagnosis and may be causes for misinterpretation are presented in Figures 1 to 4. For discussion of the manifold differences in the normal x-ray appearance of the skeleton of the growing child during the different ages and the developmental phases, see Chapter 12.

"The Borderline of the Normal and the Beginning of the Abnormal on X-rays of the Skeleton" (Köhler and Zimmer, 1968) assumes particular importance, since in the differential diagnosis one must consider, besides traumatic alterations, other possibly causative or contributing disorders.

On x-rays of the thorax and the abdomen, these individual variations are much less important, but the possibility of other nontraumatic alterations is considerably greater. Particular attention has to be devoted to evaluating the transparency of the lungs, the delineation of both diaphragms, and the size, form, position and motility of internal organs. In the abdomen, one must consider the gas and fluid content of the entire gastrointestinal canal as well as of the abdominal cavity itself. Importance must be attached to the proper knowledge of the exact position, form and size of the parenchymatous organs.

Even a normal or seemingly normal roentgen investigation may in some cases still require a follow-up or further radiologic investigations since, particularly in the case of trauma to the thorax or abdomen, the x-ray alterations may appear only after a delay of several hours or sometimes even after several days.

Technical and Roentgenographic Principles

The performance of the requested roentgenogram can usually be left to properly certified x-ray technicians, who are fully familiar with the standard views. The object of any study is initially examined at least on two perpendicular planes. The x-ray obtained in the sagittal plane is often referred to as the sagittal view or simply the a.p. view; if the rays are applied from behind, the view is designated as the p.a. view. An x-ray in the frontal plane is designated as a lateral view. With respect to additional specialized views and techniques such as tomograms or stereoscopic views, the physician in charge of the patient should not underestimate the advice and the knowledge of an experienced x-ray technician. It will benefit neither the patient nor the cooperation between physicians and auxiliary personnel if a still inexperienced physician orders special views that he thinks might be of value but that technically are impossible to obtain. If in doubt, there can always be found a technically reliable and experienced radiologist who will be available for help. Furthermore, there are sufficient books describing exposure data, techniques and guidelines for proper exposure.

On the whole, the use of a relatively soft exposure is generally accepted today for the demonstration of bony detail. This implies roentgenograms with medium exposure at 60 to 80 kV.; for the thorax and abdominal organs, high kV. technique (90 to 120 kV.); and for the soft tissues, the use of the lowest possible kV. which, in some instances, is around 40 kV. In each situation, the exposure data are dictated by the technical equipment available. In most departments, there are experienced people at work using proven and successful data. The so-called portable x-rays obtained on patients in bed demand specialized technical skill and general experience on the part of the x-ray technician. The limited capacity of portable equipment can be somewhat offset by using better amplifier screens.

X-rays of thick parts, usually from the knee upward, may require measures to remove scattered radiation by using a so-called Bucky cassette. The injured person or the injured part of the body should be positioned and repositioned carefully, avoiding pain as much as possible. The physician should decide whether the patient can be positioned on the x-ray examination table, whether the view can be better obtained with the patient in bed or on a stretcher or whether bandages, casts or extension hardware should be removed or need to be left on. X-rays of the pelvis, abdomen and spinal column, however, can only be performed with sufficient technical quality on a Bucky table. Special stretchers with Bucky cassettes are available today. These and a detachable nonopaque top should find a much wider distribution. Such specialized transportation and initial investigation stretchers should therefore be simple and, as much as possible, ensure painless positioning and moving of the injured patient.

In the case of trauma to the thorax or abdomen, a fluoroscopic investigation with spot-filming may be particularly valuable since this may lead to a rapid and reliable diagnosis. In any case, it is important for the physician in charge of the patient to know in which position x-rays are to be obtained.

The proper markings of the right or left side should never be overlooked. It is best to position this marker laterally and distal to the part of the body that is to be investigated. In lateral views, the side of the body close to the film will be so marked. Objects such as jewelry, glasses, watches, dentures, bracelets and necklaces that have to be removed in order to get good x-rays should be placed in a plastic bag or a piece of cloth among the patient's possessions. They should never be simply put aside with materials to be discarded because of the danger of total loss. Special care is necessary if the patient has lost consciousness or is in shock. Physicians and auxiliary personnel must pay attention to the most trivial details if they want to be fully protected from suspicion or lawsuits.

Indications for X-ray Examinations After Injuries

An indication to obtain roentgen examinations after injury or trauma exists in any suspected bony injury. In the case of accidents at work or if there might be legal and insurance implications, an x-ray investigation is justified. There is, however, no doubt that today, with so many minor injuries, there are far too many unnecessary x-ray investigations. And yet in questionable injuries to internal organs there are too few instances when the radiologic techniques are properly utilized. A careful radiologic investigation, perhaps using special methods, is indicated in the following situations: injury to the central nervous system, particularly with altered sensorium; blunt or open trauma to the thorax; blunt or open trauma to the abdomen; contusions of the kidney or trauma to the pelvis with hematuria or disturbed micturition; and foreign body injury or massive injury of the soft tissues with possible concomitant involvement of internal organs.

Multiple fractures or multiple trauma by necessity require an extensive radiologic investigation in order not to overlook fractures of vertebral bodies, dislocated hips and shoulders or possible internal injuries. A serious problem is often presented by severely injured unconscious patients. One should never perform an x-ray investigation if the condition of the circulatory or respiratory system is such that the life of the patient is threatened. Therefore, the traumatized patient must first be examined by a physician who will then give his diagnosis and request the proper radiologic investigation. Particularly in view of the possibility of internal injuries, it is never acceptable to have an initial examination performed by a nurse or an x-ray technician. If, on the basis of an initial insufficient general examination, x-ray investigations are incomplete or omitted altogether, there can be far-reaching medical and medicolegal consequences. Therefore, it is also unacceptable simply and solely to perform a fluoroscopic investigation even with an image intensifier. Such an approach is totally inadequate!

Superficial injuries to the soft tissues ordinarily do not require an x-ray investigation. An x-ray is, however, needed if there appears to be a foreign body present – for example, within the eyeball, after a deep penetrating knife wound of the thorax or abdomen, or in an open joint injury; or if indirectly one suspects traumatic injury such as pulmonary infarction, fat embolism, toxic or cardiac pulmonary edema, or stress ulcer of the stomach. In such instances, the respective x-ray investigation may offer positive or negative proof. Finally, the importance of postmortem roentgenograms to establish a correct diagnosis after injuries should be acknowledged. This type of investigation can offer critical information for identification and for establishing the cause of an injury and its mechanism, which may help to solve a crime.

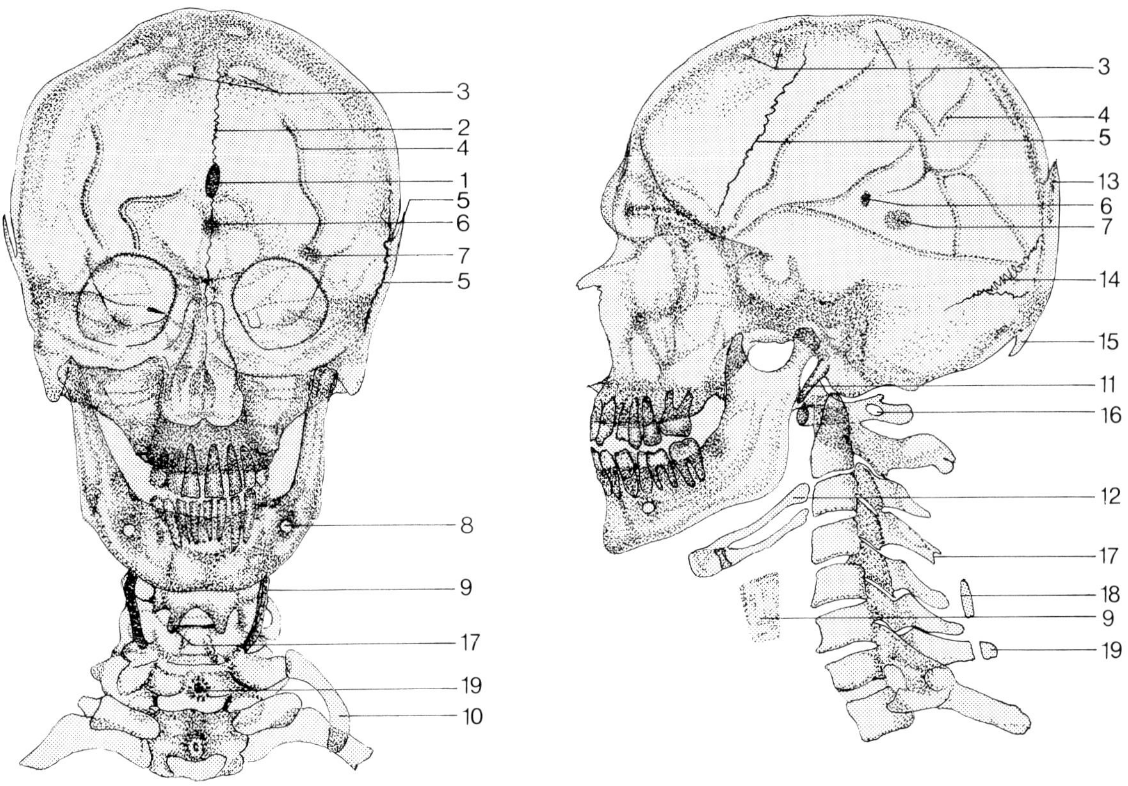

Fig. 1. Variations and possible sources for misinterpretation: skull and cervical spine.

1 Calcification within the falx
2 Persistent frontal suture
3 Pacchioni's granulations
4 Vascular grooves
5 Sutures
6 Calcification within the pineal body
7 Calcification within the plexus
8 Foramen mentale
9 Calcified thyroid cartilage
10 Cervical rib
11 Styloid processes
12 Hyoid bone
13 Parieto-occipital overlap
14 Sutures
15 Occipital protuberance
16 Foramen arcuale
17 Forked dorsal process
18 Ossification within the nuchal ligament
19 Persistent apophysis

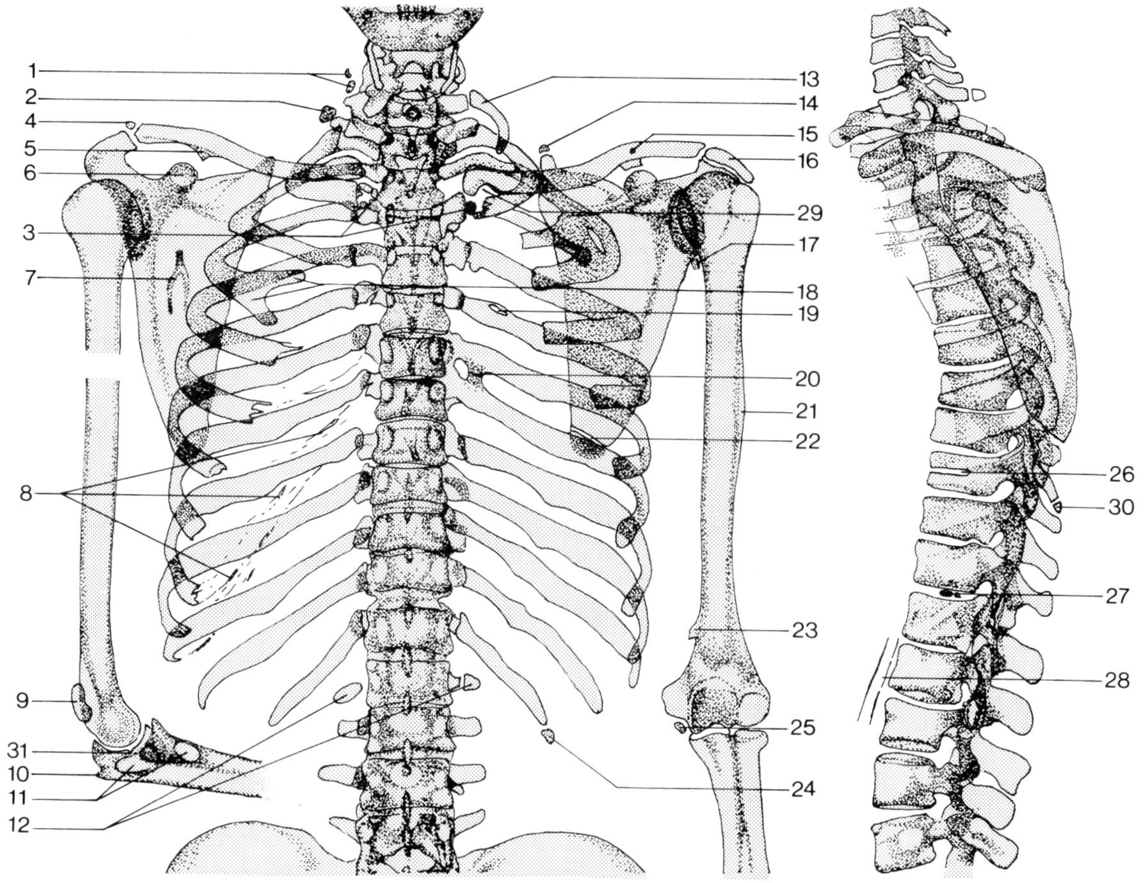

Fig. 2. Variations and possible sources for misinterpretation: thorax, thoracic spine, regions of shoulder and elbow.

1 Calcified lymph nodes
2 Persistent central ossification
3 Anterior portion of the first rib
4 Accessory ossicle
5 Protuberance of clavicle possibly forming a joint with the coracoid process
6 Coracoid process, isolated as coracoid bone
7 Vascular channels
8 Calcifications within the cartilage of ribs
9 Patella of the forearm
10 Protuberance of the olecranon
11 Normal thin zone
12 Lumbar ribs L 1
13 Cervical ribs
14 Persistent apophysis
15 Canal of supraclavicular nerve
16 Acromial bone
17 Glenoidal bone
18 Forked rib
19 Hole in ribs
20 Bridging in between ribs
21 Deltoid tuberosity
22 Persistent apophysis
23 Supracondylar process
24 Persistent center of ossification
25 Accessory ossicle
26 Vascular channel
27 Calcification of nucleus pulposus
28 Calcified abdominal aorta
29 Groove in medial portion of clavicle
30 Isolated pit of spinous process
31 Normal incisura of trochlea notch

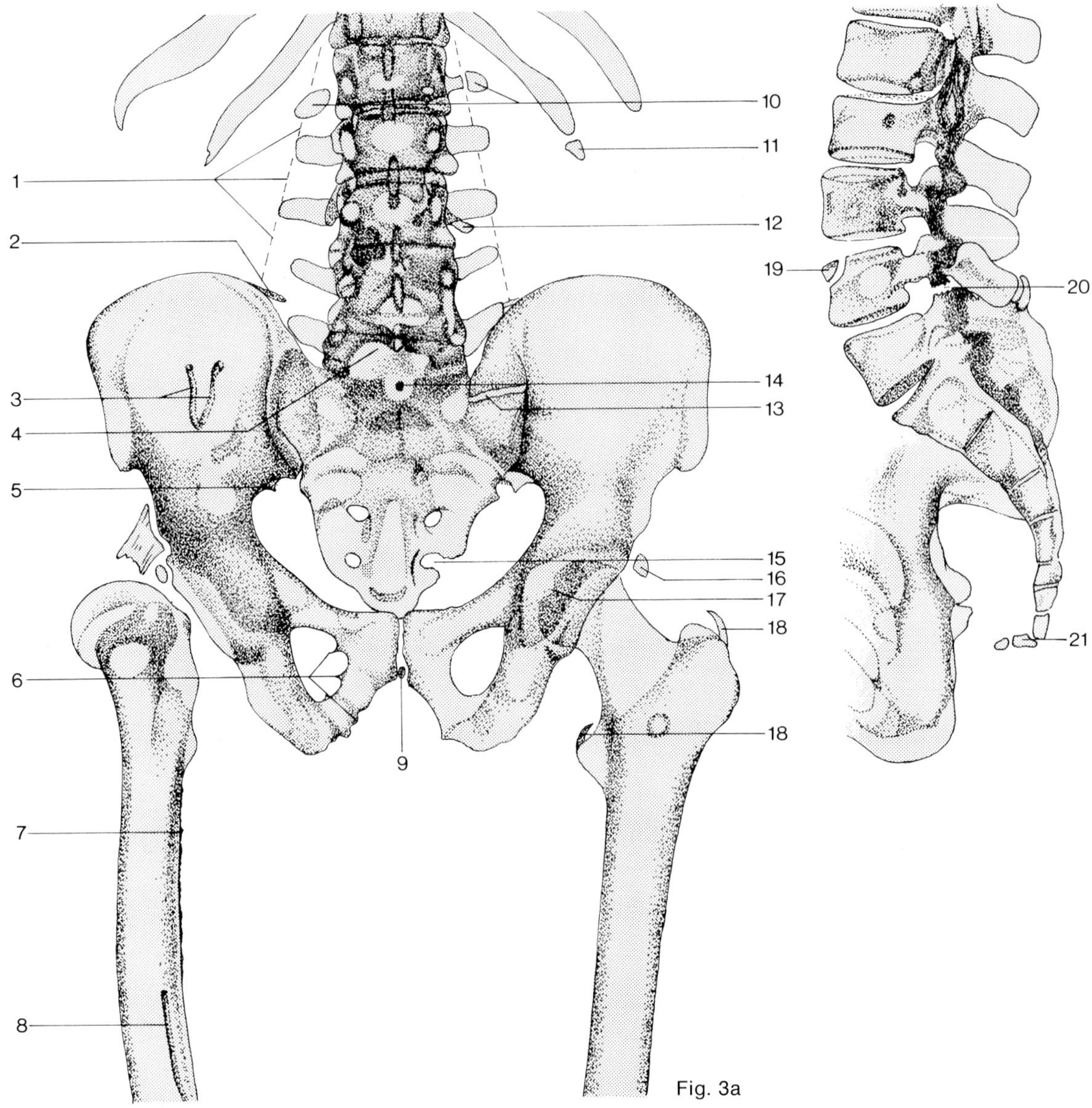

Fig. 3a

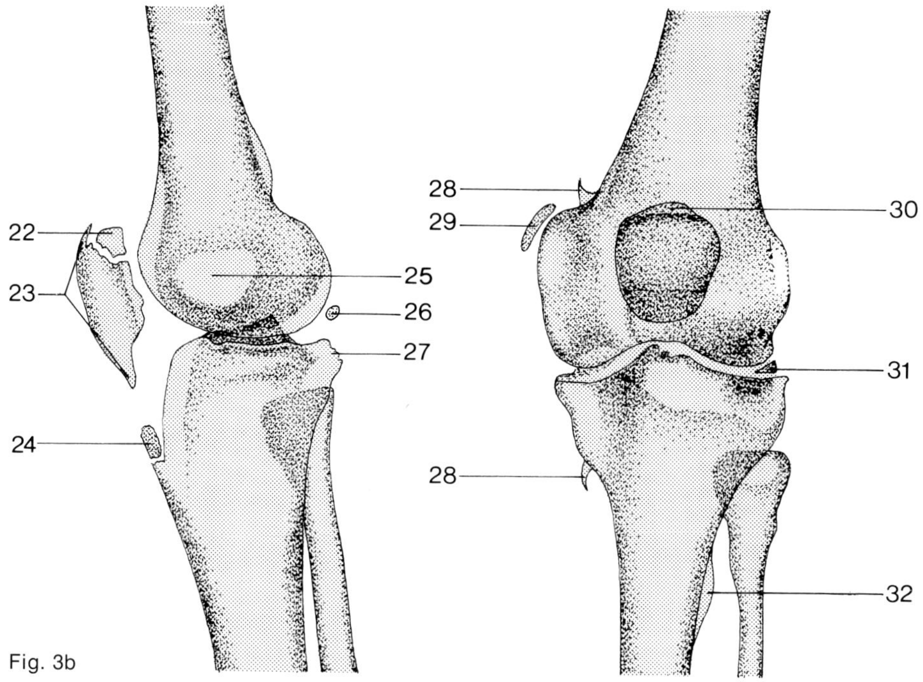

Fig. 3b

Fig. 3a and b. Variations and possible sources for misinterpretation: a) pelvis, lumbar spine, sacrum, hip joints, femur; b) knee joints.

1 Psoas contour
2 Ossified iliolumbar ligament
3 Vascular channels
4 Asymmetric closure of arch
5 Paraglenoidal sulcus
6 Normal hump and thorns
7 Linea aspera
8 Vascular channel
9 Isolated central ossification
10 Lumbar ribs (variable)
11 Persistent ossification center
12 Styloid process
13 Accessory joint
14 Isolated apophysis of spinal process
15 Congenital minor cleft
16 Acetabular bone
17 Fovea
18 Spur of trochanter
19 Nontraumatic anterior avulsion
20 Congenital cleft formation
21 Acute angle of coxitis
22 Patella partita
23 Spur of patella (ossification at origin of tendon)
24 Isolated tuberosity of tibia
25 Ludloff's zone of thinning
26 Fabella
27 Normal rough contour
28 Small exostoses
29 Stieda shadow (post-traumatic)
30 Thickening of border (normal)
31 Calcification within meniscus
32 Normal protrusion

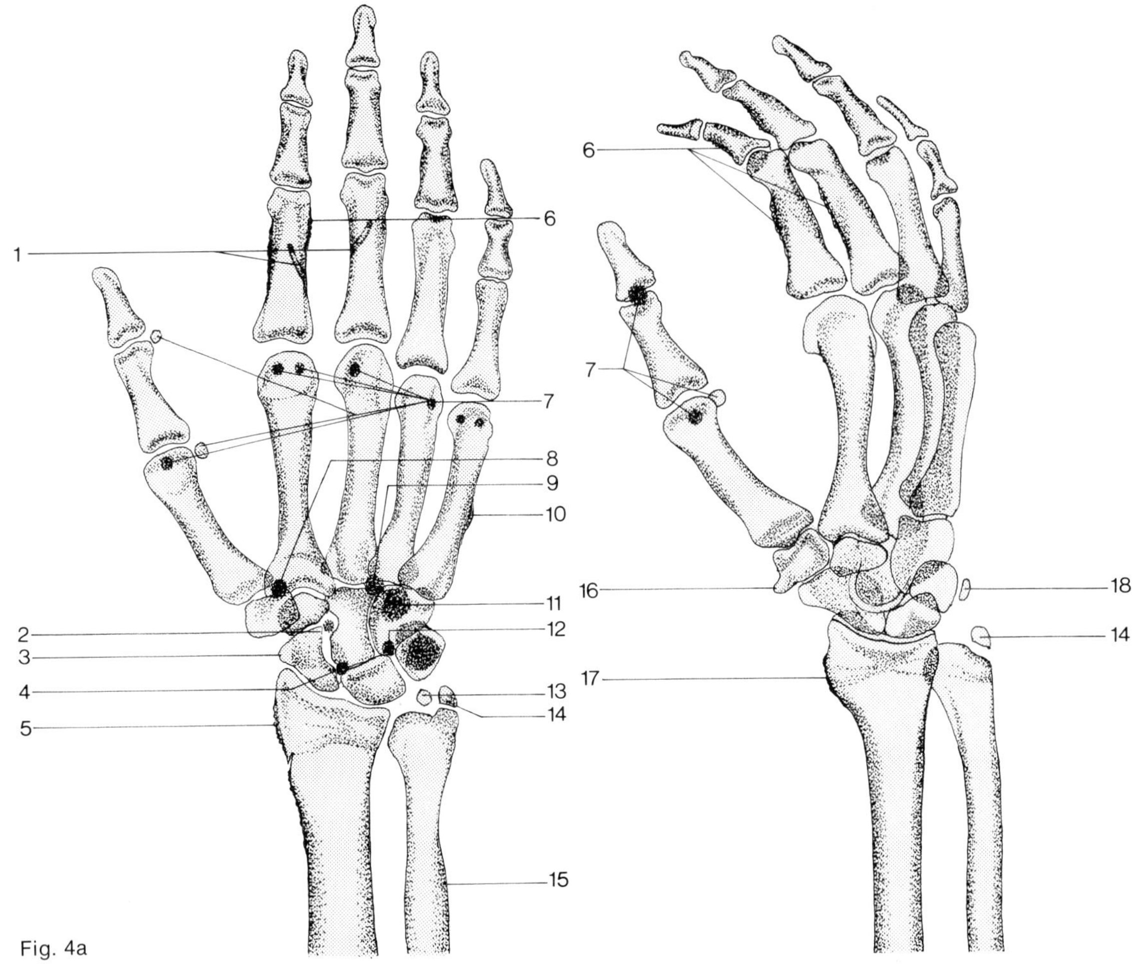

Fig. 4a

Fig. 4a and b. Variations and possible sources for misinterpretation: a) forearm and hand; b) lower leg and foot with respective joints.

1 Vascular channels
2 Os centrale
3 Tuberculum of navicular bone
4 Hypolunatum
5 Rough edge
6 Hump and rough edges – tendon insertion
7 Sesamoids
8 Secondary trapezoid bone
9 Secondary capitate bone
10 Normal hump
11 Hamulus of hamate
12 Epitriquetrum
13 Triangular bone
14 Styloid bone
15 Normal thickening
16 Turberculum of trapezoid bone
17 Normal roughening
18 Epitriquetrum (frequent avulsion)
19 Secondary calcaneus
20 Supranavicular bone
21 Rare accessory ossicles
22 Intermetatarsal bone
23 Sesamoids (may be divided)
24 Pseudofissure (Mach effect)
25 Trigonal bone
26 Insertion of Achilles tendon
27 Spur of calcaneus
28 Peroneal bone
29 Vesalian bone
30 Triangular thin zone
31 Pseudoatrophy (thin zone)
32 Subfibular bone
33 Subtibial bone
34 Sustentacular bone
35 Periosteal thickening
36 Retinacular bone
37 Subfibular bone
38 External tibial bone
39 Peroneal bone
40 Sesamoids

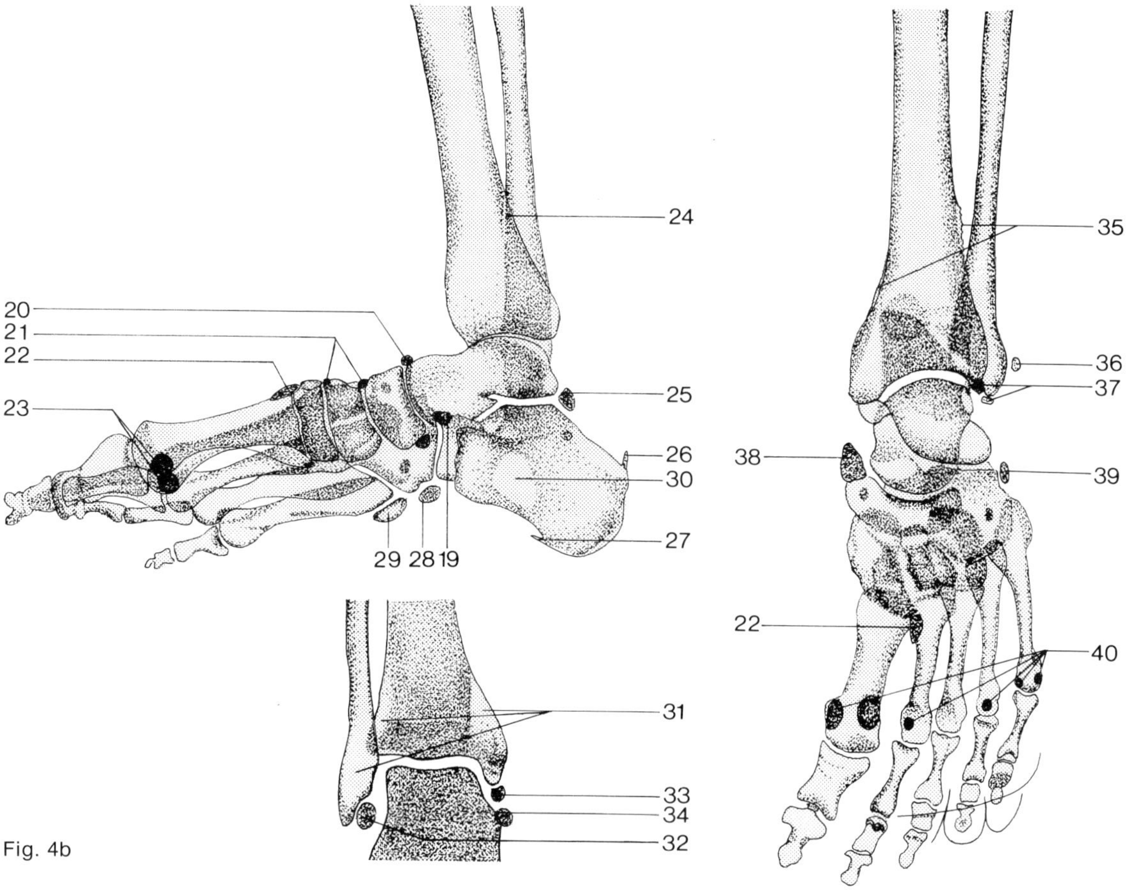

Fig. 4b

Course of Investigations

Requisition for an X-ray Investigation

In the majority of cases, it is possible after an accident to send a patient with a regular requisition form for the required x-ray investigation. On the requisition form, there should be adequate information about the history, physical examination and suspected diagnosis, and possibly a clearly defined question for the radiologist. The more thorough the initial investigation and the clearer the questions asked, the better it will be for the radiologist and his investigation.

Pertinent information about the person injured is important in order to avoid the serious consequence of confusion of films and to ensure adequate and proper film marking and billing. In cases where the patient has lost consciousness, information must be obtained from the accompanying person. Its content may have to be corroborated later. X-rays of unconscious traumatized patients must be marked as clearly as possible and in a permanent fashion so that they cannot be confused with others. If a new traumatized patient has to be sent to another institution or to another division of the hospital, the latest posttrauma x-rays should accompany the patient and be marked as clearly as possible as to their origin, identity and date.

In cases of x-ray investigation of the skeleton of patients with severe injuries, there should always be a physician present. Open complicated fractures require particular attention during the examination in the x-ray department. They must be treated and remain covered with sterile bandages if this has not been done previously. If there are visible bony elements outside an injury, they should never be retracted. No disinfectant agents should be put on open wounds, particularly with visible bony particles. During the investigation for injuries to internal organs, the cooperation of the primary physician is mandatory during fluoroscopy and particularly while contrast studies are performed. If several different investigations are needed, he will have to decide on the sequence. Furthermore, he has to decide whether bandages can be removed or should remain in place and if and how the patient can be positioned. It is valuable in many instances, after the first x-rays are obtained, to review the problem of a given patient. Possibly there are further special views necessary to fully clarify an inconclusive finding. This can then be done immediately. Close cooperation between physician and x-ray technicians will result in greater speed in performing the investigation, which is in the patient's best interest.

X-ray Analysis

In order to fully and competently evaluate an x-ray or a series of x-rays, one needs concentration, a good view box, adequate time and a considerable amount of experience. The view box should have the proper degree of luminescence and should be controllable as to the area illuminated and covered by film. In addition, there should be a so-called iris spotlight with an adaptable round field of vision in order to better visualize areas of intensive film blackening. If a spotlight is not available, one can also use a simple desk lamp with a strong enough light bulb. The significance of a sufficient period of observation is frequently underestimated. Rapid diagnoses often are misdiagnoses or at least incomplete and unreliable ones. For the majority of investigators, a complete x-ray analysis will involve three complete steps. Many will perform these subconsciously and in differing sequences:

1. A comparison with a normal case from one's individual memory when the question is asked: What is *not* normal here?
2. A deliberate search for an x-ray finding that can be expected on the basis of known clinical information.
3. An organized investigation of all the visualized details of structure and contour.

An exhaustive x-ray analysis, therefore, is not simply a cursory evaluation but systematic work comparable to that involved in acquiring the anamnestic data or in a clinical investigation.

The Report

The x-ray report should be as simple and clear as possible. In principle, it should contain a descriptive part with a subsequent concise evaluation which would correspond to the diagnosis. In simple cases and in follow-up examinations, one need not adhere to this rule. Very busy physicians will prefer to use an abbreviated style in their reports.

The different forms of fractures are designated in the x-ray report according to their radiologic appearance (Fig. 5). In many instances, the cause and mechanism of the fracture are also given, since they can be fully recognized from the radiologic appearance. Often from the x-ray it may also be possible to tell whether a fracture is open or closed.

The most frequently occurring abnormal positions for fractures are given in Figure 6. Dislocations near the palm of the hand and the sole of the foot are designated as volar angulation or displacement and plantar angulation or displacement, respectively. With regard to the mode and direction of the dislocations, there are all sorts of possible combinations.

Even though the x-ray report does not form the basis for therapy, since the physician at the time of a fracture reposition will always rely on the original x-rays, it should still fully reflect the facts. The report, just like the x-ray itself, is a document that may have to be used when the x-ray is lost, for the follow-up evaluation, for scientific investigation or for expert opinion. A short and concise description of a fracture and of the follow-up x-rays can be expected from every clinically active physician. In the evaluation of the follow-up examinations, particular attention should be directed to comments about the position of the fragments, callus formation, atrophy of bone, bony consolidation and, finally, the proper trabeculation in the area of the fracture. The various metallic devices now used for internal fixation should be properly designated (see Figs. 13.19–13.25).

An x-ray analysis and report in the case of injuries to internal organs may be much more difficult to make and therefore require more experience since the traumatic alterations are much less obvious and are frequently only recognized by indirect findings. The report on the thorax should first refer to the form of the thoracic cage, the transparency and air content of the lungs, the appearance of the mediastinum and the position and delineation of both diaphragms. In evaluating the abdomen, special at-

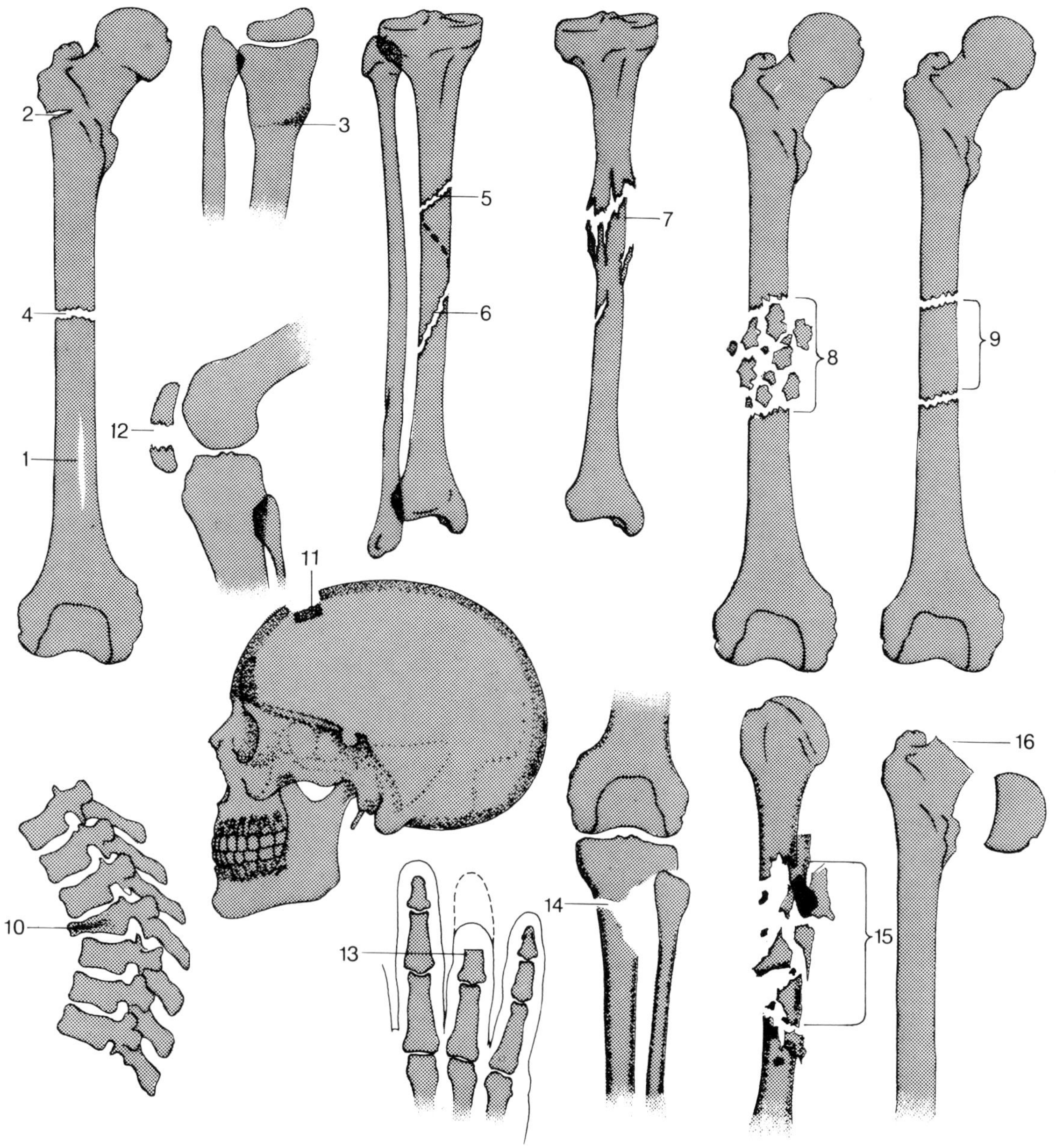

tention should be given to the form, size, position and delineation of the internal parenchymatous organs. In case of suspicion or a clinical question, it is necessary to comment on the abnormal x-ray findings that could be expected in this situation.

Fig. 5. Types of fractures.

1 Fissure
2 Infraction
3 Greenstick fracture
4 Transverse fracture
5 Oblique fracture (short, long)
6 Spiral fracture
7 Splinter fracture
8 Comminuted fracture
9 Piece fracture
10 Compression fracture
11 Depressed fracture
12 Avulsion fracture
13 Amputation
14 Pathologic fracture
15 Gunshot fracture
16 Traumatic epiphyseolysis

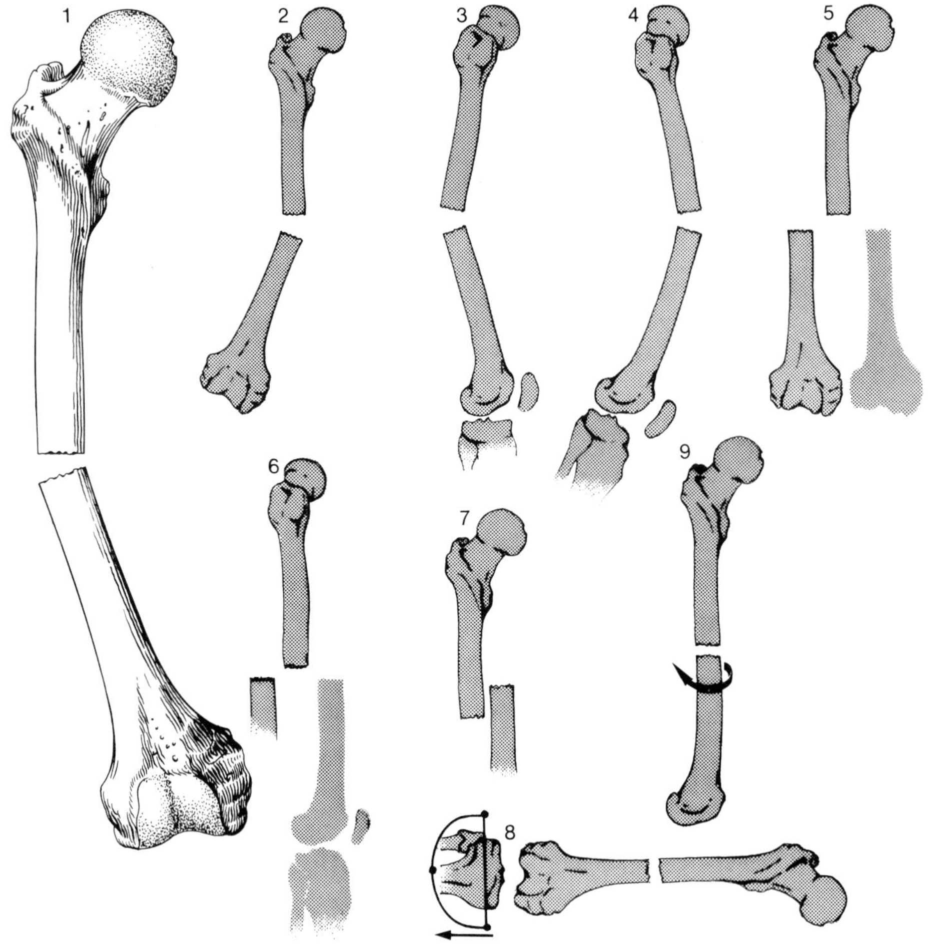

Fig. 6. Abnormal position of fracture fragments.

1 Angulation of the distal fragment medially: varus position
2 Angulation of the distal fragment laterally: valgus position.
3 Angulation of the distal fragment anteriorly: incurvation or ventral angulation
4 Angulation of the distal fragment posteriorly: antecurvation or dorsal angulation
5 Lateral position of the distal fragment medially or laterally
6 Displacement of the distal fragment anteriorly or posteriorly (ventrally or dorsally)
7 Abnormal position due to shortening
8 Abnormal position due to distraction or lengthening
9 Abnormal position due to rotation

1 Skull

During peacetime, skull and brain injuries are largely the result of traffic accidents. According to studies of large numbers of cases, the skull is involved in 65 per cent of all injured persons and in 71 per cent of all people killed in accidents (Ricklin, 1958). Less frequently, the following causes are listed: accidents in shafts, during the performance of sports (skiing, tobogganing, mountaineering) and during daily activities (such as a fall from a ladder or from a chair); being hit by objects; injuries due to violence by means of projectiles during fights and as a result of criminal actions. The amount of skull and brain injuries sustained in accidents of all sorts is roughly 25 per cent (Friedmann and Frowein, 1966a).

The increase in the number of severe skull and brain injuries during the last two decades is the result particularly of the increased speed of vehicles. The average mortality of skull and brain injuries is around 6.5 per cent (Lorenz, 1966). In traffic accidents, skull and brain injuries are the leading cause of death. In about 25 per cent of all victims of traffic accidents, there cannot be found any signs of fracture of the skull (Zatzkin, 1965). This fact is an indication that the traumatization of the brain, particularly the brain stem, is of primary importance and that a fracture of the skull as well as its radiologic demonstration are of only secondary importance to the fate of the injured person. Very frequently, there is no direct correlation between the severity of the brain damage on one side and the degree of an existing skull fracture on the other. In spite of this, it will frequently be possible to evaluate the significance and degree of trauma to the brain on the basis of the survey film of the skull according to the type and severity of an existing fracture and its localization (Göhring and Weber, 1962).

If there is no primary need for measures directed against edema of the brain, hemorrhage, shock, central respiratory depression, aspiration and disturbances of temperature regulation, an x-ray investigation will be conducted as rapidly as possible particularly when an impression fracture, a penetrating injury or intracranial hemorrhage (see Chapter 3) is suspected. In all other situations, the radiographic investigation can be postponed until several days after the actual injury, since the greatest danger to the patient stems not from the fracture but from shock, edema of the brain and intracranial hemorrhage.

Obtaining good-quality early roentgenograms of a patient with a recent skull and brain injury can be most difficult and tedious. Loss of consciousness, the restlessness and excitation that frequently follow alcoholic intake or result from accompanying severe injuries, superficial hemorrhage and vomiting often cannot be controlled and may make it impossible to obtain useful roentgenograms.

A routine investigation consists of x-rays of the skull on two planes, together with a p.a. or a.p. projection of the facial structures. In addition, there may be need for special views of the nasal bone, the zygomatic arch, the petrous bone and the base of the skull, the mandible, the mandibular joint and the teeth. Atypical half-axial or tangential views may also be required (Schoen, 1956; Clementschitsch, 1951). Good-quality survey films of the skull undoubtedly contain the best and most reliable information. In special

cases (for instance, with penetrating foreign bodies), it may be helpful, in addition, to obtain stereoscopic views or tomograms.
For stereoscopic views, the lateral projection is preferable.
During the evaluation of skull films, the following points need special consideration:

1. External form, shape and symmetry.
2. External and internal contours, structure and density of the tables of the skull as well as the normally present sutures, vascular channels, venous emissaries and their numerous variations (compare Figure 1, Introduction). There are possible causes for confusion. Fractures may be simulated by the squamosal suture, the mendosal suture, the parietomastoid suture and the occipitomastoid suture as well as the rarely seen frontal suture. Among the vascular channels, particular attention must be given to the medial meningeal artery (epidural hematoma), because of possible crossing over with a fracture line.
3. Form and delineation of the most prominent anatomic landmarks such as the sella turcica, the petrous bones, both orbits and the mastoids.
4. Delineation and transparency of the paranasal sinuses (opacification, free air-fluid level on the basis of exudate or hematoma).
5. Form and contour of the bones of the facial skeleton including the joints of the jaw.
6. Appearance of all the surrounding soft tissues (investigate with the spotlight).

Skull fractures are grouped according to their localization – as fractures of the skull, of the facial structures and of the base of the skull.
According to the mechanism of its origin, a fracture can be further characterized as a bending fracture, a bursting fracture, a penetrating injury of the skull due to projectiles or the direct result of a forceful event and, finally a special type of growing fracture during childhood.
In describing the radiologic findings, it is best to choose a classification according to the different types of fractures and add details about the localization:

Fractures of the Skull

Linear fracture (fissure, fissure-type fracture, splint or cleft fracture, splintering type fracture), fracture of an individual piece, comminuted fracture, depressed fracture, fracture due to projectiles.

Fractures of Facial Structures

Fracture of the nasal bones (fissure, transverse fracture, comminuted fracture), nasomaxillary fracture, zygomaticomaxillary fracture, palatoalveolar fracture, combined facial fractures, fracture of the orbit, fracture of the jaw (fracture of the body, the ramus or the processes of the mandible).

Fracture of the Base of the Skull

Fractures can be localized according to the exact area within the anterior, middle or posterior fossa.

Fractures of the Skull

Among fractures of the skull, it may be most difficult to recognize and demonstrate a linear fracture with a very narrow cleft. The actual fracture is more readily visible on the side close to the film since its delineation is clearer there, whereas on the side away from the film it is less well defined and of poor contour (Fig. 1.1). A fracture line can have a course that may appear short and straight, slightly curved or, as in the case of the relatively long fracture line, slightly kinked (Fig. 1.2). As the result of a similar mechanism (bursting), there can be a traumatic widening of the suture with or without an accompanying fracture (Fig. 1.3). A widened suture as well as a widened burst fracture must be considered the result of severe trauma in the presence of normal bony structures (Fig. 1.4). Comminuted fractures are usually the result of direct massive trauma. Because of their continuation into the base of the skull or the paranasal sinuses or their crossing with vascular grooves, the different fracture lines must be evaluated with great care (Fig. 1.5). The eggshell type of fracture (Fig. 1.6) is the result of circumscribed direct trauma due to minor force and somehow represents a mild form of a depressed fracture.
Correct and rapid recognition of depressed fractures is of great importance because this type of fracture needs surgical intervention. In order to fully determine the position and extent of a depressed fracture tangential views may be necessary. It is critical to thoroughly evaluate the relationship of this type of fracture with the paranasal sinuses and vascular structures. Depressed fractures are always the result of direct localized force and, in many instances, of criminal actions (Figs. 1.7 and 1.8). Depressed fractures with

overlapping of the fracture fragments represent a severe type of injury also requiring surgical intervention (Fig. 1.9).

Even during peacetime, the vast majority of fractures appearing as rounded defects are the result of penetrating injuries due to projectiles from shotguns and, occasionally, the result of foreign bodies such as splinters or bolts from dangerous machinery, as in hunting accidents, attempts at suicide, work accidents. In the wider sense, we should also consider here penetrating wounds due to deliberate traumatization with instruments (such as a hammer or knife) or a fall against hard pointed objects so that, to give an accurate definition, there is an overlap with depressed fractures. Penetrating injuries of the skull are quite unusual since knives or similar objects, in most instances, will break off before they can penetrate the skull. To determine the type and extent of injury, besides the proof of the presence and localization of a projectile or foreign body, further questions should be answered, such as the place of entry, usually appearing as a clean hole possibly marked by fine metal splinters (Fig. 1.10) and, in contrast, the exit of the projectile, which appears as a larger irregularly delineated defect. Are there several projectiles? What type of projectile is present? (See Chapter 10). If localized within one of the ventricles of the brain or within an intracranial necrotic cavity, the foreign body will change localization according to the positioning of the head. Stereoscopic views may be of help.

In all fractures of the skull, it will be very difficult to evaluate the age of the fracture. It is only possible to comment that if the edges of the fracture fragments are rounded in appearance as a result of resorptive phenomena and bony atrophy in the immediate vicinity of the fracture, its age must be several weeks to months. Usually the bony reparation of a linear fracture will take 6 to 12 months. Larger rounded defects may persist. During childhood, as a result cerebrospinal fluid of an accompanying injury to the dura, cystic accumulation of CSF may lead to a continuous widening of a fracture, resulting in a very large oval bony defect, the so-called growing fracture of the skull (see Fig. 12.9).

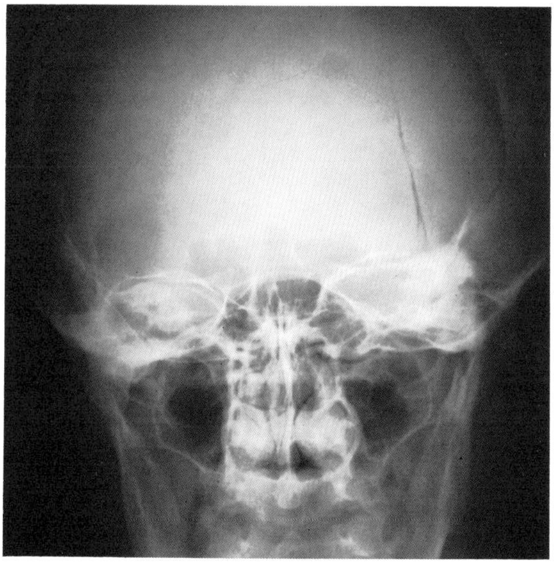

a

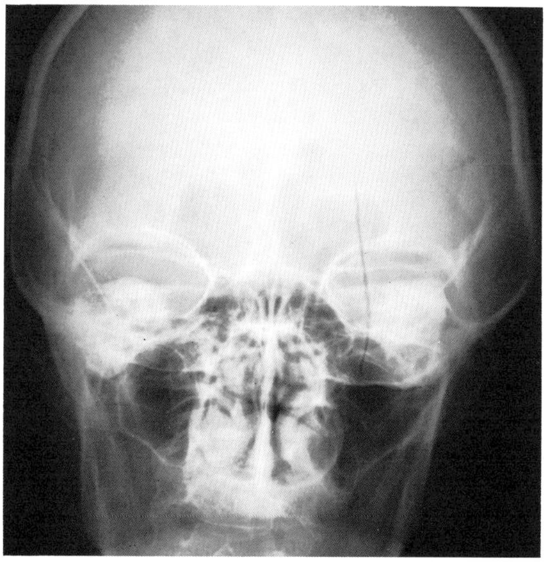

b

Fig. 1.1a and b. A 49-year-old woman after a fall onto the occiput. Linear fracture of the occipital bone on the left.

a) P. a. view: the fracture shows little contrast and is not sharp.

b) A. p. view: the fracture is well defined.

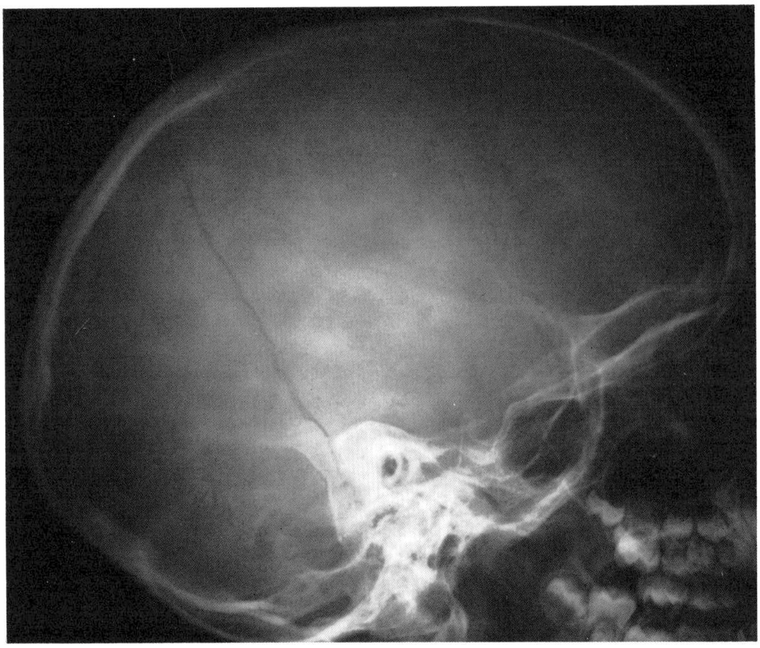

Fig. 1.2. A 7-year-old boy after a fall from some stairs. Long fracture line within the parietal bone with several areas of slight kinking.

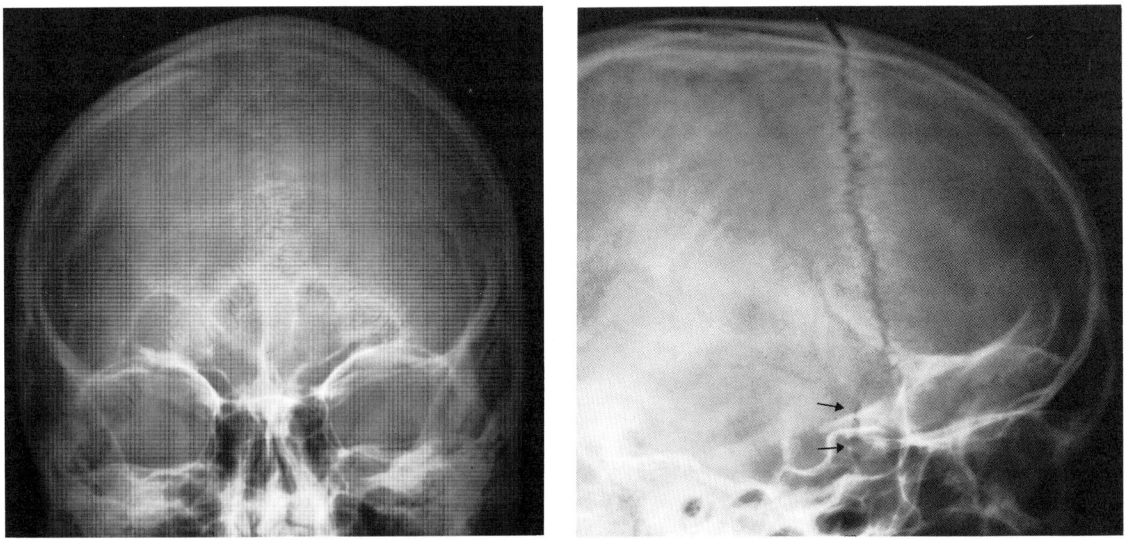

a

b

Fig. 1.3a and b. A 22-year-old student with traumatic widening of the coronary suture in the presence of a bursting fracture of the right parietal bone. There is a fissure extending from the frontal suture into the parietal bone.

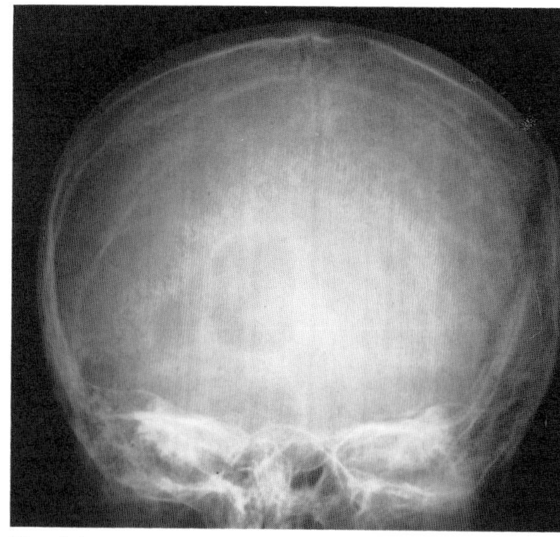

Fig. 1.4a

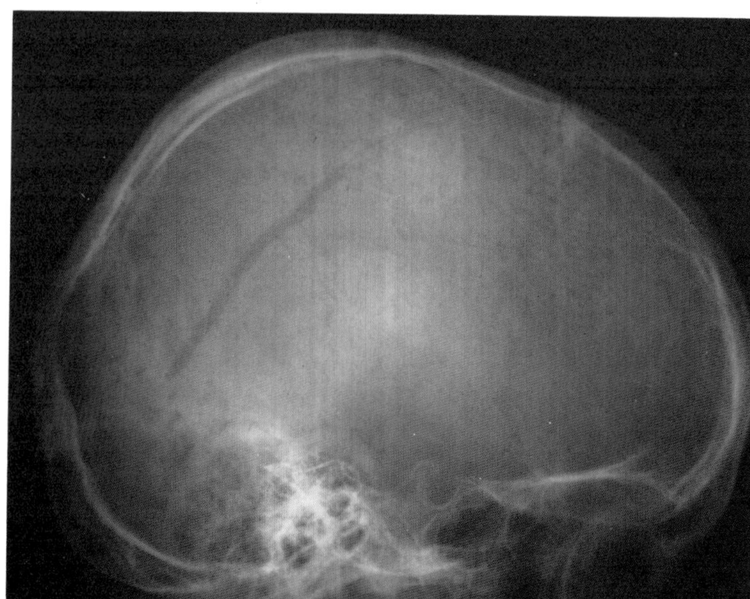

b

Fig. 1.4a and b. A 12-year-old boy. A workman was sweeping materials from the top of a high-rise building under construction. Inadvertently, a large piece of material the size of a brick hit the boy on the head. Broad left parietal bursting fracture.

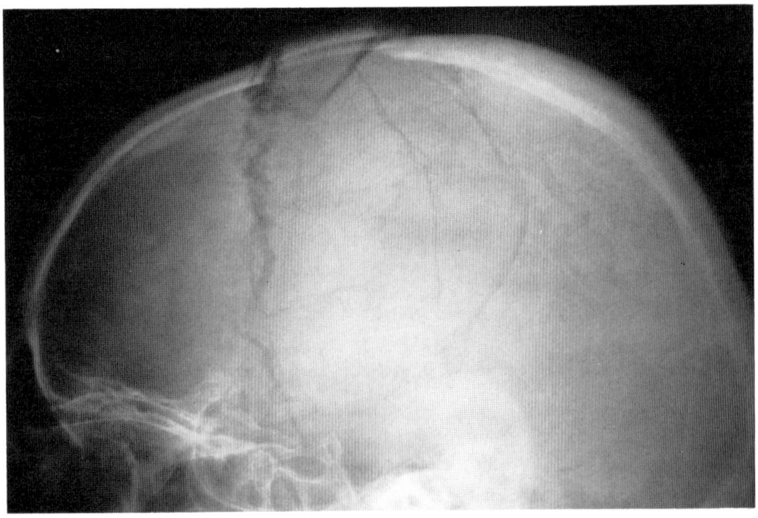

Fig. 1.5. A 24-year-old man who was a front-seat passenger in a car in a head-on collision with a tree. Ten hours after the accident, the patient expired. Splinter fracture of the middle skull.

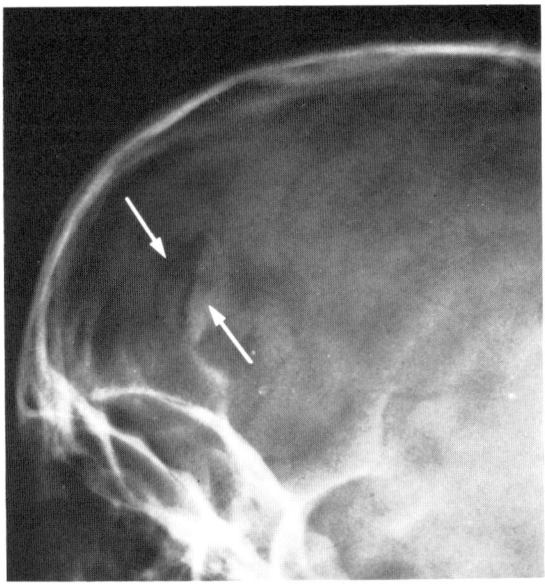

Fig. 1.6. So-called eggshell fracture of the right frontal bone. Must be properly distinguished from a depressed fracture.

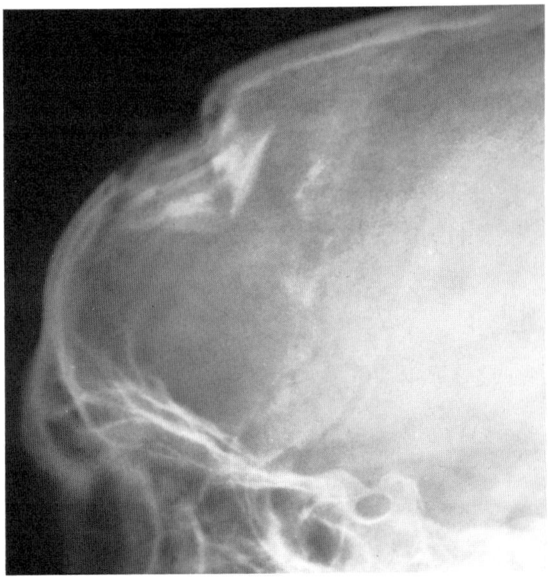

Fig. 1.7. Massive depressed fracture of the frontal bone.

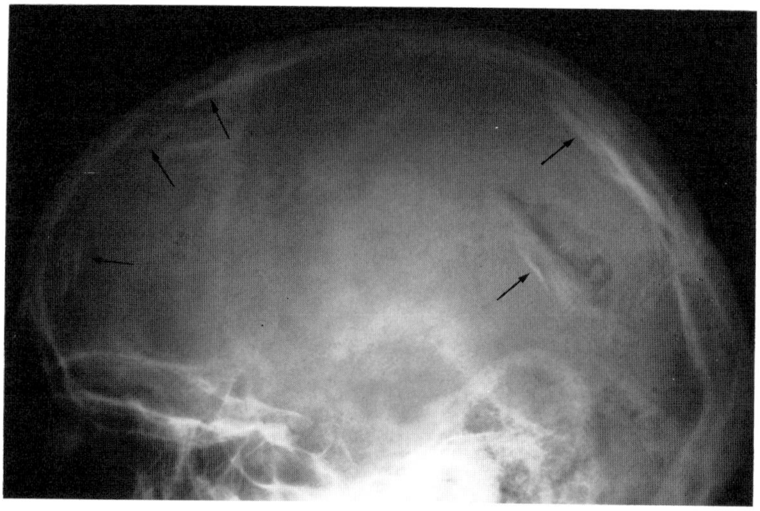

Fig. 1.8a

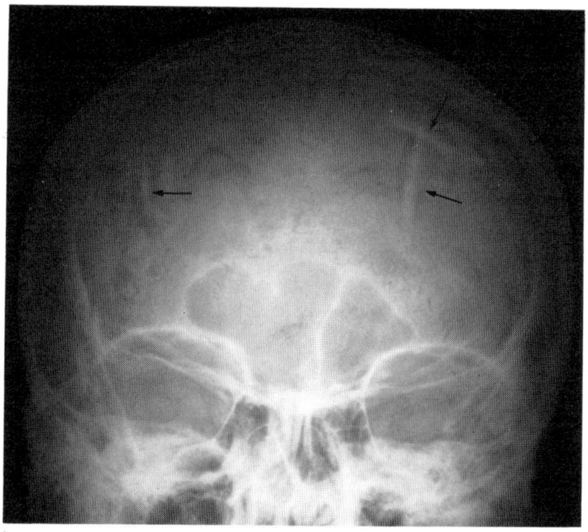

b

Fig. 1.8a and b. A 22-year-old man. 10 days after surgery, he was discharged from the hospital. There are at least five depressed fractures of the skull caused by multiple injuries with a hammer during an attempted robbery and homicide. He also had fractures of several fingers because he tried to protect himself by holding his hands over his head.

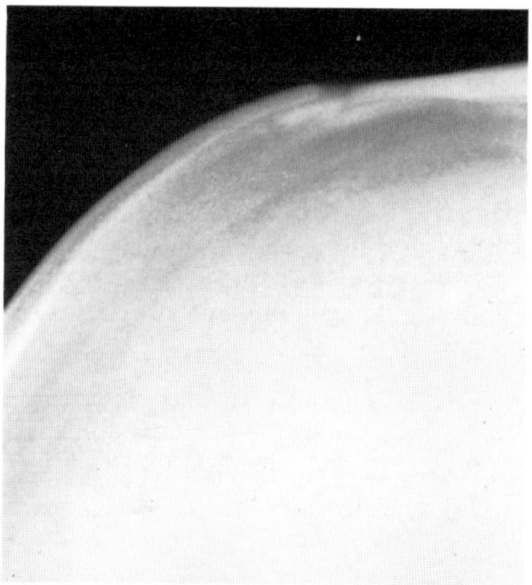

Fig. 1.9. A 22-year-old man who was a front-seat passenger in a car accident. Depressed fracture with overlapping of borders.

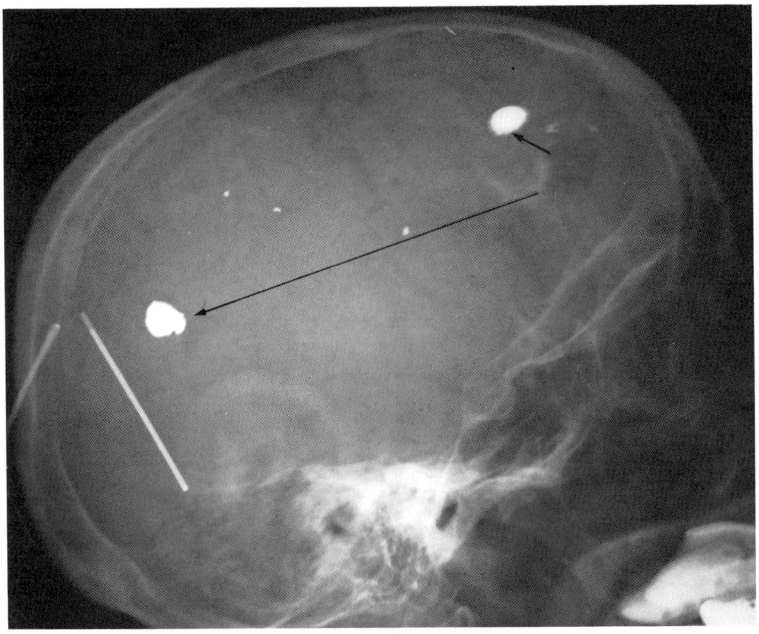

Fig. 1.10. Projectile fracture of the skull as a result of attempted suicide. Round entry of projectile in the right frontal region. There are metal splinters around the point of entry of the projectile.

Fractures of the Facial Structures

A list of the most common fractures of the face seems appropriate here in view of their frequent occurrence and potential for complications:

1. Isolated fracture of the nasal bone.
2. Isolated fracture of the zygomatic arch or the wall of the maxillary sinus.
3. Fracture of the nasal maxillary bones (Fig. 1.11a): unilateral; bilateral (in the form of a pyramid); and high transverse fracture (Le Fort III) (Fig. 1.11b).
4. Zygomaticomaxillary fracture (Fig. 1.11c): unilateral or bilateral.
5. Palatoalveolar fracture (Figs. 1.11d, 1.11e).
6. Combined fracture of the facial structures and the skull.
7. Fracture of the wall of the orbit and depressed fracture of the orbital floor.

In addition to special views of the facial bony structures, tomography is valuable and necessary in demonstrating bony injuries in the area of the middle ear and its surroundings (Frey, 1965). Details of this region can be properly recognized only on x-rays of the highest quality. In such situations, special views requiring the full cooperation of the patient are obtained only a few days after the accident. Still, it may be impossible to recognize fractures of very thin bony structures such as the ethmoid, sphenoid or lacrimal bones, the vomer, the palatine process and the nasal conchae. Even those who limit themselves to the x-ray diagnosis of the skull will be unable to perform properly without repeatedly referring to the basic anatomic data of the bony elements of the face and skull and devoting particular attention to all the necessary details of projection and exposure data in demonstrating the individual elements of this region (Clementschitsch, 1951). Injuries of the facial bones most frequently occur in traffic accidents or may be the result of fist fights and sports mishaps.

In the region of the nasal bone, fissures as well as comminuted fractures can be observed (Figs. 1.12 and 1.13). Usually, the lateral view of the nasal bone is adequate for making a diagnosis. The lateral view of the skull, however, will not be sufficient since, in this view, the area of the very fine nasal bone will be overpenetrated. Without an additional axial view, many a minimally dislocated fracture of the nasal bone will be overlooked. The suture lines toward the frontal bones and maxilla should not be misinterpreted as a fracture line. A true fracture can usually

be recognized by the disrupted contours of the back of the nasal bone and also by an elevation or depression of the distal fracture fragment. If one does not pay particular attention to the anterior nasal spine, a fracture in this location can be easily overlooked (Figs. 1.14 and 1.15).
Clouding of one or both maxillary sinuses is an important indirect sign of a nasomaxillary and zygomaticomaxillary fracture (Figs. 1.16 and 1.17). A very careful investigation of the *soft-tissue* contours is mandatory because frequently there is only a minimal step effect or angulation. In a combined fracture of the face and skull, the number and course of difficult-to-follow lines can be very confusing (Fig. 1.18). The maxillary sinuses and zygomatic arches can best be evaluated on half-axial (Waters' view) (occipitonasal or occipitomental) views of the facial structures. A depressed fracture of the orbital floor (a so-called "blow-out fracture") can best be seen on these views (Fig. 1.19). In this type of fracture, the mechanism is as follows. As a result of blunt trauma to the eyeball, there is a pressure effect on the very thin bone of the floor of the orbit with a consequent local fracture inferiorly or sometimes in the medial wall of the orbit (Brown et al., 1965; Fueger et al., 1966; Tänzer, 1966). Quite frequently, there is also emphysema of the orbit due to transfer of air from the maxillary sinuses or the ethmoid cells (Lloyd, 1966) (Fig. 1.20). The key symptoms of this particularly important type of fracture, which carry the danger of loss of visual acuity, are enophthalmos and diplopia.
The following fractures are usually best seen on lateral views, particularly if the focus is on the facial structures:

1. Fractures of the nasal bones and the anterior nasal spine.
2. Fractures of the anterior wall of the frontal sinus (Fig. 1.21).
3. Fractures of the hard palate and of the alveolar process (Fig. 1.22).
4. Fractures of the pterygoid process.

In order to demonstrate fractures of the zygomatic arch, a special tangential projection is almost always required from the angle of the mandible directed toward the upper parts of the skull (Fig. 1.23).
In spite of its massive architectural structure, the mandible is quite frequently the site of fractures (about 80 per cent of all fractures of the mandible and maxilla). The causes are the same as in fractures of the maxilla. These fractures are the direct result of trauma. With very few exceptions, fractures of the mandible offer no clinical or radiologic diagnostic difficulties. Radiologically important and impressive within the mandible is the combined channel for vessels and nerves passing through the mental foramen. A continuation of the median suture line should not be misinterpreted as a fracture.
Fractures of the body of the mandible and of the ramus (Fig. 1.24) can be differentiated as can fractures of the articular process (Fig. 1.25) and the muscular process and luxation fractures (Fig. 1.26). The schematic distribution pattern of fractures of the jaw according to Ueno (Fig. 1.27) also indicates the areas of predilection: the midline, deep alveolar area of the canine and of the wisdom teeth, ant the neck area of the articular process of the mandible. Unless a special investigation is conducted, it is quite easy to overlook fractures of the articular process owing to overlap by soft-tissue injury and hematoma. It is possible to further subdivide fractures of the articular process into fractures of the neck, fractures of the capitulum and luxation fractures (Fig. 1.28).
In general, a.p., lateral and oblique views are sufficient. The temporomandibular joint, particularly the mandibular head, is best demonstrated by lateral projections according to Schüller, by contact radiography according to Parma and in the p.a. direction according to Clementschitsch. Fractures of the muscular process are best seen in oblique projection. If there is doubt, and particularly when a fracture of the temporomandibular joint is suspected, tomography is recommended. If a dislocation is suspected, additional views with the mouth as wide open as possible, as well as the mouth closed for comparison, may add important information.
Intraoral views are indicated in order to better delineate fractures in the area of the alveolar processes and to demonstrate dental lesions, as well as in every case in which, from the clinical findings or the initial x-ray studies, these conditions are suspected. Dislocations of teeth must be differentiated from fractures. One can distinguish between dental crown fractures and dental root fractures (Fig. 1.29). In order to demonstrate fractures of dental roots, views different from the routine dental technique are needed (Fig. 1.30). It is not sufficiently well known that fractures of dental roots can heal completely and that reimplanted teeth after dislocation can heal fully, particularly if reimplantation can be performed within one hour (Talim and Anita, 1966). Fractures most frequently involve the incisors of the maxilla. Fractures of the alveolar process also occur most commonly in the maxil-

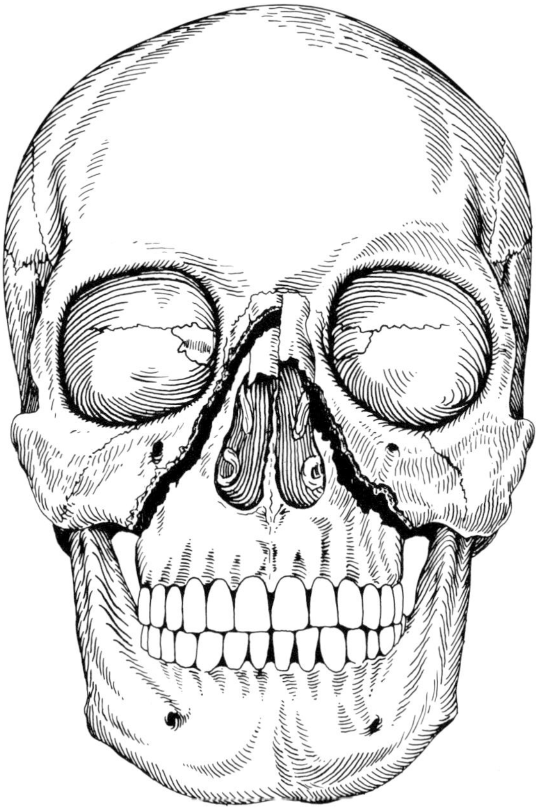

a

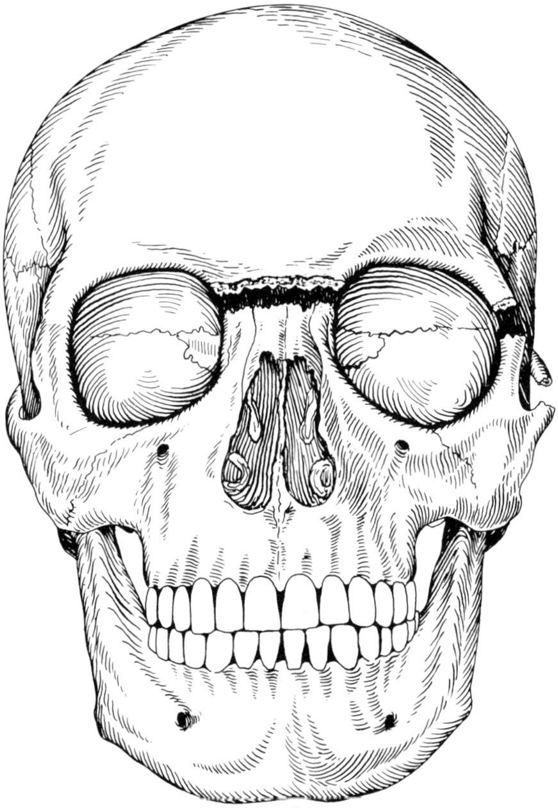

b

la, especially the medial region. In the mandible, fractures of the alveolar process usually occur in canine teeth 2–3 and in their immediate neighbors. If here are fractures of the alveolar processes, one must be very careful to investigate the possible concomitant occurrence of dental fractures, and vice versa.

To document the very unusual fracture of the hyoid bone, it is necessary to obtain a lateral view with low kilovoltage x-rays.

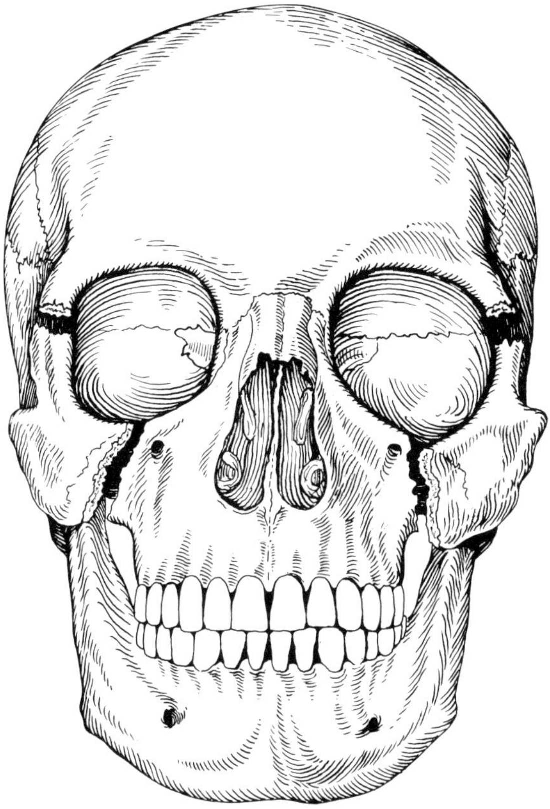

c

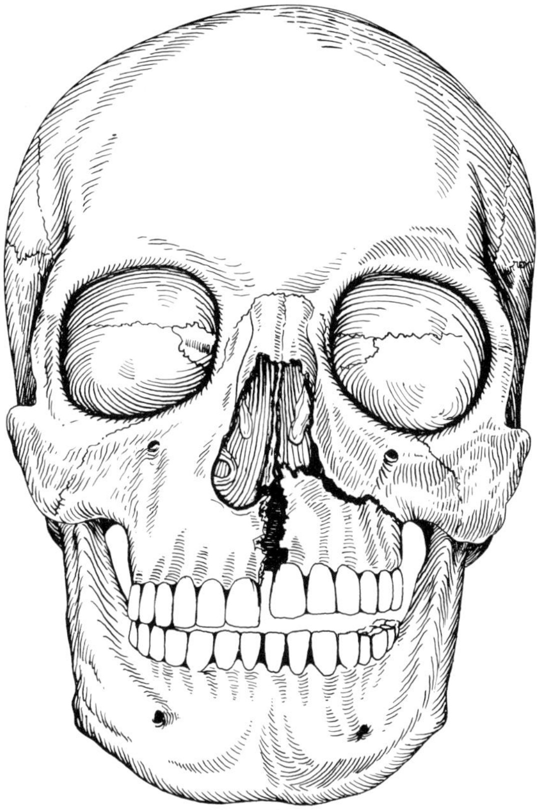

d

Fig. 1.11a–e. Schematic representation of the different types of fractures of the facial bones (after Zatzkin).
a) Nasomaxillary fracture in the form of a pyramid.
b) High transverse fracture. The fracture runs through the frontal sinuses or the dorsum of the nose, the zygomaticofrontal suture and the zygomatic arch (Le Fort III).
c) Zygomaticomaxillary fracture. Unilaterally or bilaterally, dislocation of the zygomatic bone superiorly or inferiorly, with an opening up of the zygomaticofrontal suture (Le Fort II).
d) Palatoalveolar fracture.
e) Palatoalveolar transverse fracture, with eventual involvement of the zygomatic arch or a fracture of the pterygoid process (*d* and *e* correspond with Le Fort I).

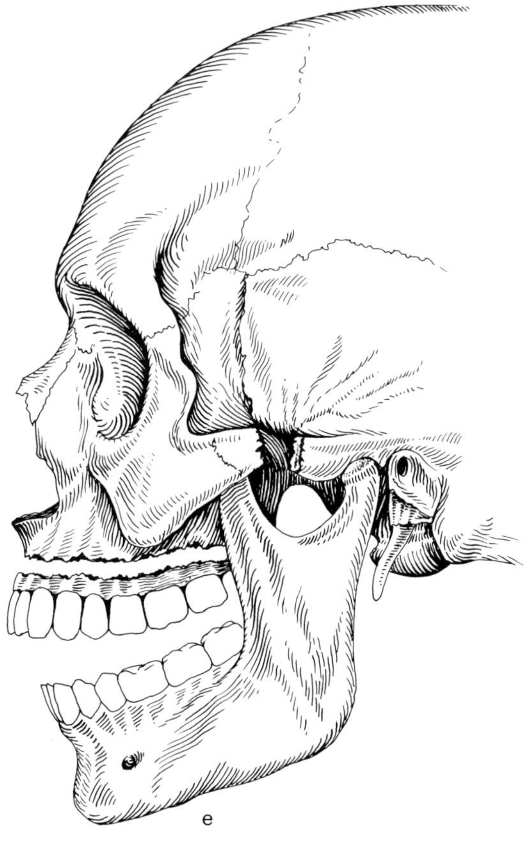

e

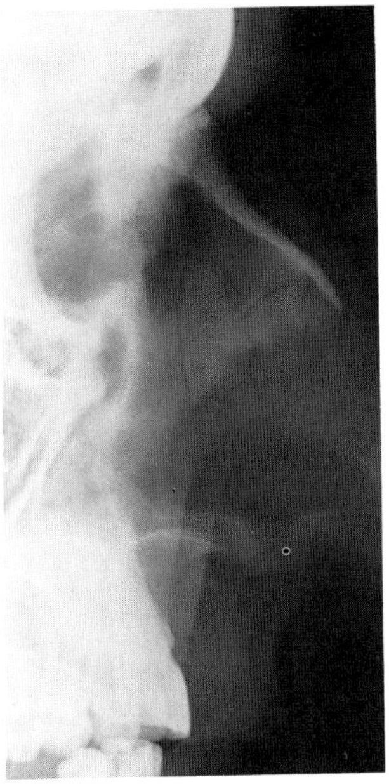

Fig. 1.12. Transverse fissure of the nasal bone.

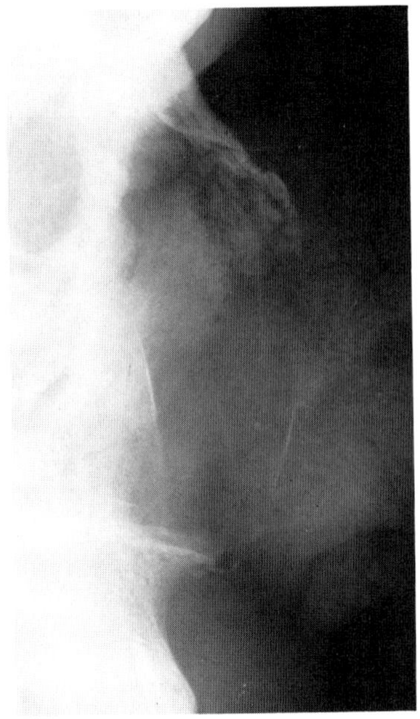

Fig. 1.13. Comminuted fracture of the nasal bone.

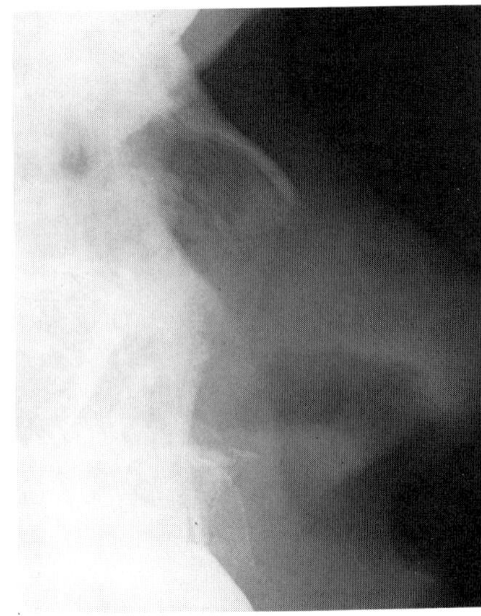

Fig. 1.14. Isolated fracture of the anterior nasal spine.

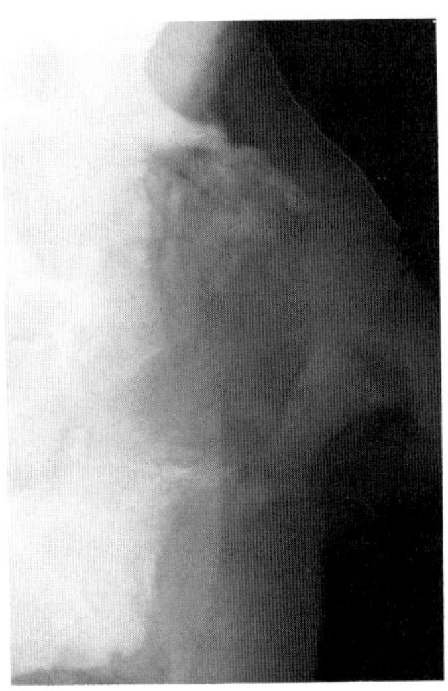

Fig. 1.15. Fracture of the anterior nasal spine at the base, with multiple chip fractures of the nasal bone.

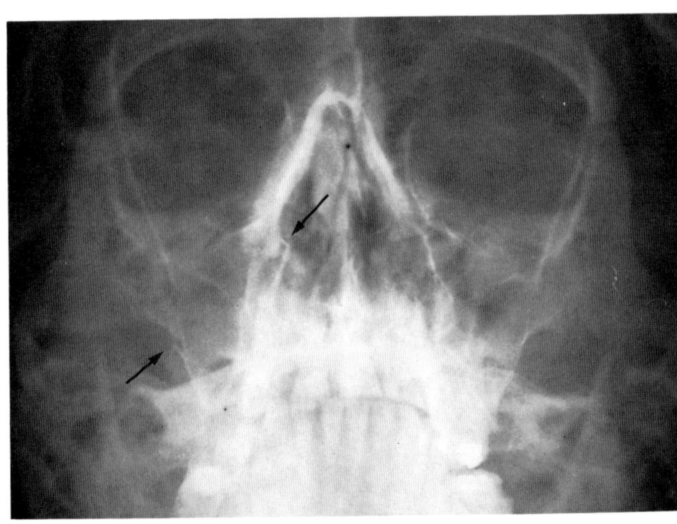

Fig. 1.16. A 28-year-old man after a traffic accident. Nasomaxillary fracture involving both maxillary sinuses. The fracture on the right is better visualized.

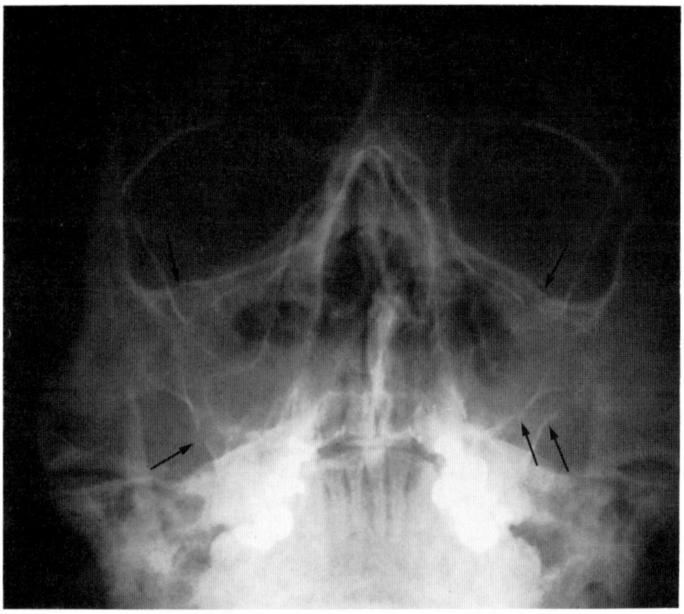

Fig. 1.17. A 21-year-old man after a traffic accident. Bilateral zygomatico-maxillary fracture involving both maxillary sinuses.

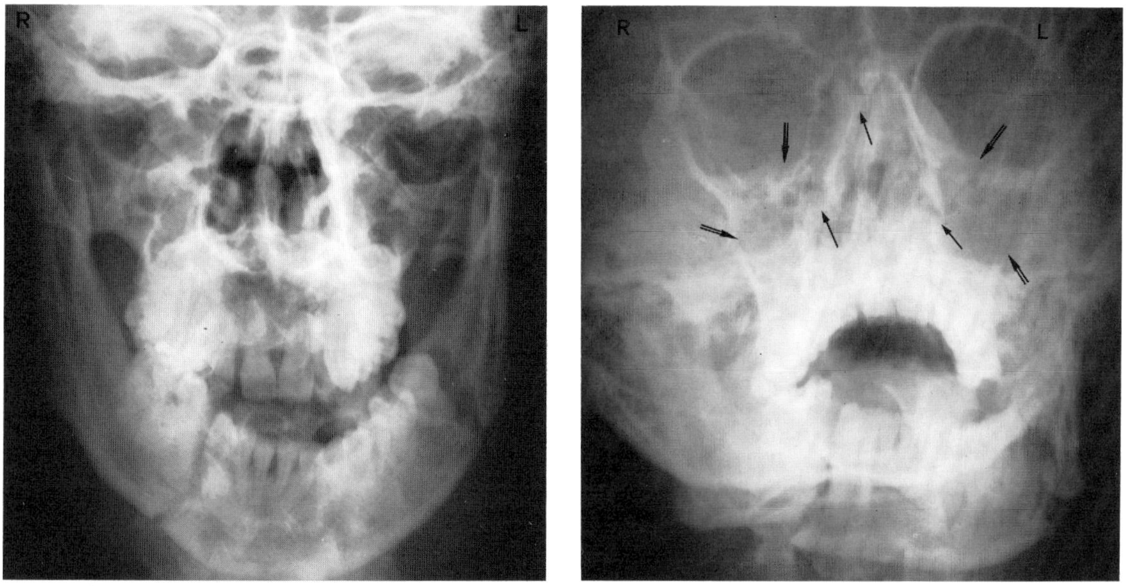

a

b

Fig. 1.18a and b. A 24-year-old man after a traffic accident. Combined fracture of facial structures. Note nasomaxillary fracture. (*Arrow,* bilateral zygomatico-maxillary fracture; *double arrow,* involvement of both maxillary sinuses). Fractures of the mandible on the right through the alveolar process of the canine and on the left through the alveolar process of the wisdom tooth. Fracture of the base of the right articular process.

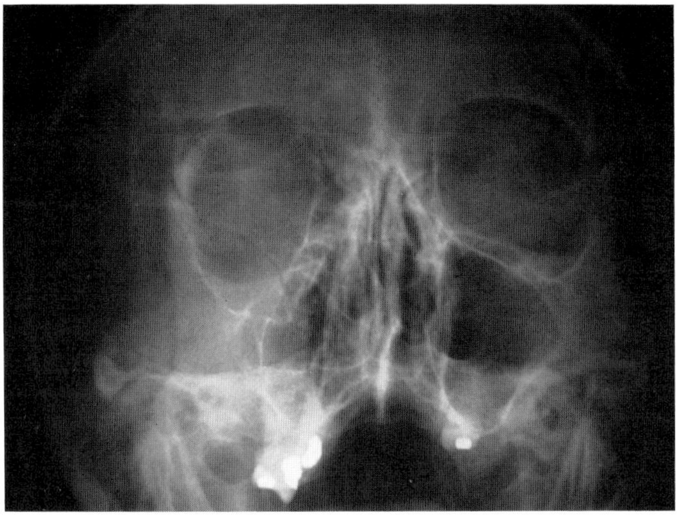

Fig. 1.19. An 83-year-old woman who was hit by a car. Depression fracture of the orbital floor on the right (blow-out fracture). Classic appearance of the fracture segments depressed into the right maxillary sinus. In addition, there are fractures of the zygomaticomaxillary and frontal orbital type.

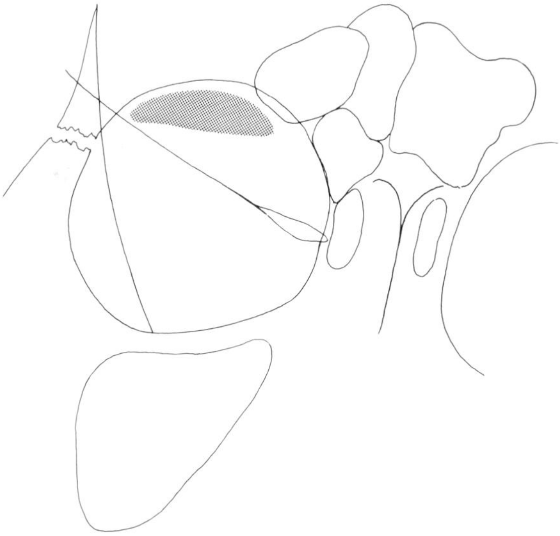

Fig. 1.20. Emphysema of the orbit in the presence of a fracture of the medial wall of the orbit (according to Lloyd).

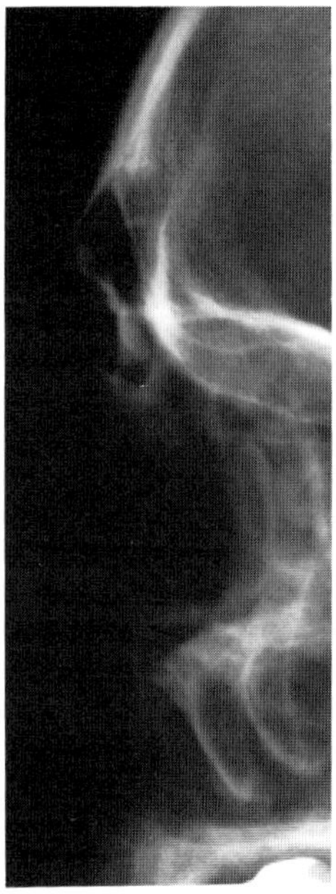

Fig. 1.21

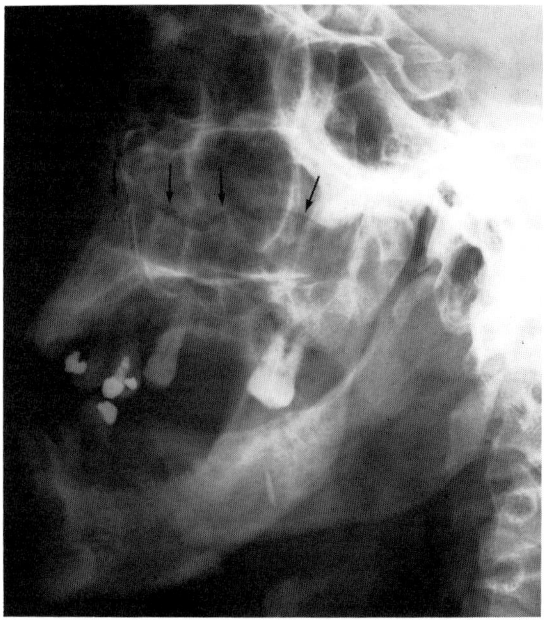

Fig. 1.22

Fig. 1.21. Depressed fracture of the anterior wall of the frontal sinus.

Fig. 1.22. A 58-year-old man with a palatoalveolar fracture as well as naso-maxillary and mandibular fractures.

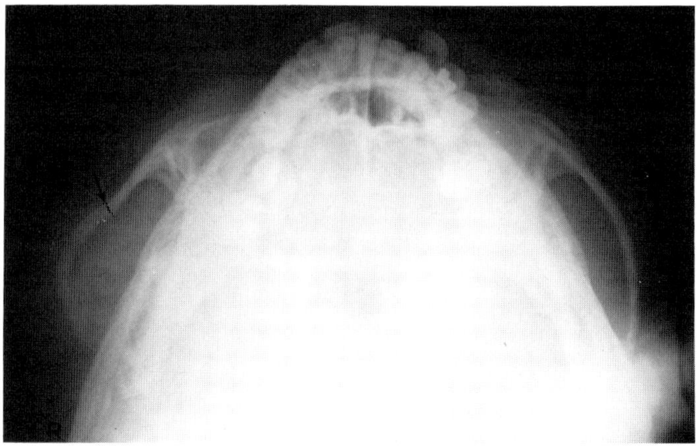

Fig. 1.23. A 40-year-old housewife with a fracture of the right zygomatic arch without significant displacement of fragments.

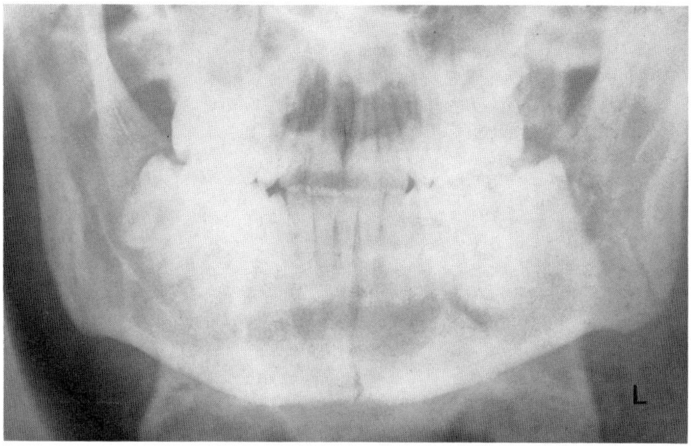

a

Fig. 1.24a–f. A 22-year-old man after a car accident (case of Dr. Zappe, Müllheim). Multiple fractures of the mandible.
a and b) Fractures of the body of the mandible in the midline: a) regular a. p. view; b) axial view.
c) Fracture of the left mandibular angle going through the alveolar process of the wisdom tooth.
d) Fracture of the left articular process at its base; zygomaticotemporal suture marked by arrow (this is not a fracture!).
e and f) Intraoral views of the fracture through the alveolar processes before and after wiring.

b

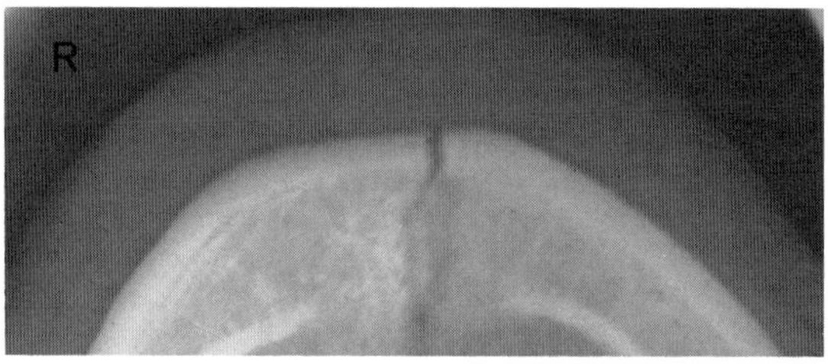

c

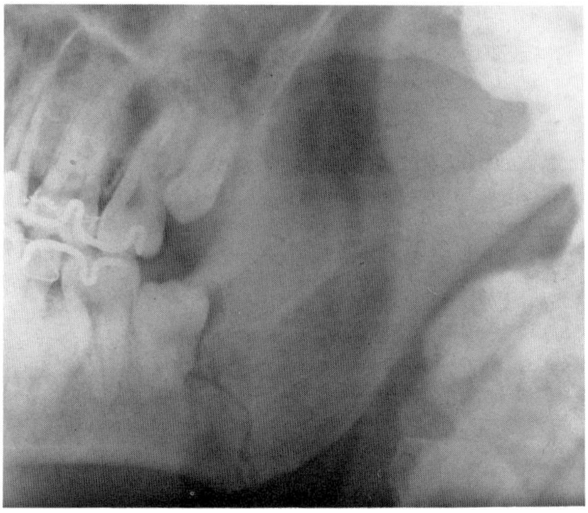

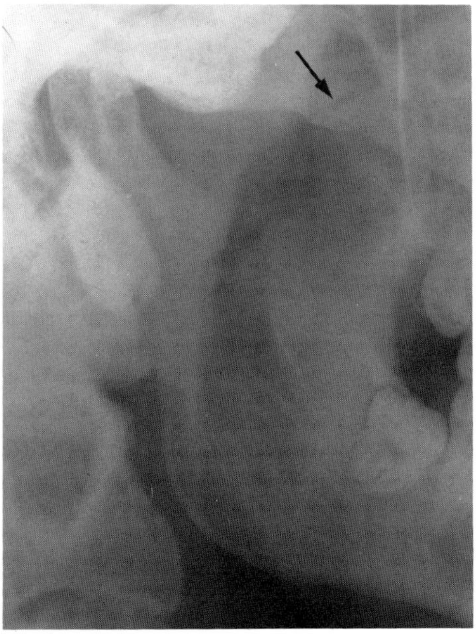

d

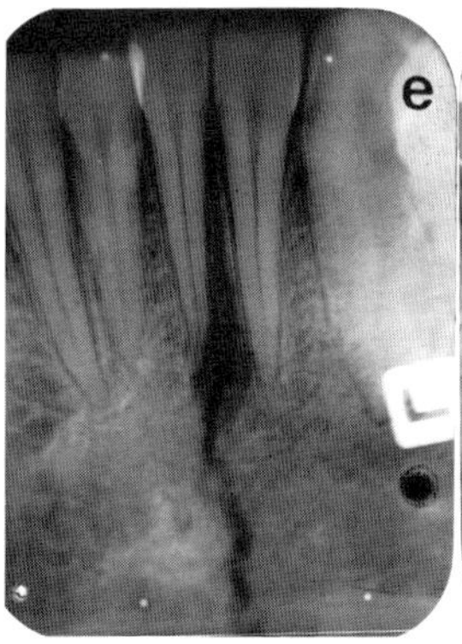

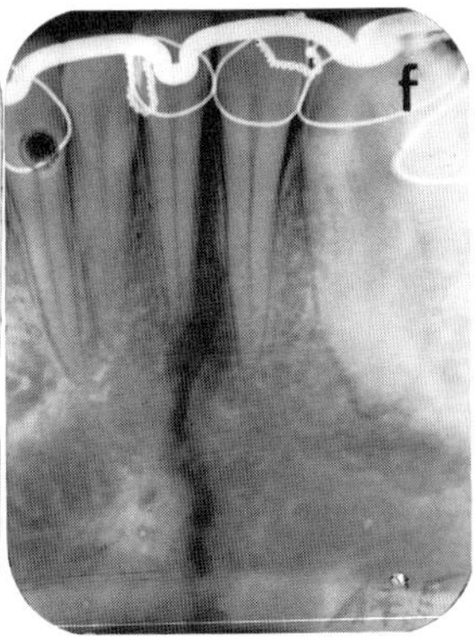

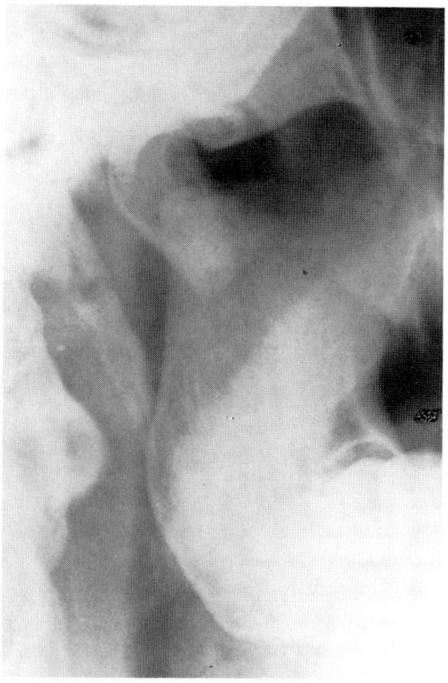

Fig. 1.25. A 21-year-old man after a traffic accident. Fracture of the articular process of the mandible (*contact view*).

a
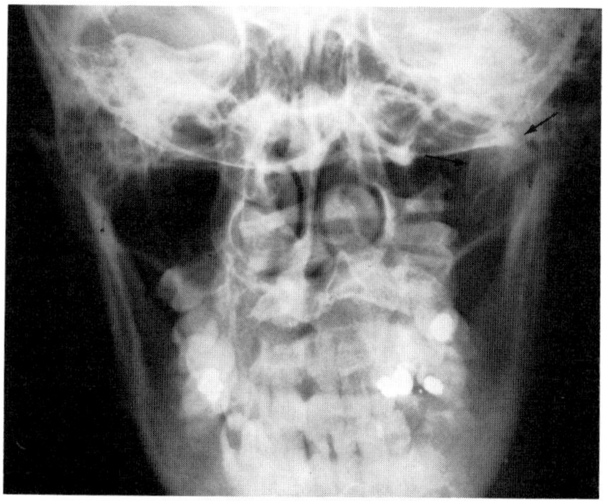

b
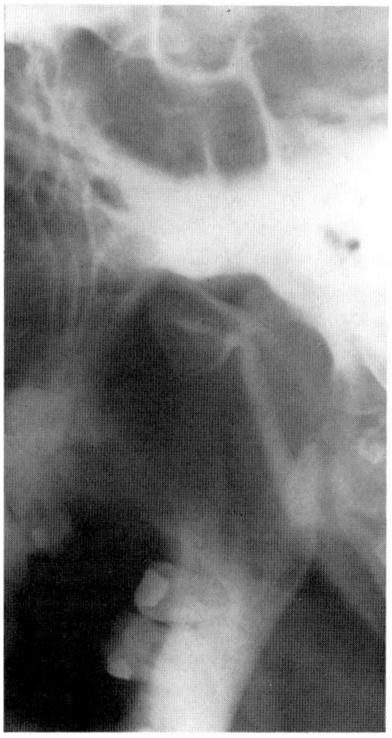

Fig. 1.26a and b. A 31-year-old woman after a traffic accident. Dislocation and fracture of the left articular process of the mandible.
a) A.p. view.
b) Contact view.

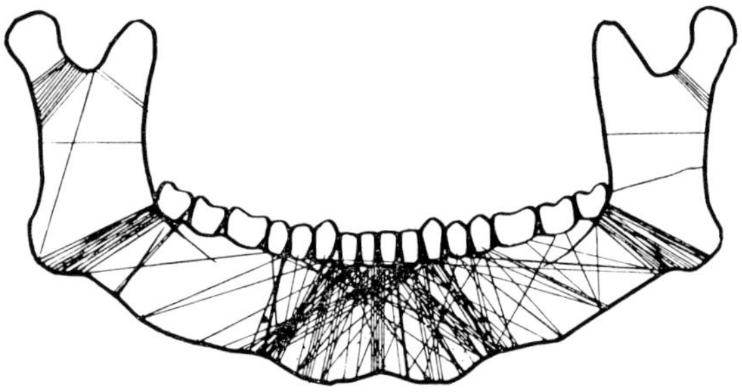

Fig. 1.27. Distribution of fracture lines within the mandible, according to Ueno (From E. Sonnabend: Traumatische Zahnschäden, Frakturen des Alveolarfortsatzes und des Unterkiefers. *In:* Deutscher Röntgenkongreß 1965. Stuttgart, Teil A. Thieme, 1966).

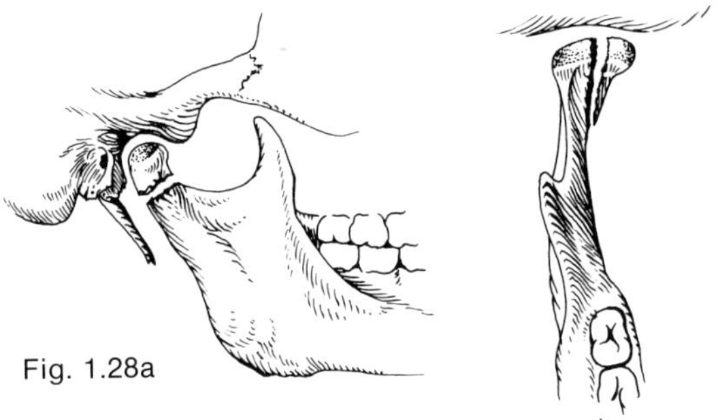

Fig. 1.28a

b

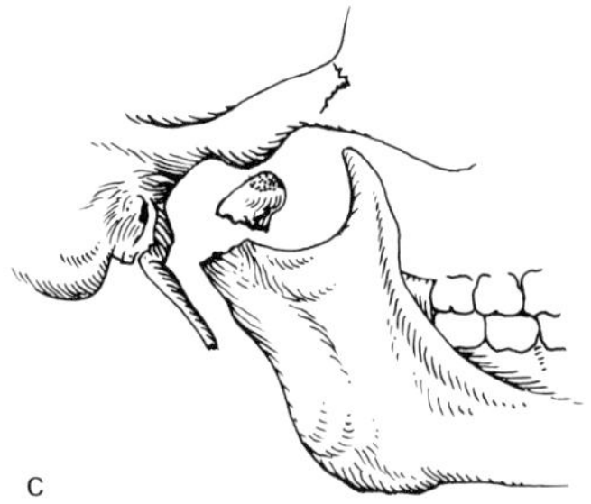

c

Fig. 1.28a–c. Fractures of the articular process of the mandible.
a) Fractures through the neck *(lateral view).*
b) Fracture of the capitulum *(p.a. view).*
c) Luxation fracture *(lateral view).*

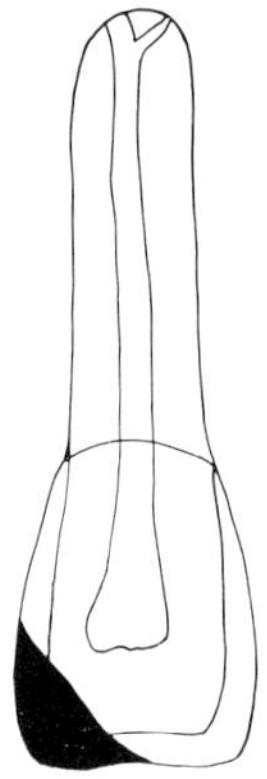

a 1 2 3

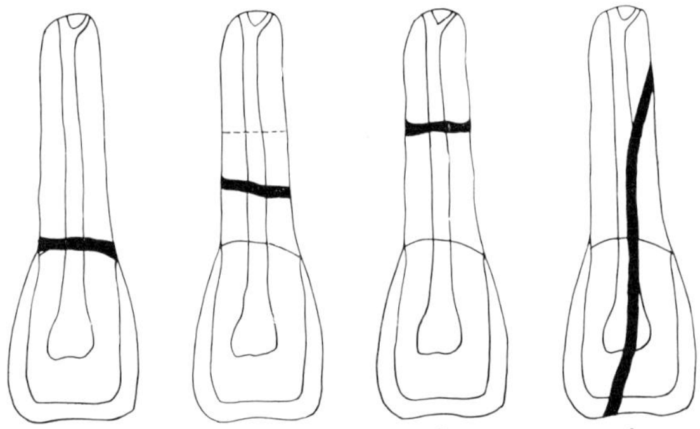

b 1 2 3 4

Fig. 1.29a and b. a) Types of fractures of the crown of the tooth: 1. Enamel-dentine fracture. 2. Fracture through dentine and pulp. 3. Fracture of crown (middle or transverse).

b) Types of fractures through the dental root: 1. Fracture from transition crown to root. 2. Fracture between neck of root and middle of root. 3. Fracture between middle and tip of root. 4. Longitudinal fracture (see Fig. 1.27).

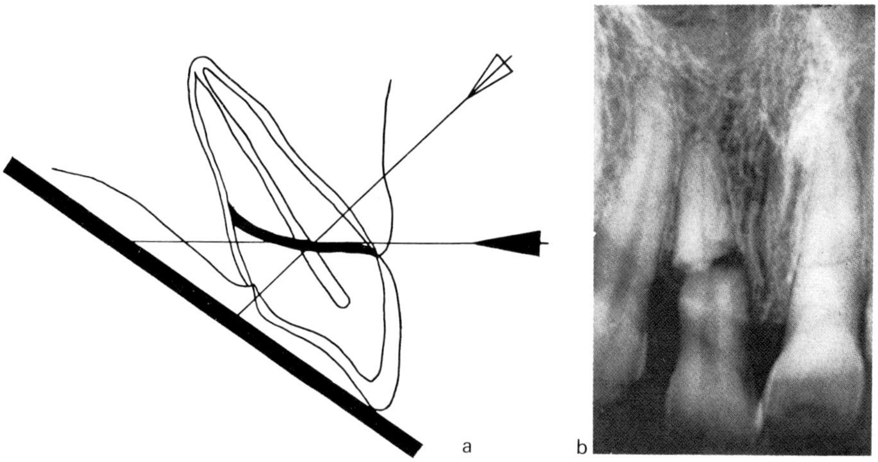

Fig. 1.30a and b. a) Preferred projection for dental root fractures. b) Dental root fracture of both upper median incisors (see Fig. 1.27).

Fractures of the Base of the Skull

Fractures of the base of the skull are the most difficult to determine radiologically. It is quite difficult to find the proper special projections. These may be inconsistent in their results and, in many instances, it may be virtually impossible to properly demonstrate the fractures; in addition, it may be particularly hard to recognize a fine fracture line where there is only minimal dislocation of the fracture fragments and where there is overlap by denser bones. Despite the fact that often there is clinically no doubt about the diagnosis – for instance, if CSF is dripping from the nose or auditory canal (a periorbital hematoma alone is no proof for the existence of a fracture at the base of the skull) – it may be impossible to prove the existence of a fracture or to localize it fully. Accompanying a fracture of the base of the skull, there may often be a coexisting fracture of the adjacent parts of the skull.

Fractures involving the frontal bone, the ethmoid and the anterior fossa can also be called frontobasal fractures (Fig. 1.31). Bleeding into the nose and the epipharynx, together with vomiting, increases the danger of aspiration. Because of a defect in the dura, there may be passage of air and infectious material from the involved paranasal sinuses into the intracranial region, leading to a spontaneous accumulation of air within the superficial CSF spaces (Fig. 1.36). In fractures in the area of the frontal sinus and the upper facial structures, one should always ascertain that there is not also a fracture of the posterior wall of the frontal sinus or the base of the anterior fossa (Fig. 1.32). Fractures of the roof of the ethmoid usually can only be recognized on sagittal tomograms (Fig. 1.33).

About three-quarters of all fractures of the base of the skull affect the middle fossa. In cases in which there is no visible fracture, the existence of an air-fluid level within the sphenoid sinus offers indirect proof for the existence of a fracture of the base of the skull and is a sign of severe skull and brain trauma with the real danger of death or permanent neurologic deficit in at least 50 per cent of all such cases (Robinson et al., 1967) (Fig. 1.34). In about one-third of all cases with a surgically demonstrated or proven accumulation of fluid at autopsy, there is also a fracture of the sphenoid. In the remaining instances, the accumulation of fluid within the sphenoid sinus is the result of damage to the mucosa or of migration of blood or cerebrospinal fluid from the nasoepipharyngeal region, as demonstrated by Etter (1963) using a contrast agent. A level within the sphenoid sinus, however, can be demonstrated only where there is liquid, blood or CSF. This is not the case where blood has coagulated.

Within the petrous bone, one can distinguish between transverse and longitudinal fractures. Frequently there is concomitant involvement of the middle ear, internal ear, labyrinth and canal of the facial nerve. If there is leakage of CSF or brain substance into the auditory canal, there must be a fracture of the petrous bone. Only rarely is it possible to prove the existence of such a fracture on plane films of the skull (Fig. 1.35). The following special views may be necessary: Stenvers, tomographic cuts a.p. or in the Stenvers view (Fig. 1.36). A simple hemorrhage from the external ear can be the result of a fracture of only the temporal bone, involving the external auditory canal (Fig. 1.37). It is always reasonable to assume that the extent of the fracture is actually greater than visible on a roentgenogram.

Occasionally there occurs, as a result of direct trauma, an isolated fracture of the mastoid process.

Fractures of the body of the sphenoid can be most easily recognized because of the interrupted contour and step formation affecting the sella turcica or the sphenoidal surface (Fig. 1.38).

In the posterior fossa, the fractures are usually longitudinal in their course, extending toward the foramen magnum or the jugular foramen. It is not possible to make a definite diagnosis based on regular skull films. A Townes' view is needed to demonstrate the area of the foramen magnum (Fig. 1.39).

A ring fracture of the base of the skull is an extremely rare type of fracture resulting from indirect trauma in the horizontal or axial direction.

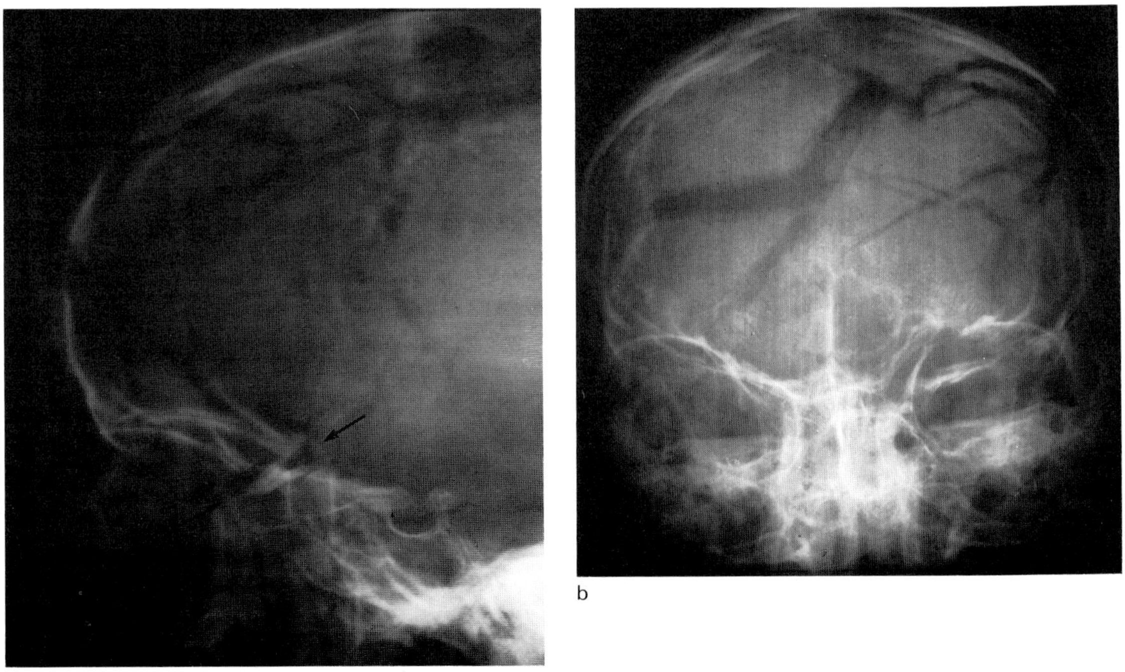

a b

Fig. 1.31a and b. A 16-year-old boy after a head-on motor scooter collision with a telephone pole. Death on the day after the accident. Massive frontobasal fracture. Wide fracture line and step formation at the base of the anterior fossa. Multiple fracture fragments in the area of the frontal and temporal bones. Fracture of the left orbit. Fracture of the facial structures. Periorbital hematoma and hemorrhage from the nose and mouth.

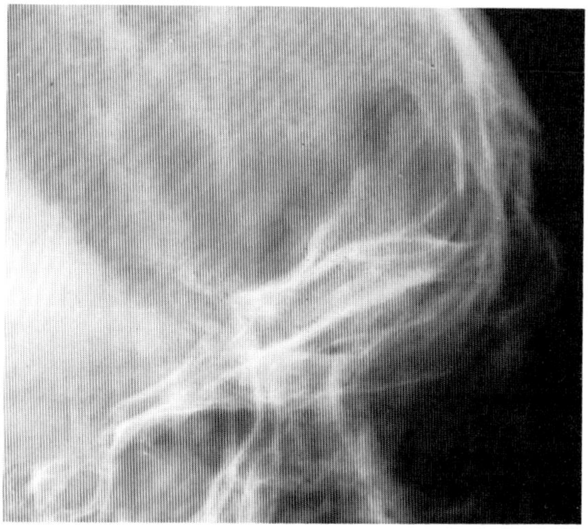

Fig. 1.32. An 18-year-old man after a car accident. Depressed fracture of the anterior and posterior walls of the frontal sinuses. Death on the day of the accident.

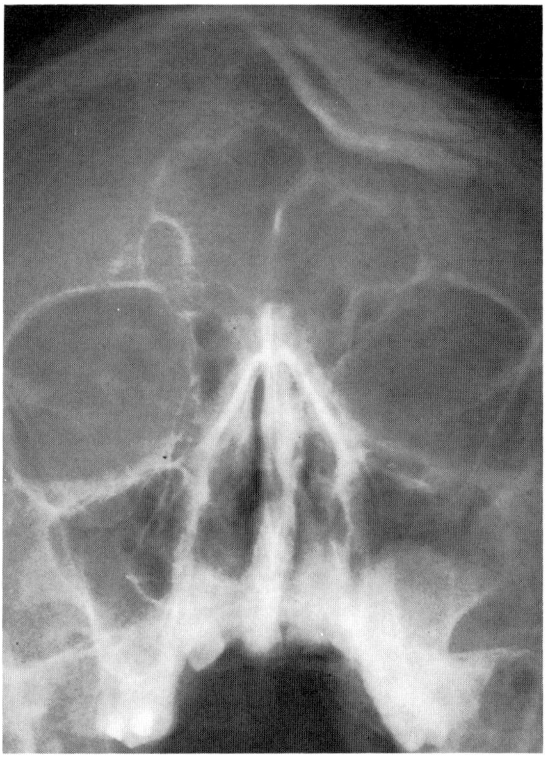

Fig. 1.33a

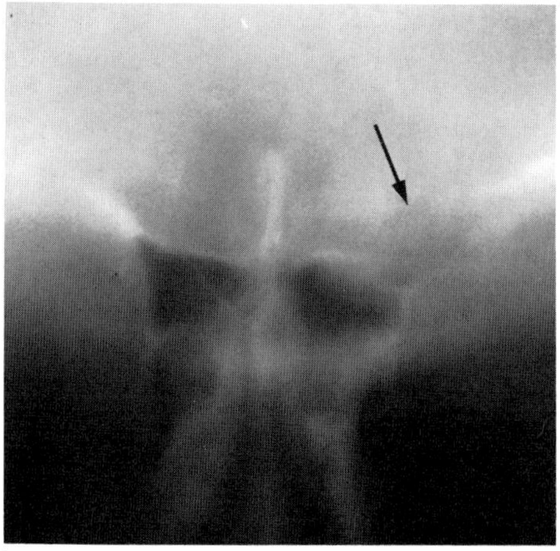

b

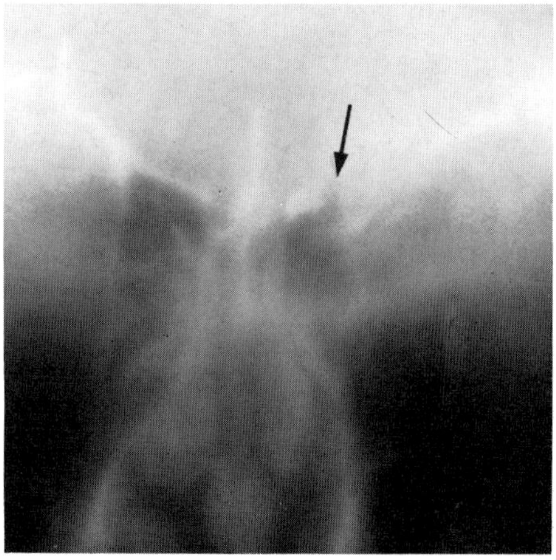

c

Figure 1.33a–c. A 32-year-old man with CSF leak through the nose since the accident. Fracture of the roof of the ethmoid cells at the level of the crista. Old depressed fracture of the frontal bone (no surgical correction!).

a) Townes' view without clear visualization of the fracture of the ethmoid.

b) and c) Tomograms: fracture of the roof of the ethmoid on left side laterally to the crista.

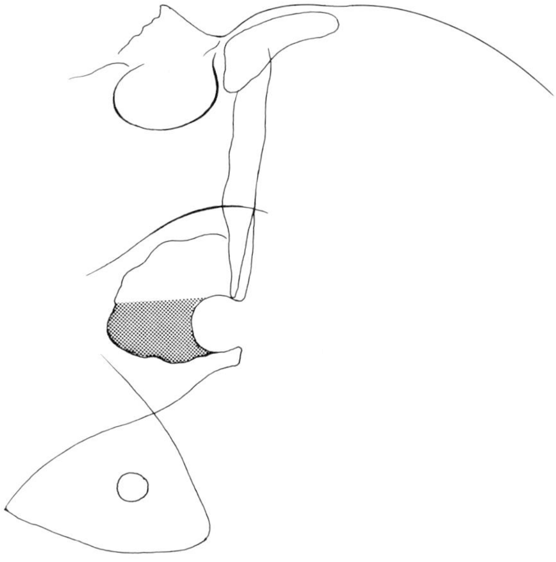

Fig. 1.34. Traumatic hemorrhage into the sphenoid sinus after a car accident. No fracture at autopsy. Demonstration of an air-fluid level on the lateral view in the dorsal decubitus (according to Robinson et al).

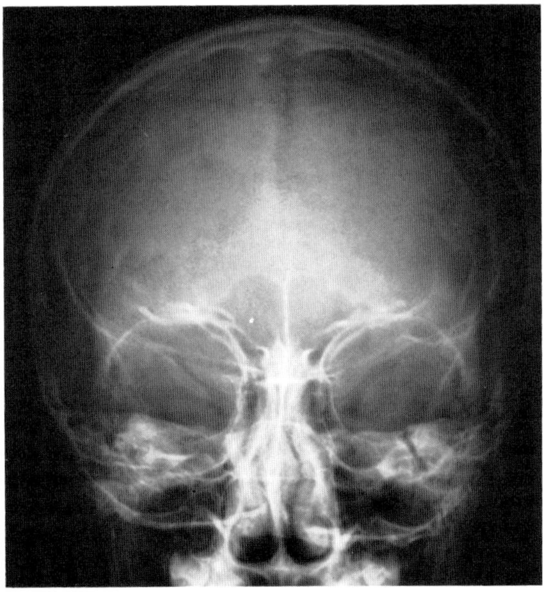

Fig. 1.35a. A 10-year-old boy who was hit by a car. Immediate loss of consciousness and bleeding from the left ear. A. p. survey film: transverse fracture of the left petrous bone; suspicion of fracture of the greater wing of the sphenoid.

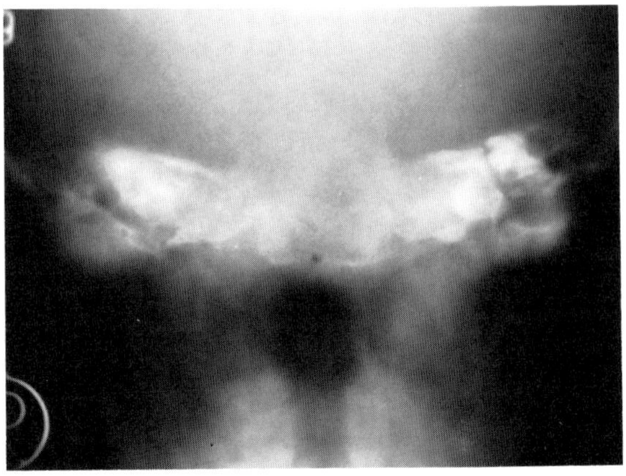

Fig. 1.35b. Tomogram in a. p. projection: transverse fracture of the left petrous pyramid medial to the ampule, with a minimal caudal displacement of the tip of the pyramid.

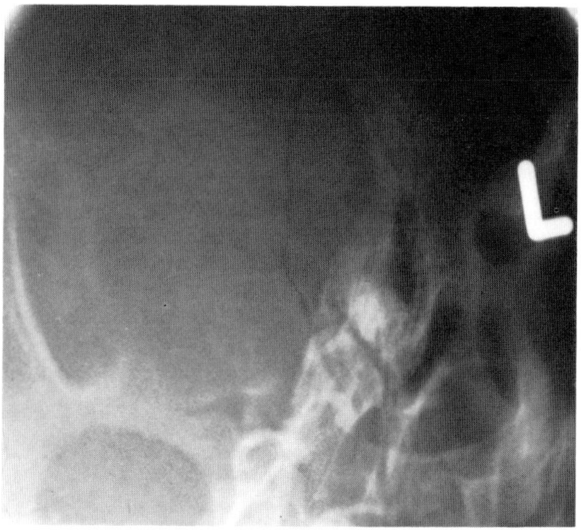

Fig. 1.36a. Same case as in Figure 1.35a. Modified view of the mastoid process. View according to Mayer. In addition to the transverse fracture of the petrous bone, there is also an extensive temporoparietal left skull fracture.

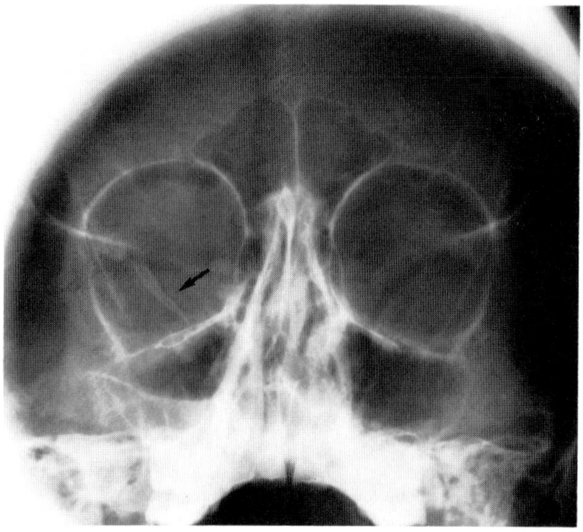

Fig. 1.36b. Same case as in Figure 1.35a. A. p. view for paranasal sinuses. Townes' view: transverse fracture of the left petrous pyramid; fracture of the greater wing of the right sphenoid, with caudal displacement of the fragment *(arrow)*. Bleeding with air-fluid level within the right maxillary sinus.

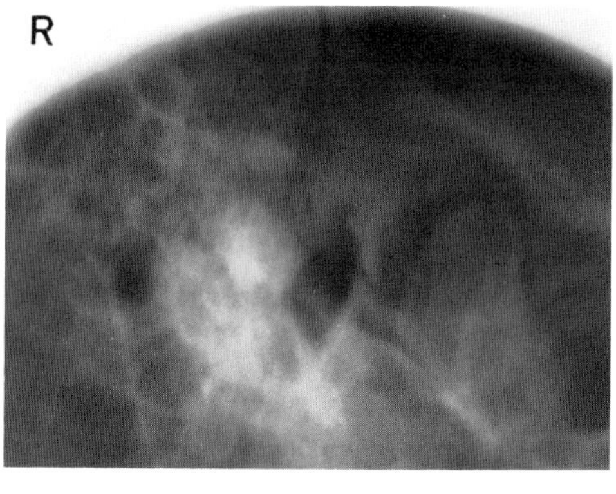

Fig. 1.37. A 31-year-old man after a traffic accident. Bleeding from the right ear. Fracture of the temporal bone through the external auditory canal.

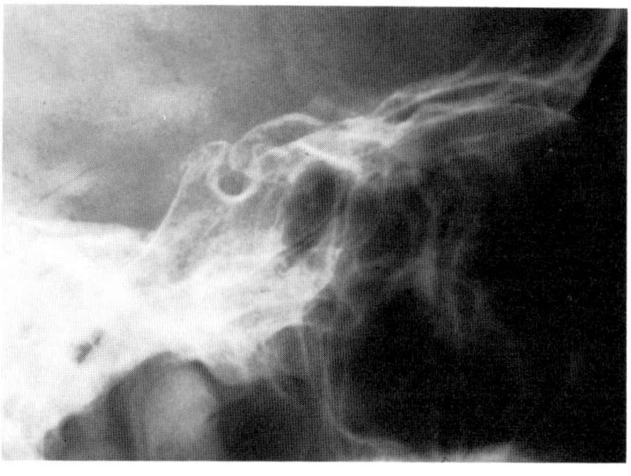

Fig. 1.38. A 17-year-old pedestrian hit by a car. Fracture of the planum sphenoidale. Dislocation within the area of the small processes. Opacification of the sphenoid sinus without a fluid level (incomplete pneumatization?).

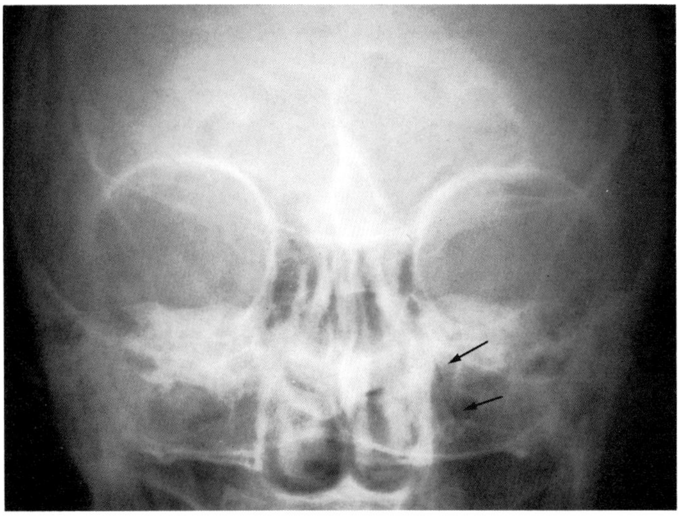

Fig. 1.39a. A 49-year-old man ejected from a car during a collision. Fracture of the posterior fossa extending toward the jugular foramen on a routine a.p. projection of the skull.

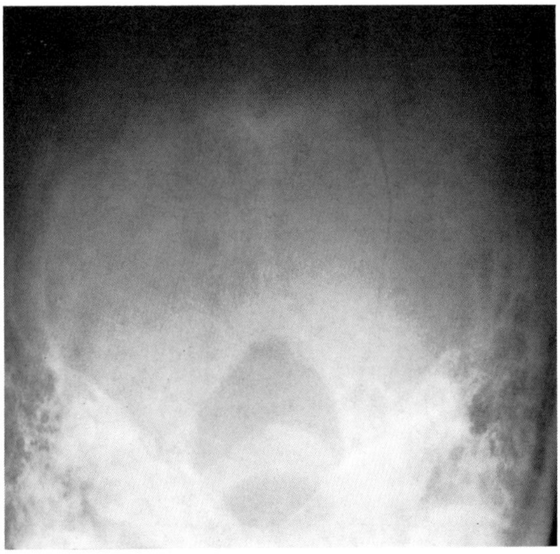

Fig. 1.39b. Special projection of the occipital bone (Townes' view).

2 Spinal Column

About 50 per cent of all spinal injuries are the result of traffic accidents. Another 40 per cent are caused by work-related accidents, particularly in mining, agriculture and the heavy metal industry. Accidents around the home and during sports activities comprise the remaining 10 per cent.

The majority of spinal injuries result from direct trauma, the mechanism being compression, flexion, hyperextension or forced rotation. There are direct traumatic effects as a result of a blow, a fall or being run over. There are no typical fractures corresponding to the type of trauma. Atypical fractures may result from direct trauma.

For practical purposes, one can distinguish between a pulled spine, spinal contusion, spinal fracture, spinal luxation, spinal subluxation and luxation-fracture of the spine. Since clinically it is impossible to differentiate properly between these types of injuries, an x-ray investigation is indicated in every one of these cases. It is important to be aware that, in cases of localized spinal injury, pain is often localized at a lower level (i.e., in a caudal direction) than that of the actual lesion. Thus the x-ray field must always be large enough. The following list of spinal injuries was suggested by Lob (1941) on the basis of anatomic alterations:

1. Isolated injury of the disk.
2. Isolated fracture of a vertebral body.
3. Fracture of a vertebral body with injury to the disk.
4. Complete fracture of the spine (fracture of the vertebra involving its arch and processes; lesion of the disk, tendons and musculature; and malalignment of vertebral bodies with fractures).
5. True dislocation of the spine.
6. Isolated fracture of the vertebral arch or processes.

The characterization of vertebral fractures as being a compression fracture, a bending fracture, a hyperextension fracture or a fracture by rotation is of practical significance when one is dealing with fractures of the cervical spine. Otherwise the descriptive terminology based on the radiologic appearance is recommended.

- Traumatic fracture
- Infraction of the upper or lower plate
- Fracture of the edge of the vertebra
- Compression fracture
- Longitudinal fracture
- Transverse fracture
- Comminuted fracture
- Luxation fracture
- Transverse or dorsal processes or posterior arch fracture

At least for use in x-ray diagnosis, the term isolated vertebral fracture should be dropped, since this describes a pathologic condition that cannot be properly evaluated from the x-ray. The problem of reliable diagnostic interpretation of lesions of the spine has several causes:

1. Contrary to fractures of the extremities with immediate functional sequelae and complaints, there may be no suspicion of the possible existence of a vertebral fracture. Therefore, no x-ray investigation is ordered.
2. It is difficult as well as demanding to secure qualitatively good roentgenograms of the spine.
3. A reliable interpretation of x-rays of the spine requires much more experience and more time than is the case in the evaluation of other fractures.
4. Old traumatic and other lesions may be misleading.
5. Other injuries may be more prominent.

The diagnostic reliability in recognizing injuries of the spine is considerably lower than for fractures of other skeletal regions. Brocher (1944)

maintains that more than half the fractures of the spine are not immediately recognized.
Survey films on two planes of the involved parts of the spine are basic for x-ray diagnosis. They should be obtained carefully with coning, using x-rays in the 70–80 kV range. In addition, it is often recommended to use detailed views, particularly of the cervical spine, as well as oblique views. If the quality of the standard views is not satisfactory, it is more sensible to repeat these rather than to immediately get special views. It is surprising how often vertebral fractures can be easily recognized on a second set of films with a slightly different projection or exposure. It is difficult to obtain technically good views, particularly lateral views of the transitional areas – cervical to thoracic spine and lumbar spine to sacrum. To this day there is no way to obtain technically good lateral views of the transitional area – the cervical to thoracic spine. Diagnostically reliable and useful films can only be obtained in patients who are cooperative and reasonably nimble. The best result often can be expected from tomograms. This also refers to investigation of the upper cervical spine. If there has only been a slight injury, it is recommended that investigation of the cervical spine be performed with the patient in a sitting position.
In all instances of severe injury to the spine, particularly those with neurologic symptoms, it will only be possible to perform the investigation with the patient remaining supine and without changing position. Such an investigation is best conducted with the patient on a movable stretcher with an undertable cassette and a lateral detachable cassette.
As a result of marked differences in anatomy and function, there are special types of injuries affecting the different parts of the spine. By the same token, there are marked differences in resistance to pressure, in extension and rotation of the vertebral bodies and intervertebral disks in the cervical, thoracic and lumbar areas (Sonoda, according to Schmorl and Junghanns, 1968).

Cervical Spine

In the region of the cervical spine, there is a frequent occurrence of luxation, subluxation and injuries to the intervertebral disks. These injuries are somehow due to the marked mobility of the neck and the considerably reduced tolerance to forces exerting pull on the intervertebral disks. The best known types of trauma to the cervical spine are injury caused by diving into shallow water (Fig. 2.1) and the whiplash injury (Fig. 2.2). The radiologically recognizable changes consist of a deformity in posture and a so-called blockage of joints due to subluxation (Fig. 2.3). A subluxation can also be the result of forced rotation. If the location of a traumatic injury to the intervertebral disk cannot be recognized on standard views of the cervical spine, it may well be achieved with a special functional study (Buetti-Bäuml, 1955). Frequently, however, such a special study of the functions of the cervical spine is avoided because six additional views are necessary (flexion, extension, tilting toward right and left, and rotation toward right and left). In view of the frequently reduced mobility due to pain, this type of study is not always feasible. Even young people may show overlapping degenerative changes. In such a situation, the results of trauma can be fully recognized only in follow-up studies (e.g., the disappearance of abnormal posture, the appearance of localized reactive findings and the reduced height of the intervertebral disk within a few months).
Dislocation of the atlas can be seen in conjunction with fractures of the dens and atlas (Figs. 2.6 and 2.7). The most frequently seen fracture of the atlas is localized in the posterior arch (Fig. 2.4). In the differential diagnosis, congenital clefts in particular must be considered. These, however, are mostly located medially, whereas fractures are frequently paramedially located, unilateral or bilateral, and often also show ragged congruent fracture edges. Falling or being hit by a heavy object, with the primary impact to the head, can result in bursting of the atlas, the so-called Jefferson fracture (Fig. 2.5).
In spite of the fact that fractures of the dens occur relatively frequently (about 10 per cent of all fractures of the cervical spine versus 1–2 per cent of all vertebral fractures), its existence is often overlooked. If there is a dislocation of the dens anteriorly (hyperflexion fracture) or posteriorly (hyperextension fracture), the lateral roentgenogram will demonstrate this unequivocally (Figs. 2.6 and 2.7). In unclear situations such as in follow-up examinations with the question of bony consolidation or the appearance of a pseudarthrosis of the dens and in suspected narrowing of the spinal canal, additional tomograms will be necessary – particularly lateral tomograms (Fig. 2.8). Fractures of the dens can be isolated or associated with a fracture of the posterior arch of the atlas. Finally, a fracture of the dens can continue into the body of the second cervical vertebra. In the differential diag-

nosis of pseudarthrosis of the dens, one must consider a persistent congenital variant, an odontoid bone. A luxation or subluxation between the dens and atlas is recognized by an increase in distance between the anterior arch of the atlas and the dens. The subluxation can occur only in the presence of a lesion of the tendons, whereas a dislocation usually requires the existence of a dysplastic dens (habitual luxation) (Fig. 2.9). If this type of dislocation occurs as a result of trauma, it is said to always result in death.

In spite of the strong structure of the body of the second cervical vertebra, it is not infrequently the site of fractures. Usually these affect the pedicles as a result of car accidents in which the vehicle somersaults (Fig. 2.10). According to Schneider and others (1965), fractures of the pedicles of the second cervical vertebra occur typically in hangman's fracture. The subluxations and dislocations occurring further down in the cervical spine are localized most frequently at the level of the 5th and 6th cervical vertebrae and are often combined with avulsion fractures (Figs. 2.11 and 2.12). Fractures of the bodies of cervical vertebrae also occur regularly in the lower cervical spine. Therefore it is very important to emphasize the significance of being able to accurately interpret each region on roentgenograms (Fig. 2.13).

Fractures of the spinous process, known in the old days as shoveler's fractures, today are most frequently the result of traffic accidents (Fig. 2.14).

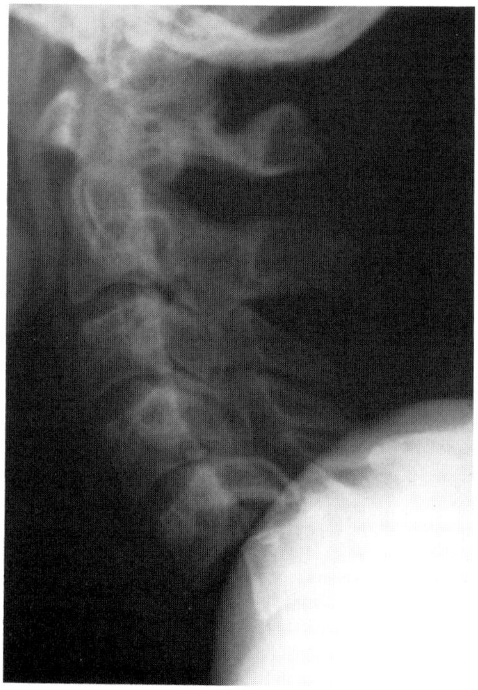

Fig. 2.1. A 21-year-old man, while diving into a swimming pool, hit another swimmer. Luxation of cervical spine 5/6; paralysis below this level.

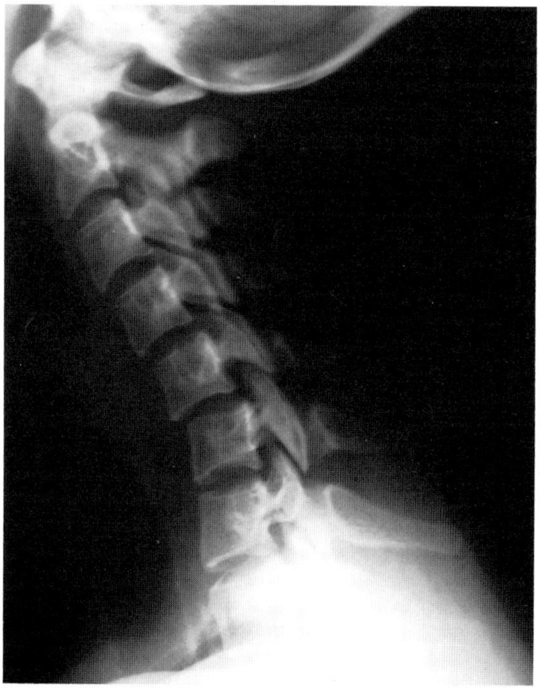

Fig. 2.2. A 21-year-old woman with subluxation of the cervical spine 5/6 and a fixed kyphotic position after whiplash injury of the neck.

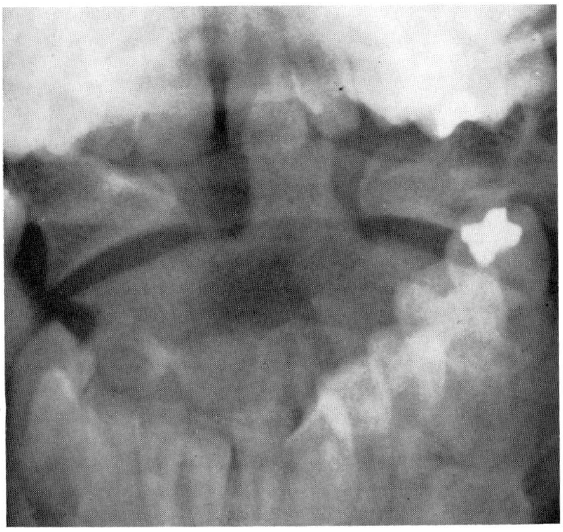

Fig. 2.3. A 17-year-old boy after an accident with a motor scooter. Fixed atlas due to subluxation.

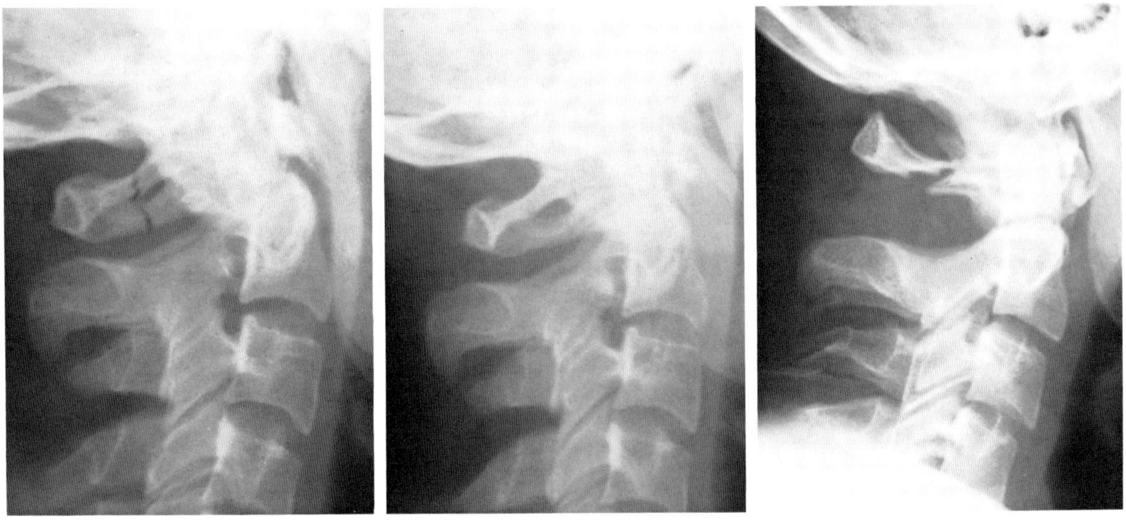

Fig. 2.4.a–c. a) A 21-year-old man with a fracture of the posterior arch of the atlas without dislocation; also fracture of the dens.

b) After six months, both fractures have healed without visible sequelae; complete bony consolidation.

c) A 20-year-old man after a car accident. Fracture of the posterior arch of the atlas with marked dislocation.

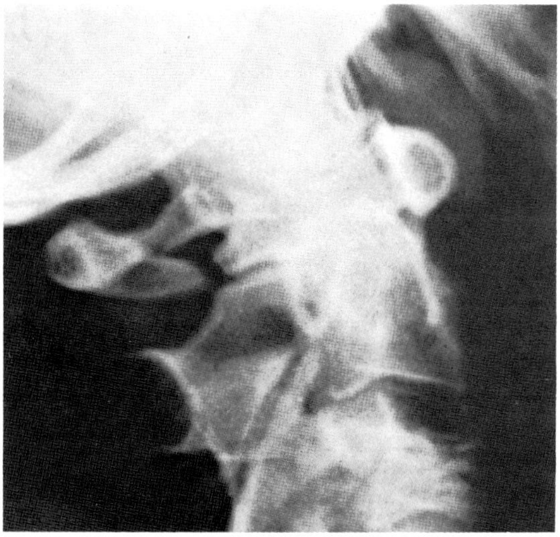

a

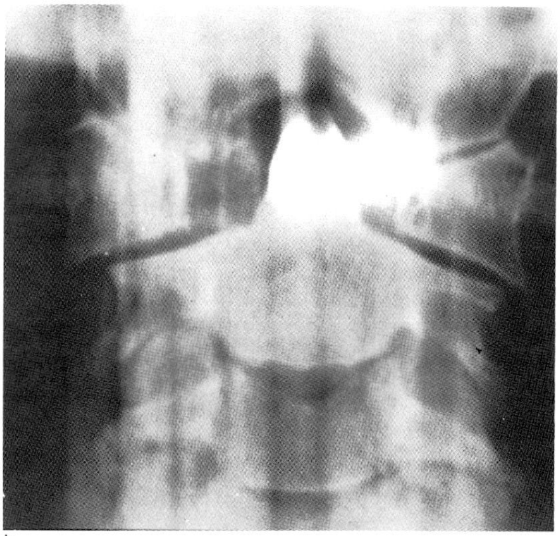

b

Fig. 2.5a and b. Compression fracture of the atlas – Jefferson fracture. Lateral dislocation of both fragments of the atlas. (From G. Schmorl and H. Junghanns: Die gesunde und die kranke Wirbelsäule in Röntgenbild und Klinik. 5. Aufl. Thieme, Stuttgart, 1968).

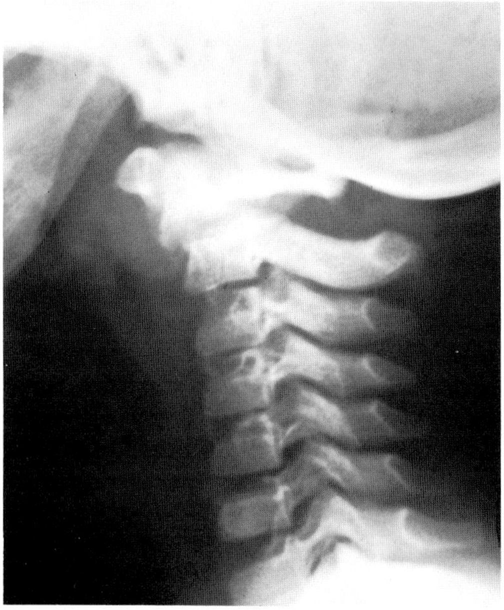

Fig. 2.6. A 3-year-old child with a fracture in hyperflexion of the dens.

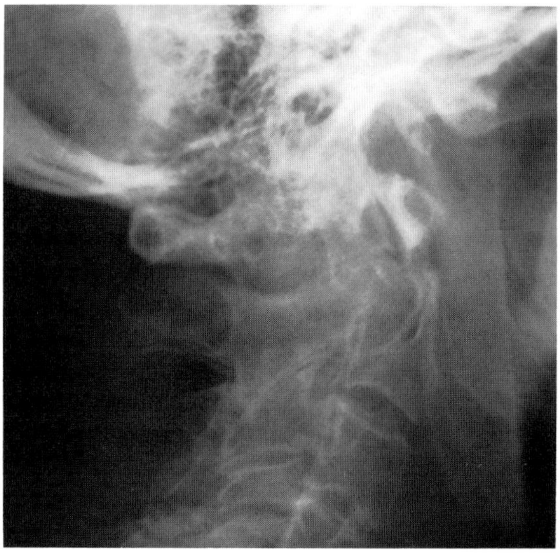

Fig. 2.7. A 61-year-old farmer with no recollection of any trauma due to severe alcoholism. Fracture in hyperextension of the dens with posterior luxation of the atlas. Fracture continues into the body of the second cervical vertebra.

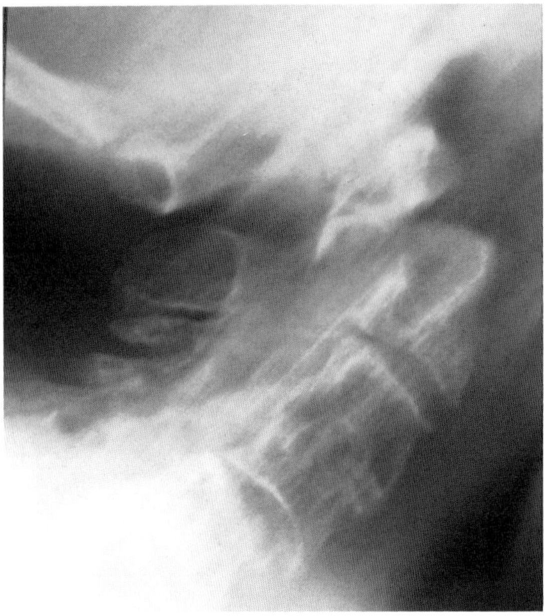

Fig. 2.8. Fracture in hyperextension of the dens in an 83-year-old woman. Dislocation of the pointed fragment of the dens into the spinal canal. This finding can only be recognized on a tomogram. The patient died.

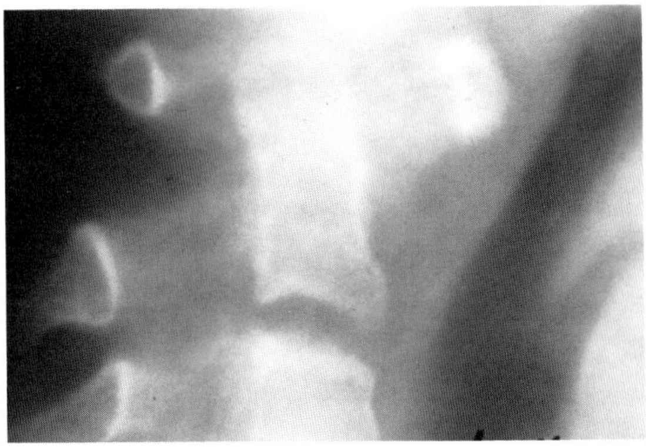

Fig. 2.9. A 16-year-old boy after repeated dislocation of the neck during clumsy movements. Luxation between the atlas and dens in the area of the transverse ligaments (tomogram).

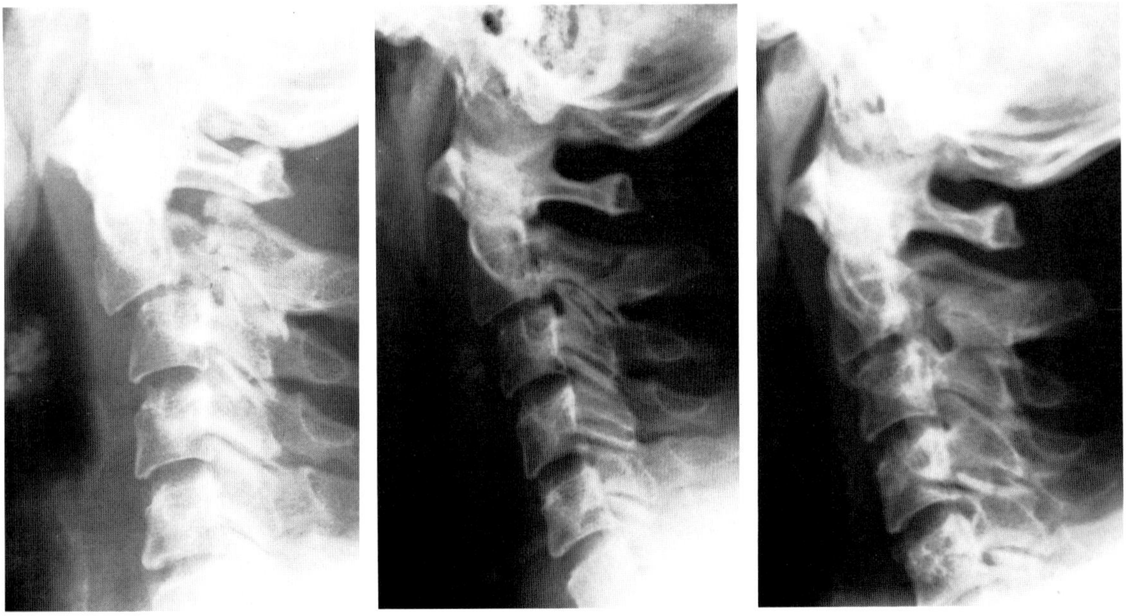

a b c

Fig. 2.10a–c. A 17-year-old girl after a car accident. Fracture of the pedicles of the second cervical vertebra.
a) Immediately after accident.
b) After reposition.
c) Fully healed local findings two years later.

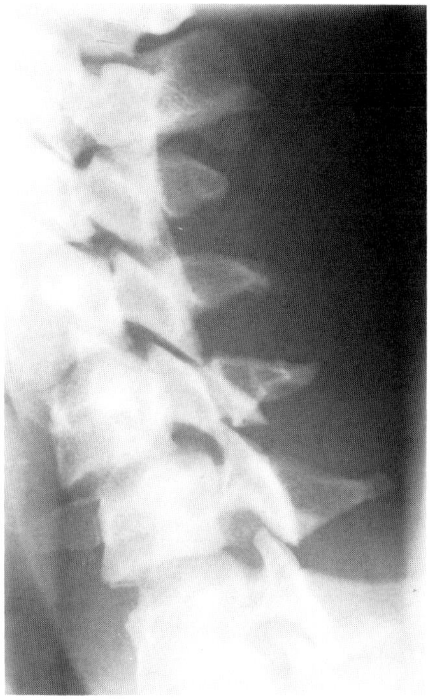

Fig. 2.11. A 15-year-old girl after a traffic accident. Right-sided luxation of the cervical spine 5/6, with a fracture of the inferior tip of the articular process 5.

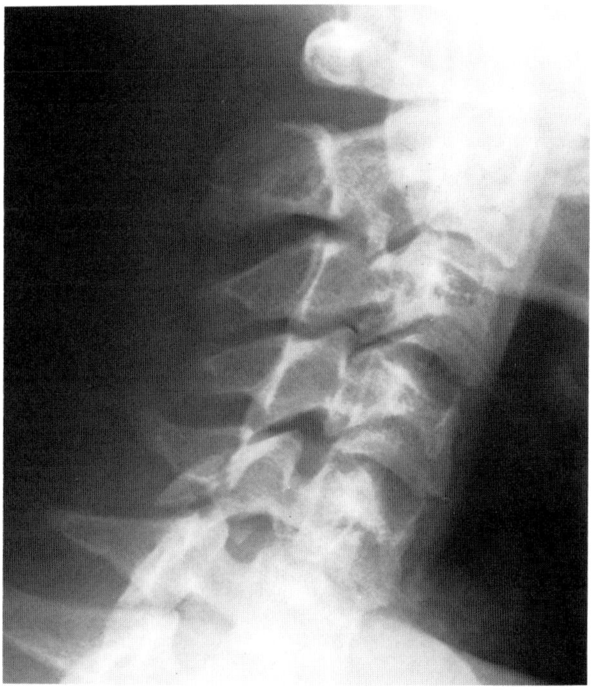

Fig. 2.12. A 19-year-old woman after a traffic accident. Subluxation of cervical spine 5/6, with avulsion fracture of the articular processes 5 and 6. Oblique view.

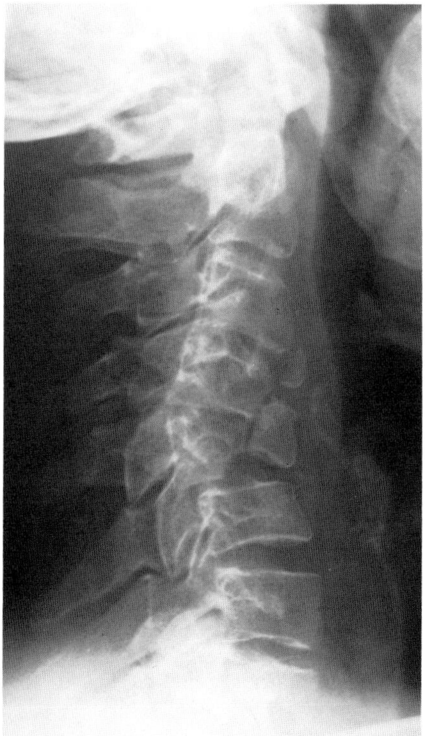

Fig. 2.13. A 42-year-old man with trauma due to a fall from a tree. Hyperflexion fracture of cervical vertebrae and respective arches. Subluxation of cervical spine 5/6.

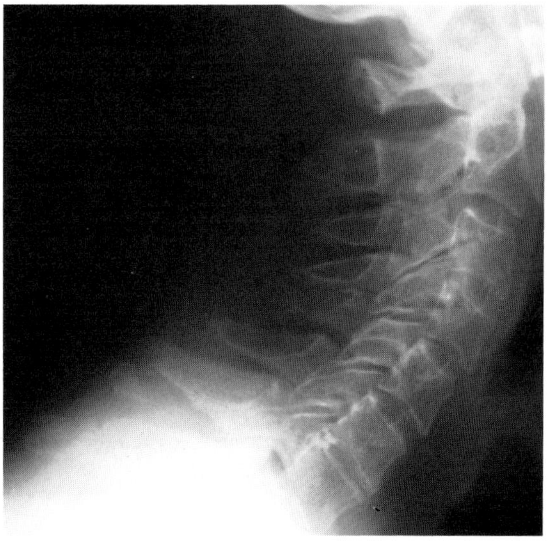

Fig. 2.14. A 58-year-old man after an accident in which the car somersaulted. Fracture of the spinous processes of the 7th cervical and 1st thoracic vertebrae.

Thoracic and Lumbar Spine

Within the areas of the thoracic and lumbar spine, luxations and luxation fractures are seen comparatively rarely. They are always the result of very severe trauma. The diagnostic changes are almost always visible on radiographs even if the film quality is inferior owing to the accident situation (Fig. 2.15). In all instances of dislocated vertebrae, there are of necessity also luxations in the small joints of the spine or fractures in the posterior elements of the vertebrae or the articular processes. All types of vertebral fractures are seen in the area under discussion, particularly avulsion fractures and compression fractures. Since 50 per cent of all fractures of vertebral bodies occur here, the most frequently involved area is that of the thoracolumbar transition zone (Figs. 2.16 and 2.17).

Fractures involving several vertebral bodies are usually located in the middle or lower 3rd of the thoracic spine. In patients with a mild compression fracture, there is a characteristic x-ray finding – gibbus formation with a wedge-shaped reduction of the ventral height of the fractured vertebral body. Occasionally this also involves the lateral half. In addition, one frequently sees anterior displacement of the upper parts of the involved vertebral body, with local step formation of the anterior vertebral contours, as well as compression, overlapping and widening of the superior portion of the injured vertebral body (Fig. 2.17). Sometimes a break in the contour can be recognized only on one side or affects one of the base plates, usually the upper one. In cases of preexisting spondylosis, special care should be devoted to recognizing normal contours and step formation (Fig. 2.18). A clear differentiation should be attempted between traumatic fracture of the base plates, avulsion fracture of the apophysis and the existence of Schmorl bodies in the lumbar area; there may also be a separate developmental ossification center (Fig. 2.19). A fracture of a vertebral body may result in a so-called traumatic Schmorl body (Schmorl and Junghanns, 1968) (Fig. 2.20). Congenital wedging or hemivertebra can be confused very easily with a vertebral fracture due to recent trauma (Fig. 2.21). Spondylolisthesis occasionally is misinterpreted as a fracture of an articular process.

In the area of the lumbar spine, there is a high incidence of fractures of the transverse processes often occurring at several levels and bilaterally (Fig. 2.23). There is not always a significant dislocation of the fracture fragments (Fig. 2.22). A fracture can be simulated by overlapping soft-tissue structures and gut as well as the psoas shadow. A possibility of misinterpretation is also presented by the so-called joints in the location of lumbar ribs at the level of the 1st lumbar vertebral body, particularly where this is unilateral (Fig. 2.23).

Isolated fractures of the posterior arches or the articular processes are hardly ever seen; this is in direct contrast to the situation in the cervical spine. They are usually present in addition to severe fractures of vertebral bodies or luxation fractures (Fig. 2.23).

Additional Injuries

The most important coexisting injuries involving vertebral fractures are those to the spinal cord, particularly with neurologic symptoms. Inconsistent data from the literature indicate an incidence of 5 to 50 per cent (Junghanns). Half of all injuries to the spinal cord occur at the level of the 12th thoracic and 1st lumbar vertebrae. Roughly 20 per cent of injuries to the spinal cord are located in the cervical area. The main causes are accidents at work and in and around the home. It appears remarkable that accidents around swimming pools and traffic accidents occur with roughly equal frequency. In traffic accidents, there is in rare instances injury to the cervical spinal cord due to a whiplash injury, with or without cervical spine fracture (Meinecke, 1970). Besides the area directly traumatized, there are also other conditions such as hematoma or edema as well as secondary protrusions or spike formation (Fig. 2.24), resulting in damage to the spinal cord. There is no consensus as to whether a more conservative or a surgical approach is best in the treatment of traumatic lesions of the spinal cord. There are special units for the treatment and rehabilitation of patients with transection of the cord.

An immediately manifest, simultaneous injury is a paravertebral hematoma. This can be very large in serial fractures involving several vertebral bodies. Frequently such a lesion is thought to be the cause of gastrointestinal symptoms such as an ileus.

Open injuries usually result from shooting accidents, always with the danger of injury to the spinal cord. Projectiles or metal splinters may be embedded for years without any symptoms within or close to a vertebral body. However they may manifest themselves at any time by a local reaction to infection or simply by mechanical irritation (Fig. 2.25).

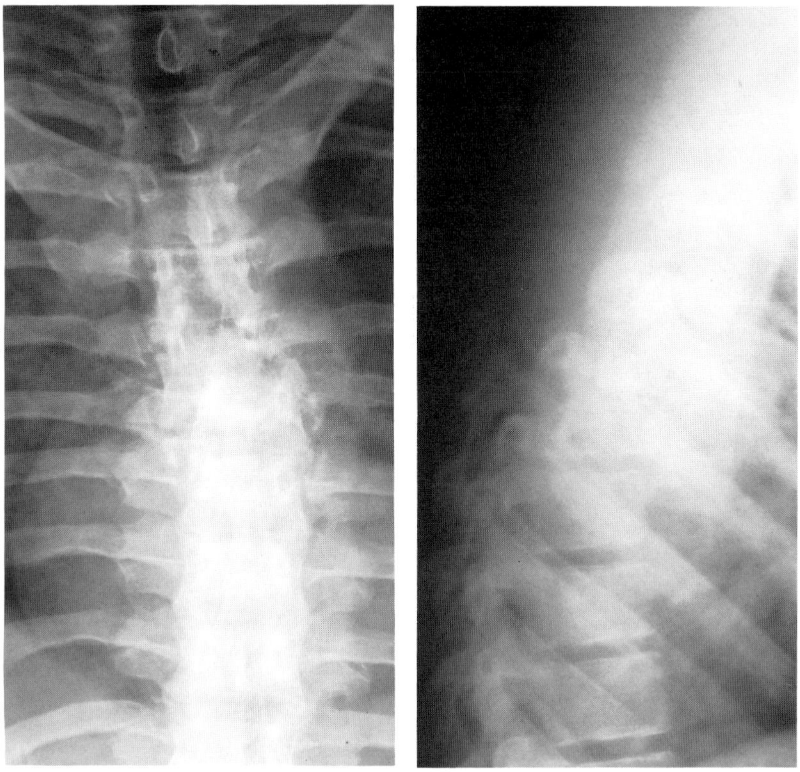

a b

Fig. 2.15a and b. A 17-year-old skilled laborer after an accident with a motor scooter. Luxation fracture of the thoracic spine 5/6. Transsection of the cord.

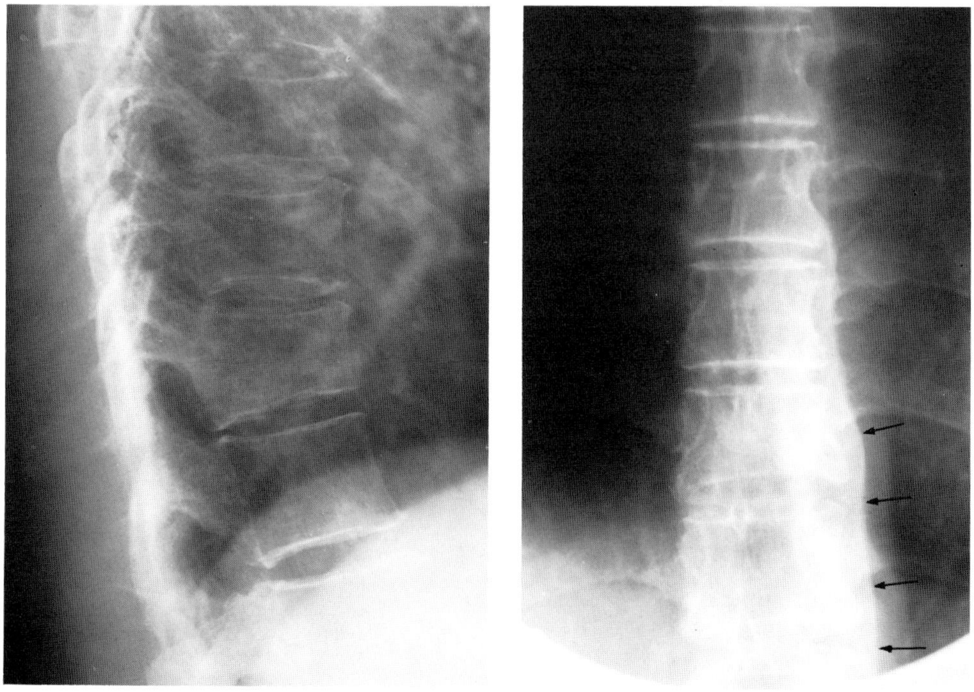

a b

Fig. 2.16a and b. Atypical compression fracture of the 10th thoracic vertebral body. Fracture through the ground plate and dislocation of the left anterior region and lower corner. Extensive paravertebral hematoma *(arrows).*

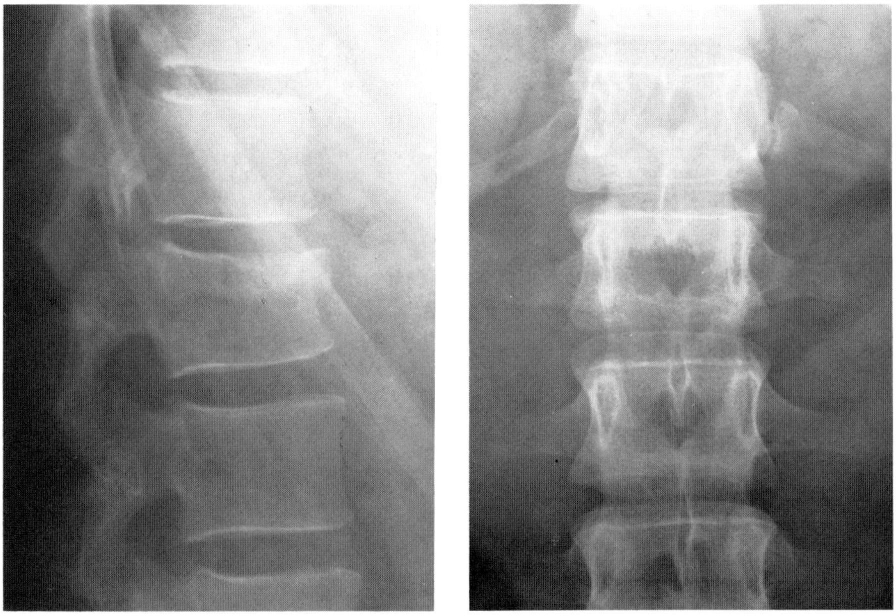

a b

Fig. 2.17a and b. A 28-year-old man after a car accident in which he ran into the car in front. Typical compression fracture of the 1st lumbar vertebral body. Slight gibbous, wedge-shaped appearance of the vertebral body anteriorly; displacement of the anterior upper vertebral contour with a step effect. Serpentine condensation due to compression.

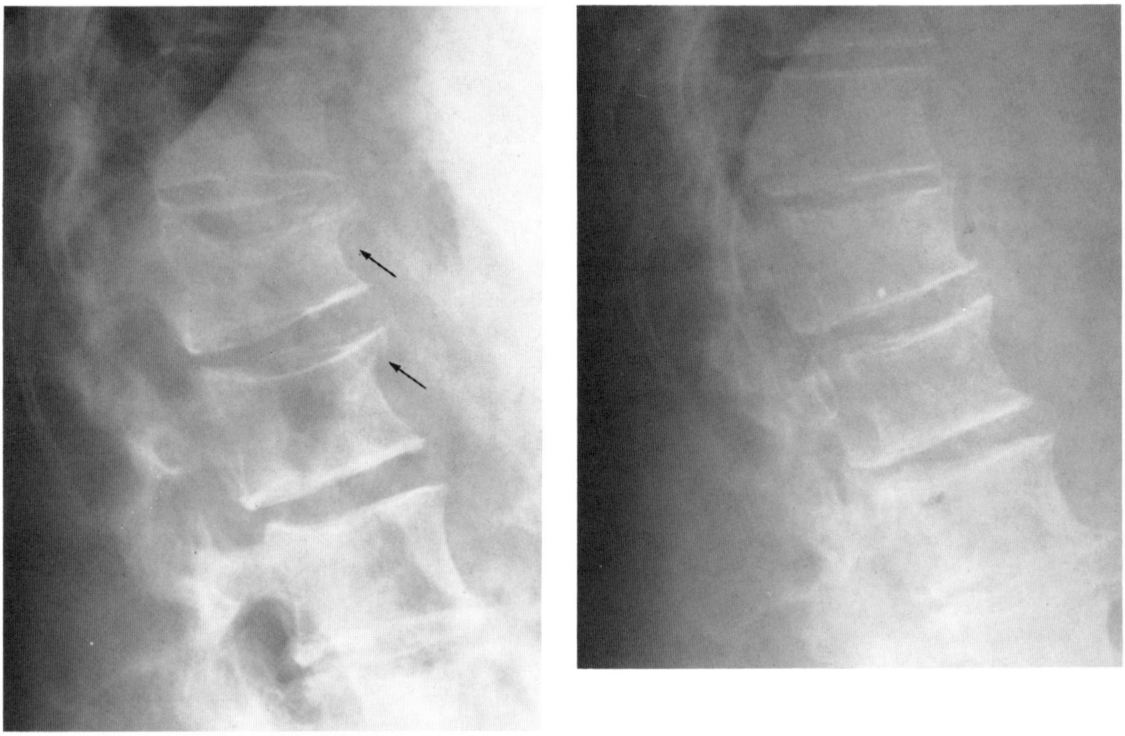

Fig. 2.18a and b. Compression fracture of the 1st and 2nd lumbar vertebral bodies.
a) Disrupted contours and step effect reliably give the diagnosis.
b) 15 months later, the residual changes cannot be differentiated from degenerative alterations.

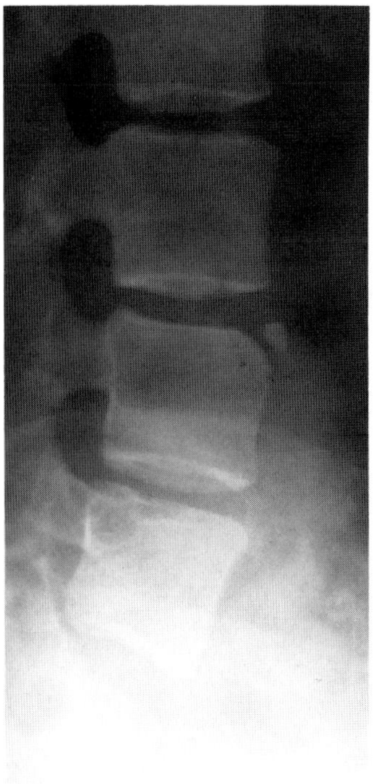

Fig. 2.19. Isolated ossicle; normal variant of the anterior upper rim; this is no fracture.

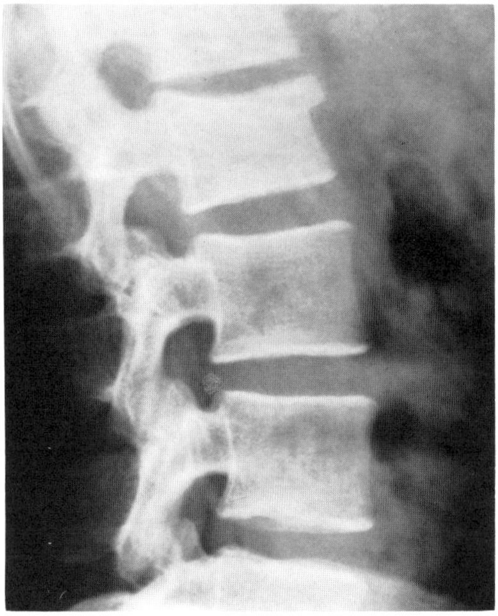

Fig. 2.20a and b. A 20-year-old man with post-traumatic Schmorl body after a fracture of the 2nd lumbar vertebral body.
a) X-ray after the accident.

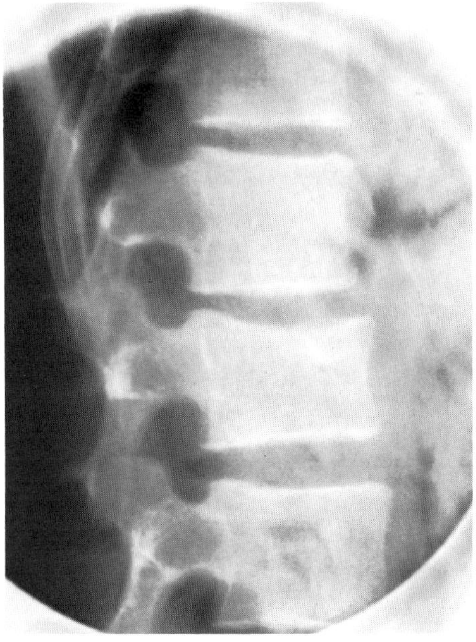

b) After 16 months.

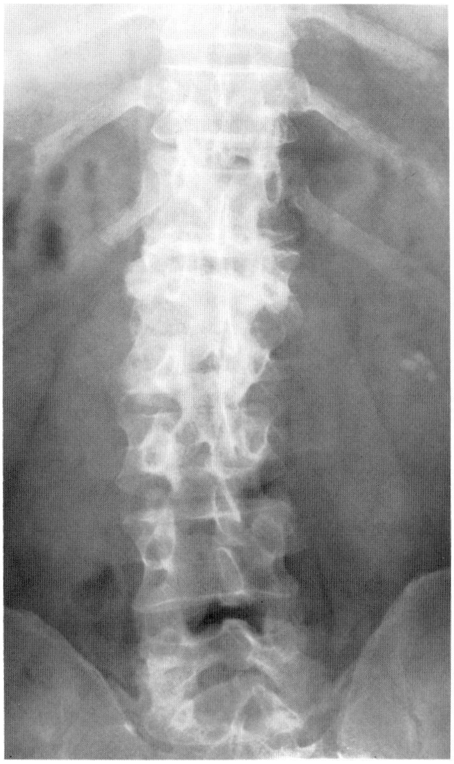

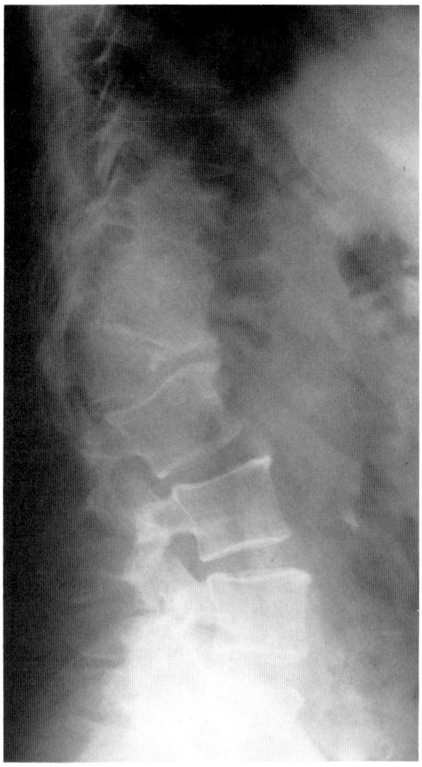

Fig. 2.21a and b. A 53-year-old man with congenital malformation. Wedge formation of the first lumbar vertebra.
a) On this a.p. view, there is an impression of a possible fracture, with deformity of the area of the 1st lumbar vertebral body.

b) On the lateral view, the dorsal hemivertebra can be fully appreciated with compensatory growth of the adjacent vertebral bodies.

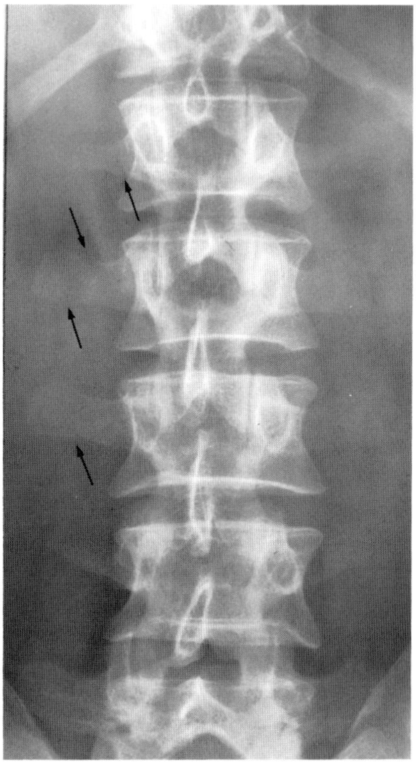

Fig. 2.22. A 40-year-old construction worker who was hit on the head by a falling board. Minimally dislocated fracture of the transverse processes of L 2 and 3 on the right; questionable fracture of the 1st lateral process of the lumbar spine.

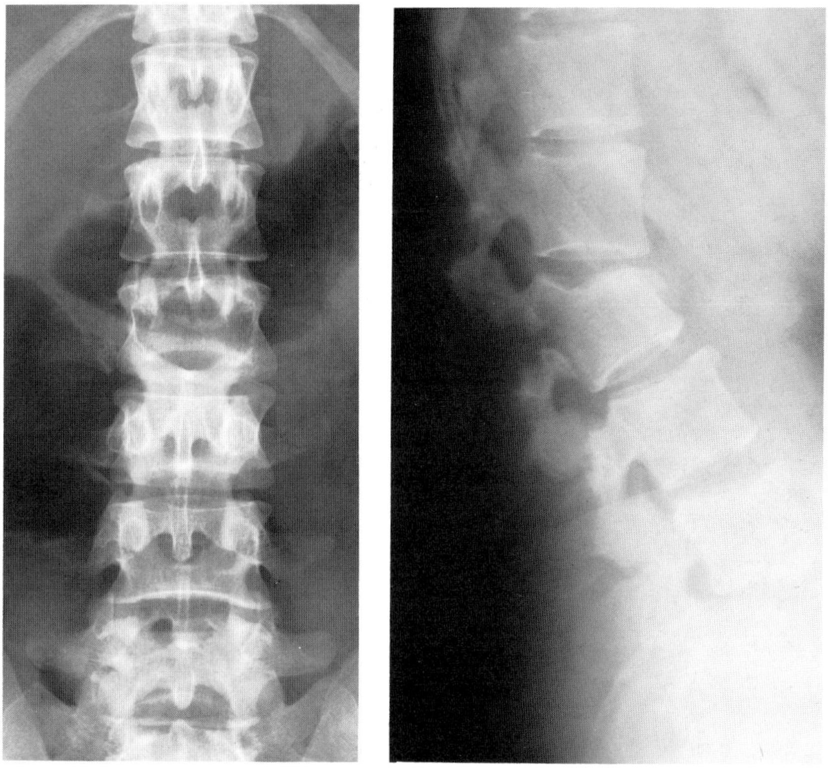

a b

Fig. 2.23a and b. A 21-year-old woman who was run over by her own car when her three-year-old child managed to loosen the hand-brake. Fracture of the dorsal arch and of the spinous processes of the lumbar vertebral body 2, with a severe compression fracture. Less dramatic similar involvement of the 3rd and 4th lumbar vertebral bodies. Fracture of the lateral processes 2 and 3 bilaterally. The 12th thoracic vertebra has lateral processes with articulation (transitional vertebra).

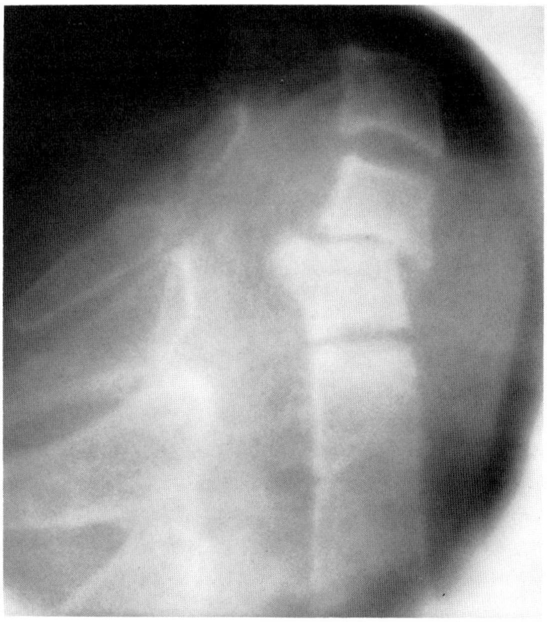

Fig. 2.24. A 38-year-old man who fell head first from a tree. Secondary formation of a marked local swelling at the posterior and upper region of the 7th cervical vertebra ten weeks after a fracture with luxation. Symptoms of compression of the spinal cord with neurologic manifestations (tomograms).

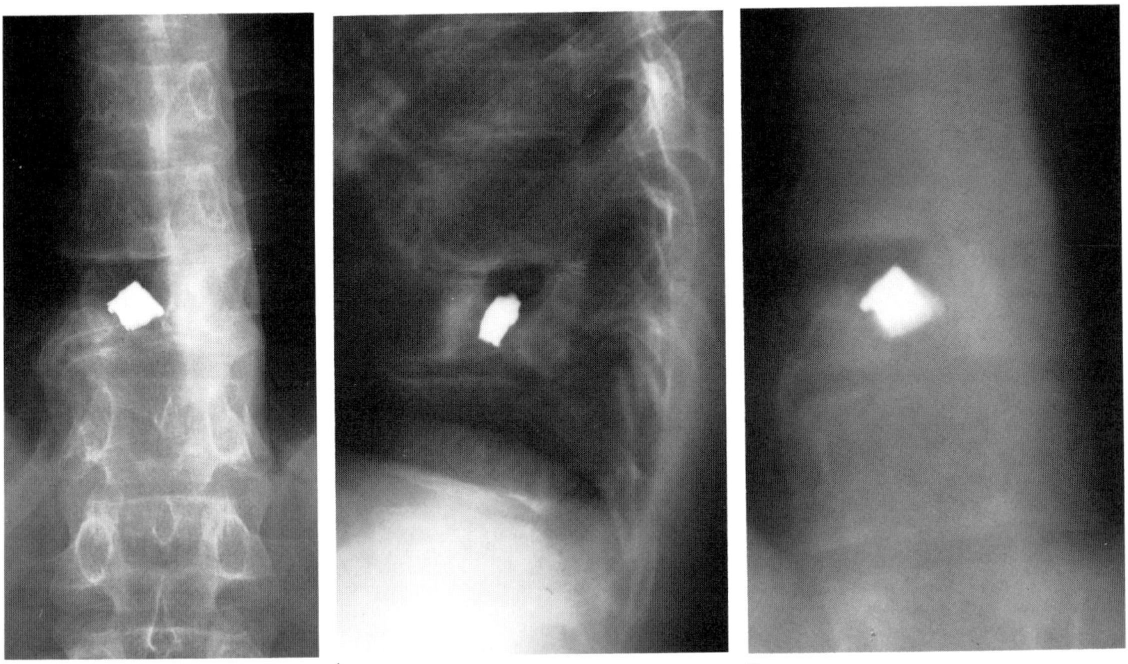

a b c

Fig. 2.25a–c. A 46-year-old man who never had any symptoms since the end of World War II; however, when driving his tractor he now has intolerable back pain. He is known to have had a shrapnel splinter located in the 11th thoracic vertebral body for 26 years. a and b) A. p. lateral survey. c) Tomogram. There is a marked area of resorption around the splinter, almost complete loss of height of the intervertebral disk area and a defect of the right part of the vertebral body.

3 Neuroradiologic Special Studies with Contrast Media After Skull and Brain Trauma and Injuries to the Spine

Skull and Brain Trauma

Irrespective of the radiologic findings on standard views, there must be an exhaustive neuroradiologic investigation if there are clinical indications for the presence of increased intracranial pressure and when the condition of the patient justifies the performance of specialized procedures.

It may be clinically impossible or only minimally probable to try to differentiate between hemorrhage of the skull and brain, edema of the brain without hemorrhage, and contusion of the brain stem. The danger of additional damage to the patient and the cerebral circulation resulting from the investigation has to be viewed as being less than the possibility of losing the patient because of an undiagnosed hematoma. It is recommended that neurosurgical expertise be involved early in the investigation. A basis for such interventions, however, must be the objective demonstration of hemorrhage and its localization.

An indication for angiography is given only if it is suspected that there is a hematoma that can be approached surgically with a good chance of success (Huber, 1969). If a patient already shows signs of severe functional central nervous system loss (decerebration), therapeutic and diagnostic measures do not make sense. Still, there are two reasons for advocating such procedures: on the one hand, there are neurosurgeons who will base their decision on whether there is still cerebral circulation; on the other hand, it is an accepted procedure to stop further respirator treatment of a patient with proven brain death if angiography demonstrates complete stasis of the cerebral vessels (Fig. 3.1).* It can be assumed that nontherapeutic indications will become even more important in our age of organ transplantation and because of the still unsettled question of an exact definition of clinical death. (The respective present criteria are: absence of spontaneous respiration, flat EEG and complete stasis of cerebral circulation. It has already been postulated that during angiography all four main vessels must be fully investigated.) All these precautionary measures are required before making the serious decision to stop all resuscitation efforts.

Percutaneous carotid angiography is used most frequently to demonstrate the cerebral circulation. Angiography of the vertebral arteries is of minimal importance in the treatment of traumatic brain injuries. Vertebral angiography is technically difficult and more dangerous. Furthermore, there is very little information to be gained, even if there is bleeding within the posterior fossa. In every instance, there must be rapid seriography since, in addition to a static finding, this will also offer information on the dynamics of cerebral perfusion. In an emergency, it is still possible to limit the recording to three films (arterial, capillary and venous phases).

It is usually impossible to differentiate between an epidural and a subdural hematoma even on high-quality angiograms. This differentiation must be made preoperatively on the basis of the clinical course.

---

* This attitude is apparently widespread in Western Europe. Caution is indicated in the United States in light of the Quinlan case in New Jersey.

On a sagittal angiogram, both types of hemorrhage will show a displacement of the vessels away from the skull, with a space free of vasculature between contrasting vessels of the surface of the brain and the inner table. Frequently there is an associated displacement of the anterior cerebral artery toward the opposite side (Fig. 3.2). If this deviation is absent despite the proven presence of a subdural or epidural hematoma, another hematoma on the opposite side must be seriously suspected (Fig. 3.3).

Hematomas of a more frontal, parietal or parieto-occipital location can sometimes not be recognized on orthograde, a.p. angiograms, since there may be overlap by adjacent parietal vessels or by the borders of the diploë. If there is a deviation of the anterior cerebral artery or, during the venous phase, a displacement of the inner cerebral veins without definite proof of a subdural hematoma, the investigation must be continued. It is then necessary to obtain two runs with the head rotated about 20 degrees around the longitudinal axis toward the right and left sides (Fig. 3.4). Among traumatic intracranial hemorrhages, the distribution is as follows: subdural hematomas – 65 per cent; epidural hematomas – 25 per cent; and intracerebral hemorrhage – 10 per cent. If of sufficient size, the last two are characterized by an arching of arteries surrounding a usually rounded avascular area (Fig. 3.5).

The most important sign on an angiogram is the lateral displacement of the anterior cerebral arteries. If the location of the hemorrhage is anterior regardless of whether it is epidural, subdural or intracerebral, the artery is displaced and forms an arch toward the other side; if, however, the hemorrhage is located more posteriorly, this vessel is simply displaced in a parallel fashion.

Lateral displacement also can be caused by unilateral edema of the brain due to trauma. After dehydration therapy and abatement of the symptoms of increased intracranial pressure, follow-up angiography will reveal that, because of the reversal of edema of the brain, the anterior cerebral artery has returned to its midline position. The choice of side in angiography is dictated by the clinical symptoms (contralateral hemiplegia, ipsilateral mydriasis, etc.). The greatest significance has to be attached to the finding of unilateral mydriasis. A hemiparesis can also be the result of a simple contusion, whereas subdural or epidural hematomas are located on the contralateral side. Fractures of the skull are even less reliable findings in the attempt to determine the involved side of the brain. In 65 to 70 per cent of all cases, there is a subdural hematoma contralateral to the skull fracture. In fractures crossing the course of the meningeal artery, one can expect an epidural hematoma on the side of the fracture. This is also possibly the case in fractures extending into the middle cerebral fossa (temporobasal epidural hematoma).

Statistically, it can be shown that, in cases of temporobasal epidural hematoma, there is most frequently an epidural hematoma caused by an injury to the branch of the medial meningeal artery (Fig. 3.6). On a lateral angiogram, one notes an arched curving of the medial vessels. In addition, these may be compressed and displaced frontally. In the a.p. view, the group of vessels of the medial meningeal artery may also be abnormally located. They are displaced superiorly, the main branch taking a right course upward and laterally from its origin at the internal carotid artery. The avascular area of the hemorrhage, however, is not as clearly visualized as in parietal hemorrhage, since there is overlap by bony structures of the pyramid and orbit. In rare instances, one can also recognize an accumulation of blood originating from the medial meningeal artery (Fig. 3.7).

In a patient in whom, immediately after severe skull and brain trauma or shortly thereafter, an audible bruit is heard with the further appearance of pulsating exophthalmos after some time, together with marked dilatation and arterialization of the veins in the eyeground, there must be an arteriovenous fistula between the internal carotid artery and the cavernous sinus. Angiographically, this short circuit can be demonstrated by the fact that during the injection of the contrast agent there is almost simultaneous opacification of the internal carotid artery and the usually dramatically enlarged cavernous sinus, together with the petrous sinus and the interior jugular vein (Fig. 3.8). Frequently one can recognize during the arterial phase large veins leading toward the frontal, parietal and occipital areas, together with opacification of the veins of the external circulation. In order to be able to demonstrate fully all the involved vessels, it is important to perform rapid sequence angiography with two to three pictures per second.

Formerly, a traumatic arteriovenous fistula between the carotid artery and the internal jugular veins (extremely rarely between the vertebral artery and the jugular vein) (Fig. 3.9) was most frequently the result of stabbings. Today, however, this complication does occur with increasing frequency after traffic accidents. This condition is recognized by the presence of the well-known pulse synchronous engine murmur. Immediate angiography of the aortic arch with demonstration of all vessels supplying the neck is indicated before the short circuit with the reduced supply of oxygenated blood to the brain leads to irreparable damage to the central nervous system or to cardiac decompensation.

Traumatic saccular aneurysms of the cerebral vessels are rarely seen; also rare is similar involvement of the medial meningeal artery.

Extreme caution is advised in the diagnosis of a traumatic vascular occlusion, be it of the internal carotid artery after trauma to the neck or of the media after skull and brain trauma (Fig. 3.10). Quite frequently in such cases there are preexisting alterations of the arteries, and the trauma will lead to shock, disturbed circulation, edema of the brain and coagulation defects. Frequently trauma – not only due to a fall but also to traffic accidents – is not the cause but rather the consequence of an acute vascular occlusion, with resulting short periods of loss of consciousness.

Fat embolism of cerebral vessels after extracranial fractures can be demonstrated during angiography as occlusion of smaller arterial branches. It cannot be differentiated from an embolism of other origin.

Posttraumatic late sequelae to the brain can be evaluated by pneumoencephalography. It is important that the investigation by instillation of gas not only demonstrate all the parts of the ventricular system but that all the areas of the subarachnoid space above the hemisphere be examined. Only after all posttraumatic sequelae such as edema and loss of brain substance have fully abated will it be possible to determine the amount of brain damage. On the average, this will take six to eight weeks after the trauma.

After generalized edema of the brain and loss of consciousness have persisted for days or weeks, pneumoencephalography will reveal varying degrees of enlargement the ventricles; this as an expression of loss of parenchyma. In cases of unilateral involvement, one occasionally finds a unilateral marked enlargement of the lateral ventricle, with displacement (e vacuo) of the ventricular system toward the side of the deformation (Fig. 3.11). Local deformation of the lateral ventricle with circumscribed protrusion most frequently is the result of a strictly local trauma (rarely without an open skull injury or depressed fracture). A pointed contour of an enlarged area of a ventricle is indicative of scarring of the brain, extending all the way toward the internal wall.

In local foci of contusion, the subarachnoid spaces will show up as large furrows of coarse accumulations of gas. It must, however, be considered that organizing hematomas of the cortex, even after local formation of scar tissue in the degenerated cortical area, can fill these spaces. A radiologic diagnosis of the underlying pathology is thus impossible.

The formerly often utilized air insufflation of the subdural spaces in the diagnosis of posttraumatic epilepsy to demonstrate the presence of brain and dura scars is largely abandoned today. This is the result of the fact that neurosurgical excision of the scars done some years ago usually leads to further postoperative brain and dura scars. This operative approach has been abandoned because of poor results.

As the result of open skull and brain trauma, brain abscess is a much feared complication that may manifest itself sometimes only after a very long interval, up to several years after the trauma. In the majority of cases, such an abscess is observed clinically as an intracranial space-occupying lesion and can be demonstrated accurately by angiography. Accompanied by a lateral displacement of the anterior cerebral arteries and the adjacent vessels, the abscess is seen as a round area free of contrast agent (Fig. 3.12). During the late stages, there is development of a thin wall with newly formed vessels. This can be recognized occasionally as a very faint rim of vessels around a completely contrast-free area. In cases in which an abscess has penetrated into the CSF spaces, with acute neurologic and psychiatric symptoms, patients may occasionally survive. If so, and after the acute symptoms have abated, it will be possible to demonstrate the old abscess by gas ventriculography (Fig. 3.13).

Posttraumatic CSF leaks from the nose and ear without exception are proof of a severe skull and brain injury. This symptom is always the result of a fracture extending through the anterior base of the skull or the posterior wall of the frontal sinus, with resultant seeping of CSF from the nose, into the epipharynx or from the medial fossa into the ear. In all cases, there must be a tear of the dura. Pinching of parts of the dura within the fracture will prevent the normal healing process and the spontaneous closure of the fistula. The fistula, however, may close by local adhesions but will still be the "opening" for repeated ascending meningitis; if there is to be surgical closure of the fistula, prior accurate localization is mandatory. Its radiologic confirmation can be very difficult and is a relatively un-

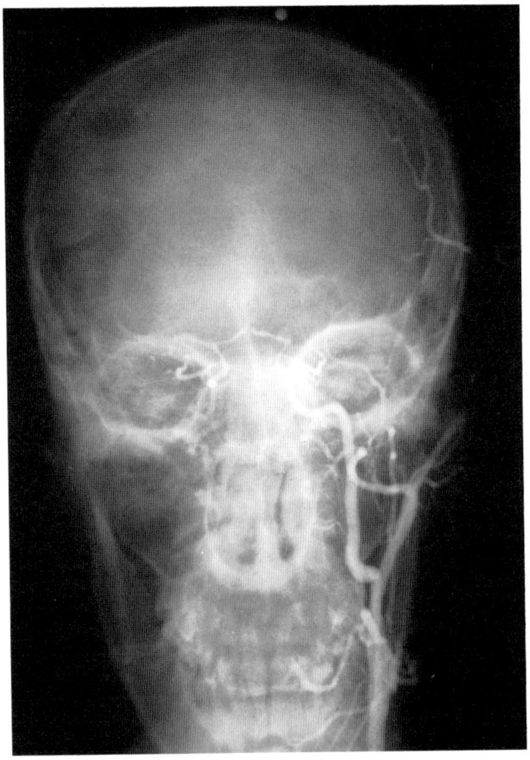

rewarding task. Without tomography on different planes, a study will be always incomplete; also, it is often impossible to accurately demonstrate the fistula. Somewhat better results are obtained by CSF scintigraphy. Here the radioactive isotope is injected into the CSF space in the suboccipital cistern, and subsequently appears on a piece of cotton placed in the nostril or the external auditory canal.

Fig. 3.1. A 17-year-old boy with skull and brain trauma after a traffic accident. In spite of craniotomy on the left, there is loss of consciousness for the last 10 days. Transfemoral carotid angiography; the majority of contrast agent is passing through the external carotid artery. Intracranially, there is filling of only the carotid syphon bilaterally, the circular part of the anterior cerebral artery bilaterally and both ophthalmic arteries. There is no contrast agent visible within the area supplied by the anterior and medial cerebral arteries. There is thus a total arrest of the cerebral circulation.

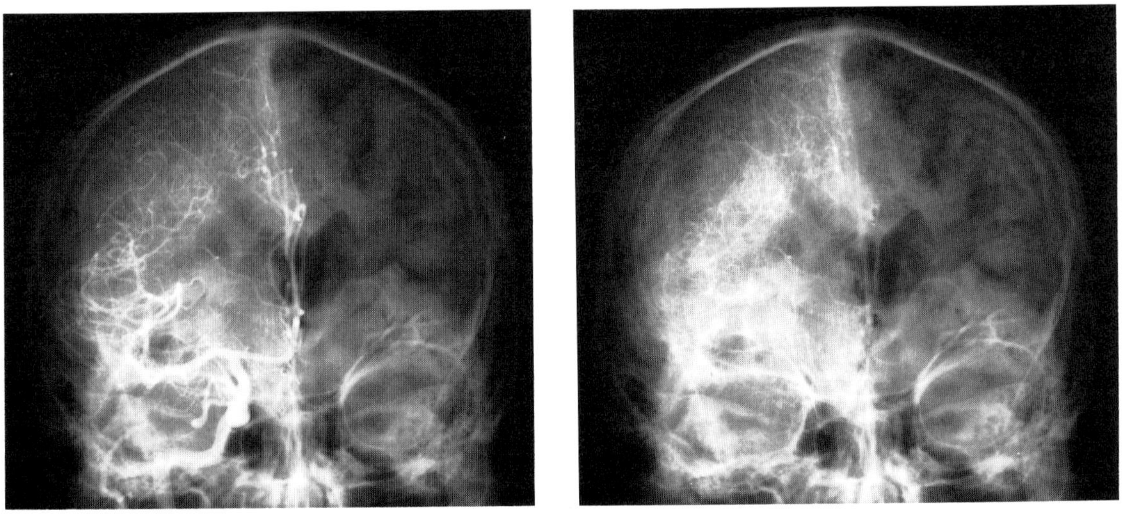

Fig. 3.2a and b. Six weeks ago, the patient suffered trauma of the head by hitting a stair in a stable. No loss of consciousness. Minimal weakness on one side. Three days prior to admission, there was a seizure involving the left side in particular. Therefore, pneumoencephalography was performed. Because of deviation of the ventricular system, the next step was angiography of the right internal carotid artery.
a) View during injection; parallel displacement of the anterior cerebral arteries. Compression of the medial vessels and displacement downward; arching of the marginal vessel of the media.

b) Roentgenograms 3 seconds after completion of injection; biconvex contrast-free space in the right parietal region.

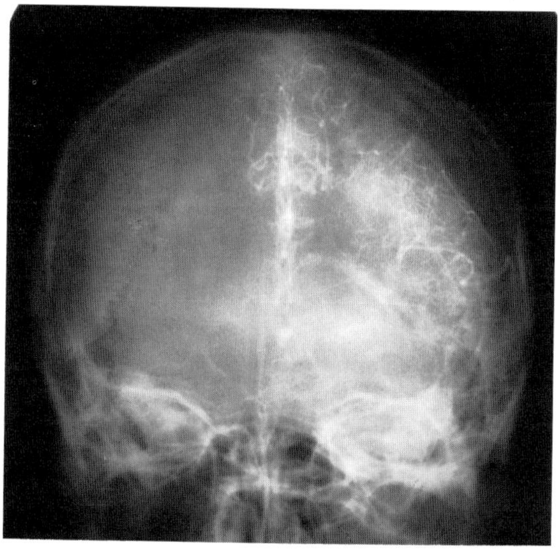

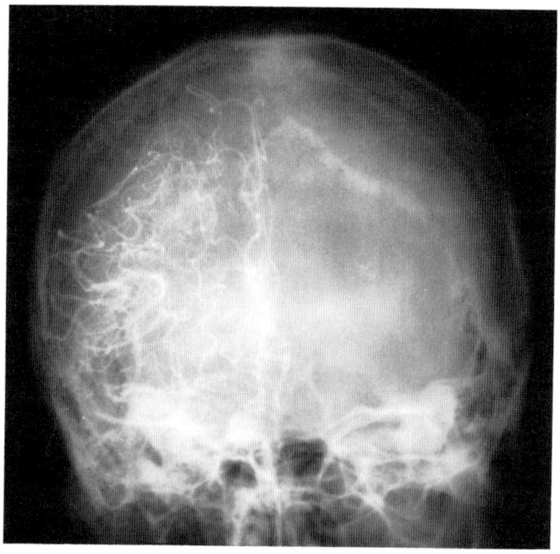

Fig. 3.3a and b. Bilateral carotid angiography in the presence of bilateral subdural hematoma in the parietal area.
a) Roentgenogram 3 seconds after completion of injection; medially positioned anterior cerebral artery with anterior sclerotic kinking. Biconvex avascular space in the left parietal region.
b) Roentgenogram 3 seconds after injection terminated; medially placed anterior cerebral artery. Flatly delineated deviation of the medial branches in the right parietal region, with an avascular space.

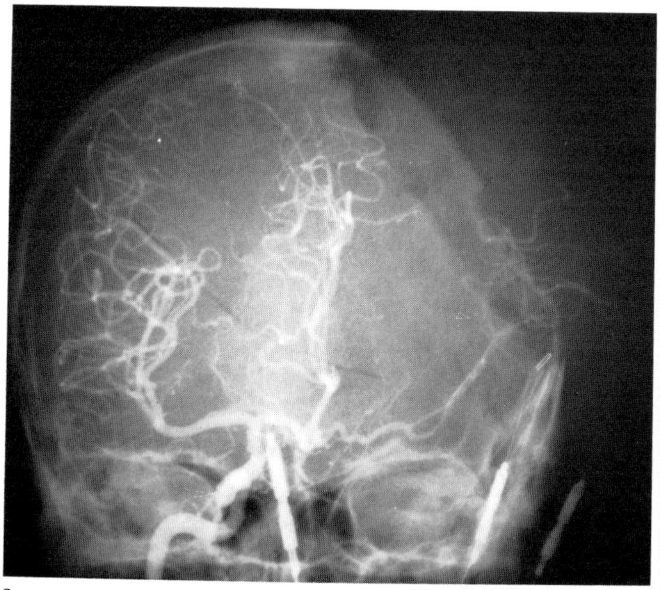

a

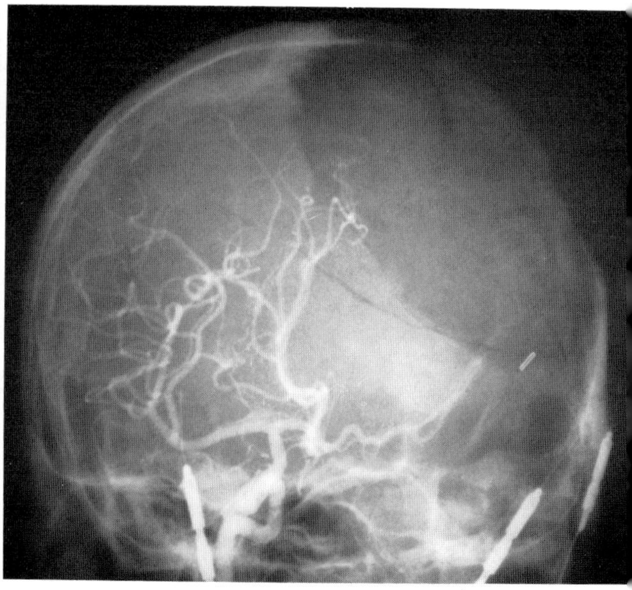

b

Fig. 3.4a–c. Internal carotid angiography on the right in the presence of a mostly occipital epidural hematoma. Ringlike fracture on the right extending from the temporal over the parietal to the occipital region. Condition after an extensive craniotomy of the left frontoparietal region, with removal of a subdural hematoma on the preceding day.
a) Massive prolapse of the brain from the bony defect, with protrusion of the opacified left group of medial vessels. Mild parallel displacement of the anterior cerebral arteries. Narrow avascular space in the right temporoparietal region.
b) Twenty-degree rotation toward the right in order to demonstrate the frontoparietal area; the branches of the medial cerebral artery all reach the inner table.

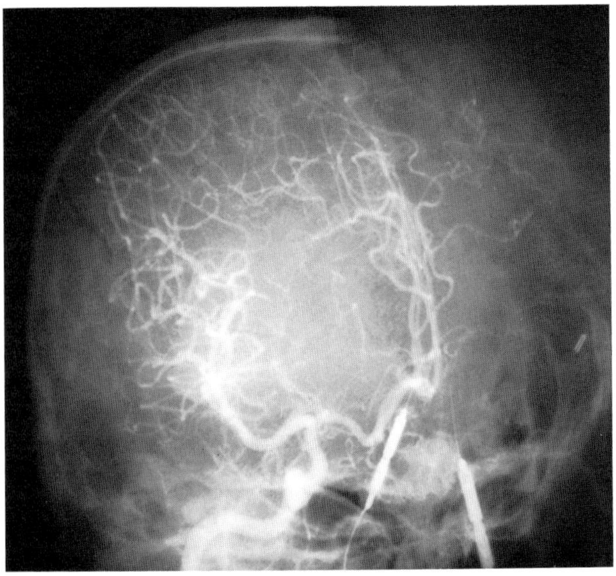

c

Fig. 3.4c. View with 20-degree rotation toward the left demonstrating the parieto-occipital cortical-wall areas; 25 mm wide avascular space in the right parieto-occipital region. Massive epidural hematoma probably extending into the left frontal region. Extension possibly occurred after operative intervention.

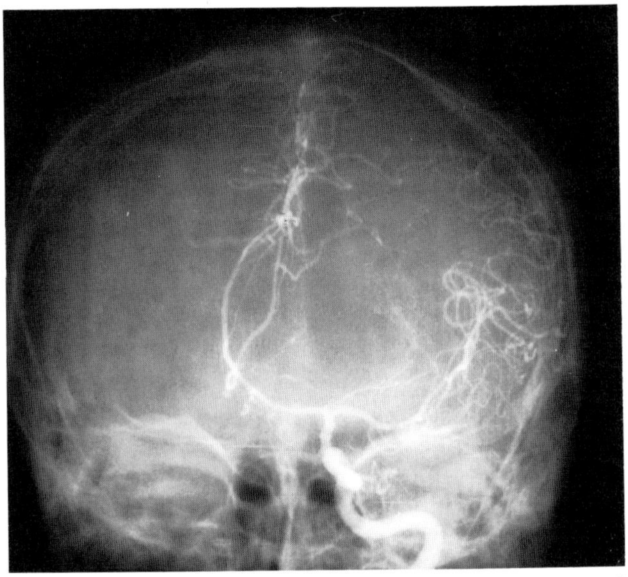

a

Fig. 3.5a–c. Internal carotid angiography (left) 1 day after severe covered skull and brain trauma, with continuous and persistent loss of consciousness. Large intracerebral hematoma of the left frontal area.

a) A. p. view during injection; high degree of arching and lateral displacement of the free portion of the anterior cerebral arteries. There is generalized narrowing of the cerebral arteries.

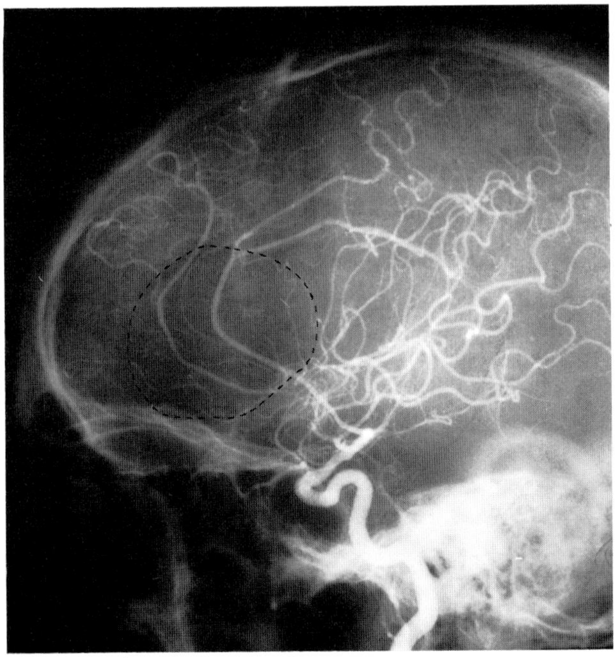

b

b) Lateral view during injection; compression of the branches of the medial cerebral artery posteriorly and downward. Avascular area in the frontobasal region.

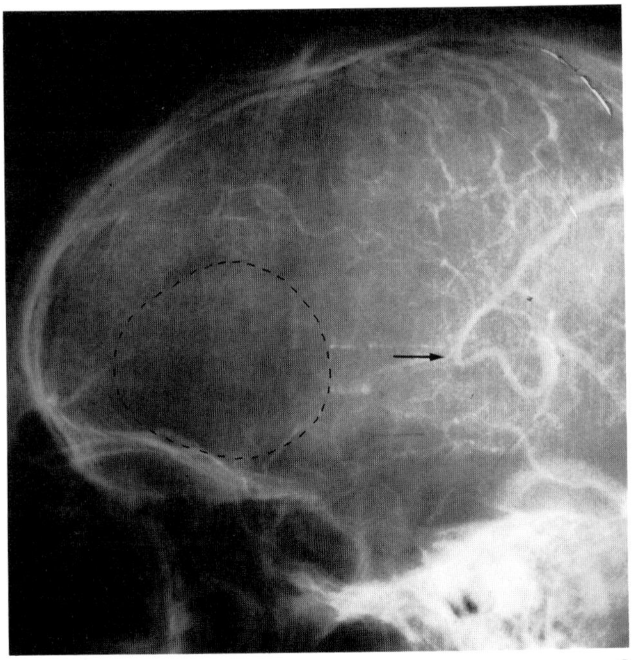

c

c) Lateral view 7 seconds after injection; avascular area in the frontobasal region. There is marked compression of the inner cerebral vessels with displacement posteriorly (→).

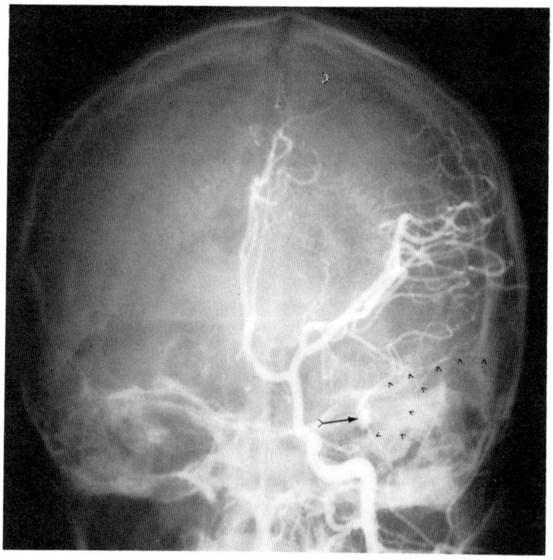

a

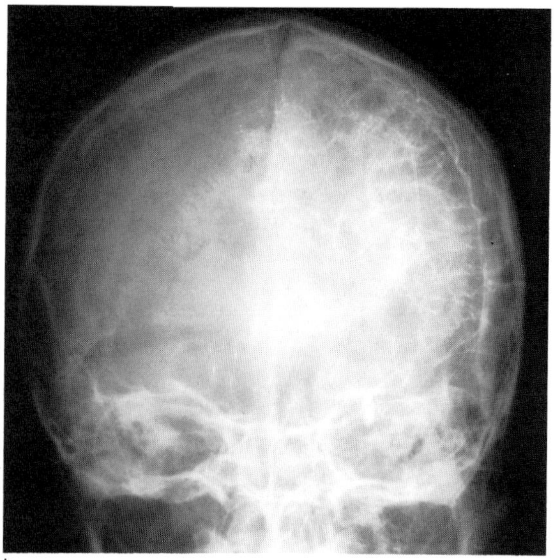

b

Fig. 3.6a–c. Angiography of the left common carotid artery 2 hours after a traffic accident resulting in severe skull and brain trauma and immediate loss of consciousness. On the left, there is a wide pupil unresponsive to stimulation.

a) A.p. view during injection; lateral displacement of the anterior cerebral artery toward the right. Elevation of the main branches of the medial cerebral artery. Elevation and arching of the medial meningeal artery toward the midline (/\). Extravasation of the contrast agent from the medial meningeal artery. There is an almost avascular space in the temporobasal region (→).

b) A.p. view 4 seconds after injection; extravasation projecting itself onto the upper third of the orbit. Branches of the medial meningeal artery still contain contrast.

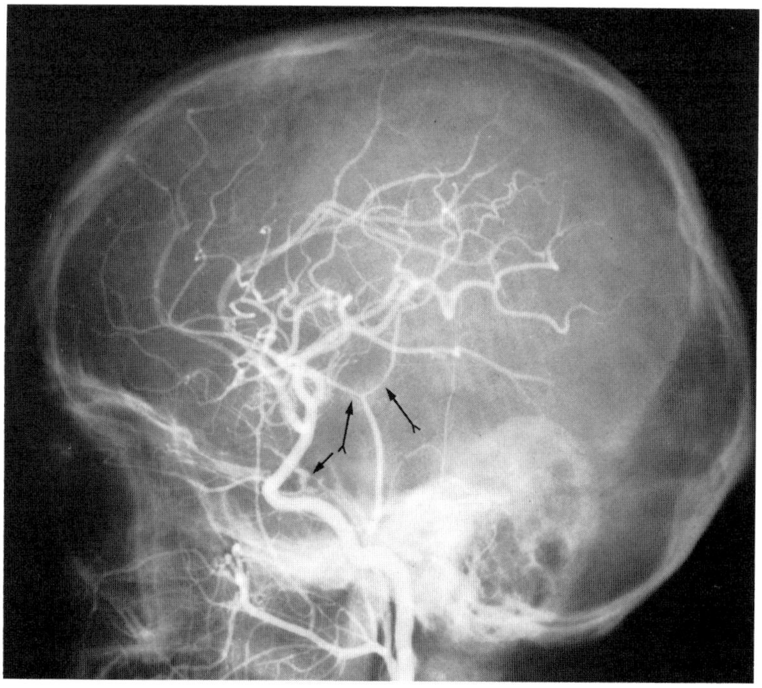

Fig. 3.6c. Lateral view during injection; arching of the carotid syphon. Arching and displacement of the medial group. Extravasation (↓). Marked narrowing of the caliber of the branches of the meningeal artery (↑).

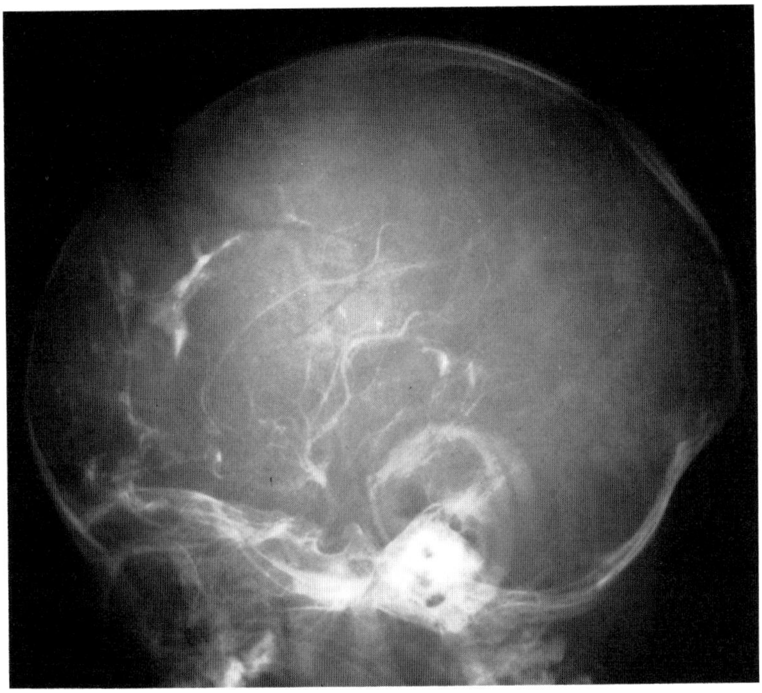

Fig. 3.7. A 2-year-old child with extensive fractures of the skull after a traffic accident. Late phase of angiography of the internal carotid artery. Multiple areas of extravasation of contrast agent from several injured branches of the cerebral arteries (frontopolar artery, callosomarginal artery and posterior cerebral arteries).

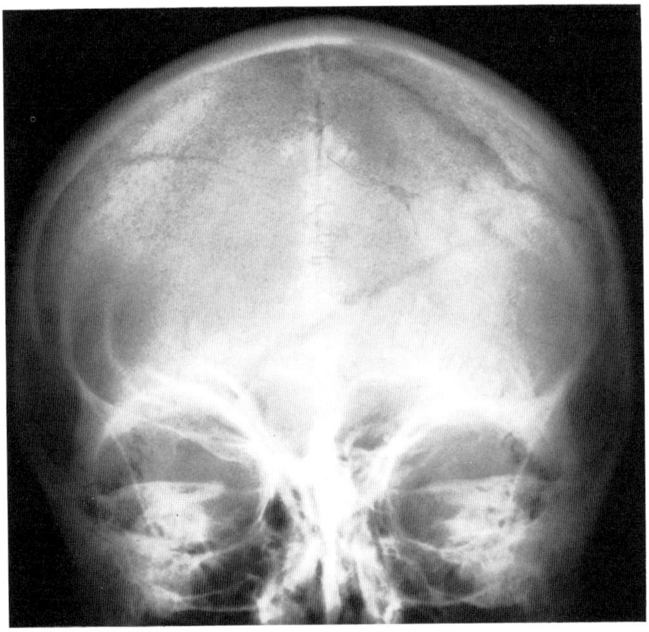

a

Fig. 3.8a–d. Internal carotid angiography. Arteriovenous fistula between the internal carotid artery on the left and the cavernous sinus. Ten days ago, the patient was in a traffic accident resulting in multiple fractures of the skull. Marked pulse–synchronous engine bruit over the left temple. Pulsating exophthalmos on the left.
a) A.p. view of the skull with multiple fractures.

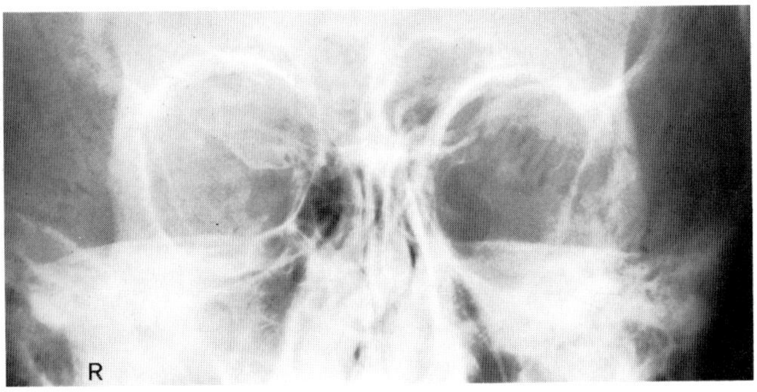

b

Fig. 3.8b. View of the orbit with fracture of the lesser and greater wings ot the sphenoid on the left, and small bony fragments above the sella turcica.

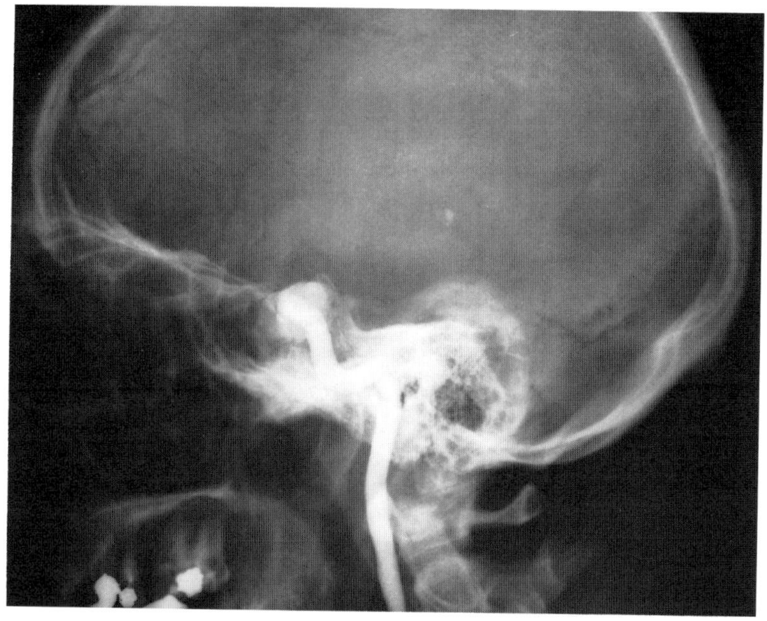

Fig. 3.8c. Internal carotid angiography *(left)*. X-ray during injection; saccular enlargement of the vessel in the area of the cavernous sinus.

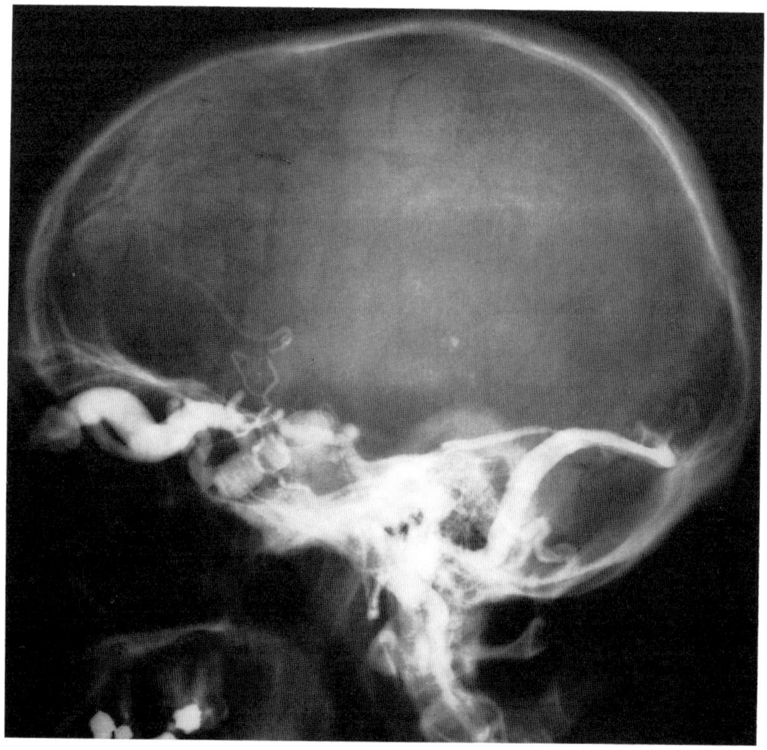

Fig. 3.8d. Roentgenogram 1 second after completion of injection; huge arterialized vein arising from the cavernous sinus and leading toward the left orbit, the inferior petrous sinus, the transverse sinus and the external veins.

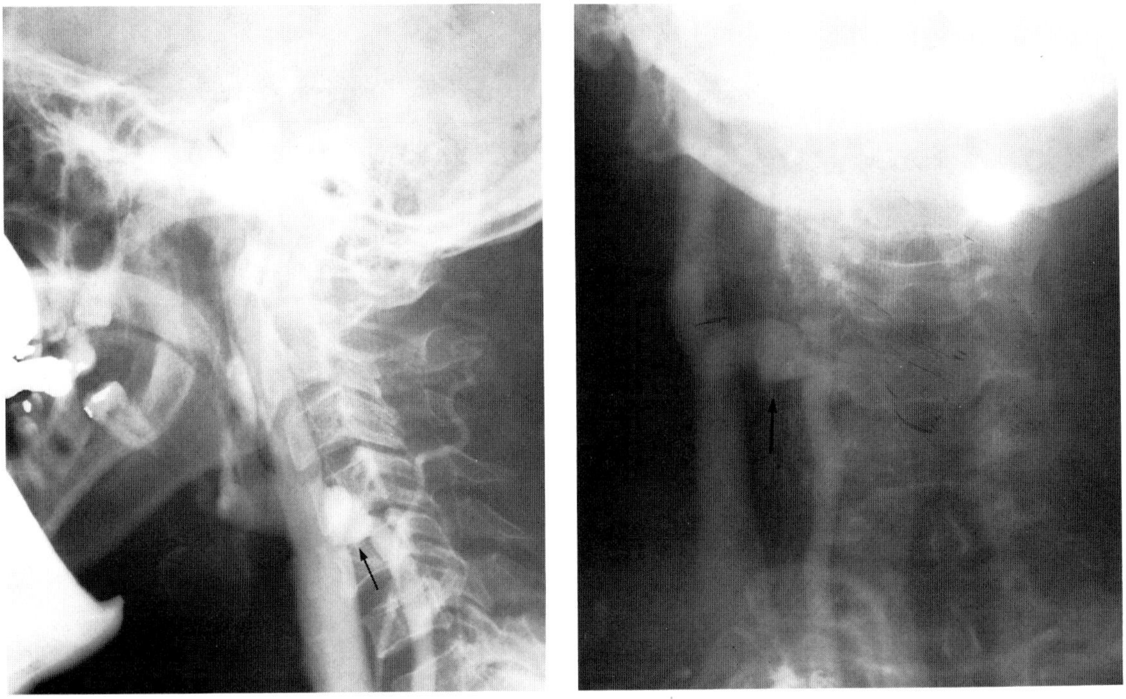

Fig 3.9a. Text see page 61

Fig. 3.9b

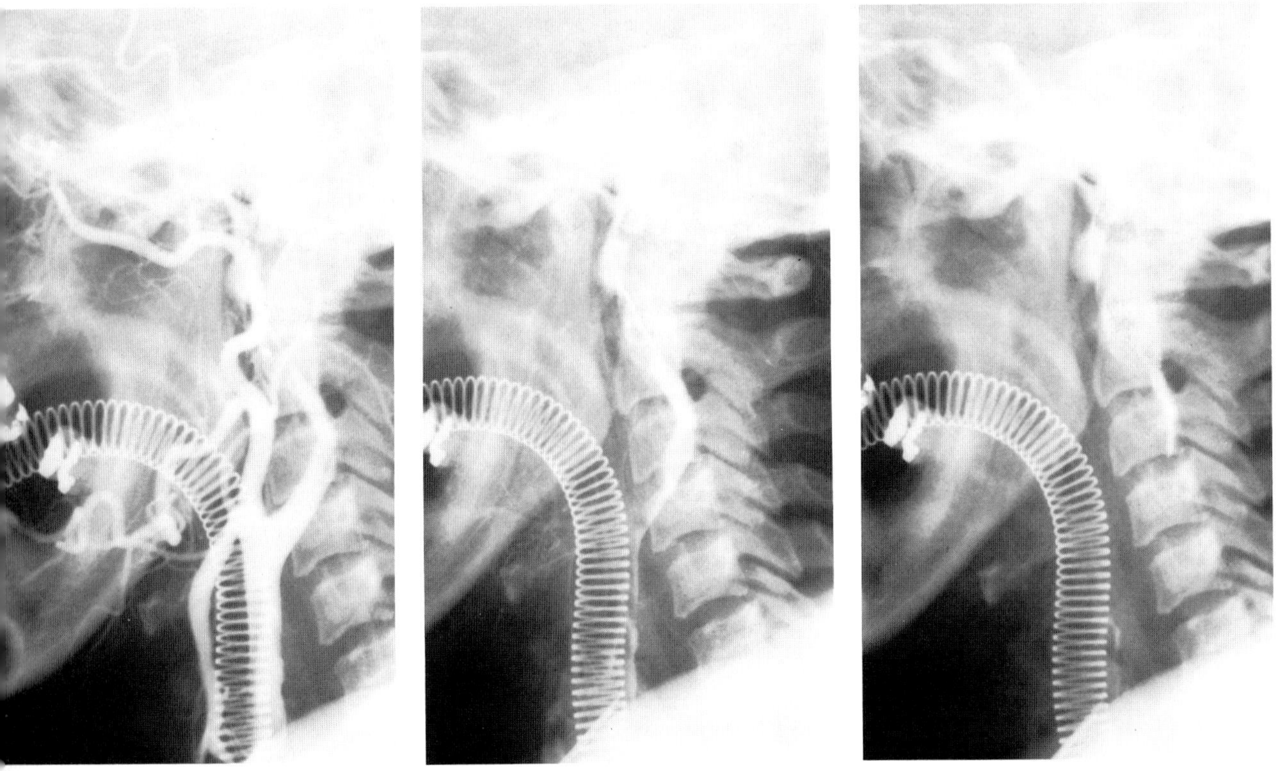

Fig. 3.10a b c

◀ Fig. 3.9a and b. Arteriovenous fistula between the vertebral artery and the internal jugular vein. Eight days after being stabbed at the level of C3/4 with root damage and increasing pulse–synchronous tinnitus first on the right, then also on the left.
a) Lateral view during injection into the right vertebral artery; filling of vertebral artery up to the 4th cervical vertebra. At this level, there is a saccular enlargement of the vessel with immediate transfer of the contrast agent into the internal jugular vein. The latter is arterialized up to the base of the skull.
b) A.p. view during injection into the right vertebral artery; filling of the right vertebral artery up to the 4th cervical vertebra. At this level, there is a fistula into the jugular vein.

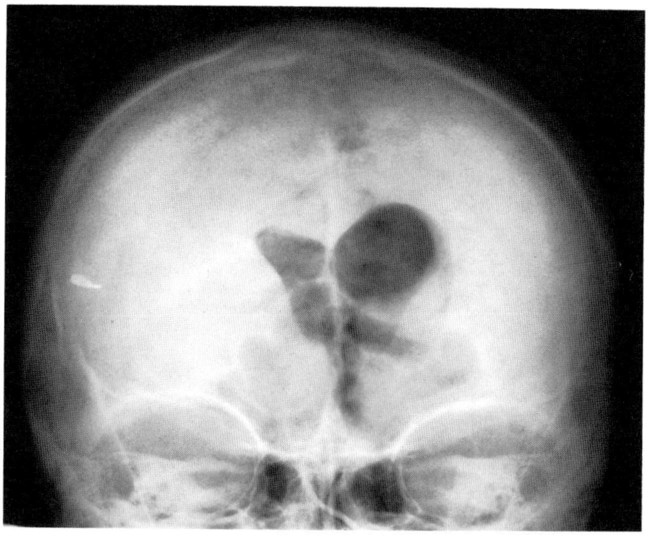

Fig. 3.11a

◀ Fig. 3.10a–c. Common carotid angiography on the right 2 days after a traffic accident resulting in concussion and blunt trauma to the neck. 24 hours after the accident, hemiplegia develops on the left as a result of thrombosis of the carotid artery.
a) Lateral view during injection; proper filling of the external branches. Irregular narrowing of the lumen of the internal carotid artery at the level of the 3rd cervical vertebra. At the 2nd cervical vertebra, there is a loss of internal contour of the internal carotid artery.
b) View 4 seconds after completion of injection; filling of internal carotid artery but with a large defect. Poor visualization up to the base of the skull.
c) Deposition of contrast agent at the level of cervical vertebrae 2/3. Very slow evacuation of contrast agent superiorly, with filling of the internal carotid artery up to its syphon.

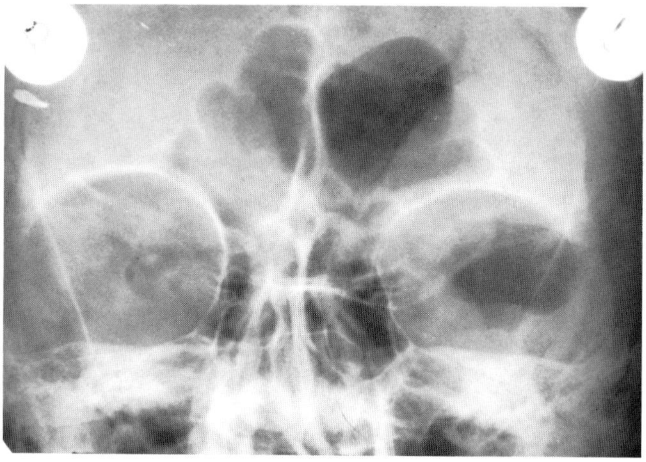

Fig. 3.11b

Fig. 3.11a and b. A 1944 left temporal injury by shrapnel.
a) A.p. view; unremarkable lateral ventricle on the right; markedly dilated, plump lateral ventricle on the left. Surgical defect in the left temporal area. Small metal splinter in the right temporoparietal region.
b) The dilatation of the left lateral ventricle is most marked in the region of the temporal horn. The right temporal horn is normal.

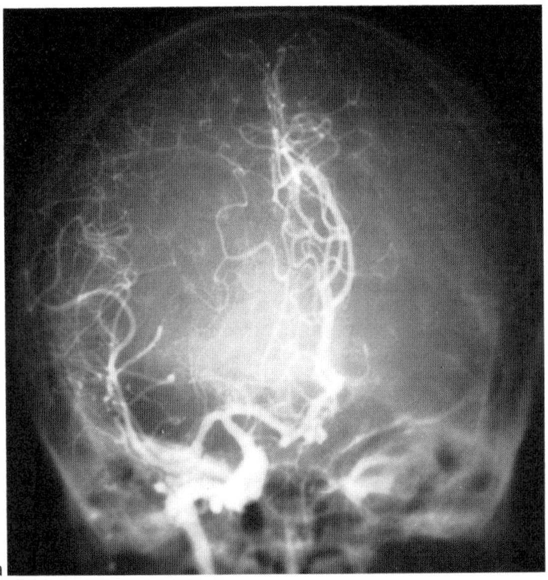
a

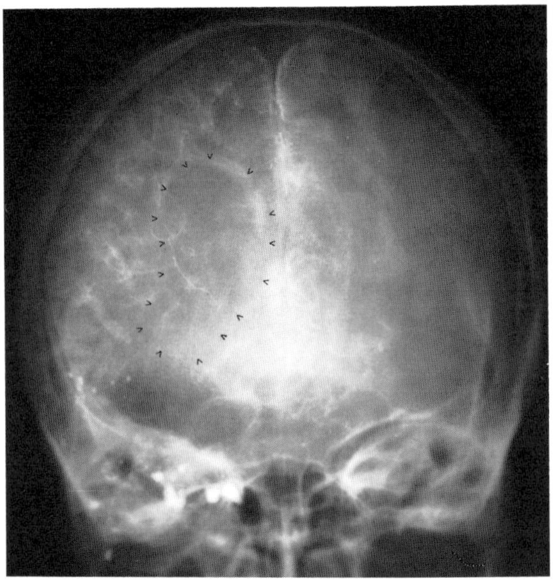
b

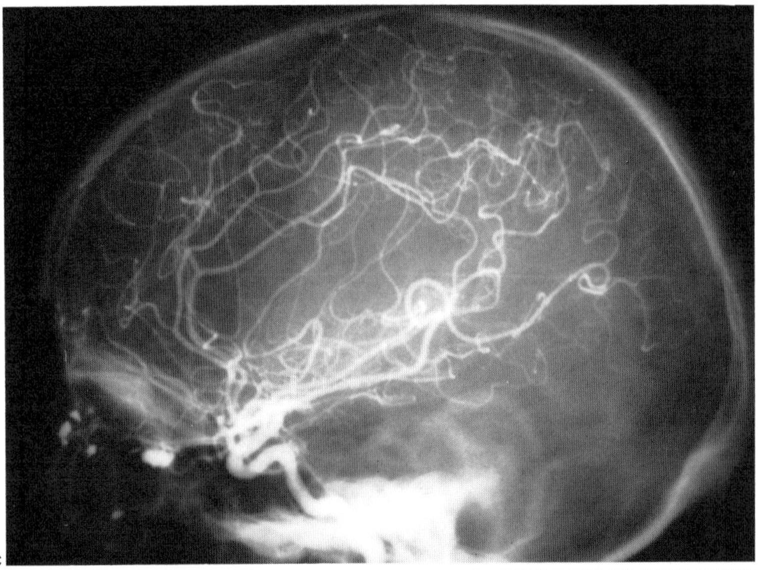
c

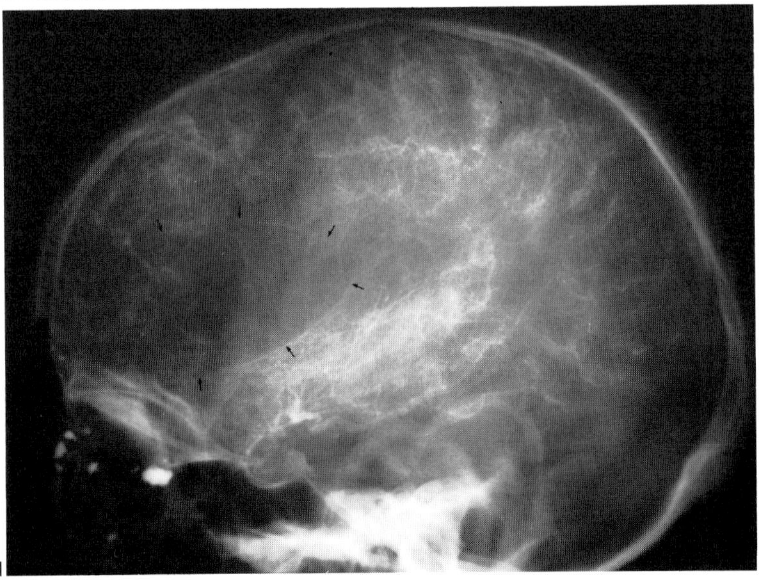
d

Fig. 3.12a–d. A 1944 right frontal grenade splinter injury penetrating the right frontal sinus; loss of the right eye; and an intermittent CSF fistula from the right nostril. Internal carotid angiography. Late abscess in the right frontal region.
a) A.p. view during injection; marked lateral displacement of the anterior cerebral artery. Impression of the main branches of the media.
b) X-ray 4 seconds after injection; during the capillary phase, there is an avascular area in the right paramedian region with a rimlike condensation of contrast agent (/\) (wall of the abscess).
c) Lateral view during injection; inferior displacement of the medial branches; humping of the anterior cerebral arteries in the area of the genu of the corpus callosum by a mass displacement below the cerebral falx.
d) View 5 seconds after injection; egg-shaped avascular region within the frontal pole and extending far posteriorly (→).

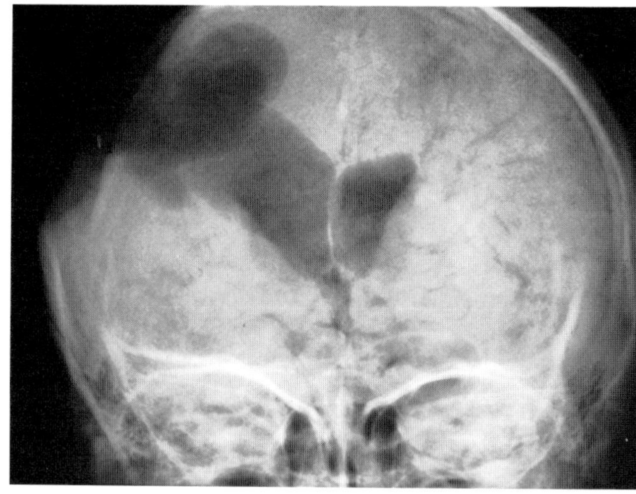

Fig. 3.13a

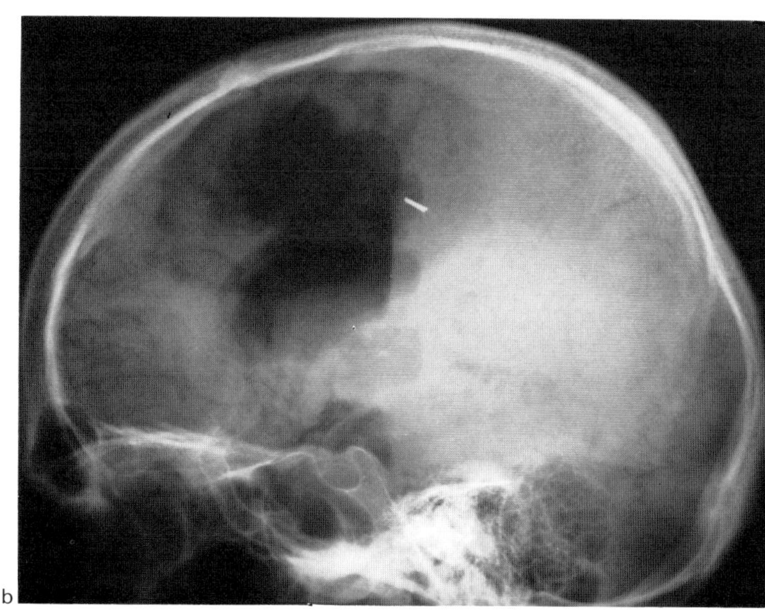

b

Fig. 3.13a and b. A 1960 penetrating skull and brain injury in the right parietal region. Since 1962, the patient suffered focal epileptic seizures involving the left side of the body. In 1964 there was acute, highly febrile meningeal infection with subsequent neurosurgical intervention and emptying of an abscess. Pneumoencephalography was performed in 1966; posttraumatic widening of the right lateral ventricle. There is a large surgically evacuated abscess cavity in the right frontoparietal region communicating with the right lateral ventricle.

Vertebral Column–Spinal Cord Trauma

When clinically marked neurological deficits appear hours or days after trauma to the vertebral column, with the absence of radiologically recognizable signs of injury to vertebrae or of dislocation, myelography is indicated.

If, immediately after trauma, the clinical examination reveals a traumatic transsection of the cord, there is no indication for any investigation using contrast agents. Experience accumulated from many neurosurgical interventions indicates that, in such instances, there is either a total transection of the cord or a massive hematomyelia with significant edema of the inner region. Chances for successful surgical intervention in the latter situation are jeopardized further by trauma during the operation. Conservative therapy, therefore, is to be preferred. In cases with a free interval, an epidural or subdural nemorrhage is often found to be a cause o compression of the spinal cord; in rarer circumstances, hematomyelia and hemorrhage into the spinal cord are other causes.

For the neuroradiologic diagnosis with contrast agent, it is important to realize that there may be a traumatic protrusion of the disk, particularly in cases of whiplash injury to the cervical spine. As a result of overexertion of the longitudinal ligament and prolapse of tissue from the disk, there may not only be neurologic symptoms corresponding to certain vertebral levels but also compression of the spinal cord, which may not necessarily coincide with the apparent clinical level as demonstrated by myelography. The lesion may well be situated 2 to 3 vertebral body levels cranial to the location of the neurologic symptoms (Fig. 3.14).

Finally, there is an absolute indication for performance of studies with iodinated oils when total avulsion of a nerve root in the area of the lower cervical spine is suspected. Such a complication is not infrequently seen after accidents with motorcycles or motorscooters.

In the diagnostic approach to traumatic lesions of the spinal cord, the most frequently used type of study is myelography with iodinated oil; the second most commonly used study is gas myelography or, in the case of a total stop in the attempt to demonstrate the upper as well as the lower extent of the space-occupying process, a combination of both methods. The choice of the region for performance of the spinal tap, whether suboccipital or lumbar, must be based on an evaluation of all the findings and the general condition of the patient. Only in the lumbar region of the spinal canal is it possible to perform myelography with water-soluble contrast agents. If there is an epidural or subdural hematoma, the obstruction will be seen on myelography as a discontinuity or a pointed narrowing of the negative or positive contrast (Fig. 3.15). It is often possible to demonstrate the displacement of the spinal cord and its being pressed toward the wall of the side opposite the hemorrhage (Figs. 3.16 and 3.17). Multiple hemorrhages can be visualized as an hourglass-shaped narrowing of the contrast column. In instances of hematomyelia, there is an almost complete stop of the contrast and a swelling of the spinal contours (Fig. 3.18).

Total avulsion of a nerve root in the cervical region (thoracic or lumbar avulsions are only rarely seen) is documented with iodinated oil myelography showing the presence of a sacular widening of the normally short, pointed and narrow region of the root pockets in the sagittal view (Fig. 3.19). The contrast agent visible beyond the ruptured root pockets can extend far laterally and inferiorly toward the cervical plexus. Such a migration of contrast, together with the saccular appearance, will be accepted by the majority of neuroradiologists as proof of total root avulsion. A negative finding, however, will not eliminate the suspicion of such a lesion. Nonvisualization of root pockets may be the result of either massive local swelling or hemorrhage into the pockets.

For confirmation of a traumatic lesion of the intervertebral disk, diskography can be applied (the injection of Conray urographic or angiographic agents into the disk). This method can be used during the acute stage as well as for demonstration of traumatic late sequelae. The seeping of contrast agent from the area of the fibrous ring is proof of a lesion of the disk. In addition, this method offers the possibility of demonstrating the displacement of tissue from the disk into the fractured vertebrae or spinal epidural space. The routine use of this procedure, however, is still under discussion. On the one hand, the method should be applied at the levels of several segments because of the frequently misleading segmental localization on the basis of the neurologic symptoms. On the other hand, the performance of the technique and the reliable reading of the obtained documents must be reserved for the experienced neuroradiologist who frequently will not be able to derive more than a suspicion from such studies.

Spinal osseous venography after injecting a spinous process with aqueous contrast agents (such as urographic or angiographic Conray, etc.) may demonstrate a lesion of the epidural space where there is displacement or interruption of the epidural veins. However, since its diagnostic value is too limited, this technique has not found much enthusiasm as an approach to traumatologic diagnosis.

If late traumatic sequelae such as arachnoiditis, adhesions or fusion after local hemorrhage are suspected, myelography with iodinated oil will produce the best results (Fig. 3.20). Within the lumbar region myelography with water-soluble contrast agents is now available. Gas myelography, however, is not suited for this purpose.

Fig. 3.14. Injury sustained after a fall on the head, with extreme extension of the cervical spine. Radiologic findings of a lesion at C5. Myelography was done on the day of the accident. Suboccipital Pantopaque myelography: top of the contrast agent at the level of intervertebral disk C 3/4 is due to a completely perforated disk with protrusion of tissue into the spinal canal.

Fig. 3.15. Result of a chain reaction car accident, with incomplete findings of transsection of the cord five hours after the accident. Suboccipital gas myelography; defect (^v) within the gas column extending from the 5th cervical vertebra to the 2nd thoracic vertebra in the presence of an epidural hematoma after whiplash injury to the cervical spine without visible fracture or luxation.

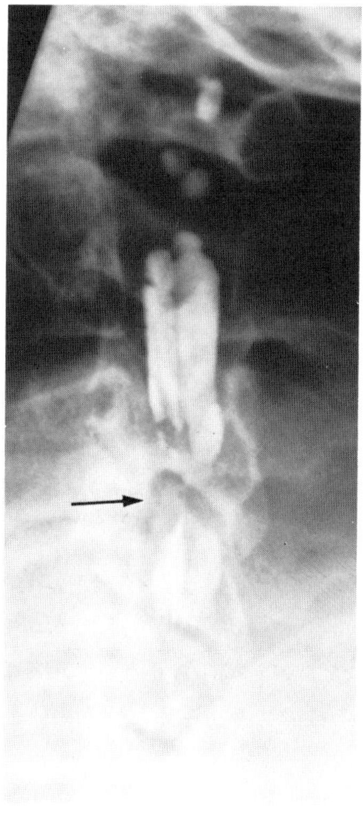

Fig. 3.14

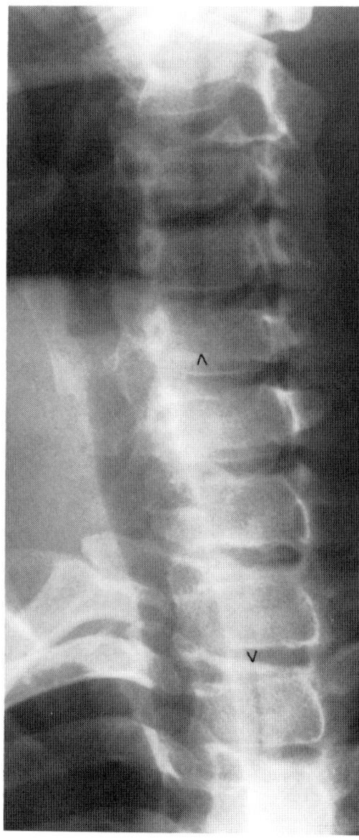

Fig. 3.15

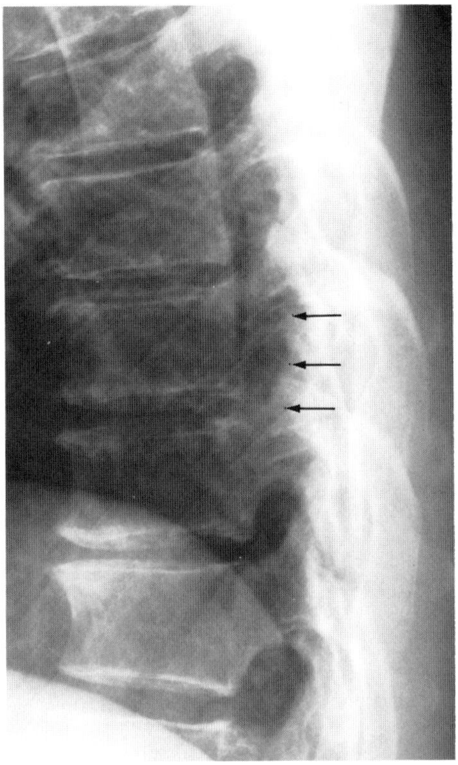

Fig. 3.16. Transsection of the cord below the tenth-thoracic vertebra three hours after a fall on the back. Suboccipital gas myelography; pressure of the spinal cord posteriorly toward the vertebral bodies. Complete stop from the level of the lower border of the 9th thoracic vertebra due to an epidural hematoma.

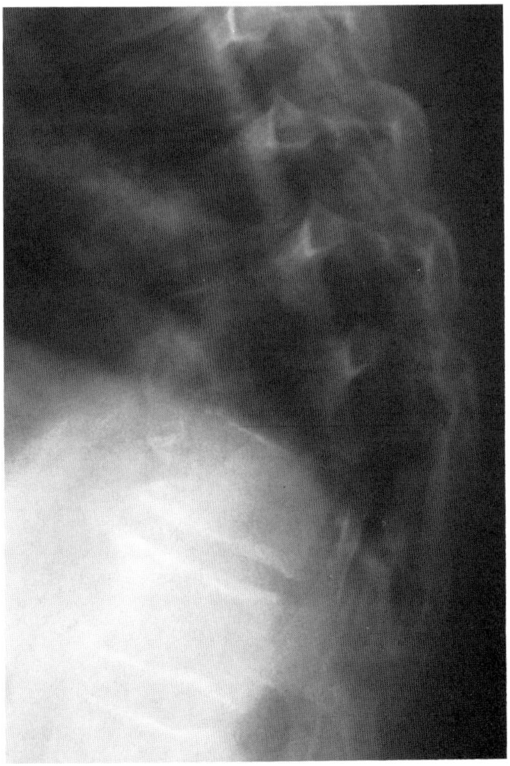

Fig. 3.17. Three months ago, the patient fell from six meters onto his feet. Fractures of both lower extremities, pelvis and immediate symptoms of transsection of the cord. After surgery, there was no improvement. Suboccipital gas myelography; compression fracture of the 10th thoracic vertebra, with local gibbus formation. Top of the gas shadow is slightly below the compressed vertebra. Pressure effect on the spinal cord toward the posterior edge of the 10th thoracic vertebra by an old organized epidural hemorrhage.

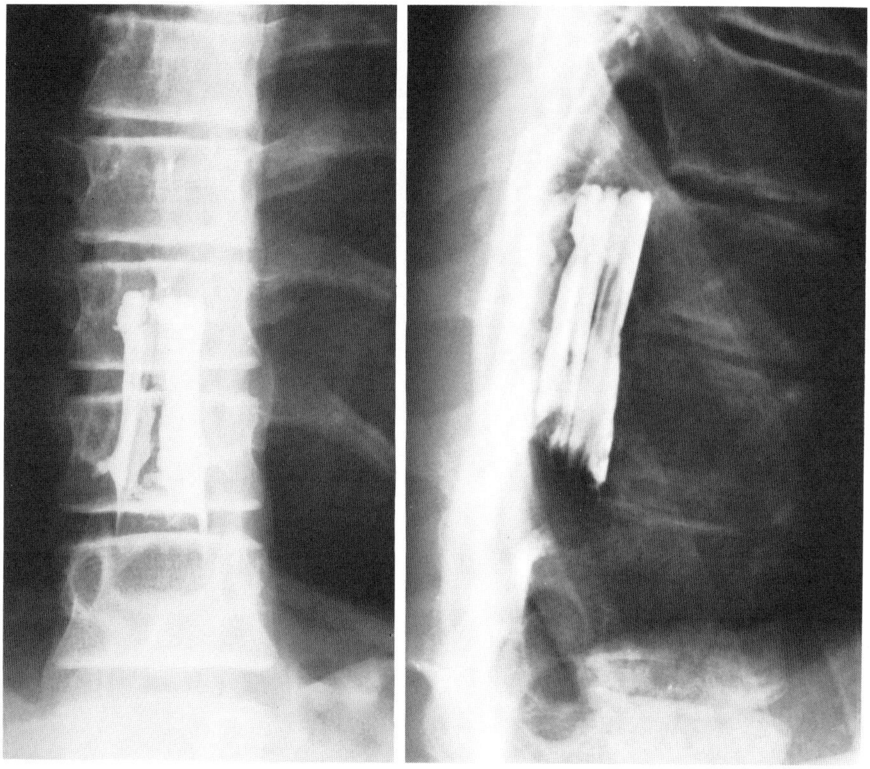

Fig. 3.18

Fig. 3.18. Shortly after trauma, there were increasing symptoms of transsection of the cord, which were fully established after 2 days. Surgery was performed three days after trauma, with only minimal improvement. Pantopaque myelography; total stop at the level of the 11th and 12th thoracic vertebrae, with displacement of the spinal cord toward the right and enlargement of its contour by hematomyelia at the level of the 11th thoracic to the 2nd lumbar vertebrae after hyperextension trauma.

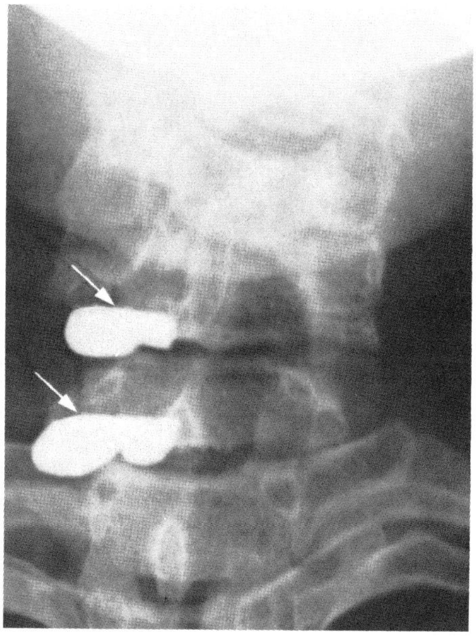

Fig. 3.19

Fig. 3.19. A.p. view of the cervical spine of a 24-year-old man. Plexus avulsion on the right after motorcycle accident. With Pantopaque myelography, accumulation of contrast agent within the intervertebral foramina allows the conclusion of an avulsion of the spinal roots at C 7 and C 8. (From P. F. Matzen and H. K. Fleissner: Orthopädischer Röntgenatlas. Stuttgart, Thieme, 1969.)

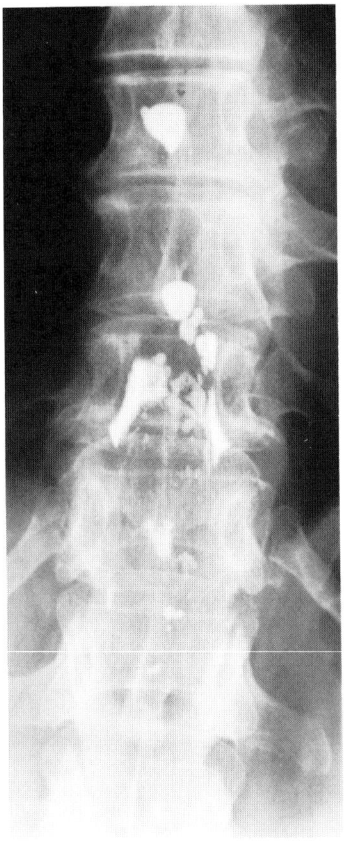

Fig. 3.20. Six months ago the patient fell on his back, with subsequent paralysis for 10 days. At that time, there was spinal subarachnoid hemorrhage. With Pantopaque myelography, there was an almost complete stop at the level of T11. Single drops of contrast agent were seen at the level of T9 and 10. Minimal droplets were present below this incomplete stop. Spinal arachnoiditis, with marked sensibility deficit and paresthesia, as well as disturbed function of the bladder and rectum, were noted.

4 Pelvis

Fractures of the pelvis are most frequently seen after a fall or a collision and rarely result from other mechanisms such as avulsion or a gunshot. Age distribution shows a rapid increase during the second decade, in keeping with the increasing exposure to dangers professionally, in sports or in traffic. A further peak occurs in the age group above 60 years, reflecting an increased risk of trauma because of the reduced ability to react fast enough. In all age groups, pedestrians run the highest risk and form 70 per cent of patients with pelvic fractures (Gilchrist and Peterson, 1967).

A survey of the different types of pelvic fractures and luxations are given in Figure 4.1. Among the isolated fractures, those of the symphysis are seen most often (Fig. 4.2a), followed in frequency by those of the acetabulum (Fig. 4.2b), the iliac bone and, much less commonly, those of the coccyx (Fig. 4.2c). For practical purposes, the many traumatic lesions of the pelvic skeleton are grouped in the following manner: combined fractures of pelvic bones (Figs. 4.3 to 4.5); avulsion fractures (Fig. 4.6); luxation and luxation fractures (Figs. 4.7 to 4.12); and rupture of symphysis and sacroiliac joints (Fig. 4.13).

A high proportion of fractures of the pelvis are associated with injuries to organs within the pelvis or the abdomen. In decreasing frequency, these complications are: rupture of the bladder; rupture of the urethra or of both organs; retroperitoneal hematoma; rupture of the diaphragm; injury to the gut; ruptured spleen; rupture of the mesentery; damage to nerves; rupture of blood vessels; tears in the vagina (after Zatzkin, 1965). Often there are several of these complications simultaneously.

Trauma to the pelvis during pregnancy will carry the risk of a ruptured uterus or of direct damage to the fetus, with the possibility of intrauterine fracture of the fetal skull (Wallner, 1969).

After traumatic deformity of the pelvis regardless of the type and degree of dislocation and the formation of callus, one must anticipate obstetrical complications during subsequent pregnancies.

Usually it is only possible to obtain a.p. views in the presence of fractures of the pelvis. Lateral views are technically feasible but require highly effective equipment and experience. Such a view may be consulted for the exact localization or dislocation of an acetabular fracture as well as for the demonstration of a well-maintained or abnormal joint relationship of the hip. Frequently, however, it is quite sufficient to elevate the involved side by 30 degrees from the a.p. view (Fig. 4.8).

If the findings are not clearly visualized, particularly in the area of the ischiopubic segment, additional views in the a.p. projection may be required, with tilting of the central ray 20 to 30 degrees cranially or eventually 10 to 20 degrees caudally.

X-ray analysis of injuries to the pelvis should always include careful attention to the soft tissues. Abnormal shadows or a displacement of the bladder are almost always expressions of a retroperitoneal hematoma or extravasation of urine. Such a suspicion must be voiced so that further diagnostic measures are undertaken – e.g., intravenous urography or urethrocystography. Injuries to the bladder and urethra are seen most often in fractures of the pubic bone and in simple or combined fractures of the anterior pelvic ring (Figs. 4.14 and 4.15), rarely in fractures of the acetabulum and hardly ever in isolated fractures of the iliac bone or in iliosacral dislocation. Occasionally, rupture of the bladder may occur in trauma to the pelvis without a visible fracture. Because of the high incidence of coexisting severe injuries, Zatzkin (1965) insists that every patient with a fractured pelvis must have the benefit of an abdominal survey film. Fractures of the sacrum usually occur together with other pelvic fractures; fractures of the coccyx, however, are frequently isolated. The radiologic symptoms vary from a hardly recognizable fracture line without any dislocation to complete avulsion with somewhat marked displacement of the fragments into the inner pelvic region (Figs. 4.16 and 4.17). Developmental variations in the form of the coccyx may present difficulties in interpretation to the beginner. Usually fractures of the sacrum and coccyx are best demonstrated on a lateral projection (Fig. 4.18). The value of the a. p. view may be significantly enhanced by an enema, thus avoiding overlap of rectal content. Other improvements may be obtained with special techniques such as zonography or tomography.

Fig. 4.1a–f. Survey of pelvic fractures and dislocations of the hip:
a) Localization of pelvic fractures: 1 = sacroiliac opening of joint; 2 = fracture of sacrum or coccyx; 3 = avulsion fracture of superior and anterior iliac spine; 4 = fracture of os pubis; 5 = fracture of os ischium; 6 = rupture of symphysis; 7 = posterior ring fracture of pelvis; 8 = fracture of iliac bone; 9 = fracture of joint socket; 10 = fracture of rim of joint; 11 = anterior pelvic ring fracture; 7 and 11 together = double unilateral pelvic ring fracture (from Malgaigne).
b) Posterior upper luxation (iliac luxation). ▶
c) Posterior inferior luxation (ischial luxation).
d) Central luxation of hip.
e) Anterior inferior luxation (infrapubic or obturator luxation).
f) Anterior superior luxation (suprapubic luxation).
(Fig. 4.1b–f: from H. R. Zatzkin: The Roentgen Diagnosis of Trauma. Chicago, Yearbook Medical Publishers, Inc., 1965. Used by permission.)

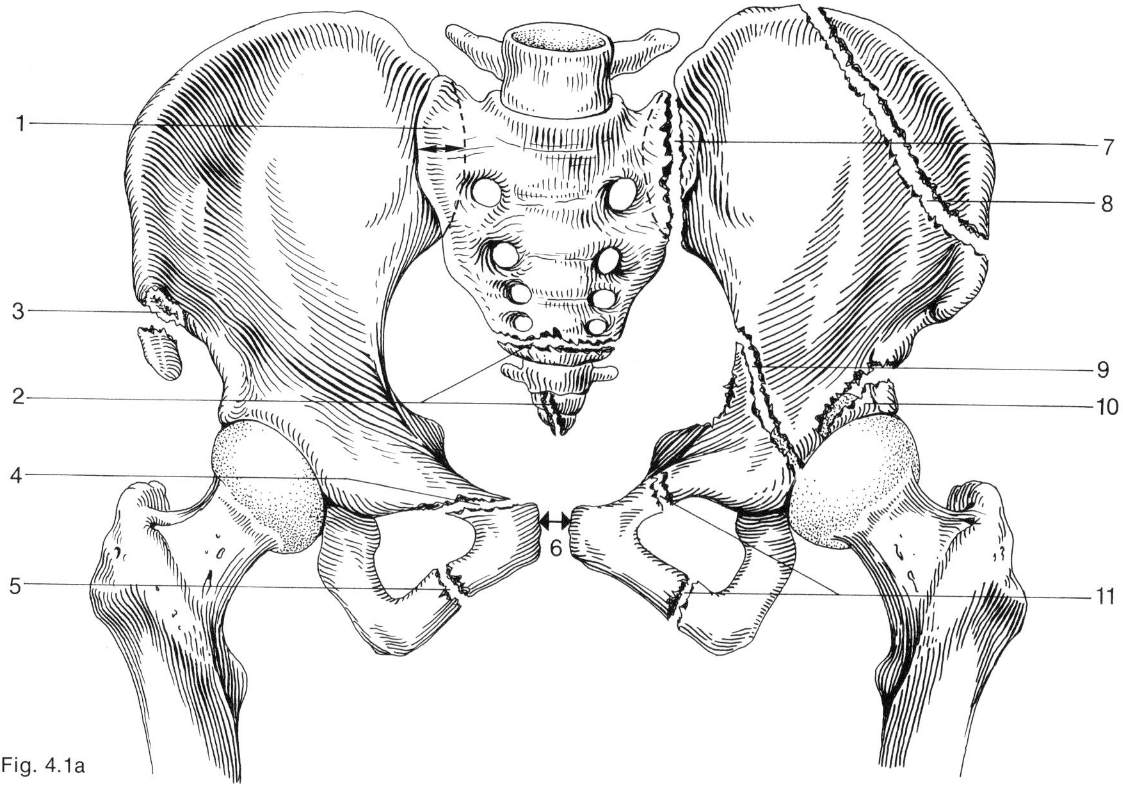

Fig. 4.1a

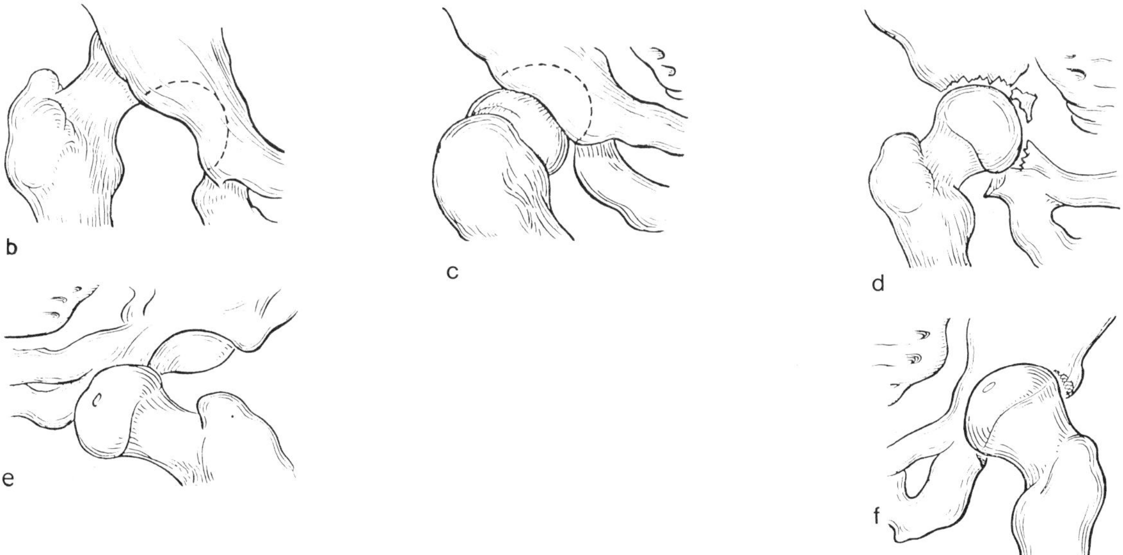

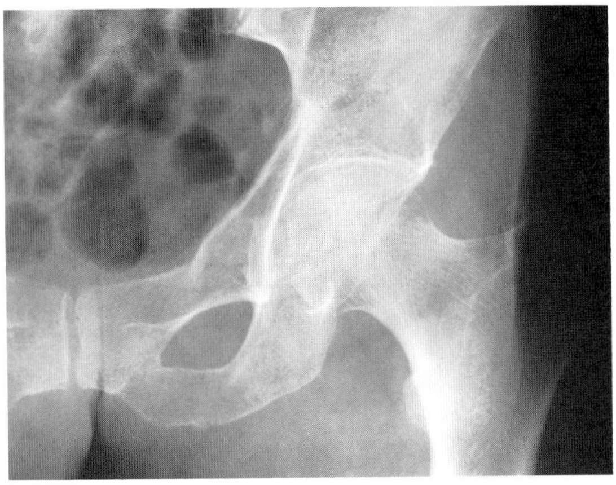

Fig. 4.2a. A. 71-year-old woman with an isolated fracture of the pubic bone.

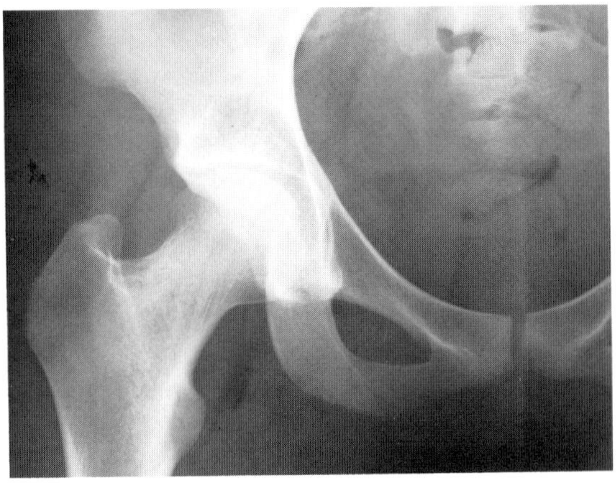

Fig. 4.2b. An 18-year-old girl after a car accident. X-ray follow-up 26 days later reveals the fracture more clearly. Isolated fracture of the joint socket on the right.

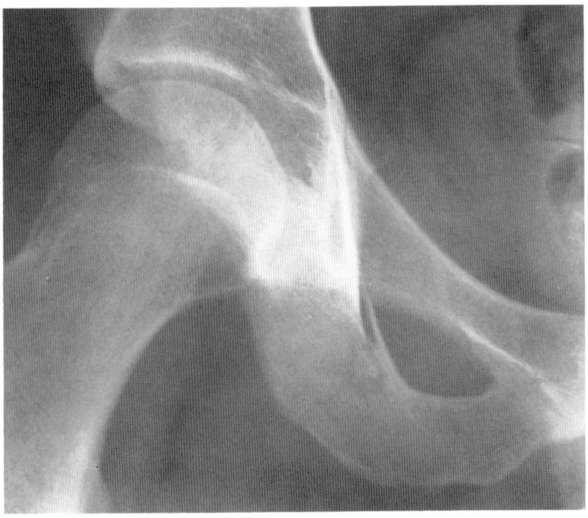

Fig. 4.2c. A 27-year-old man after a head-on car collision with a telephone booth. Isolated fracture of the ischial bone on the right.

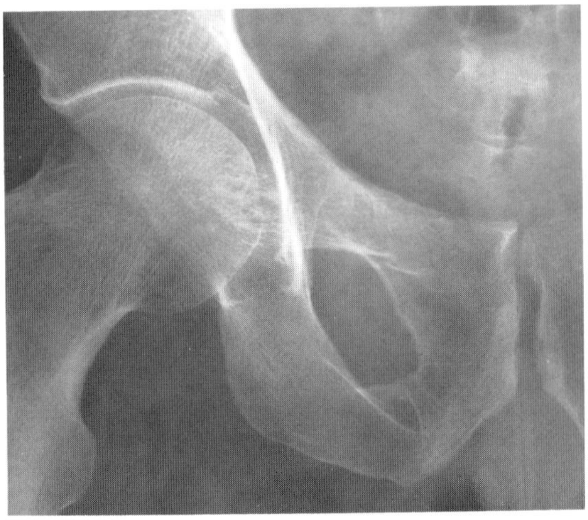

Fig. 4.3. A 51-year-old man with a contusion of the right half of his buttocks. Fracture of the anterior pelvic ring on the right; visible only on the follow-up x-ray 3 weeks after the accident.

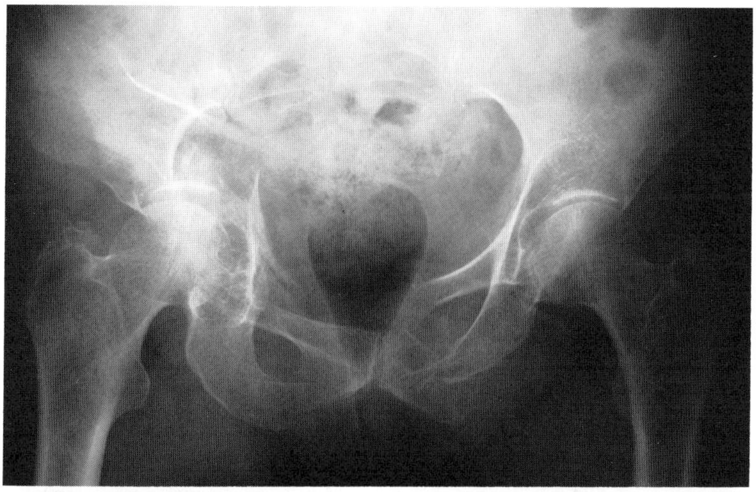

Fig. 4.4. A 77-year-old woman after a traffic accident. Combined fracture of the anterior pelvic ring with a fracture of the right femoral joint socket. Marked dislocation. Avulsion from the right major trochanter.

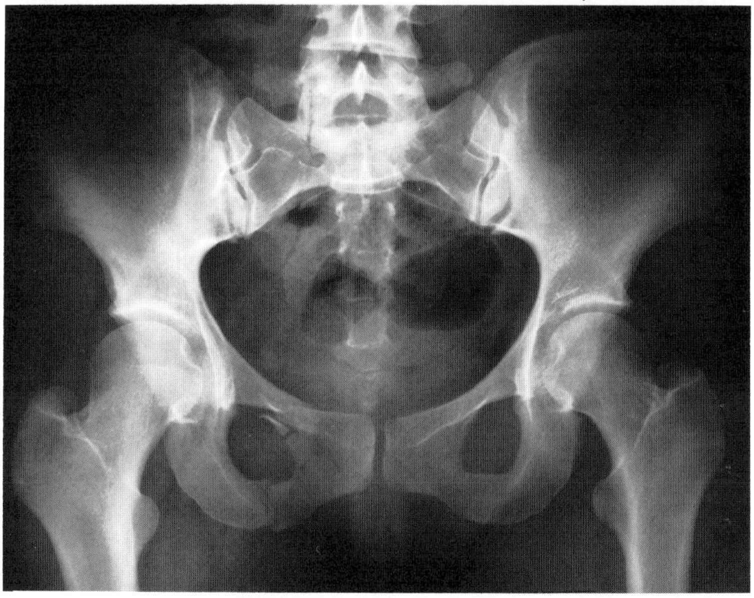

Fig. 4.5. A 35-year-old woman who was a passenger in a car in a traffic accident. Vertical fracture of the anterior and posterior parts of the pelvic ring on the same side (Malgaigne's fracture).

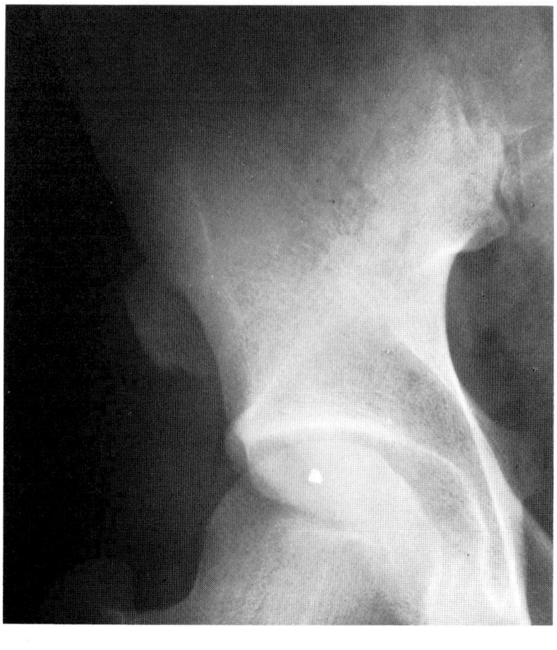

Fig. 4.6. A 17-year-old boy after being hit by a car. Avulsion fracture of the superior anterior iliac spine on the right. Bony consolidation with slight inferior dislocation of the spine.

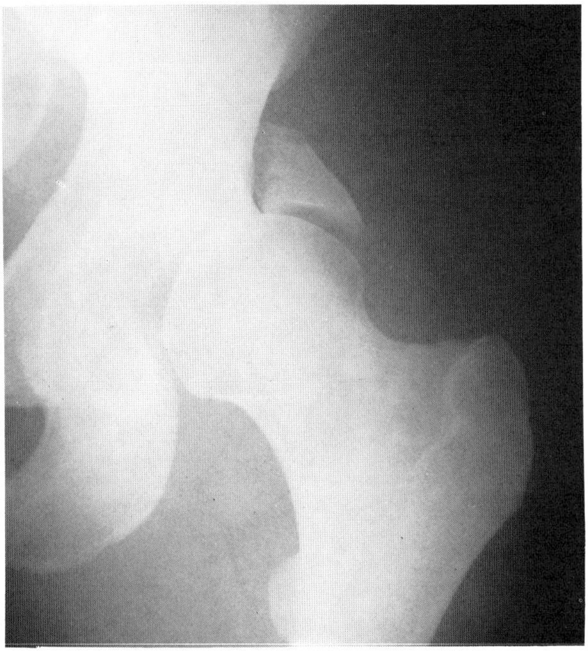

a

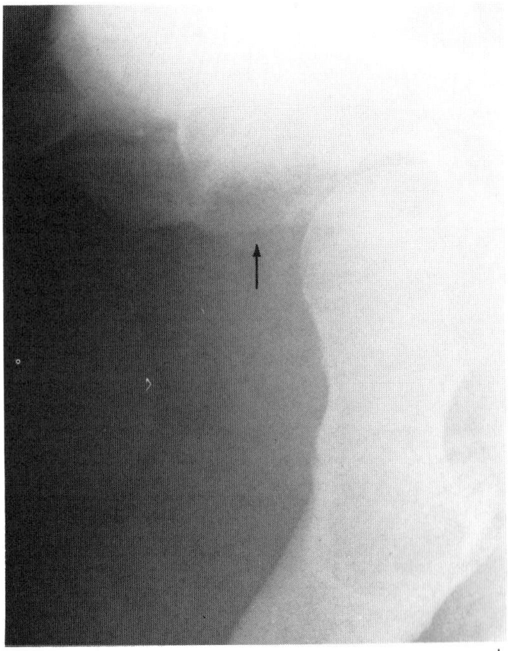

b

Fig. 4.7a and b. A 24-year-old man, after a head-on car collision. Iliac dislocation of the hip, with fracture of the articular lateral lip. Note the empty socket on the axial view (↑).

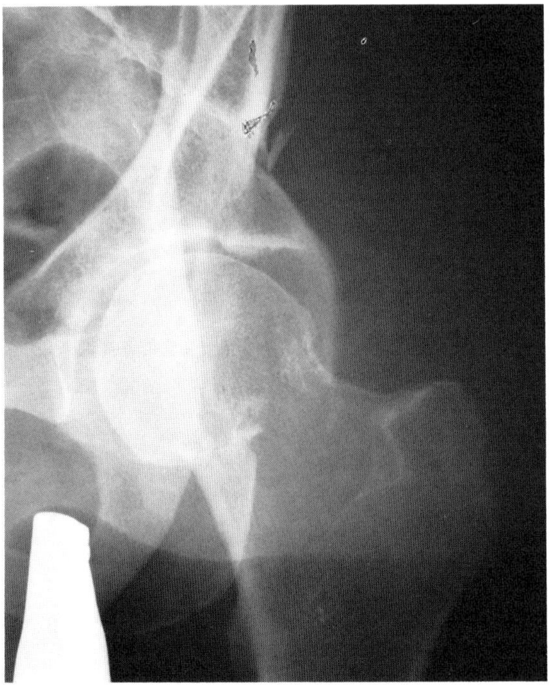

Fig. 4.8. Approximately 40-year-old man after a car accident. Iliac dislocation of the hip on the left, with fracture of the acetabulum. This view reveals an empty socket on special a.p. view, with anterior rotation of about 45 degrees on the left side. Dislocation of the fragment of the acetabulum.

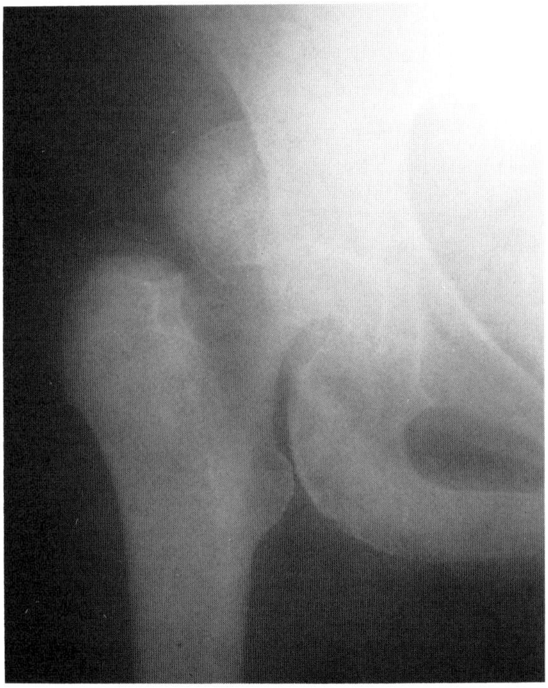

Fig. 4.9. A 60-year-old woman with dislocation of the femoral head and medial fracture of the femoral neck.

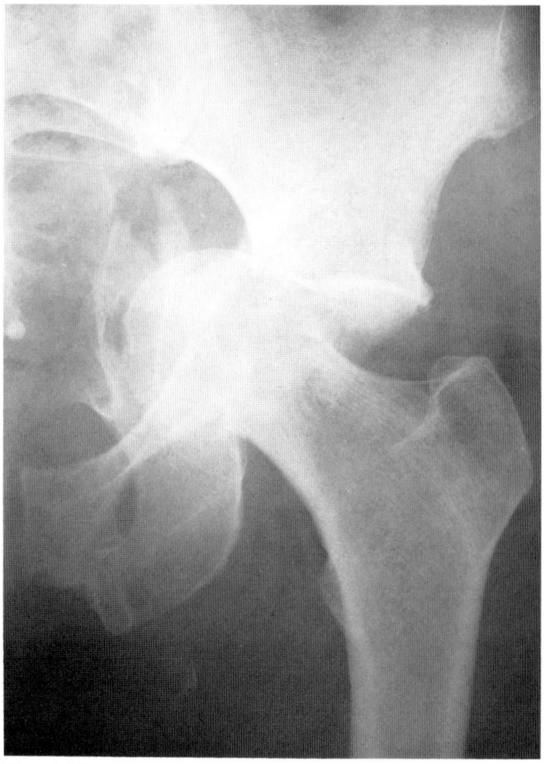
Fig. 4.10a

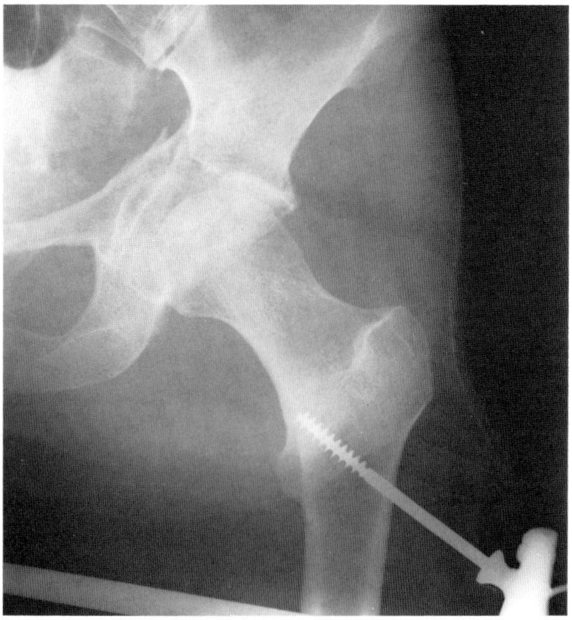
b

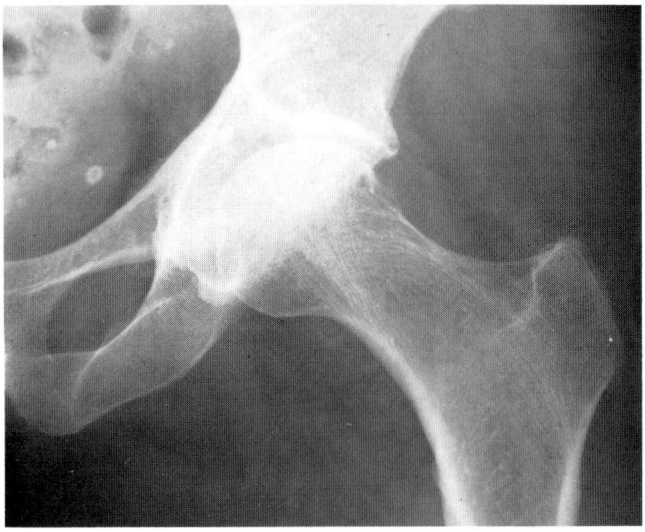
c

Fig. 4.10a–c. A 56-year-old woman hit by a car in the region of her left hip.
a) Central dislocation of the hip, with a fracture of the articular socket and of the os pubis.
b) Reposition by lateral pull after insertion of an intraosseous screw.
c) Condition 2 years later.

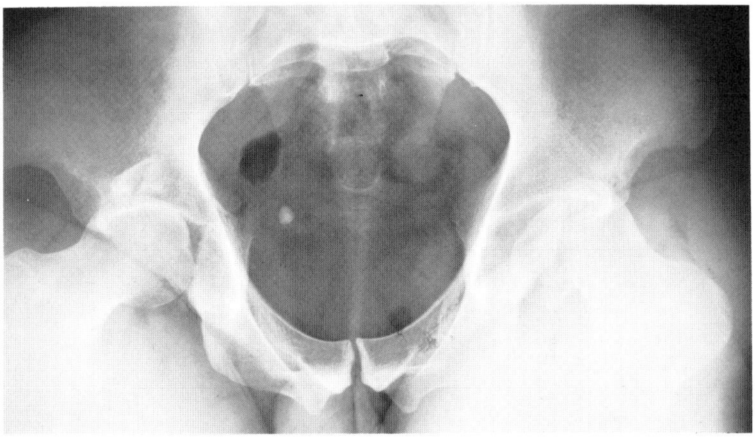

Fig. 4.11. A 29-year-old man after a car accident. Bilateral dislocation of the hips. Fracture of the articular socket and rim on the right. Fracture of the left femoral head.

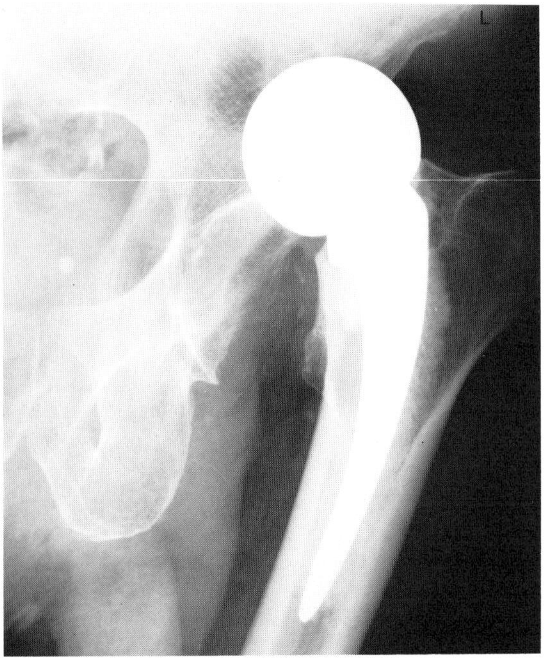

Fig. 4.12. A 93-year-old man with dislocation in the presence of a Thompson endoprosthesis.

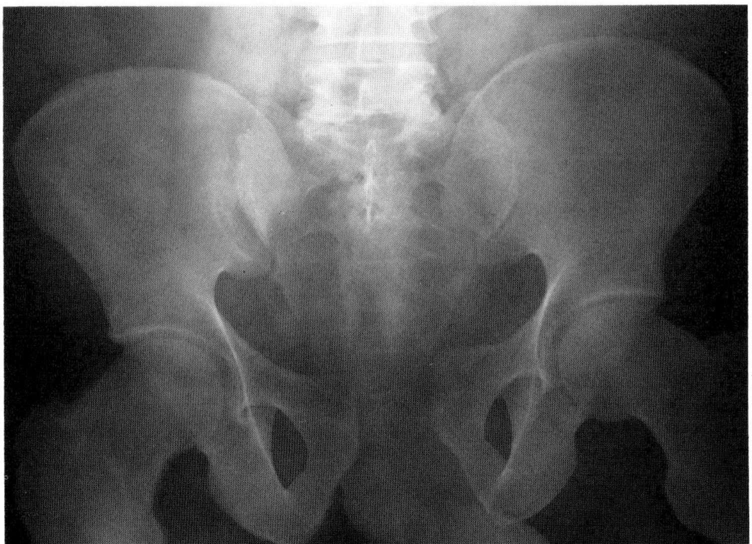

Fig. 4.13. Rupture of the symphysis; opening of the right sacroiliac joint.

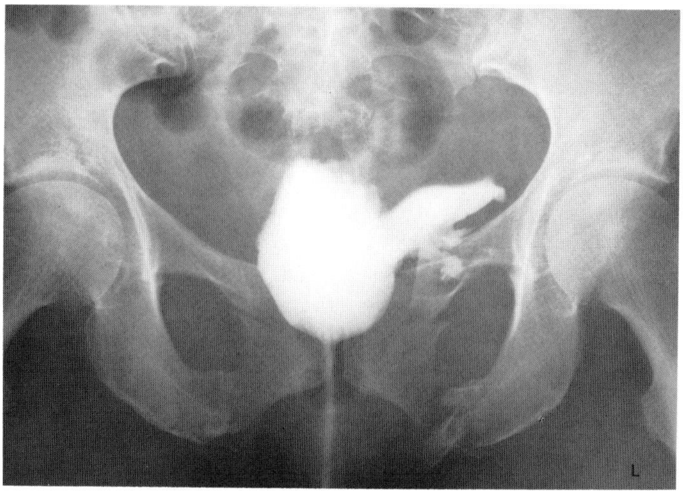

Fig. 4.14. A 60-year-old woman hit by a car while crossing the street. Fracture of the anterior pelvic ring bilaterally. Extraperitoneal accumulation of urine from the ruptured bladder. Additional injuries include cerebral concussion, lower leg fracture on the left and a ruptured diaphragm on the left.

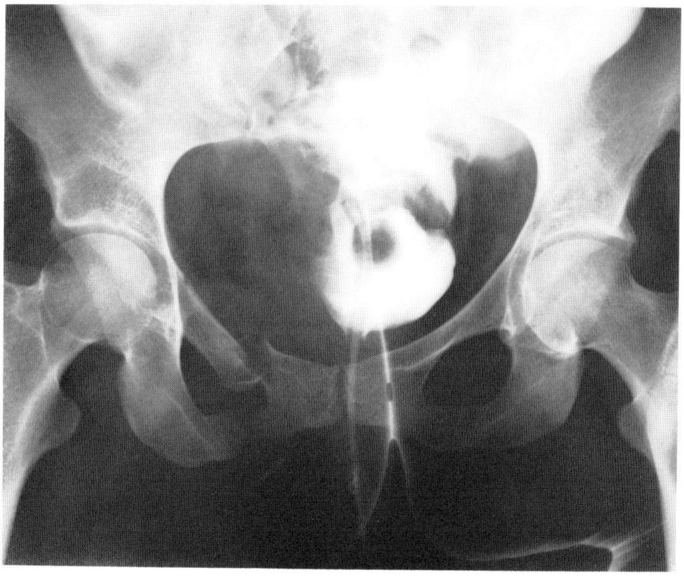

Fig. 4.15. A 29-year-old woman who was a passenger in a car in an accident. Intraperitoneal rupture of the bladder in the presence of a fracture of the anterior pelvic ring. Cystogram after insertion of a catheter into the bladder; contrast extends far into the abdominal cavity. Displacement of the bladder.

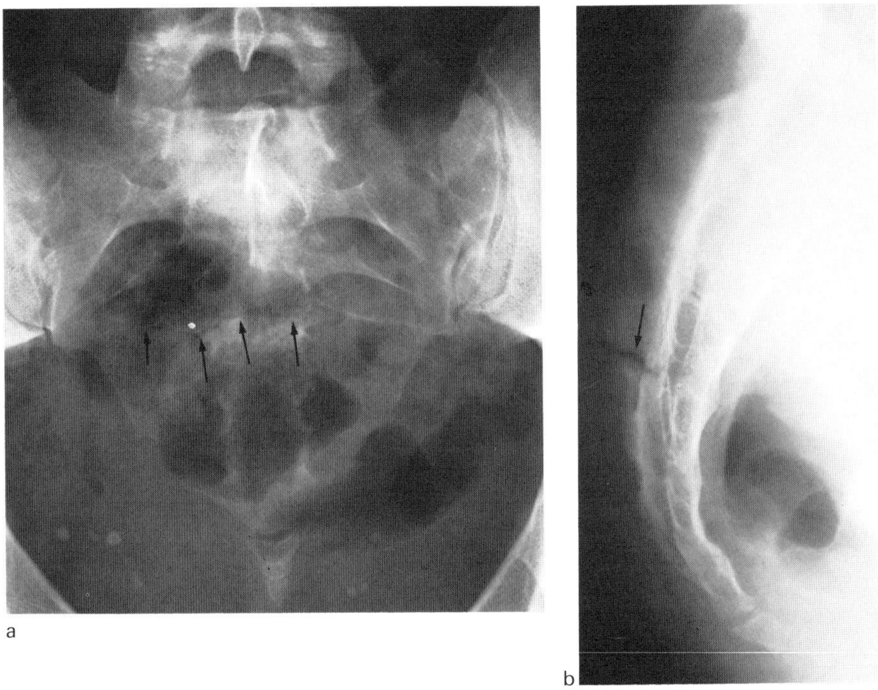

a

b

Fig. 4.16a and b. A 27-year-old woman who suffered a fall while skating. Fracture of the sacrum without significant dislocation. Fracture is visible on both views (↑).

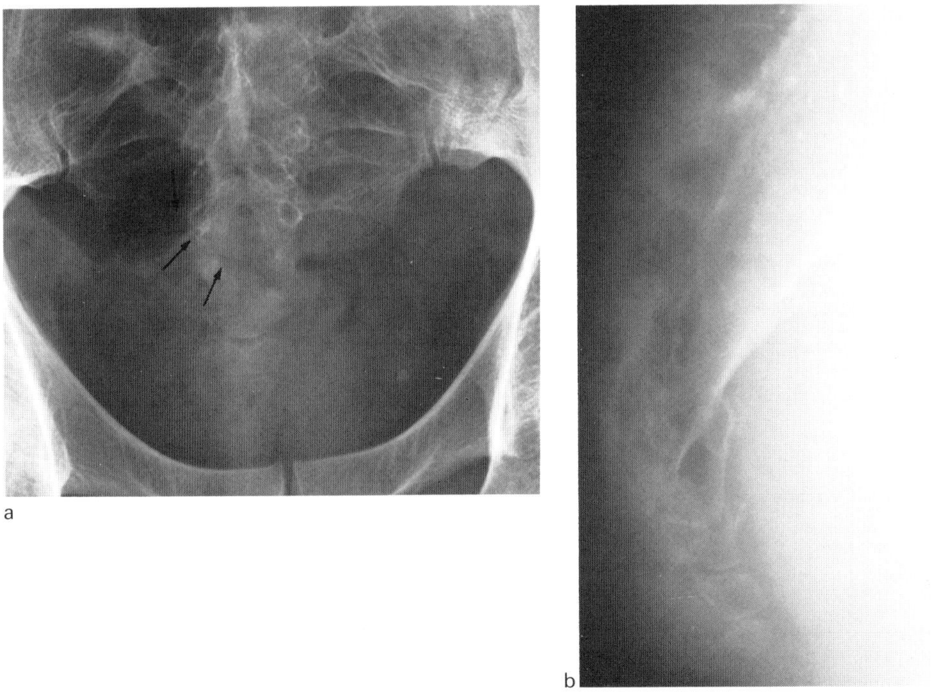

a

b

Fig. 4.17a and b. A 45-year-old man after a fall from a scaffold. Deep fracture of the sacrum, with dislocation toward the inner pelvic area. This finding can be better appreciated on the lateral view *(b)*.

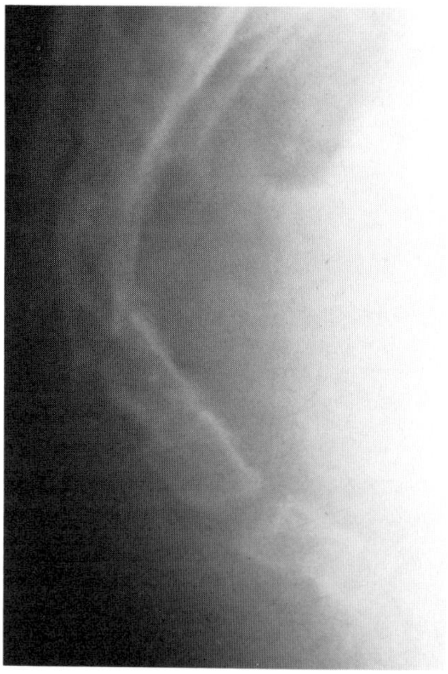

Fig. 4.18a

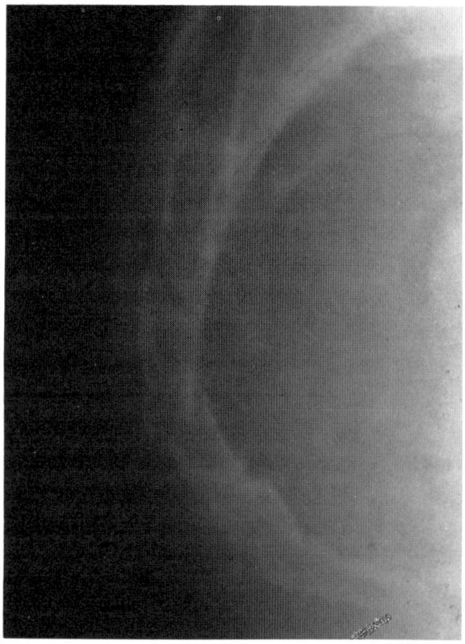

b

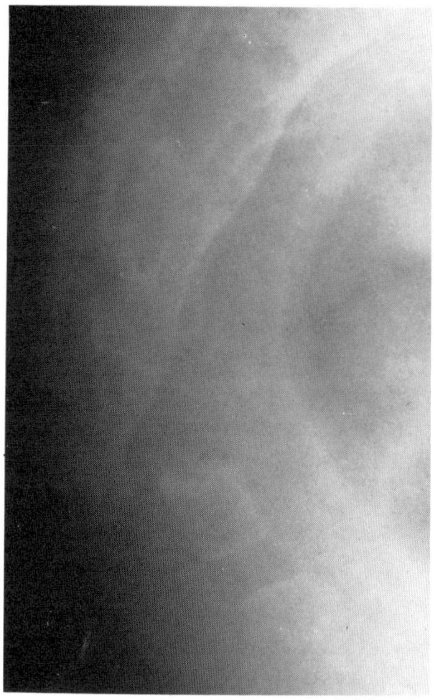

c

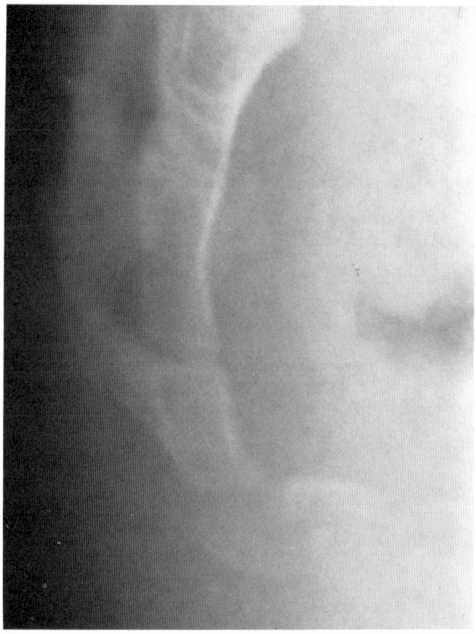

d

Fig. 4.18a–d. Isolated fracture of the coccyx.
a and b) With minimal dislocation (most frequent manifestation).
c) With marked dislocation toward the inner pelvis.
d) Comminuted fracture. All these fracture types, despite good technique on a. p. views, were only visible on the lateral films.

5 Upper Extremity

Traumatic dislocation most frequently involves the shoulder joint as a result of a fall on the hand or elbow, of the arm suddenly being caught or of a direct punch. Among different types of luxation (Fig. 5.1), the most commonly seen is the subcoracoid dislocation. The posterior and superior dislocations occur more rarely.

The typical posture of the involved arm and the reduced range of motion usually will allow only an a.p. view. An axial view should never be forced; however, if in doubt this is particularly useful to prove the existence of an often missed posterior dislocation (Fig. 5.2). The sign to be looked for in such a posterior dislocation on an a.p. view is the space between the articular surface of the humoral head and the lateral labrum of the glenoid cavity. Frequently, besides dislocation of the shoulder there is bony avulsion. Avulsion of the greater tuberosity often occurs without dislocation (Fig. 5.3). Habitual dislocation of the shoulder can be recognized radiologically if there is Hermodsson's deformity of the humeral head (compare with "hatched head" deformity in Fig. 14.32).

It should be mandatory always to obtain an x-ray after reposition of a dislocated shoulder. Control examination by fluoroscopy is totally inadequate. After fixation of the arm to the body, it is impossible to obtain axial views. If there is doubt as to a successful reduction, one should obtain a lateral transthoracic view of the shoulder.

The diagnosis of dislocation of the acromioclavicular joint does not offer any difficulties (Fig. 5.4). A subluxation is best documented if, at the time of exposure of the roentgenogram, the arm is abducted. The dislocation of the sternoclavicular joint, however, may be difficult to demonstrate. This can best be done by the use of tomography.

Fracture luxation of the shoulder is very difficult to manage and is a serious injury (Fig. 5.5); Figure 5.6 shows a variant of this. Among fractures of the humerus in close proximity to the shoulder (Fig. 5.7), fracture of the surgical neck is seen most frequently, whereas fractures of the anatomic neck occur rarely. There is often somewhat significant reduction in length. Abduction occurs much more commonly than adduction (Fig. 5.8). Frequently there is a dorsal angulation of the shaft, which can be fully appreciated only on an axial view, as well as a lesion of the lesser tuberosity.

Fractures of the medial 3rd of the clavicle may be difficult to recognize owing to an overlap with ribs and lateral processes of the vertebral bodies (Fig. 5.9). The same is true of fractures of the scapula, with the exception of a massive fracture of the neck of the scapula and its lateral border (Fig. 5.10). Fractures of the clavicle are occasionally accompanied by similar involvement of the upper ribs, which might be easily overlooked (Fig. 5.11). The humeral shaft may be affected by different types of fractures due to a fall or a direct force (Fig. 5.12). Special designations should be applied to fractures of the distal portion of the humerus (Fig. 5.13), which often occur in adults as comminuted or transcondylar fractures (Fig. 5.14). Condylar fractures usually affect the capitulum of the humerus (Fig. 5.15). In all instances of dislocation and fractures of the shoulder, the humerus or the elbow, damage to vascular or nerve structures must be anticipated. It is, therefore, important to investigate at the initial examination the possible presence of altered circulation or motility (check the innervation of the radial, median and ulnar nerves even if there is only a minor injury) (Fig. 5.16). Luxation of the elbow (Fig. 5.17) usually shows posterior dislocation of the bony elements of the forearm that form the joint (Fig. 5.18). Anterior dislocation is rarely seen. During the radiologic investigation, one should check carefully for avulsions, particularly of the coronoid process or possibly a fragment from the radial head on the volar surface (Fig. 5.19). A severe dislocation can be accompanied by rupture of soft tissue, thus forming an open luxation (Fig. 5.20). During childhood, there are also epiphyseolysis and dislocation or fracture of ossification centers (see page 237). A special type of injury is the Monteggia fracture-luxation combining a fracture of the ulna with dislocation of the radius usually anteriorly (volar Monteggia fracture-luxation). The dislocation of the radius is easily overlooked especially when the dislocation is minimal and the projection does not properly visualize the pathology (Figs. 5.21 and 5.22). The posterior Monteggia fracture-luxation occurs infrequently (Fig. 5.23). Fractures of the olecranon (Fig. 5.24) usually are accompanied by a dislocation of the proximal fragment cranially. Almost always, there is involvement of the joint (Fig. 5.25). As a result of direct trauma, there can occasionally occur a fracture of one of the spurs of the olecranon (Fig. 5.26).

Among fractures involving the head of the radius, one can distinguish between chip fractures and fractures of the neck (Fig. 5.27). With only minimal dislocation, it can be quite difficult in both types to recognize that there is a fracture (Fig. 5.28). A comminuted fracture or a marked dislocation of the head of the radius nowadays will require surgical intervention with resection (Fig. 5.29).

In the area of the forearm, isolated fractures can involve the radius or ulna. The origin of the parry fracture is well understood. Fractures of the forearm with involvement of both bones usually also show a marked dislocation (Fig. 5.30), its direction being determined by the external force or muscle pull. The disadvantageous local anatomic conditions for external fixation always result in the danger of complication, particularly pseudarthrosis in fractures of the forearm. Therefore, the position of the fragments must be checked repeatedly.

A similar combined lesion such as the Monteggia fracture-luxation occurs at the distal forearm, the so-called Galeazzi fracture-luxation (Fig. 5.31). The most common radius fracture involves a rather atypical location above its distal end. In about half of all patients with this fracture, there is simultaneously avulsion of the ulnar styloid process and, rarely, an avulsion from the dorsal surface of the triquetrum (Figs. 5.32 and 5.33). The x-ray will show a somewhat marked dorsal angulation and dislocation of the distal joint of the radius as well as radial angulation and dislocation. Almost all distal fractures of the radius have concomitant involvement of the joint (Figs. 5.34 to 5.36). In the presence of a free fracture fragment dorsally, in comminuted fracture with involvement of the joint, frequent x-ray follow-up examination is required in order to promptly recognize slipping off of this fragment. An isolated fracture of the ulnar styloid process is rarely seen (Fig. 5.37). During childhood, greenstick fractures and epiphyseolysis occur frequently (see page 238). A postreposition x-ray report should always contain a comment on the angle of the joint, with emphasis on a possible subluxation at the distal radioulnar joint, possibly the result of shortening of the radius (Fig. 5.38). In the area of the carpal bones, one should never overlook a dislocation of the lunatum (Fig. 5.39) and special attention should be given to perilunatum dislocation (Fig. 5.40; compare Fig. 5.35).

If there is a fracture of the navicular bone where the proximal fragment is luxated together with the lunatum, we are dealing with a luxation fracture of de Quervain (Fig. 5.41). Navicular fractures may be hard to recognize (Fig. 5.42). A local vascular channel and its duplication are rare as developmental anomalies. If a fracture of the navicular bone is suspected, one should always obtain a special view, with the hand held as during writing (Fig. 5.43). If the usual techniques will not allow good recognition of the local pathology, a tomogram will give clear answers (Fig. 5.44). Avulsions of the tubercle or at the level of the tubercle often occur; however, avulsions of the triquetrum are most common and are best seen on the lateral view (Fig. 5.45).

As a consequence of a navicular fracture, a resorptive cystic defect or necrosis of the proximal fragment sometimes develops. Both may occur simultaneously (Fig. 5.42). Necrosis is recognized by a thickening of the bony structures. Pseudarthrosis of the navicular bone often occurs. Its recognition may be accidental. This implies that the fracture was actually missed at the time of trauma and, therefore, no therapy was initiated. Fractures or luxations of the other carpal bones are only rarely seen. If such a finding is suspected but cannot be demonstrated on regular survey films on two planes, special views are needed (Figs. 5.46 to 5.49).

The best known fracture involving the metacarpal bones is the so-called Bennett's fracture. This refers to a fracture of the basal and ulnar corner of the first metacarpal bone which involves the joint and luxation or subluxation of the first metacarpal bone while maintaining the articular integrity of the fragment (Fig. 5.50).

Dislocation of several metacarpal bones results in a peculiar positioning of the middle hand (Fig. 5.51). Fractures of the head of the metacarpal bones are usually quite noticeable because of their volar angulation and also can be recognized if dislocation is minimal (Fig. 5.52). There is a very high incidence of traumatic lesions of the fingers. They have many different aspects and are the result of various injuries during professional sports and everyday activities (Figs. 5.53 to 5.59). Articular involvement should always be reported. In the search for small traumatic alterations, it is recommended that the contour of all fingers be viewed with special care, particularly in the region of the joints. Professional accidents and those occurring during household activities frequently lead to open fractures. These most often involve the lateral fingers, thumb, index finger and little finger (Figs. 5.60 to 5.62). Undoubtedly our hands are exposed to the greatest danger when we work with the many machines of today (Fig. 5.63). Traumatization frequently is the result of carelessly handling or playing with explosives (Fig. 5.64)

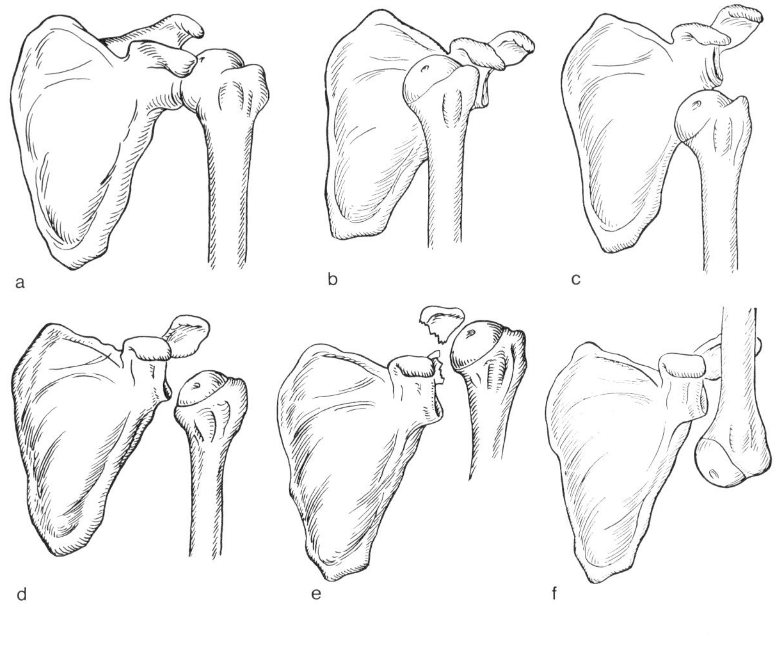

Fig. 5.1a–f. Dislocation of the shoulder. a) Normal articulation; b) anterior dislocation; subcoracoid or infraclavicular dislocation; c) anterior dislocation; axillary or subglenoid dislocation; d) posterior dislocation; e) superior dislocation with fracture of the acromion; f) luxation with elevated arm. (From H. R. Zatzkin: The Roentgen Diagnosis of Trauma. Chicago, Yearbook Medical Publishers, Inc., 1965. Used by permission.)

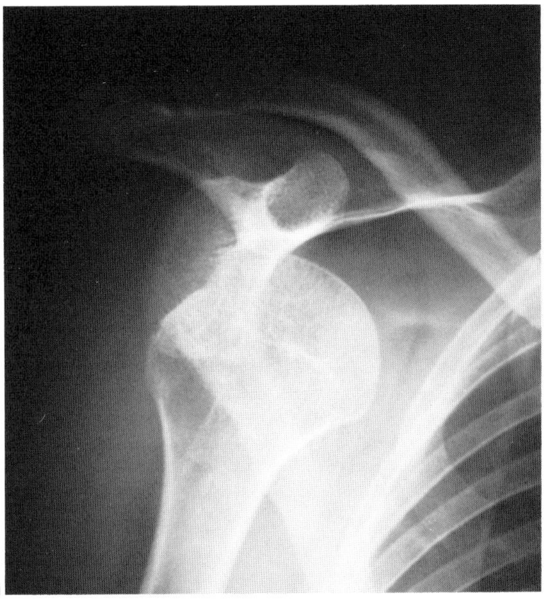

a

Fig. 5.2a–d. a) Anterior dislocation (subcoracoid dislocation).
b and c) Posterior dislocation after an accident 2 years previously and which was not recognized. Bony consolidation of clavicular fracture. Also, soft-tissue ossification and bony avulsion anterior to the empty articulation.
d) Anterior dislocation of the shoulder on axial view. Bony avulsion from the head of the humerus anterior to the articulation (1, acromion; 2, coracoid).

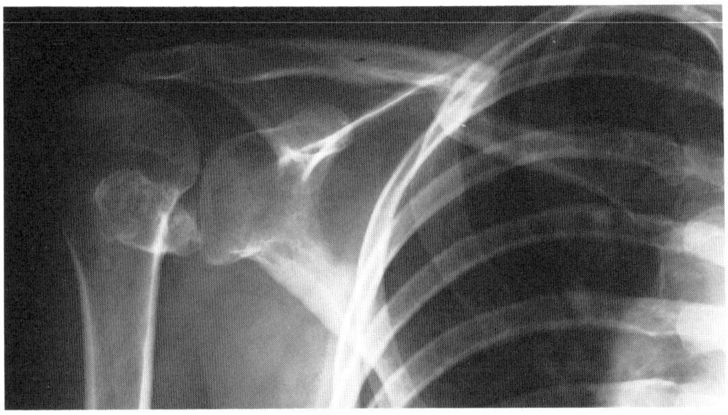

b

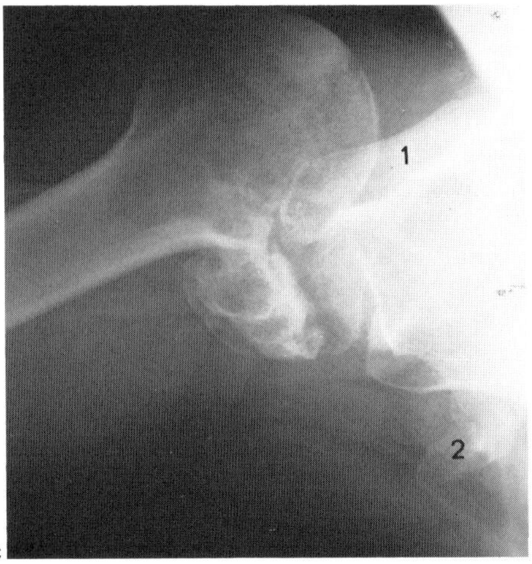

c

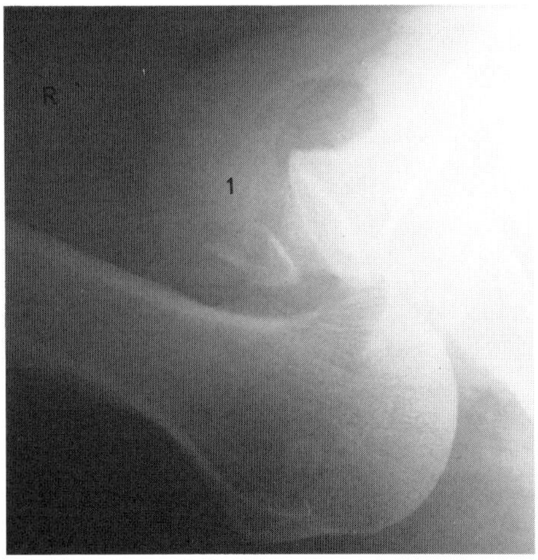

d

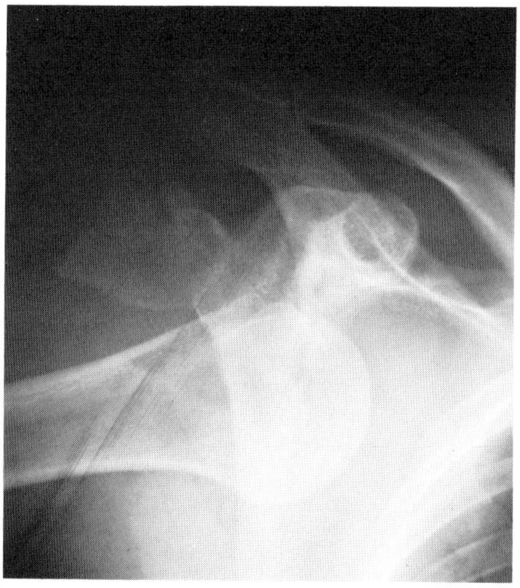

a

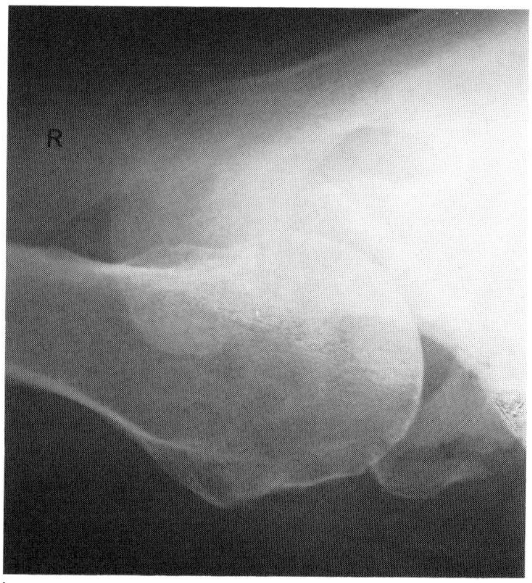

b

Fig. 5.3a–c. a) Anterior dislocation (axillary dislocation) with avulsion of the greater tuberosity, which is a frequent finding.

b) Avulsion of the tip of the coracoid process in a subcoracoid dislocation (dislocation repositioned).

c) A 28-year-old skier with an avulsion of the greater tuberosity.

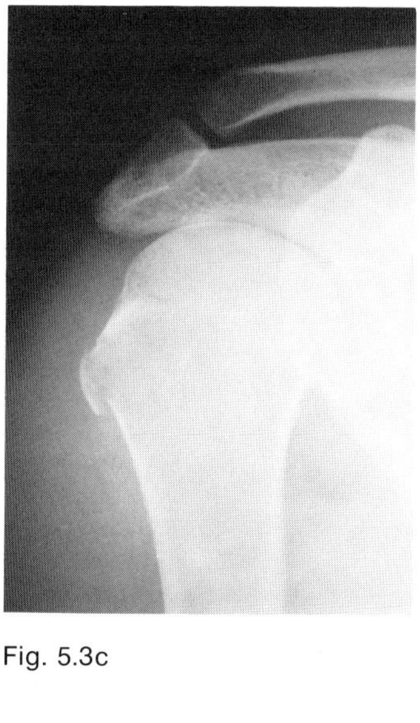

Fig. 5.3c

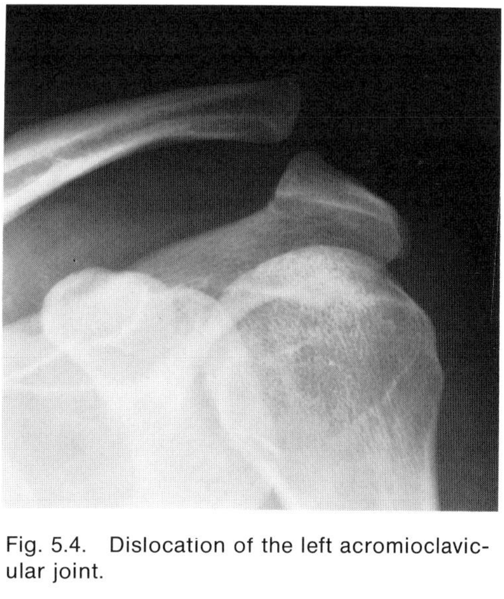

Fig. 5.4. Dislocation of the left acromioclavicular joint.

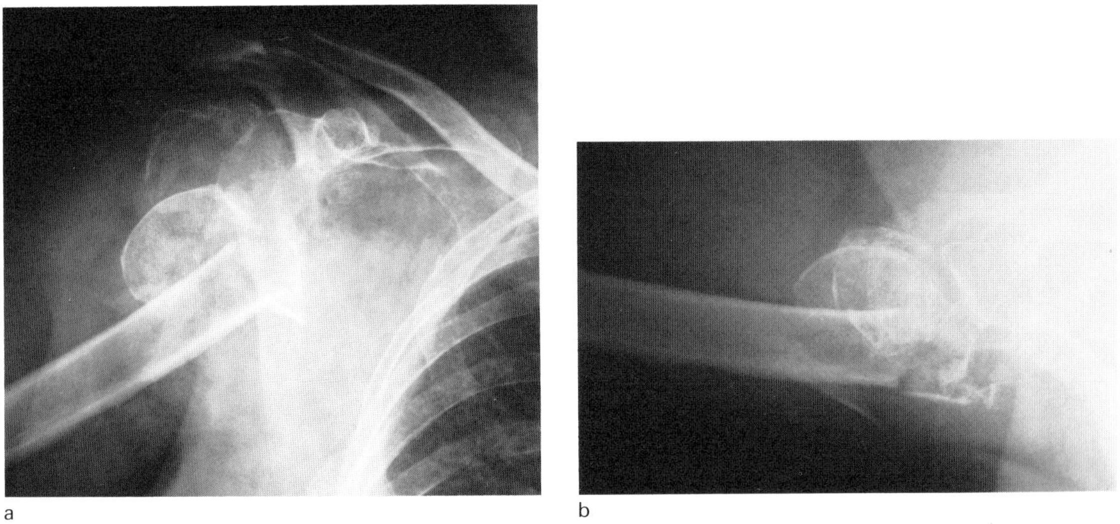

Fig. 5.5a and b. A 78-year-old woman who fell in the ladies' room because of a fainting spell. Abduction fracture with posterior and inferior dislocation of the humeral head.

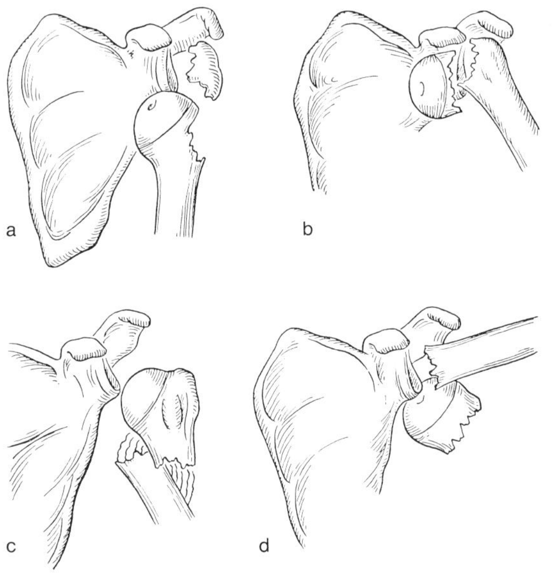

Fig. 5.6a–d. Fracture and dislocation of the shoulder. a) Anterior and inferior dislocation with avulsion fracture. b) Anterior dislocation with abduction fracture. c) Old fracture with pseudodisplacement (muscular atrophy). d) Posterior dislocation with abduction fracture. (From H. R. Zatzkin: The Roentgen Diagnosis of Trauma. Chicago, Yearbook Medical Publishers, Inc. 1965. Used by permission.)

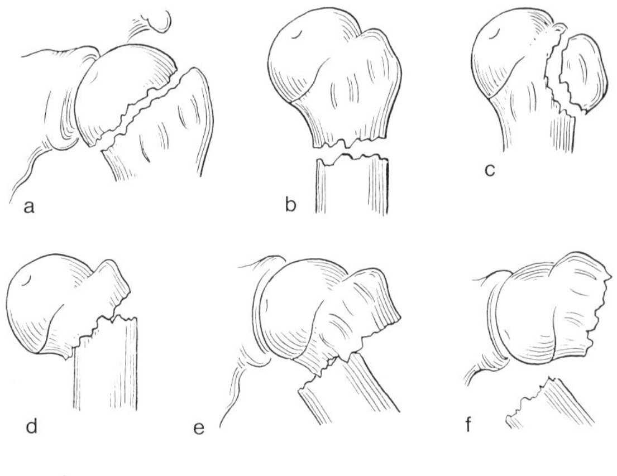

Fig. 5.7a–f. Humeral fracture close to the shoulder joint. a) Fracture of the anatomic neck. b) Fracture of the surgical neck. c) Avulsion fracture of the greater tuberosity. d) Abduction fracture with impaction. e) Abduction fracture with impaction. f) Abduction fracture without impaction. (H. R. Zatzkin: The Roentgen Diagnosis of Trauma. Chicago, Yearbook Medical Publishers, Inc., 1965. Used by permission.)

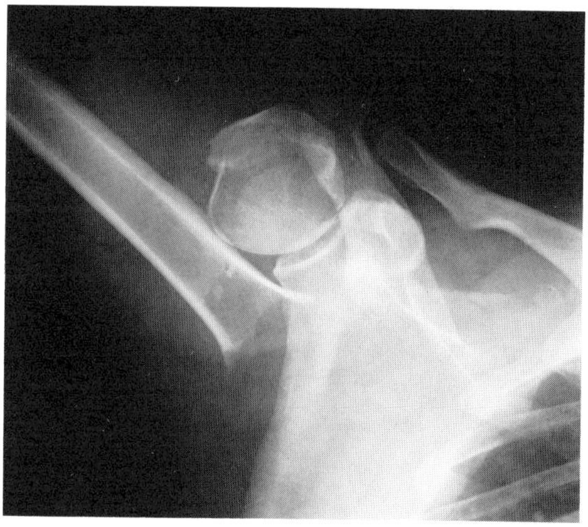

Fig. 5.8. A 40-year-old man who was run over by a tractor. Fracture of the humeral neck with abduction. The humeral shaft is displaced and located behind the rotated head. Marked shortening.

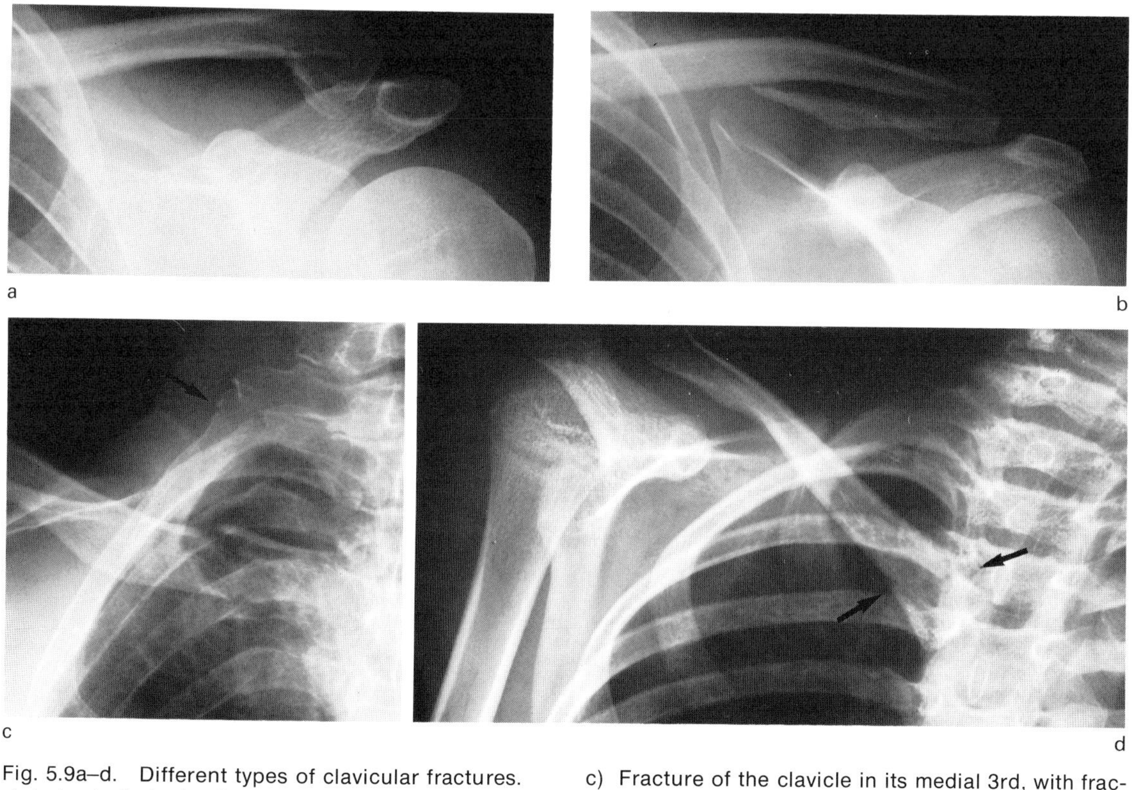

Fig. 5.9a–d. Different types of clavicular fractures.
a) Lateral clavicular fracture with involvement of the acromioclavicular joint.
b) Comminuted fracture of the lateral 3rd of the clavicle.
c) Fracture of the clavicle in its medial 3rd, with fracture of the 1st rib.
d) Fracture of the medial 3rd of the clavicle.

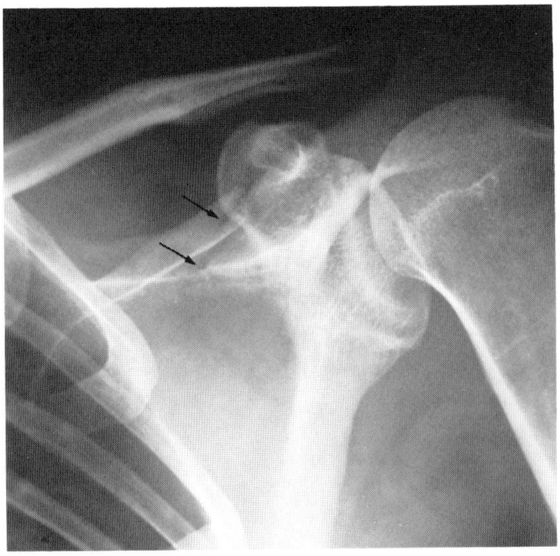

Fig. 5.10a

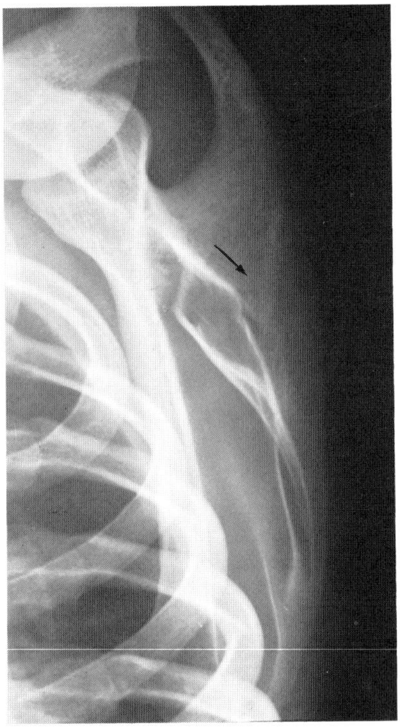

Fig. 5.10b

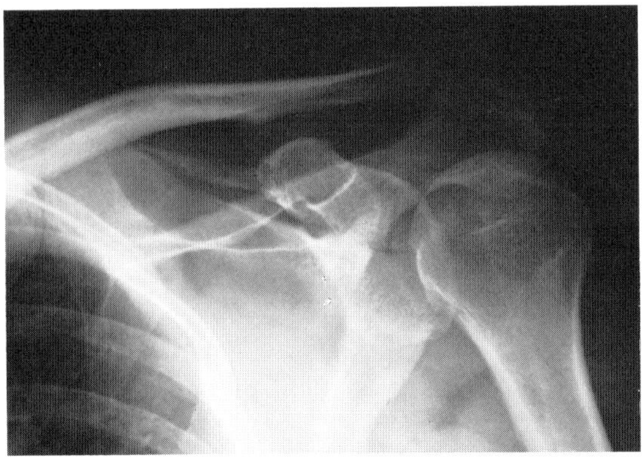

c

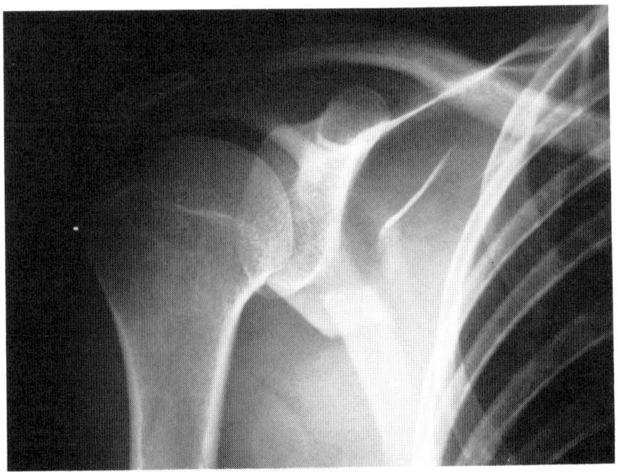

d

Fig. 5.10a and b. A 28-year-old man after a traffic accident. Fracture of the scapular spine.
c) Fracture of the upper border of the scapula extending into the joint.

d) A 26-year-old farm woman who was attacked by a cow. Fracture of the neck of the scapula and its lateral rim.

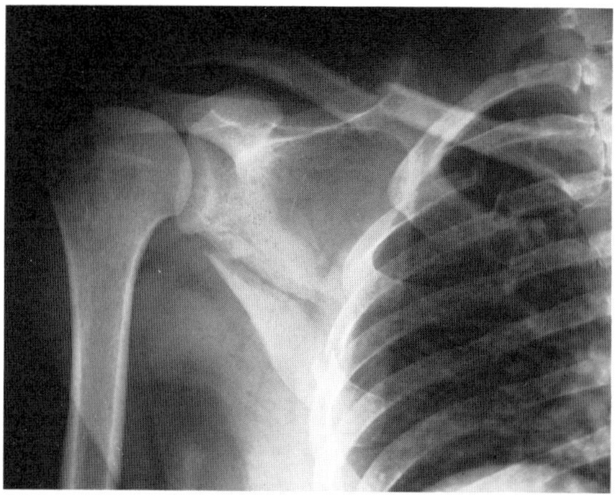

Fig. 5.11. A 33-year-old man after a car accident. Transverse fracture of the middle third of the right clavicle. Fracture of the scapula; fractures of the 2nd to the 5th ribs on the right.

Fig. 5.12. An 18-year-old man, with concussion of the base of the brain following a traffic accident. Untreated. Transverse fracture of the humerus of 5 weeks' duration. ▶

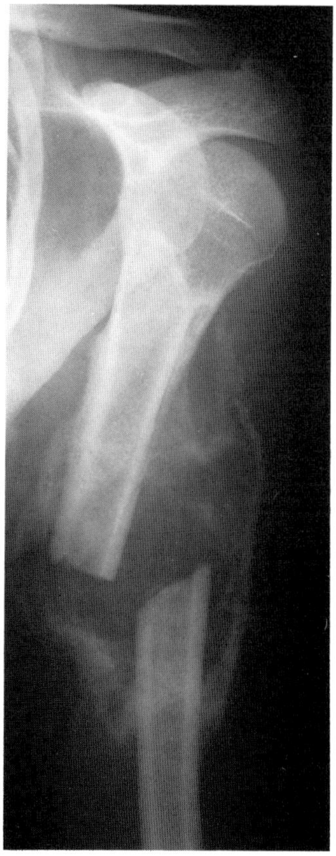

Fig. 5.12

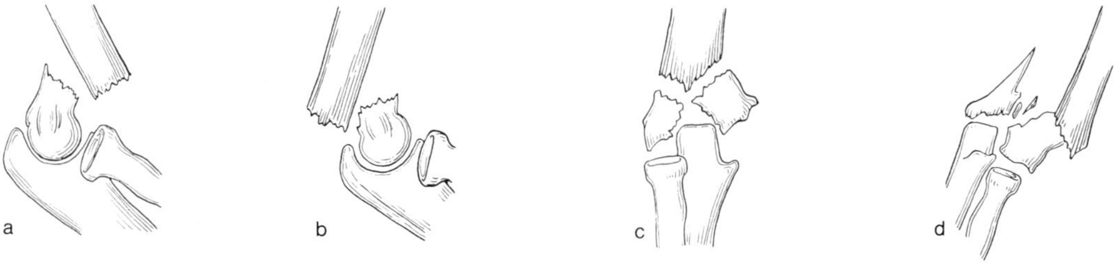

Fig. 5.13a–d. Fracture of the distal region of the humerus.

a) Supracondylar fracture after overextension; posterior (backward) displacement and angulation.

b) Supracondylar fracture with anterior (forward) flexion displacement.

c) Y-shaped intercondylar fracture; olecranon is wedged between the condyles.

d) Y-shaped comminuted fracture with lateral displacement. (From H. R. Zatzkin: The Roentgen Diagnosis of Trauma. Chicago, Yearbook Medical Publishers, Inc., 1965. Used by permission.)

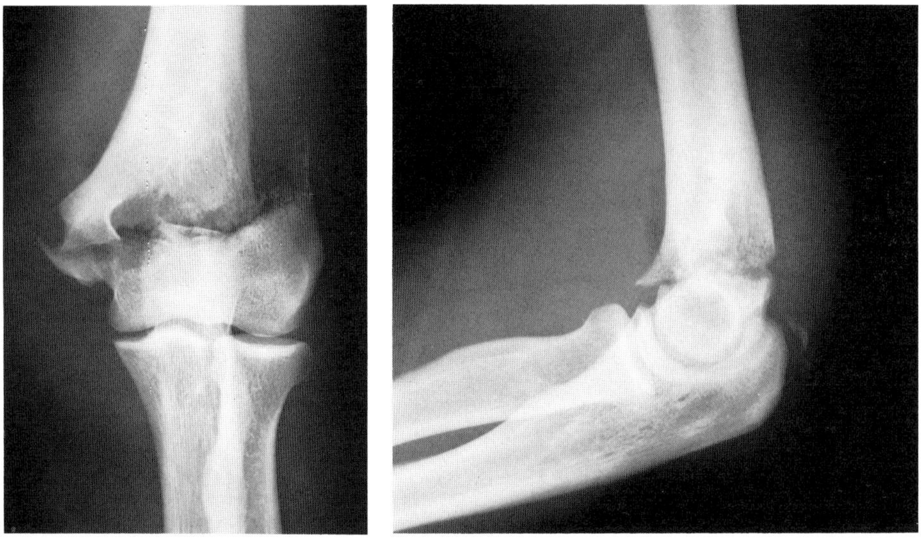

a

Fig. 5.14b

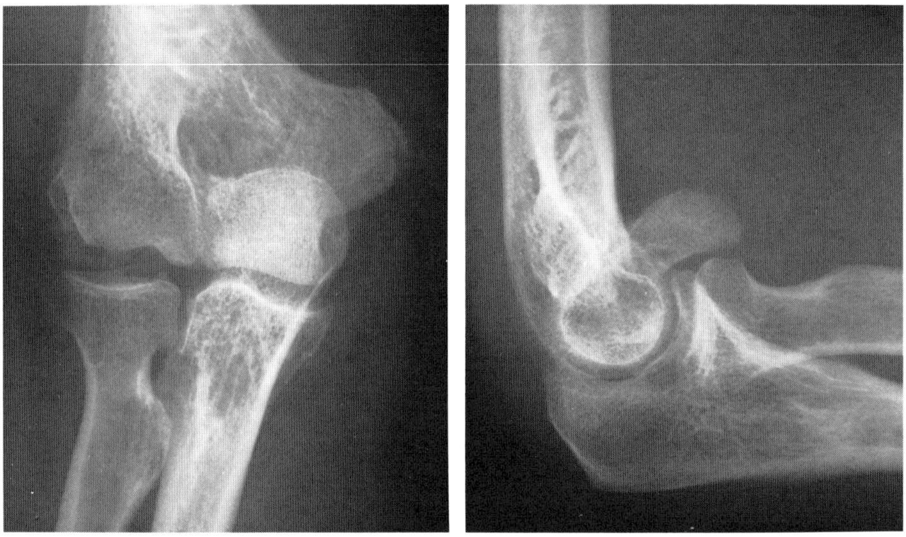

a

Fig. 5.15b

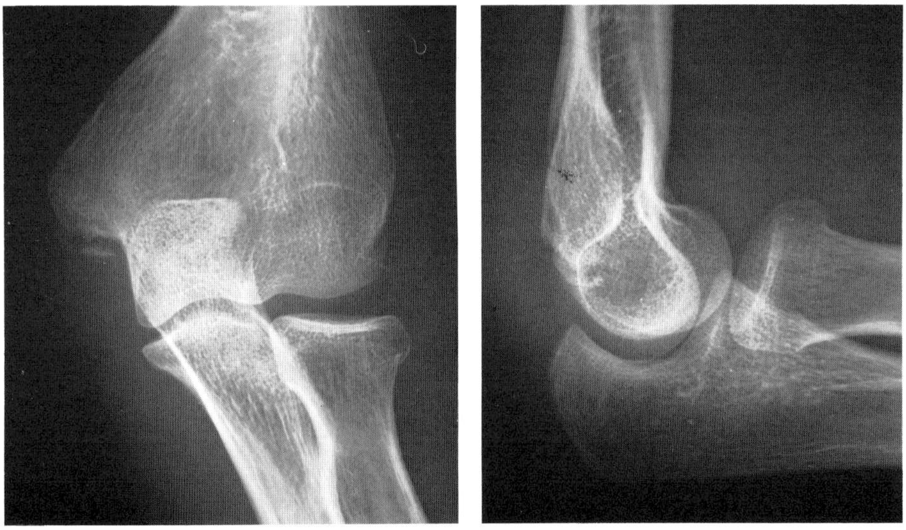

a

Fig. 5.16b

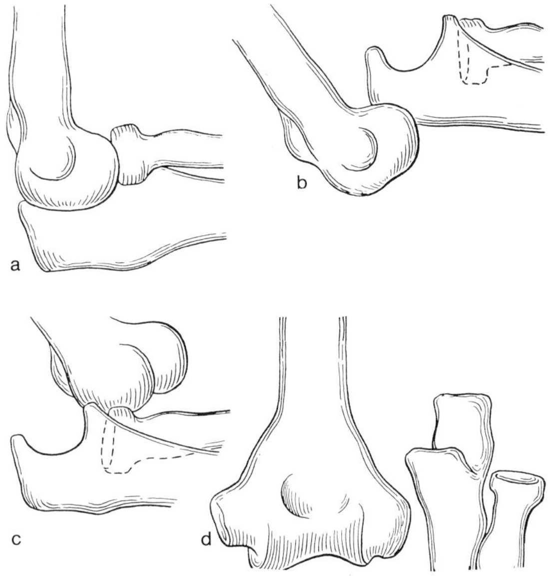

Fig. 5.17

◀ Fig. 5.14a and b. A 33-year-old man with a transcondylar humeral fracture with marginal fracture fragments. Later pseudarthrosis developed.

◀ Fig. 5.15a and b. A 66-year-old woman after a traffic accident with a motorscooter. Fracture of the humeral capitulum.

◀ Fig. 5.16a and b. A 13-year-old girl after an accident at home. Avulsion fracture of the distal contour of the medial epicondyle, with a lesion of the ulnar nerve; note also the fracture of the radial head.

▲

Fig. 5.17a–d. Dislocation of the elbow. a) Normal articulation. b) Anterior dislocation. c) Posterior dislocation. d) Lateral dislocation. (From H. R. Zatzkin: The Roentgen Diagnosis of Trauma. Chicago, Yearbook Medical Publishers, Inc., 1965. Used by permission.)

Fig. 5.18a and b. Most frequently seen type of dislocation of the elbow. Small marginal bony fragmentation within the empty articulation of the olecranon.

▼

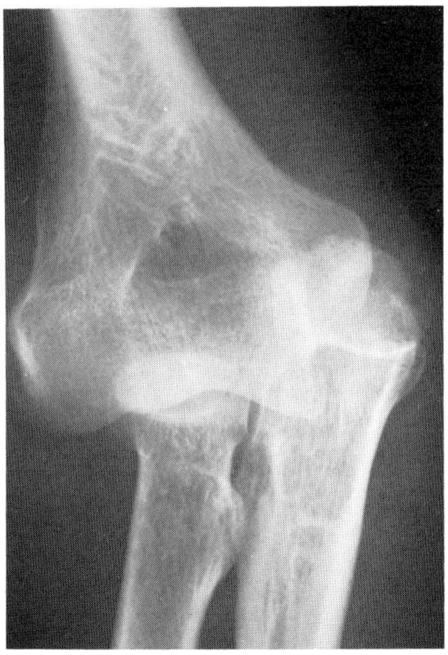

Fig. 5.18a

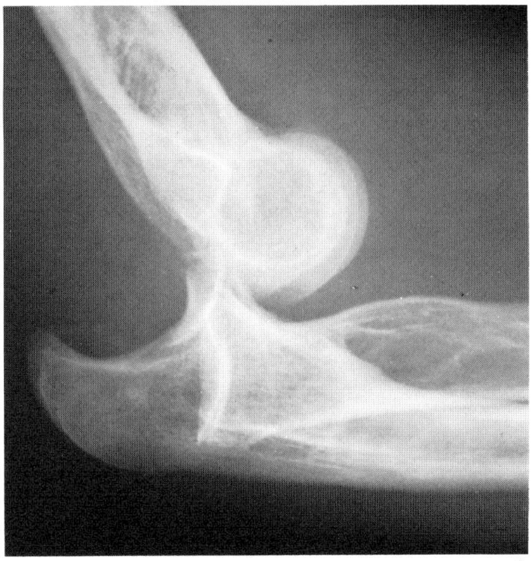

b

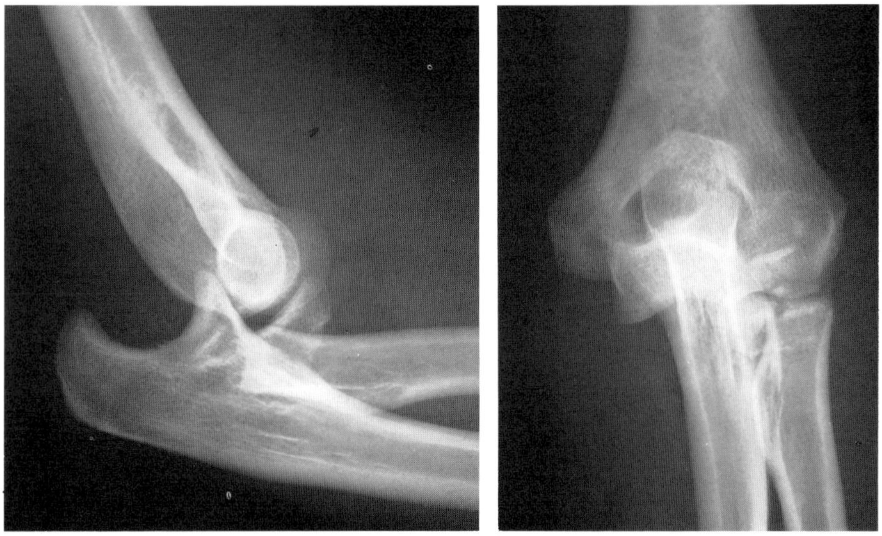

Fig. 5.19a b

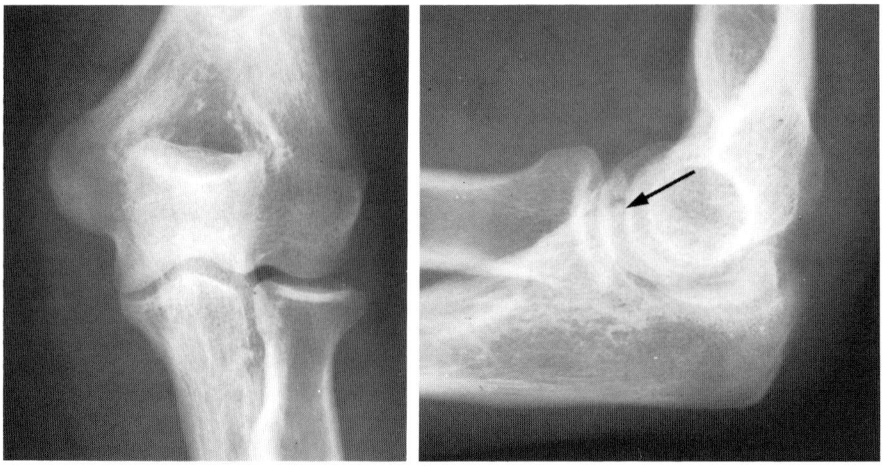

c d

Fig. 5.19a–d. a and b) A 28-year-old medical student fell from a car while under the influence of alcohol. Posterior dislocation of the elbow, with volar avulsion of the radial head. c and d) A 51-year-old woman with a fracture of the ulnar coronoid process. Dislocation reduced.

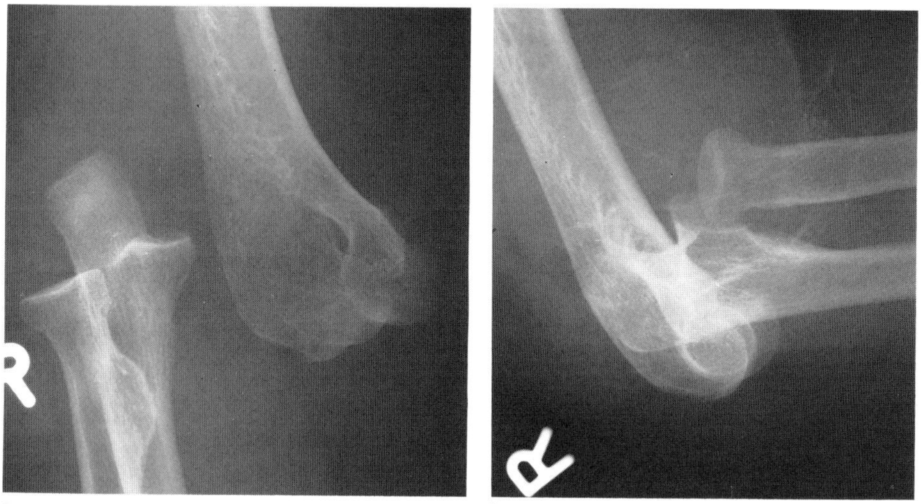

a b

Fig. 5.20a and b. An 81-year-old woman after a fall from a chair at home. Open lateral dislocation of the elbow.

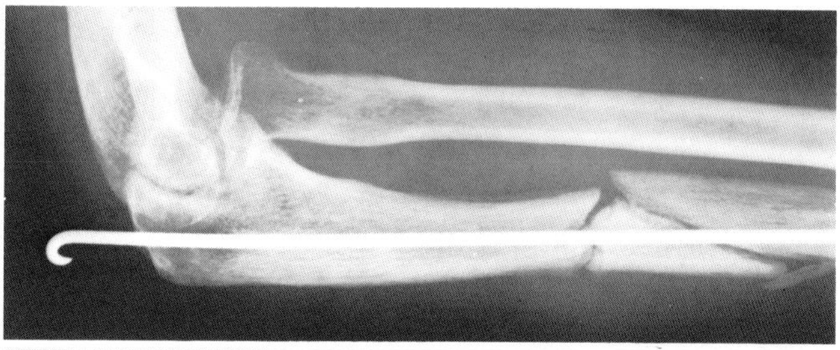

Fig. 5.21. A 41-year-old man with a Monteggia fracture. After removal of the plaster cast and on an ideally projected x-ray demonstration of the Monteggia fracture, one now recognizes the previously missed dislocation of the radius.

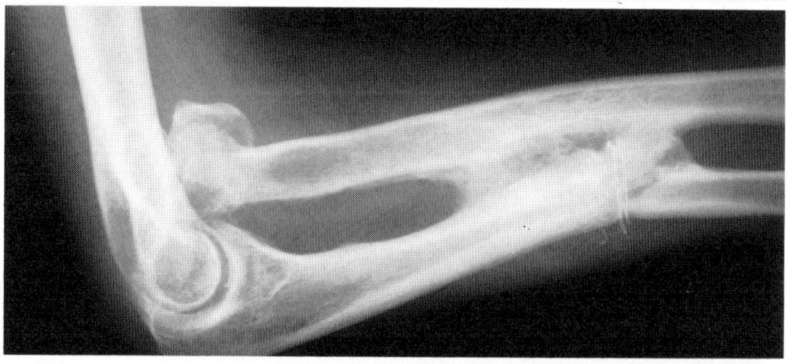

Fig. 5.22. A 65-year-old man with a local condition about 8 months after a Monteggia fracture. The luxation of the radial head could not be corrected. Abnormal position of the ulna with marked bridging callus as a result of insufficient fixation.

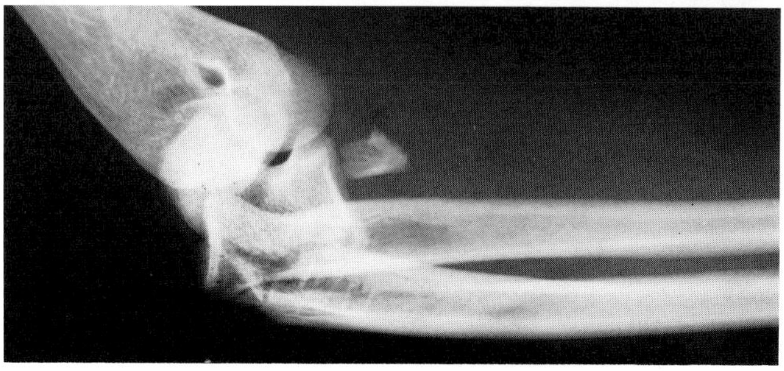

Fig. 5.23. A 38-year-old man who was hit by a car on the sidewalk. Posterior Monteggia fracture.

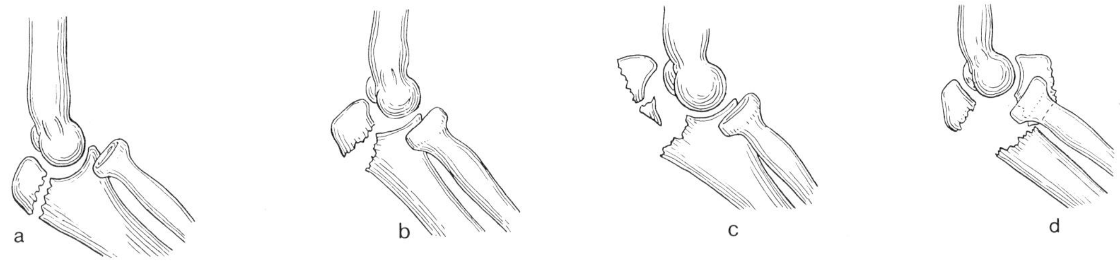

Fig. 5.24a-d. Fracture of the olecranon. a) Simple olecranon fracture without significant dislocation. b) Olecranon fracture with typical dislocation. c and d) Comminuted fractures. (From H. R. Zatzkin: The Roentgen Diagnosis of Trauma. Chicago, Yearbook Medical Publishers, Inc., 1965. Used by permission.)

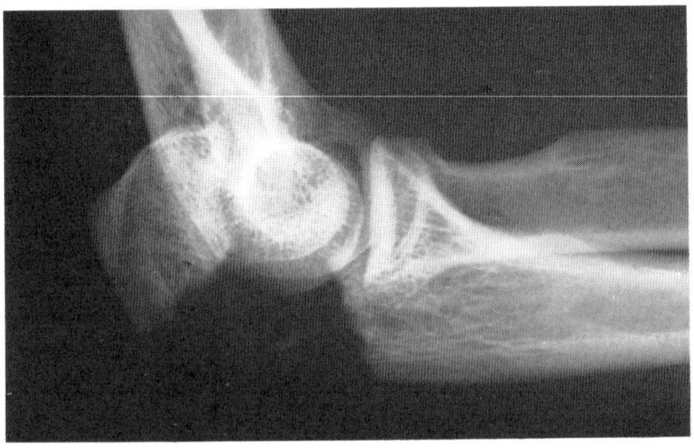

a

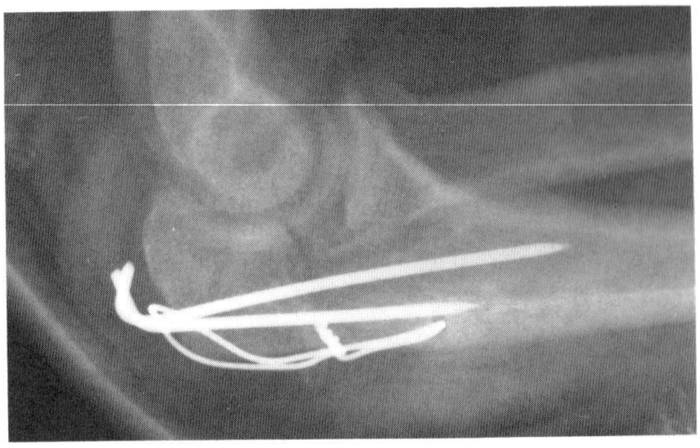

b

Fig. 5.25a and b. A 28-year-old man. a) Car driver's fracture of the olecranon, with opening of the joint. b) Follow-up film after pinning and pulling together of fracture; there is good anatomic reposition (good adaptation).

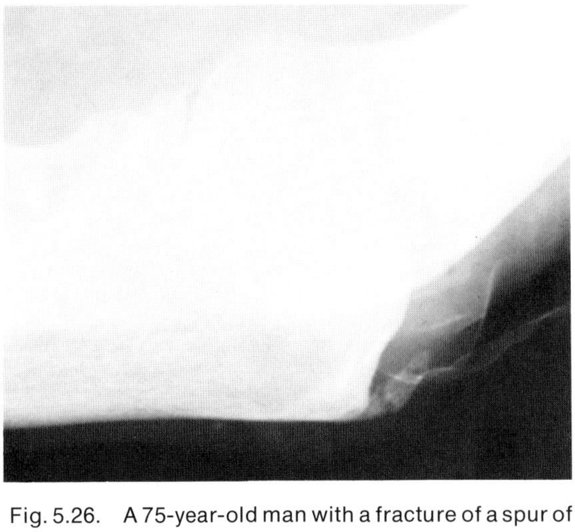

Fig. 5.26. A 75-year-old man with a fracture of a spur of the olecranon.

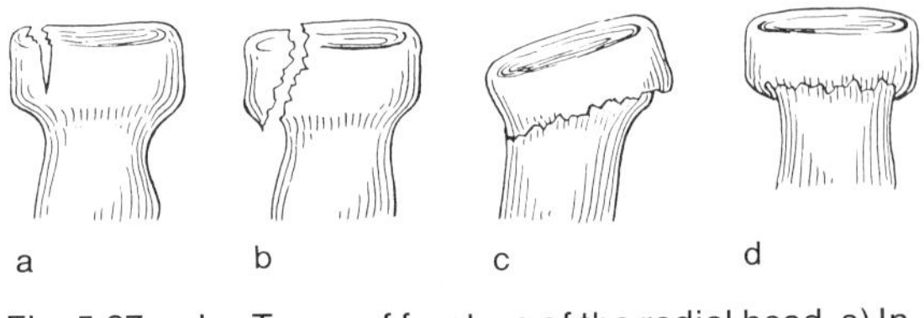

Fig. 5.27a–d. Types of fracture of the radial head. a) Incomplete wedge. b) Displaced chip. c) Fracture of the radial head in the area of the neck, with angulation. d) Fracture of the radial head in the neck area, with impaction. (From H. R. Zatzkin: The Roentgen Diagnosis of Trauma. Chicago, Yearbook Medical Publishers, Inc., 1965. Used by permission.)

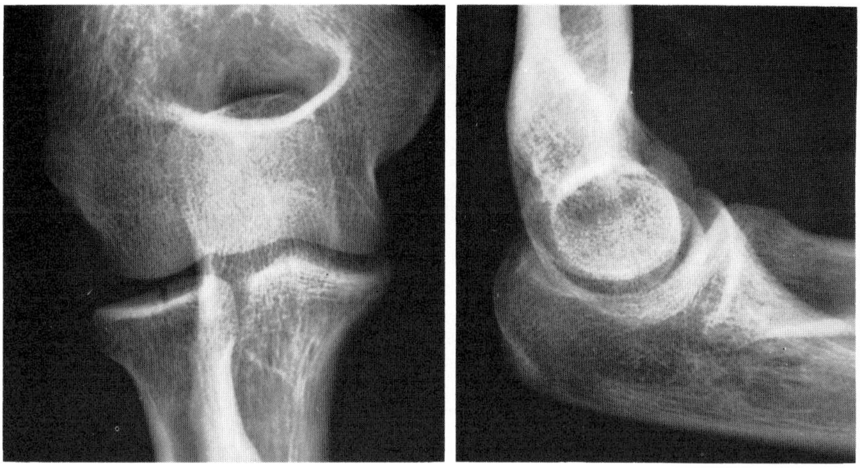

a b

Fig. 5.28a and b. Chip fracture of the radial head.

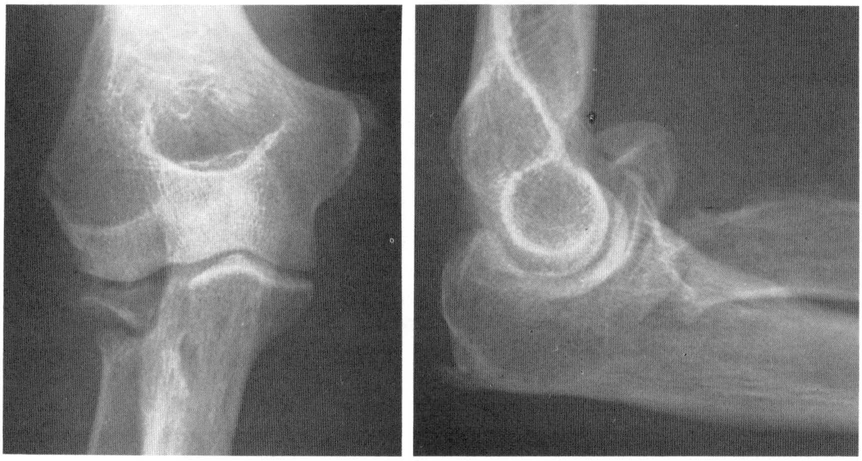

a b

Fig. 5.29a and b. Fracture of the radial neck, with 180-degree rotation of the head.

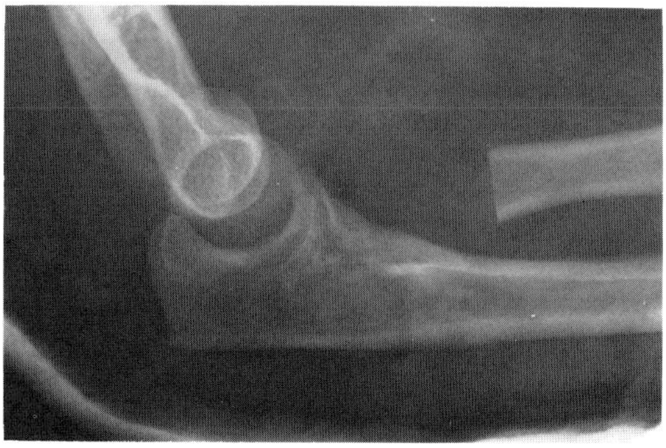

Fig. 5.29c. Condition after resection of the radial head.

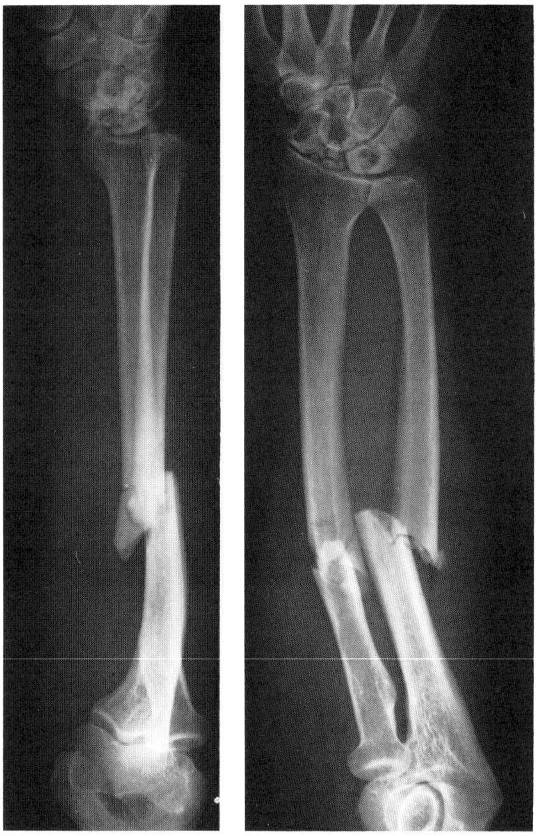

a b

Fig. 5.30a and b. A 62-year-old man injured while cranking the motor of his car and the crankshaft suddenly recoiled. Fracture of the forearm in the proximal half. Additional findings: pseudarthrosis of the navicular, lunate and capitate bones.

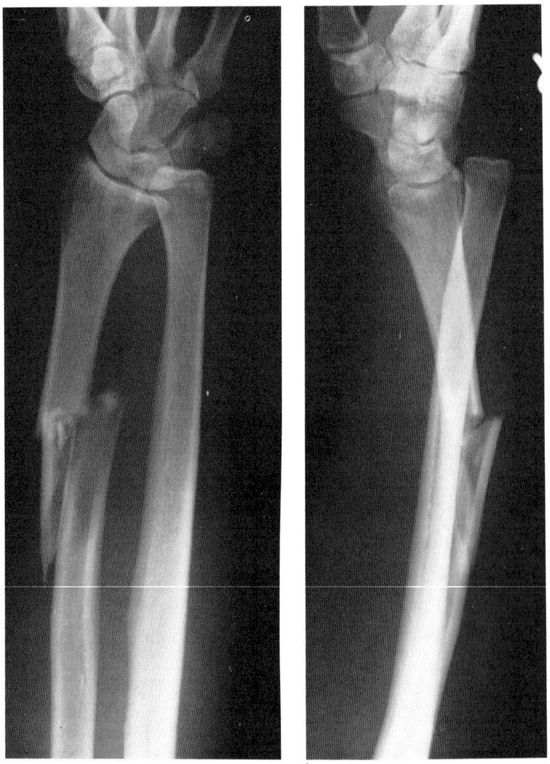

a b

Fig. 5.31a and b. A 47-year-old man after a motor-scooter collision with a car. Fracture of the radius and dislocation of the ulna from the distal radioulnar joint (Galeazzi fracture).

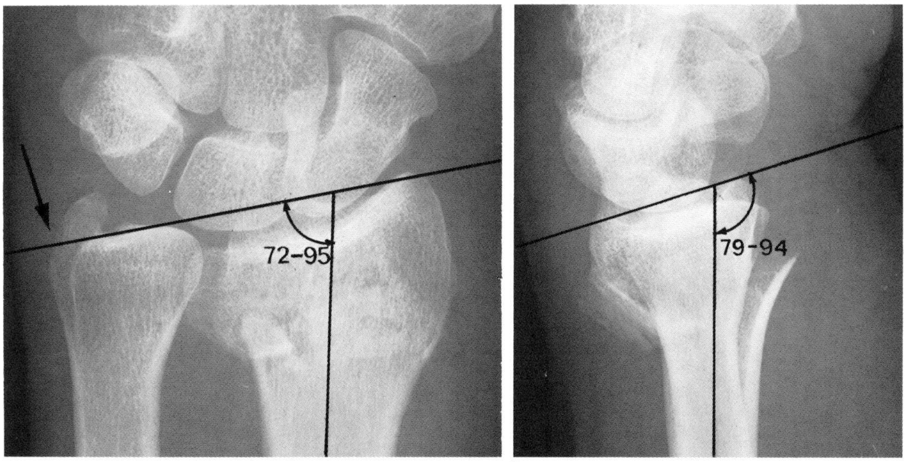

a b

Fig. 5.32a and b. A 64-year-old man with a fracture of the radius in a typical location. Dorsal angulation of the articular portion. Fracture of the ulnar styloid process *(arrow)*.

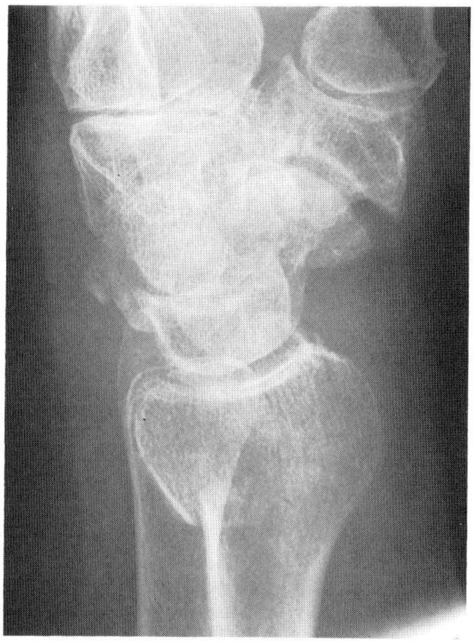

Fig. 5.33. A 68-year-old woman with an avulsion from the dorsal surface of the triquetrum; fracture of the radius.

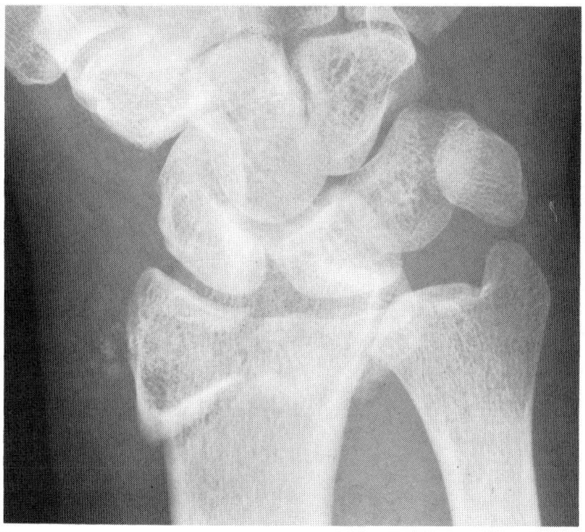

a

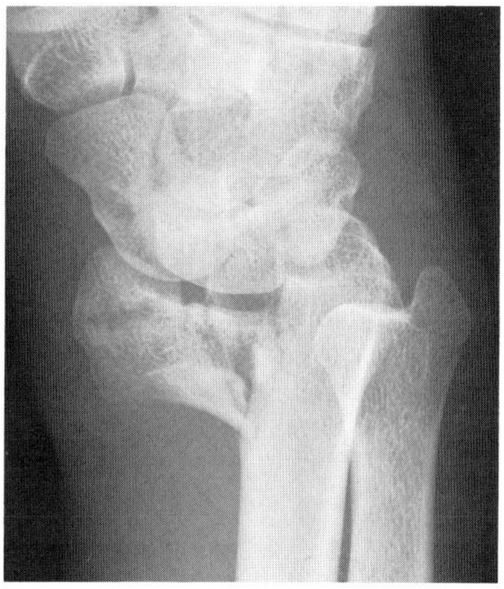

b

Fig. 5.34a and b. A 41-year-old man after a motorscooter collision with a car. Atypical fracture of the radius involving the joint. Angulation toward the volar and radial sides.

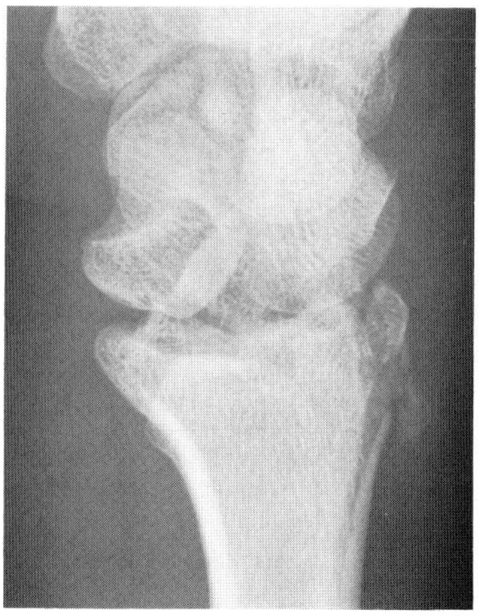

a

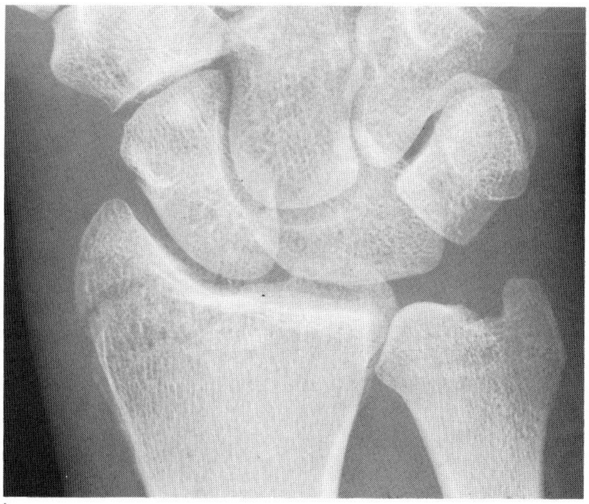

b

Fig. 5.35a and b. A 38-year-old man after a fall from a ladder. Fracture of the styloid process of the radius and of the dorsal edge of the radius extending into the joint.

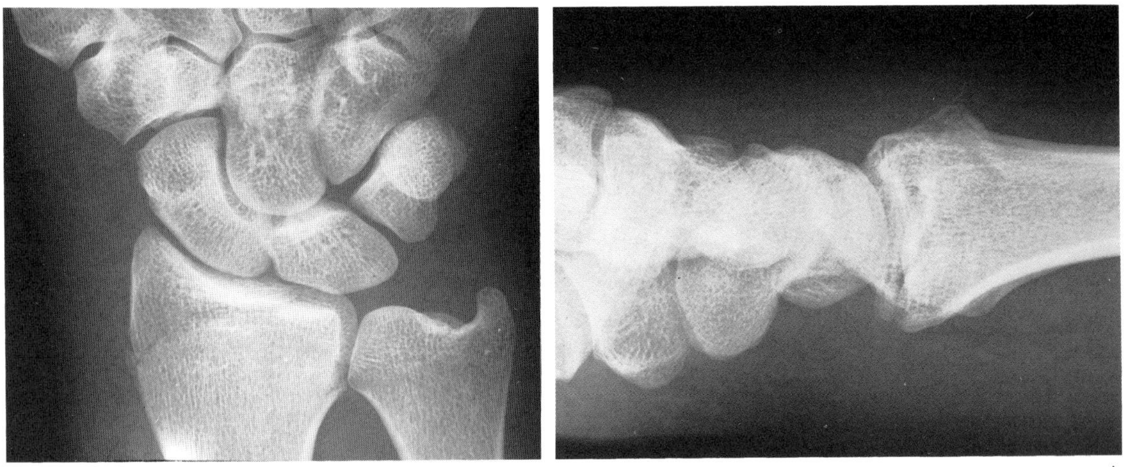

Fig. 5.36a b

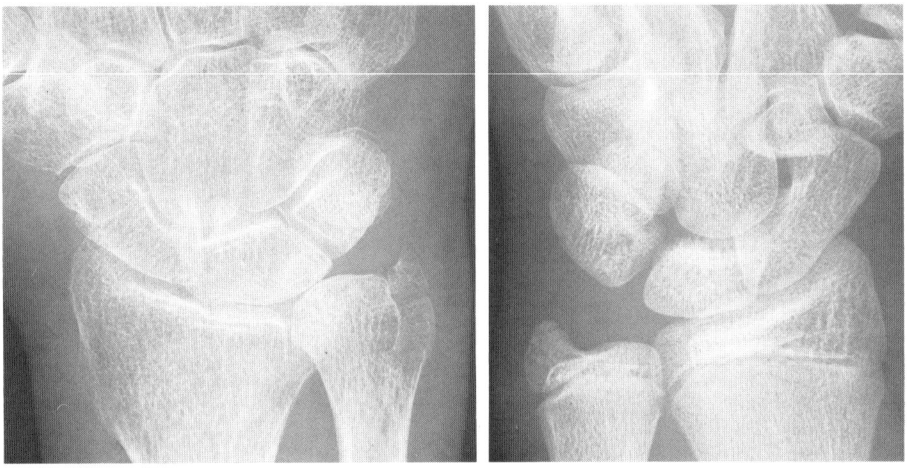

Fig. 5.37a b

Fig. 5.36a and b. Fracture of the radius extending into the joint. On a. p. view, there is an illusion of a persistent epiphysis. Dorsal hump.

Fig. 5.37a and b. A 62-year-old woman. a) Isolated fracture of the ulnar styloid process at its joint space. b) A 17-year-old girl after an accident on a bicycle. Isolated fracture of the tip of the ulnar styloid process.

Fig. 5.38a–f. A 61-year-old woman. a and b) Fracture of the radius in a typical location involving the joint. c to f) Controls after 2 and 8 months; increase in the dorsoradial angulation and in the abnormal position at the distal radial joint. Additional findings: traumatic involvement of an old ossification within the soft tissues and posttraumatic osteoporosis. Resorptive posttraumatic defect involving the ulnar styloid process. ▶

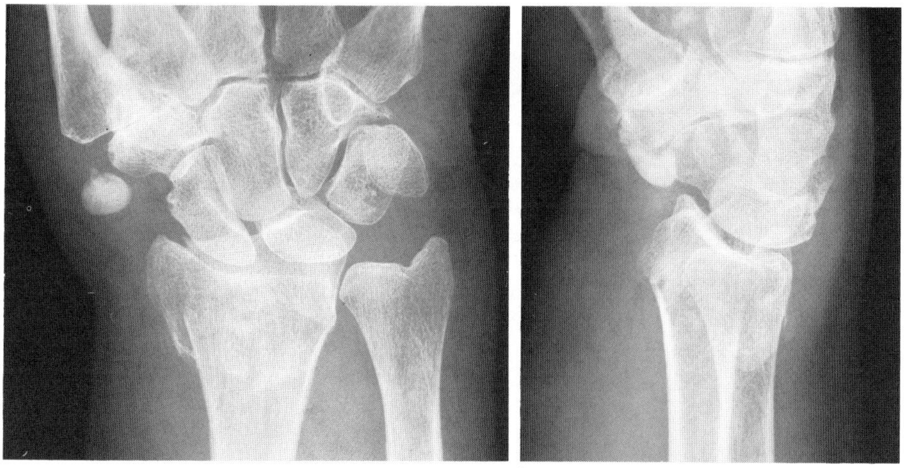

Fig. 5.38a b

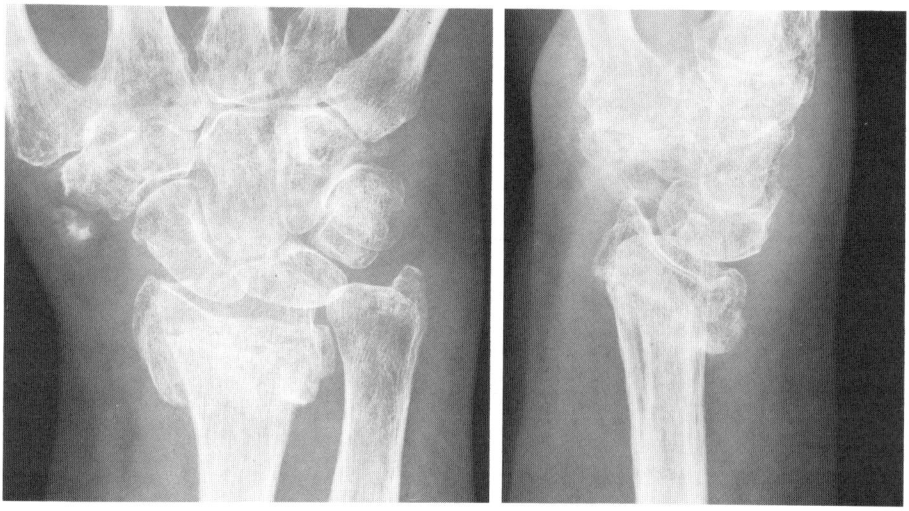

Fig. 5.38c d

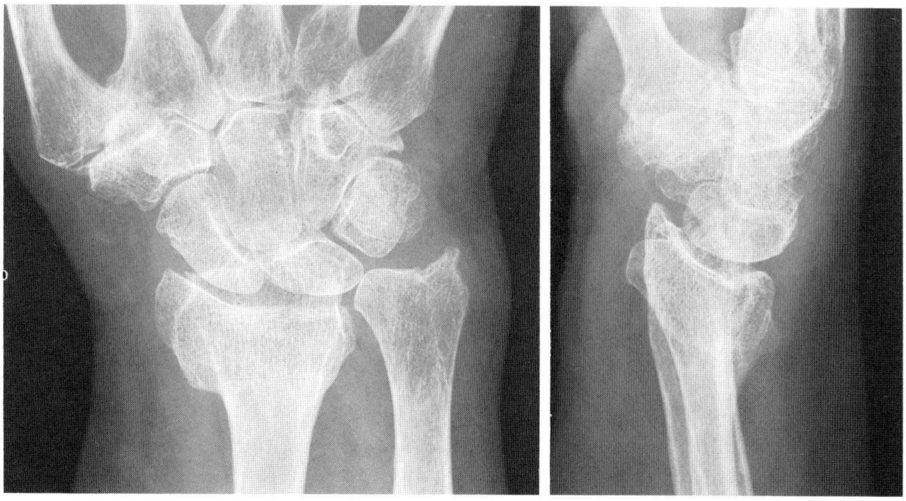

Fig. 5.38e f

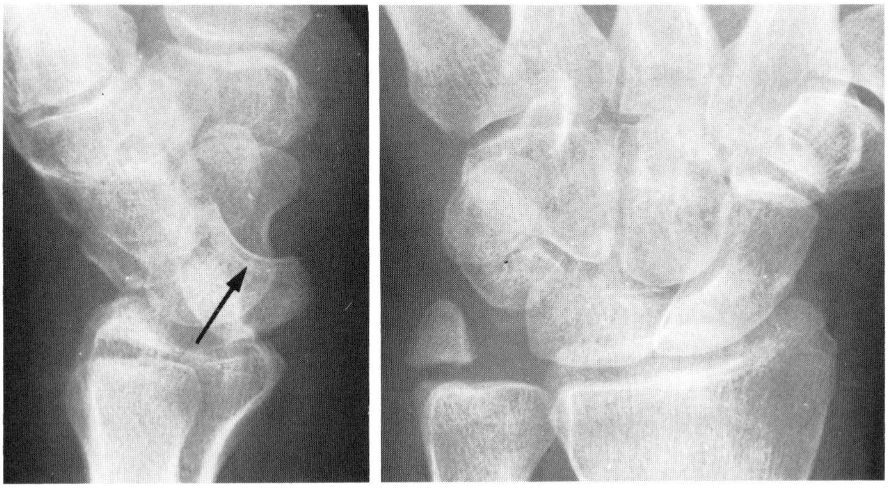

Fig. 5.39a b

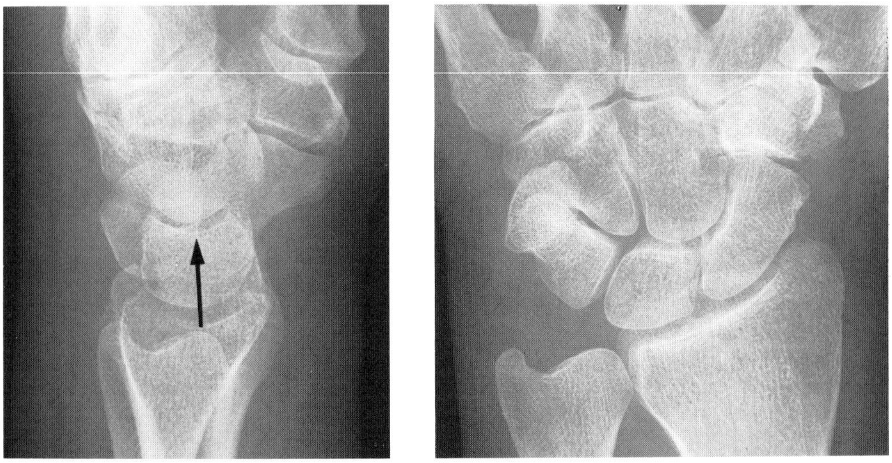

Fig. 5.39c d

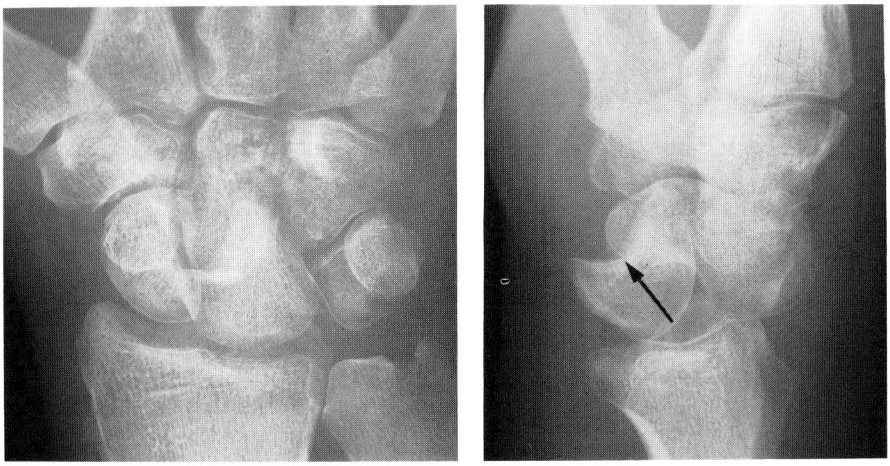

Fig. 5.40a b

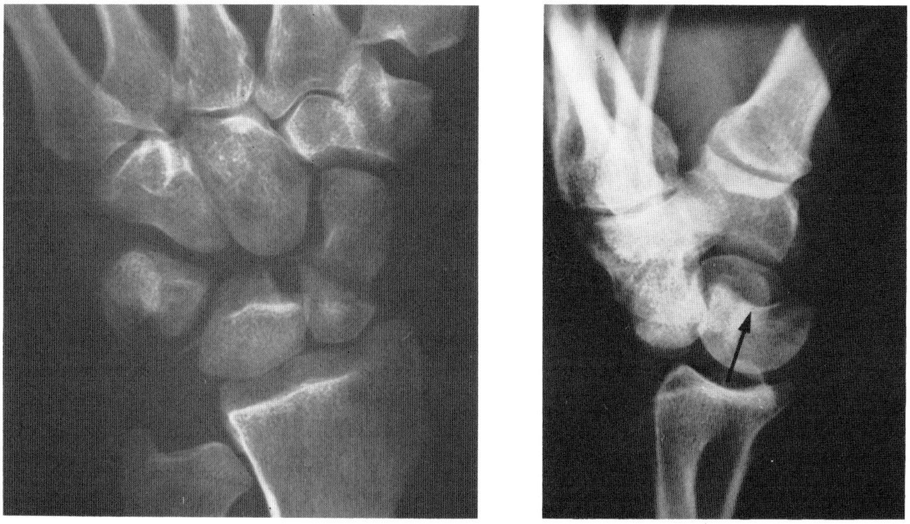

Fig. 5.41a b

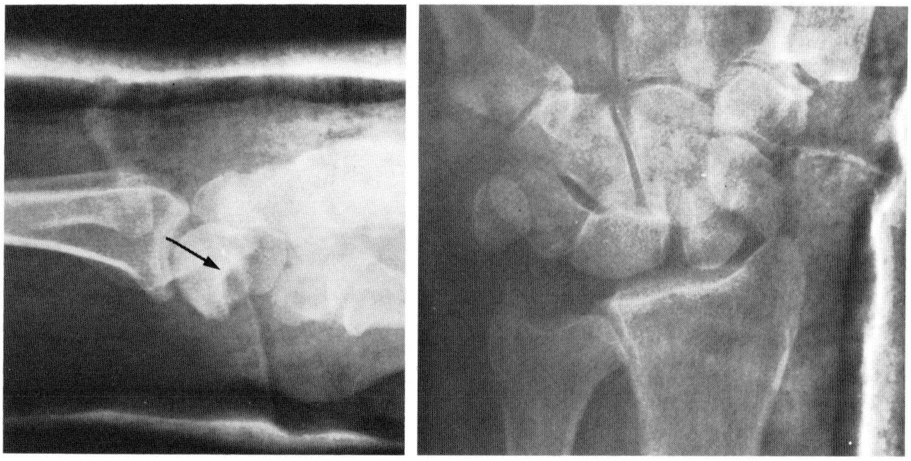

Fig. 5.41c d

◀ Fig. 5.39a–d. a and b) Simple dislocation of the lunatum (pseudarthrosis of the ulnar styloid process).
c and d) Normal articulation for comparison. The axis of the lunatum is identified by markers.

◀ Fig. 5.40a and b. A 64-year-old man with a perilunar dislocation. The lunatum is displaced in the volar direction and is also tilted. The other carpal bones have been pushed out of their normal axis in the dorsal direction.

Fig. 5.41a–d. A 50-year-old woman after a fall from a chair onto her left hand.
a and b) de Quervain type dislocation and fracture (fracture of the navicular bone, with dislocation of the lunatum together with the proximal fragment of the navicular bone.
c and d) Follow-up in plaster cast shows dislocation unchanged.

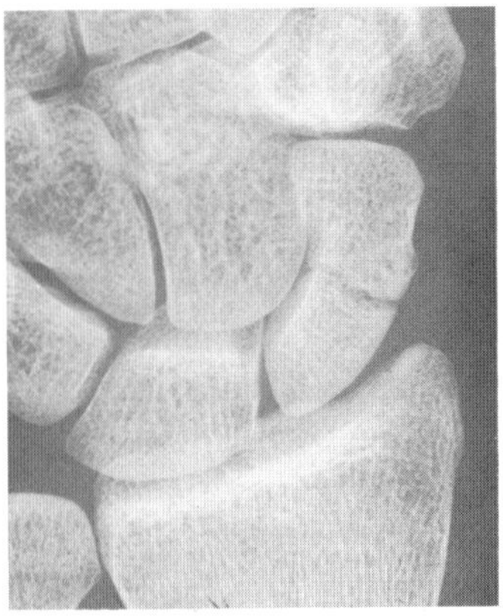

a

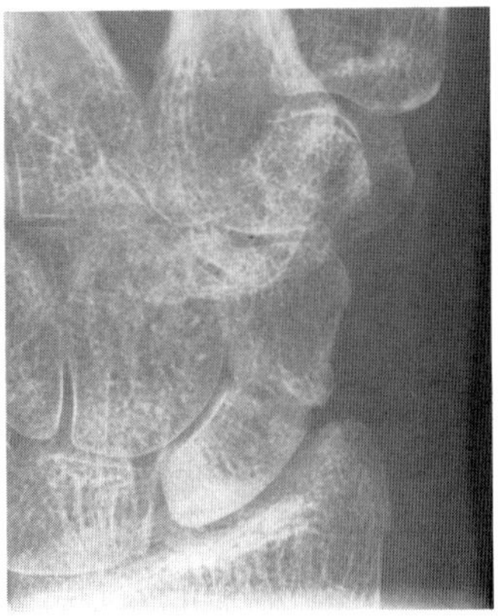

b

Fig. 5.42a and b. A 25-year-old woman after a fall onto her left hand.
a) Recent fracture of the navicular bone.
b) After 3 months, onset of cyst formation in both fragments and necrosis of the proximal corner.

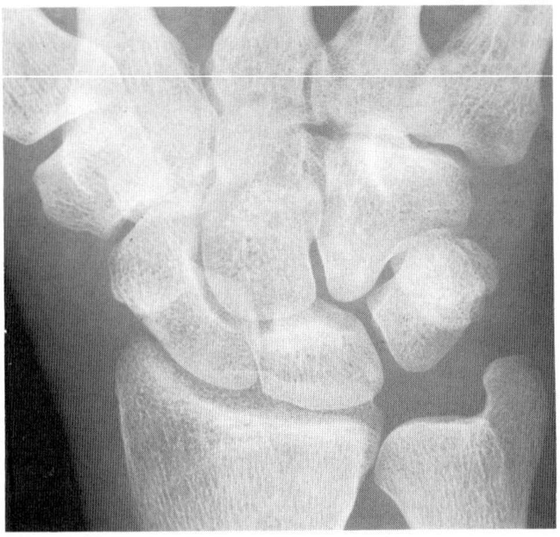

Fig. 5.43a

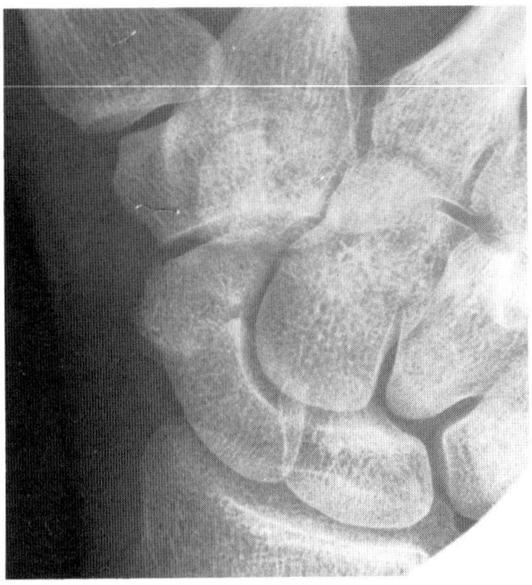

b

Fig. 5.43a and b. a) Routine view of the carpal joint. Fracture is not reliably seen.
b) View in writing position; definite proof of fracture of the navicular bone.

◄ Fig. 5.44. A 29-year-old man who 1 month ago fell on his left hand. Fracture of the navicular bone shown tomographically. Six different projections were not considered reliable proof of the existence of this fracture.

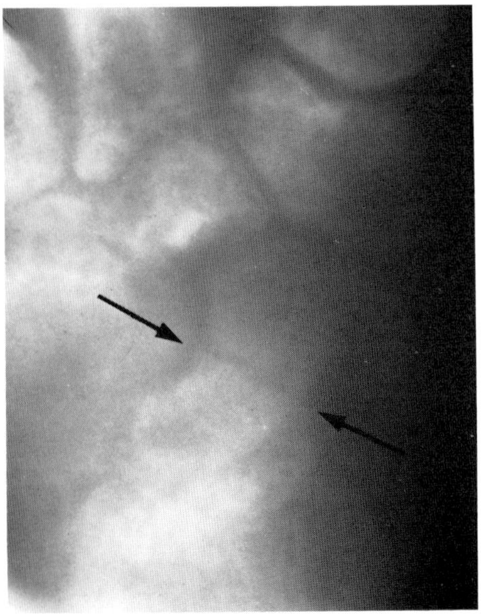

Fig. 5.44

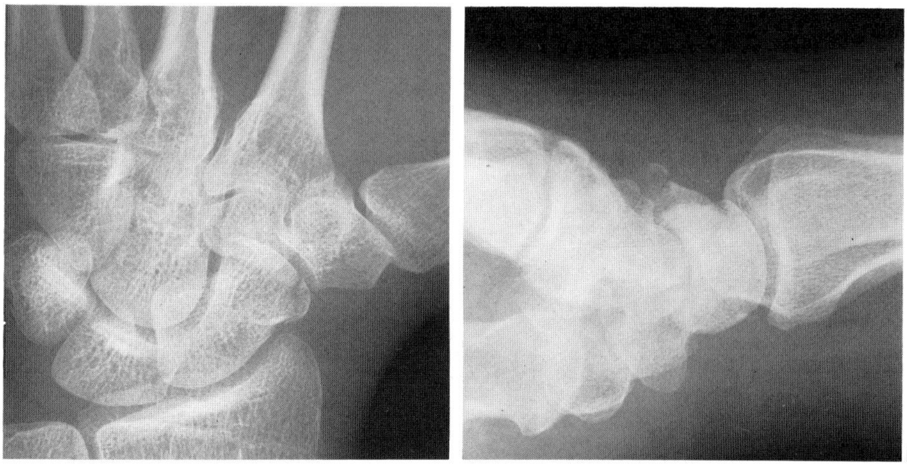

a b

Fig. 5.45a and b. a) A 26-year-old woman with an avulsion of the tubercle of the navicular bone after falling on her hand.
b) 48-year-old man who fell on his hand. Avulsion from the dorsal aspect of the triquetrum.

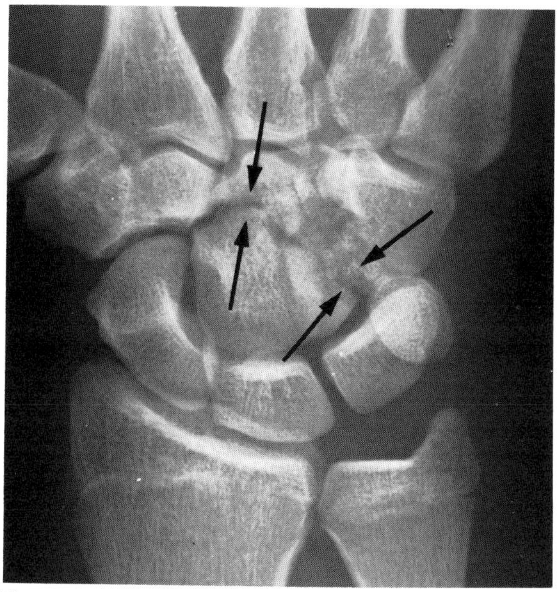

Fig. 5.46. A 17-year-old stonemason after a tombstone fell on his hand. Fracture of the capitate and hamate.

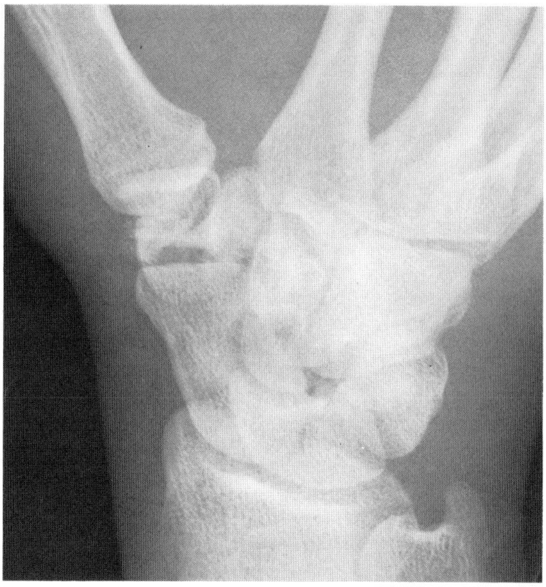

Fig. 5.47. An 18-year-old man who was a passenger in a car accident. Fracture of the trapezium.

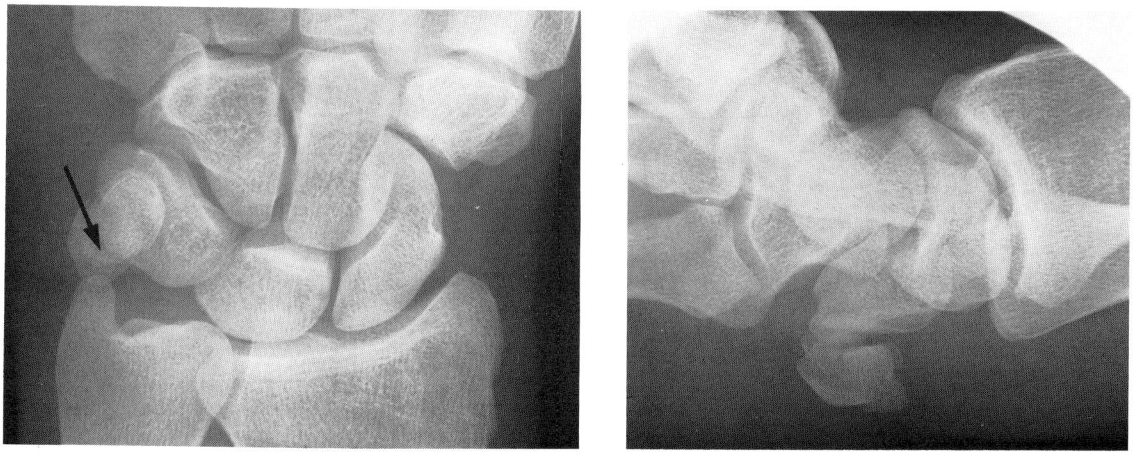

a b

Fig. 5.48a and b. Fracture of the pisiform bone. a) A. p. view. b) Special view.

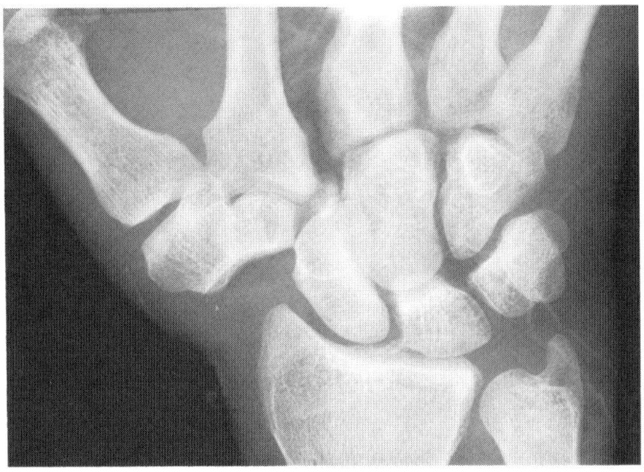

Fig. 5.49. Dislocation of the intercarpal joint with an avulsion from the capitate bone. Rupture of the ligament between the base of the 2nd and 3rd metacarpals.

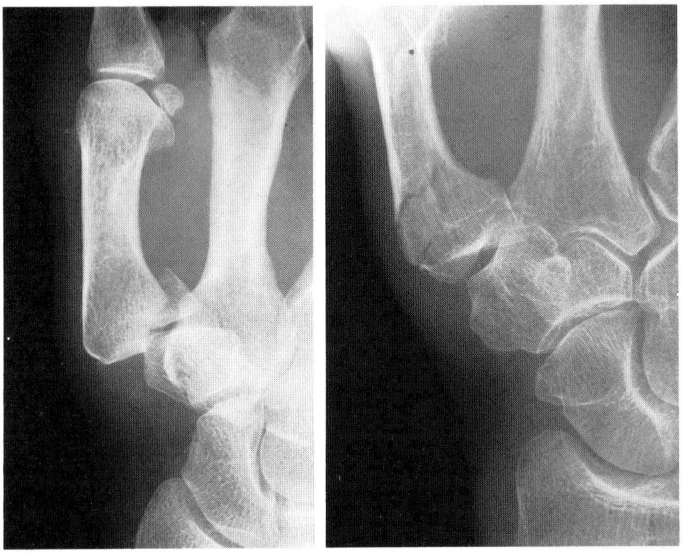

a b

Fig. 5.50a and b. a) Bennett's fracture. b) Fracture of the 1st metacarpal bone close to its base.

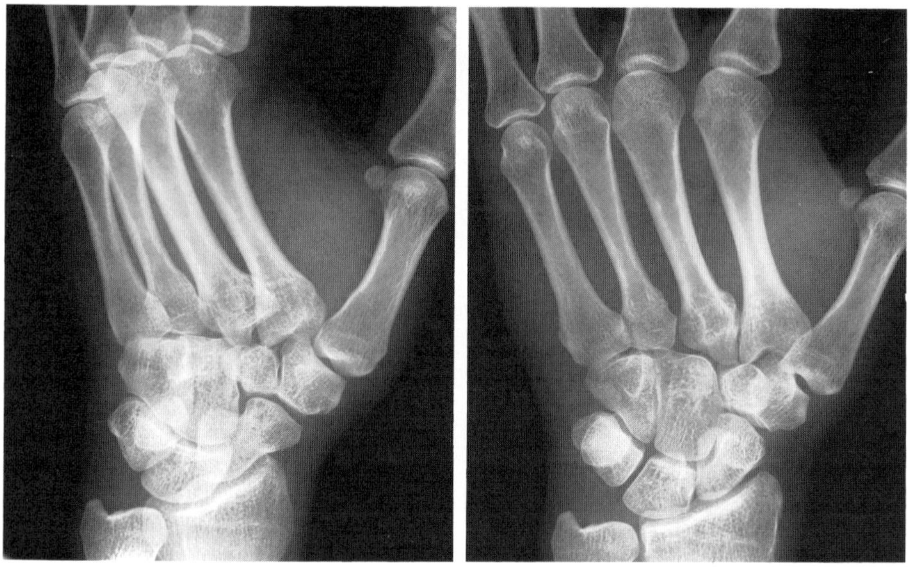

Fig. 5.51a b

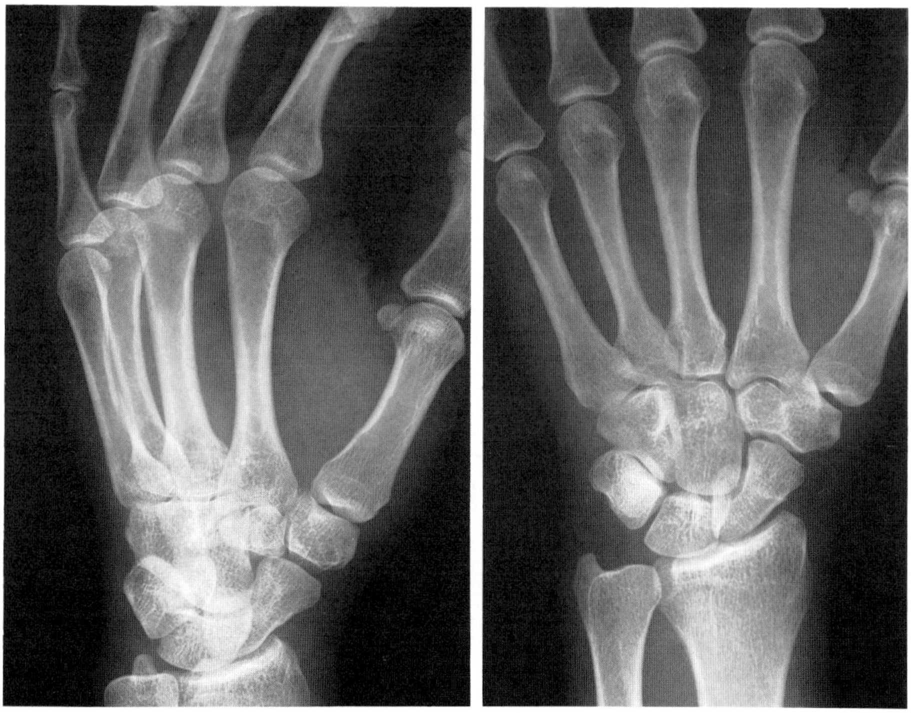

c d

Fig. 5.51a–d. a and b) Luxation of the 2nd and 4th metacarpal bones. c and d) Follow-up examination after reposition.

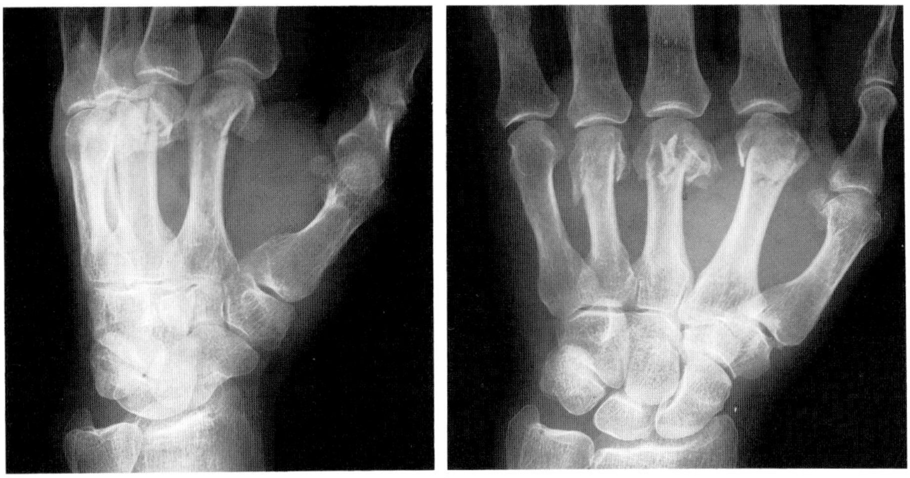

a b

Fig. 5.52a and b. A 62-year-old man after a motorscooter collision with a truck. Fracture of the distal heads of the 2nd to 4th metacarpal bones; volar angulation with impaction.

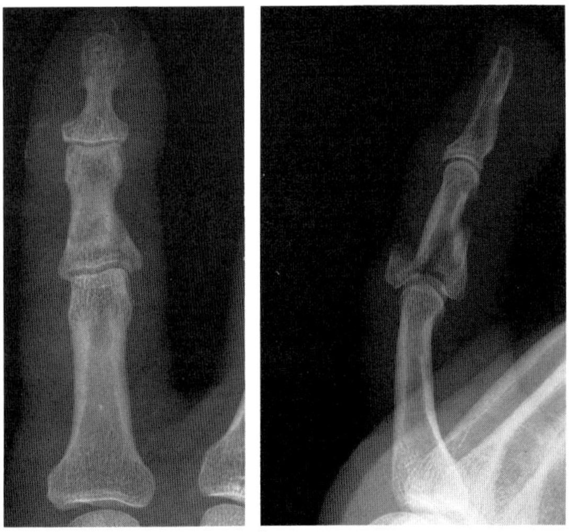

a b

Fig. 5.53a and b. A 58-year-old man after an accident at work. Fracture of the medial portion of the small finger with involvement of the joint.

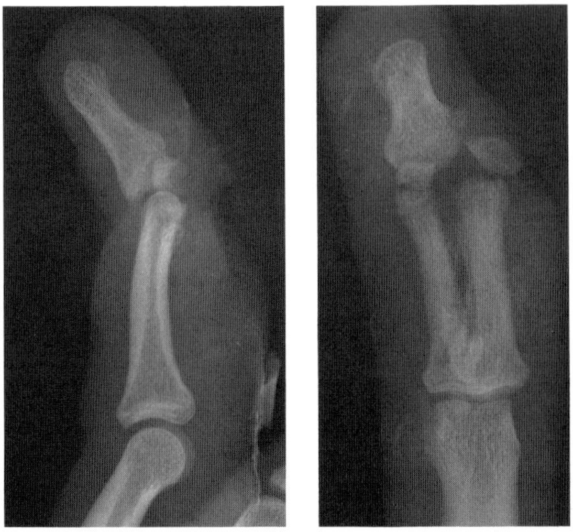

a b

Fig. 5.54a and b. A 16-year-old apprentice in a moving company, whose finger was caught between two metal bars. Longitudinal compression fracture of the midportion of the middle finger also involving the distal part (open fracture).

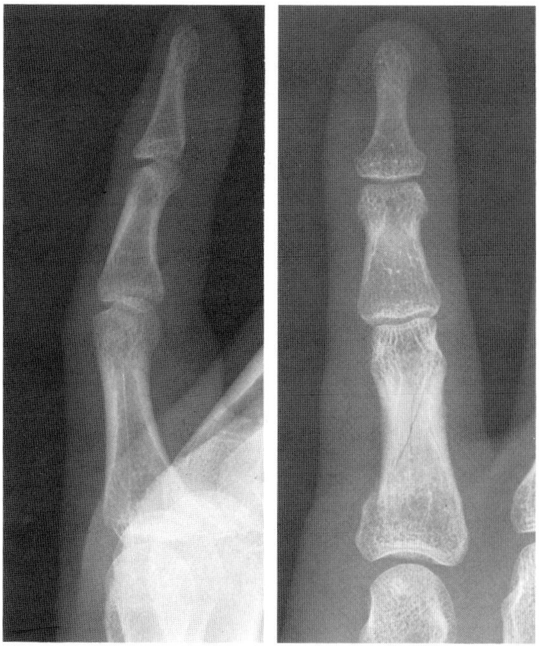

a b

Fig. 5.55a and b. A 25-year-old soccer goalkeeper with a fracture of the ground phalanx of the little finger close to its base, with a longitudinal fissure line.

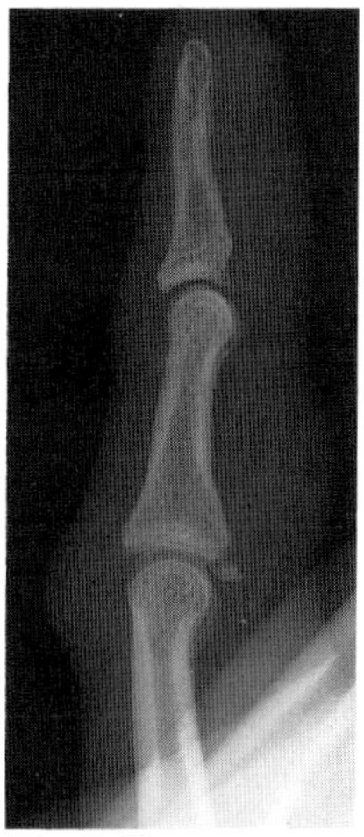

Fig. 5.56

Fig. 5.56. A 26-year-old handball player with a small avulsion from the proximal volar edge of the middle phalanx of the small finger.

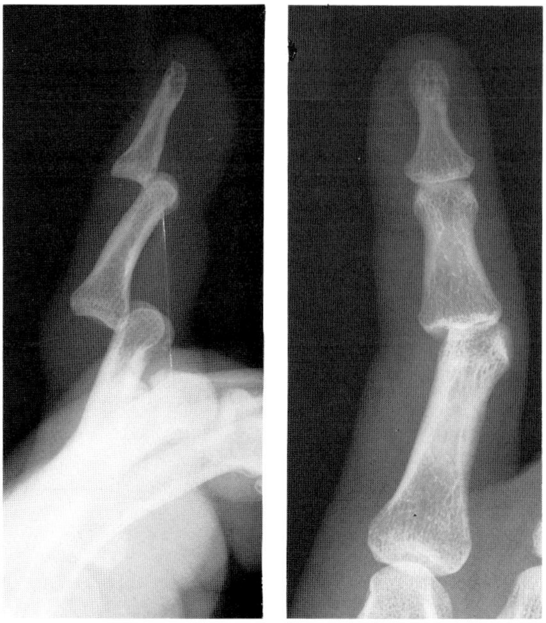

a b

Fig. 5.57a and b. A 28-year-old man after a sports accident. Step ladder effect due to interphalangeal dislocation of the small finger.

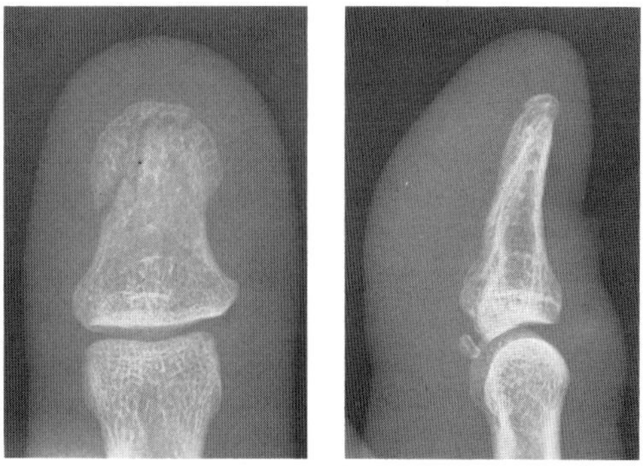

a b

Fig. 5.58a and b. A 22-year-old man whose thumb was caught in a bus door. Avulsion fracture of the distal phalangeal tuberosity of the thumb.

Fig. 5.59a and b. An 18-year-old man after an accident ▶ at work. Fracture of the tip of the distal phalanx and longitudinal fissure of the middle finger.

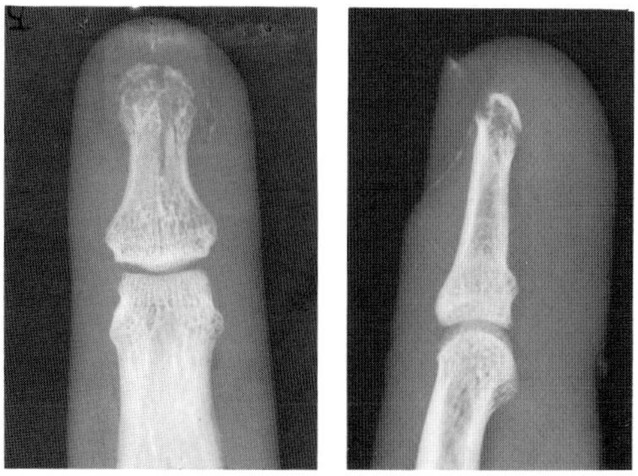

Fig. 5.59a b

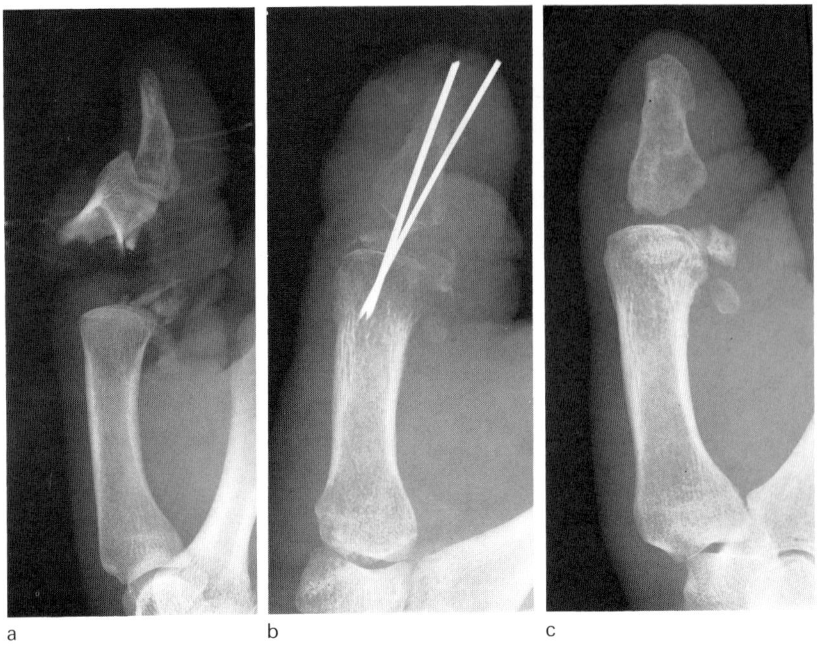

Fig. 5.60. a) Injury of the right thumb as a result of working with a circular saw.
b) After removal of the fragment of the ground phalanx and fixation of the distal phalanx to the 1st metacarpal.
c) Condition 3½ years after trauma and operation.

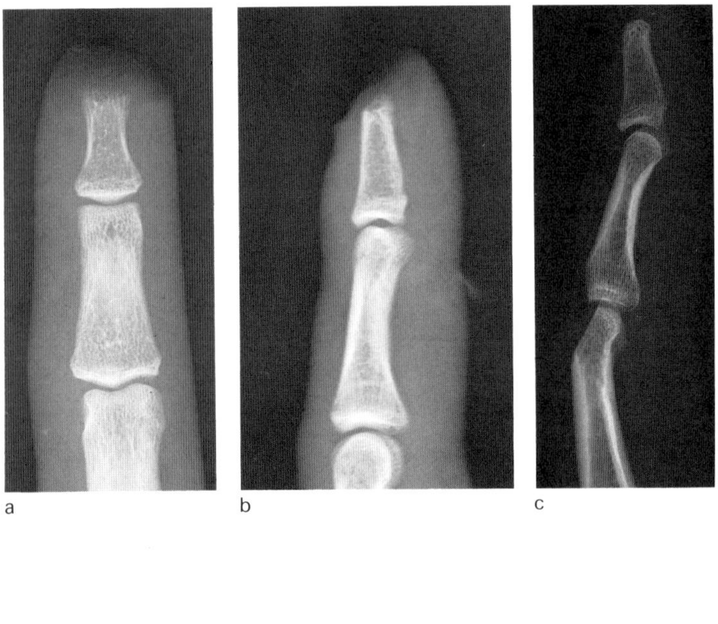

Fig. 5.61. An 18- and a 21-year-old wood worker who injured themselves while planing.
a and b) Planing injury of the tip of the right index finger.
c) 3 years later, planing injury of the right index finger ground phalanx, with separation of the flexor tendon and opening of the joint space.

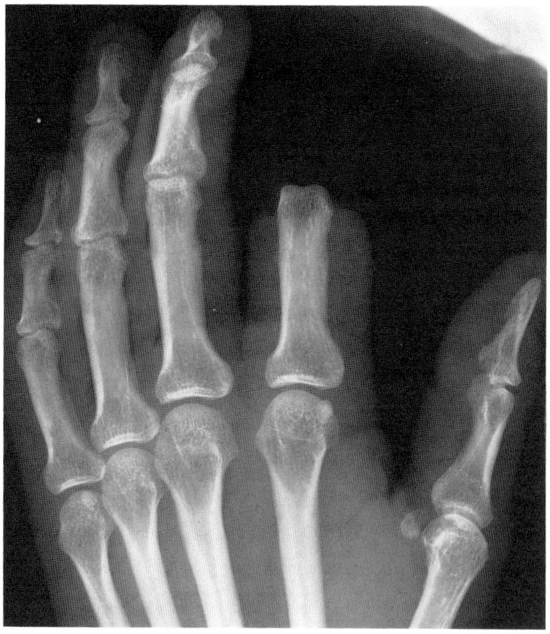

Fig. 5.62. A 40-year-old woman whose finger was caught in a machine. Shearing off of left index finger at the middle interphalangeal joint.

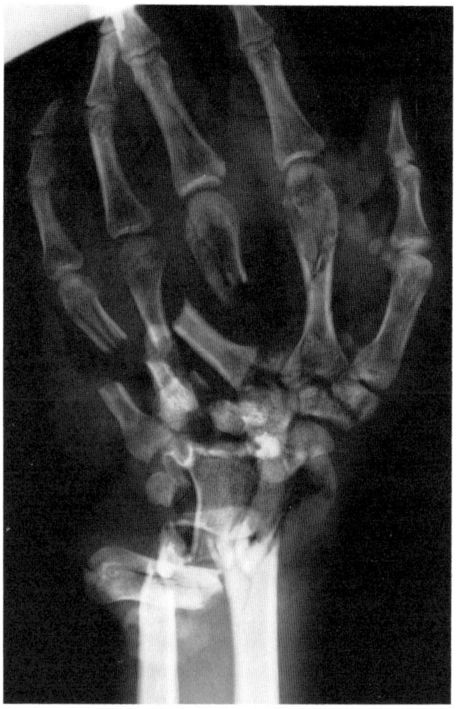

Fig. 5.63. A 20-year-old metal worker whose hand was caught in a sheet metal press. Amputation injury of the left hand.

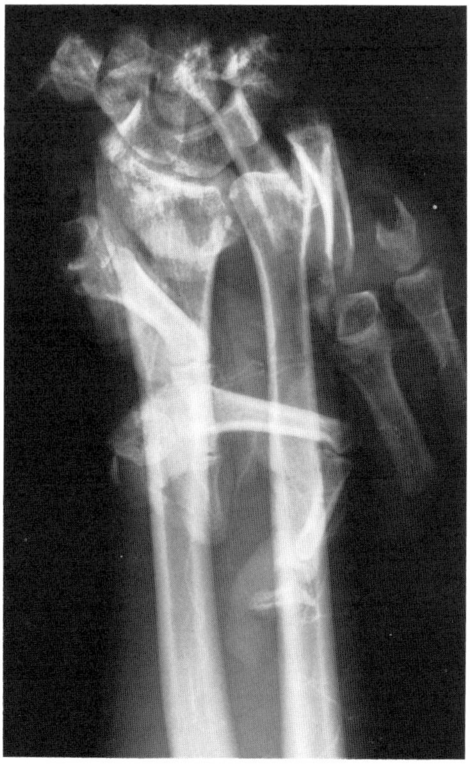

Fig. 5.64. A 23-year-old medical student involved in a premature explosion of a charge while manipulating an old gun. Amputation injury of the right hand.

6 Lower Extremity

The much feared fracture of the femoral neck affecting patients of advanced age is the result of a fall onto the hip. Depending on the direction of the forces involved, there are different types of fractures (Fig. 6.1). The abduction type of medial fracture of the femoral neck usually shows impaction, whereas all the other types of femoral neck fracture including the peritrochanteric type have an external rotation of 45 to 90 degrees (Fig. 6.2). It is not always possible to distinguish between the lateral femoral neck fracture and the peritrochanteric and subtrochanteric types. Impacted and minimally dislocated femoral neck fractures can be difficult to recognize. Fracture of the head of the femur is rare (Fig. 6.3). With today's operative approach of nailing the fractured femoral neck, along with the recent introduction of endoprostheses of the femoral neck and even further replacement of an entire hip joint, mortality among older people has been reduced from a frequently poor prognosis in the past to only about 2 per cent today. The development and introduction of the image intensifier in combination with television have spurred great advances in the performance of these operations.

In the area of the femoral shaft, all types of fractures are seen. The repeated x-ray follow-up examinations necessary for conventionel management of fractures have been largely abandoned since the introduction of the more successful method of Küntscher with stable internal fixation. Conservative management is needed today only in a few exceptional instances. Typical fractures of the distal femur are the supracondylar type, the condylar avulsion or tear or the Y-shaped intercondylar fracture. Both of the last two mentioned have articular involvement (Fig. 6.4). Because of displacement of the short distal fragment due to pull by the gastrocnemius muscle, there is always the danger, in supracondylar fracture, of an injury to the vessels or nerve (Fig. 6.5). Light trauma can result in an intercondylar fracture without significant dislocation (Fig. 6.6).

In dislocation on the knee as well as the patella, x-ray investigation is needed only for documentation and to obtain information on possible additional bony injuries (Fig. 6.7 and 6.8). Free fluid or blood can be recognized radiologically by the opacification of the superior recess (Fig. 6.9). An open injury of the joint can be demonstrated more readily on a roentgenogram. Very often they are recognized only during surgical revision (Fig. 6.10).

The avulsion of a cruciate or collateral ligament can be recognized radiologically by the increased motility in the sagittal direction (drawer phenomenon) or by the increased width of the articular space due to pulling of the lower leg during exposure to x-rays (Figs. 6.11 and 6.12). Lesions of ligaments are frequently accompanied by avulsion fractures of the intercondylar eminence, particularly the medial tip, and at the lateral corner of the tibial head and of the fibular head (Figs. 6.13 and 6.14). An avulsion of the tibial tuberosity is the result of pull at the point of insertion of the patellar ligaments (Fig. 6.15). Fresh injuries to the meniscus cannot be demonstrated directly on x-rays.

Fractures of the patella can be classified as transverse fractures, stellate fractures and comminuted fractures (Fig. 6.16). In the differential diagnosis, one must consider the developmental type of patella partita, especially when there is no trauma in a patient's history. An additional axial view usually helps to clarify the situation. Displacement of the patella distally or proximally is an indication of a complete tear of the extensor tendon or the patellar ligament (Fig. 6.17).

At the level of the tibial plateau, as the result of bending and compression forces, there may be an impression or a depressed fracture usually of one of the condyles, particularly the lateral one. There may also be a splitting type of fracture due to unusually severe forces such as a fall from a great height or traffic accidents (Fig. 6.18). Widening of the joint space of the unfractured side indicates a tear of the ligament (Fig. 6.19). There are transitions between the isolated tibial plateau fracture and the subcapital fracture of the tibia (Fig. 6.20). Rarely, one will not be able to recognize free fluid in the joint in fractures of the tibial plateau.

Isolated fractures of the tibia or fibula are seen less frequently than complete fractures of the shank. Fractures of the shank have a high incidence, particularly as the result of traffic accidents (Fig. 6.21). Contrary to this, one must expect only minimal radiologic findings in fatigue fractures of the tibia (Fig. 6.22). During the last few years, as the result of changes in gear for skiers – to high, tight boots – there is a new type of fracture of the distal 3rd of the shank, the so called ski-boot fracture (Fig. 6.23). This type of fracture is often seen among active skiers and takes the place of the old ankle fracture previously connected with this sport.

Ankle fractures with a variety of manifestations, with and without dislocation or subluxation, are among the most common injuries of the lower extremity (Figs. 6.24 and 6.25). Others include distortions, with tearing of ligaments, and dislocation – usually dorsal displacement of the talus (Fig. 6.26). Held views (with pull) to demonstrate the presence of a tear of a ligament are usually not necessary in the area of the ankle, since already minor degrees of dislocation of the talus will result in widening of the affected joint space which will be recognized (Figs. 6.27 and 6.28). A fracture of the ankle located above the articular plane always shows instability, and a supramalleolar fracture of the lateral part of the ankle usually is combined with a rupture of the tibio-fibular syndesmosis. The degree of this injury can be recognized by the lateral displacement of the fibula and talus (Fig. 6.29). Fractures of the ankle occasionally do not show significant radiologic findings. In the lateral view, a minimal displacement of the lateral part of the ankle and Volkmann's triangle are usually best visualized. Sometimes, however the avulsion of Volkmann's triangle can only be spotted on an a.p.view (Figs. 6.30 to 6.32). Since it is the purpose of all forms of therapy to get an ideal reposition and fixation, it is important to ascertain and emphasize the minimal abnormalities of position at the time of radiologic follow-up or postoperative control. When x-rays are taken through a plaster cast, good results may be difficult to obtain. There are various types of metallic devices used for internal fixation (Fig. 6.33).

In the area of the ankle, dislocation between the talus and calcaneus, as well as between the calcaneus and tibia and fibula, can occur without fractures. Fracture of the talus, especially of the neck, may easily be overlooked (Fig. 6.34). It may also be difficult to properly recognize fractures of the calcaneus. Compression fractures, particularly after a fall onto the heel, may result in a decrease or disappearance of the angle formed by the tuber and the joint, and thus a traumatic flat foot may result (Fig. 6.35). An axial view frequently will show widening of the fractured calcaneus. One can distinguish between fractures with joint involvement and extra-articular fractures (Fig. 6.35 and 6.36). Avulsion fractures are rarely seen in the area of the talus and calcaneus (compare Figs. 6.34 and 6.37). Fractures or dislocations of the other tarsal bones are seldom seen. In addition to the standard planes, one should obtain a view of the mediotarsal region if local involvement is suspected. This will best demonstrate the condition of the tarsal bones (Fig. 6.38).

It is difficult to diagnose properly dislocations and avulsions close to the base of the mediotarsal area (Fig. 6.39). Accessory bones must always be distinguished from avulsions (Fig. 6.40). Complete dislocation of the joints of Chopart or Lisfranc does not occur very often (Fig. 6.41). Fractures of the mediotarsal bones or the toes offer no problem diagnostically. They are usually the result of external trauma, of heavy objects falling on the bones or of the foot being run over by a wheel. One should always emphasize the danger of joint involvement (Fig. 6.42) as well as possible lesions of ligaments (Fig. 6.43). The local reaction at the 2nd metatarsal caused by a fatigue fracture (closed fracture) may be misinterpreted as the result of an infectious process or an early tumor formation, since there is no indication of trauma (compare with Fig. 7.2). Fracture of a sesamoid bone, especially in the area of the big toe, can occur but, in most suspected cases, there is a bipartite sesamoid.

Dislocations of the toes are frequently accompanied by minor bony avulsions. In order to document these properly and to avoid overlooking subluxation, it is helpful to obtain a lateral view on small film, possibly dental film. A fracture in a location normally occupied by a joint space is rare (Fig. 6.44).

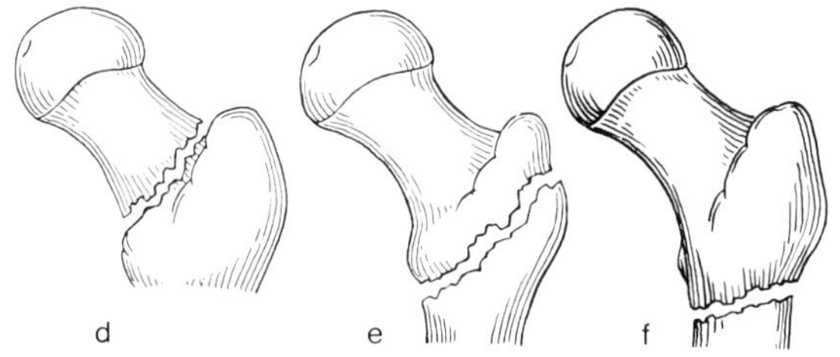

Fig. 6.1a–f. Fractures of the proximal end of the femur.
a) Subcapital or medial femoral neck fracture, abduction type (in varus position).
b) Subcapital or medial femoral neck fracture, abduction type (valgus position).
c) Transcervical fracture of the femoral neck.
d) Lateral fracture of the femoral neck.
e) Transtrochanteric fracture of the femur.
f) Subtrochanteric fracture of the femur.
(From H. R. Zatzkin: The Roentgen Diagnosis of Trauma. Chicago, Yearbook Medical Publishers, Inc., 1965. Used by permission.)

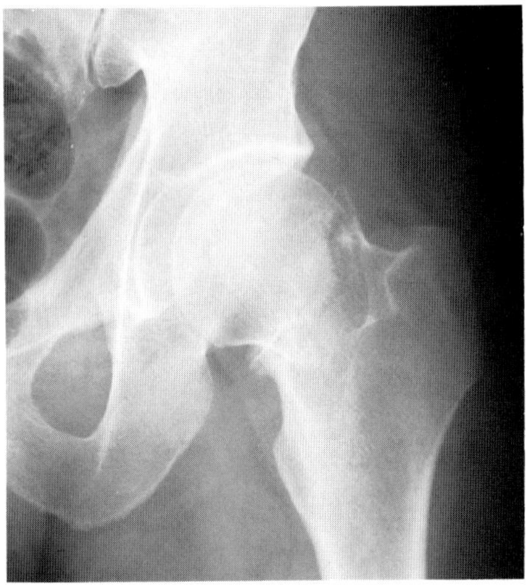

Fig. 6.2. Impacted medial femoral neck fracture, abduction type.

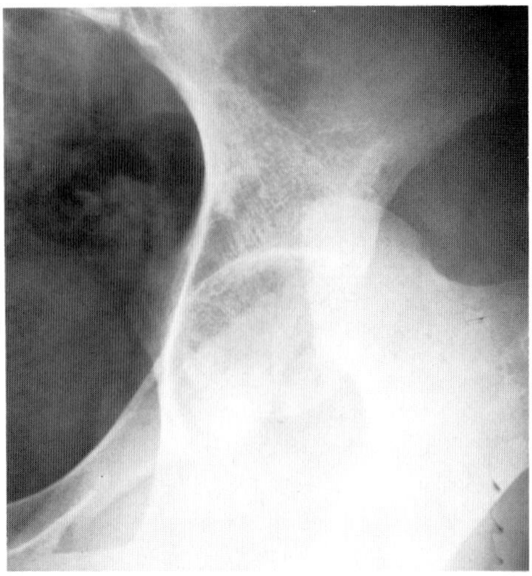

Fig. 6.3. A 22-year-old man, while drunk, hit a wall with his car. Knocking off of femoral head.

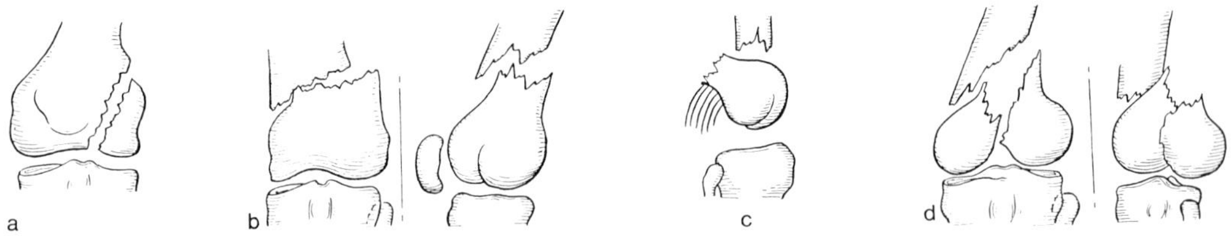

Fig. 6.4a-d. Fractures of the distal femoral region.
a) Fracture of the lateral condyle.
b and c) Supracondylar fracture of the femur, with typical dislocation of the distal fragments.
d) Y-shaped intercondylar fracture.

(From H. R. Zatzkin: The Roentgen Diagnosis of Trauma. Chicago, Yearbook Medical Publishers, Inc., 1965. Used by permission.)

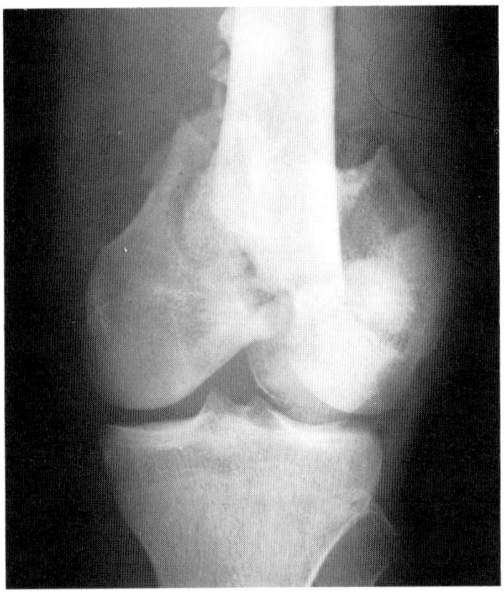

a

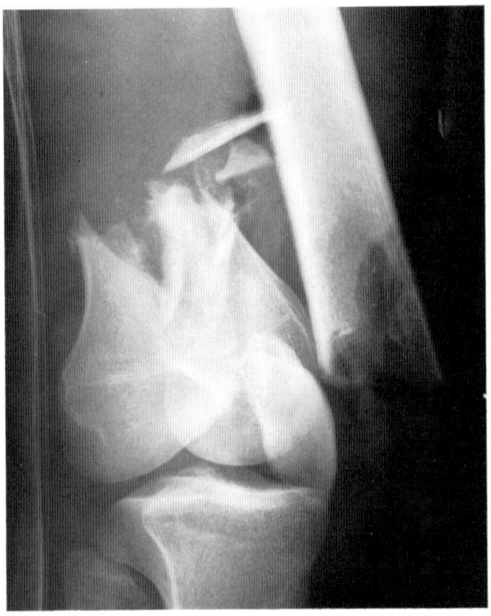

b

Fig. 6.5a and b. A 23-year-old man with open intercondylar fracture of the femur, with typical dislocation.

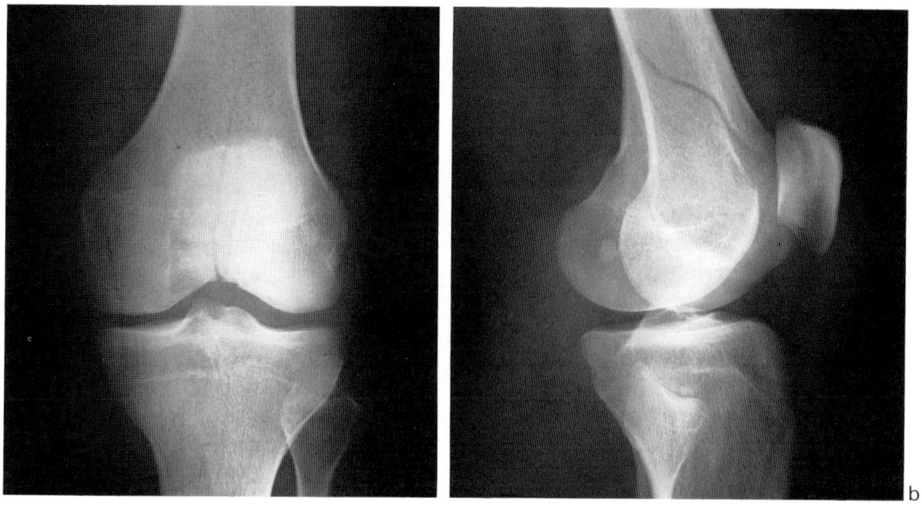

a b

Fig. 6.6a and b. A 28-year-old man after a fall on his left knee. Admitted with the diagnosis of patellar fracture. Intercondylar fracture without significant dislocation.

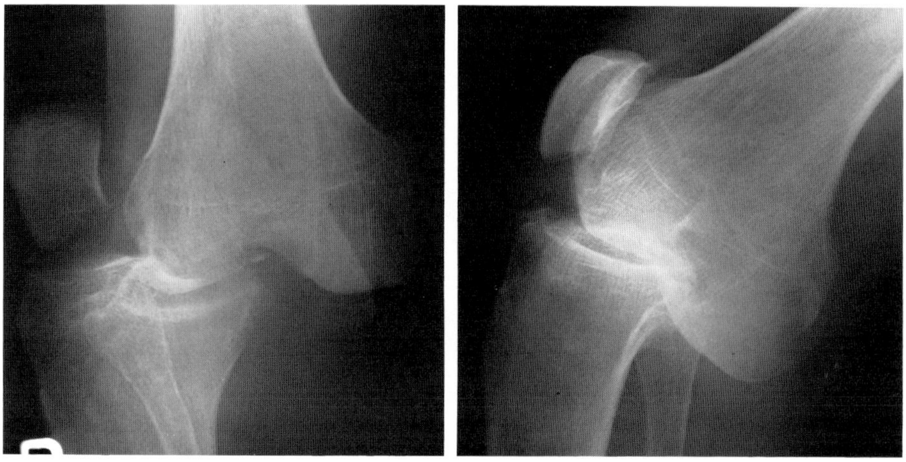

a b

Fig. 6.7a and b. A 52-year-old man who was hit by a car as a pedestrian. Dislocation of the knee with small bony avulsions.

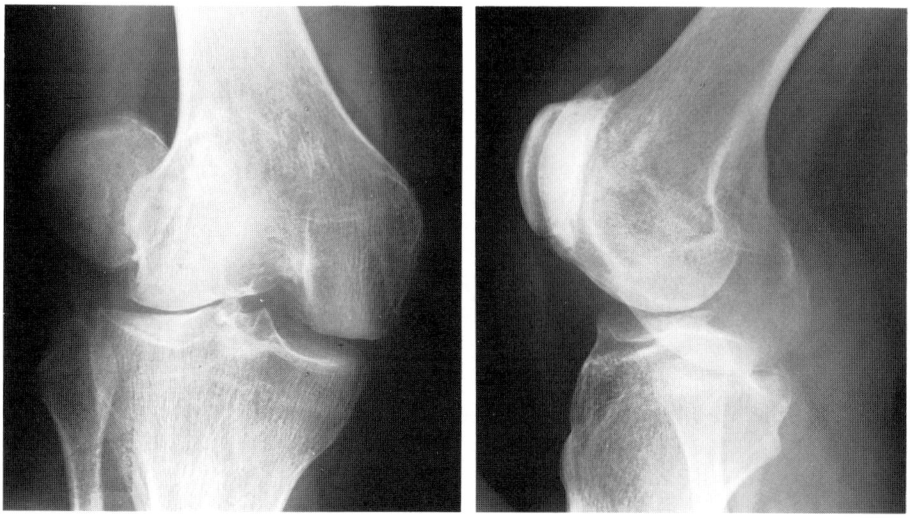

a b

Fig. 6.8a and b. A 64-year-old woman who fell while walking downstairs. Dislocation of the patella.

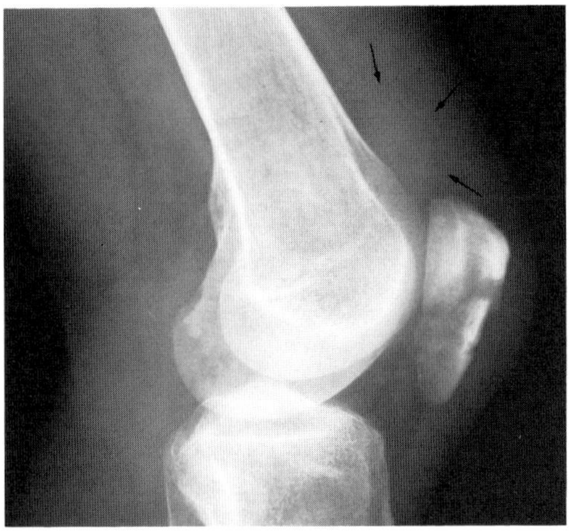

Fig. 6.9. A 53-year-old man with opacification of the superior recess by hemarthrosis *(arrows).* Fracture of the patella.

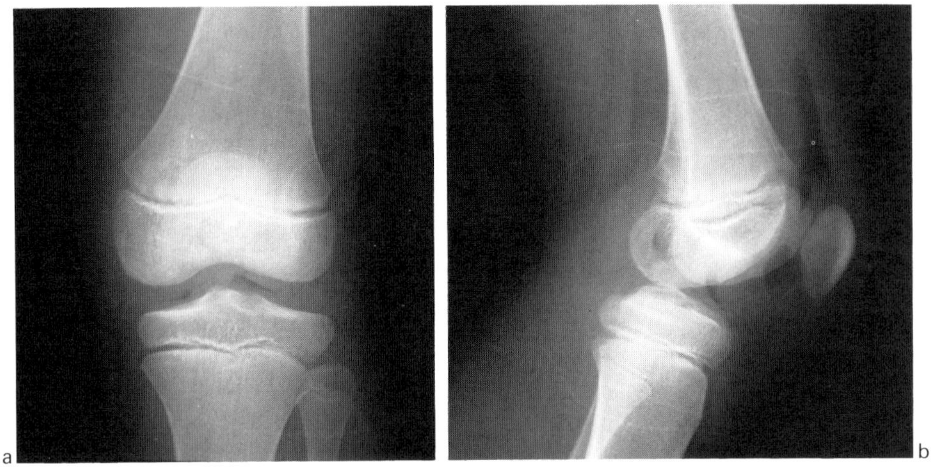

Fig. 6.10a and b. A 9-year-old boy after a collision with a car while riding a bicycle. Open injury of the knee joint, with air in the space and recess.

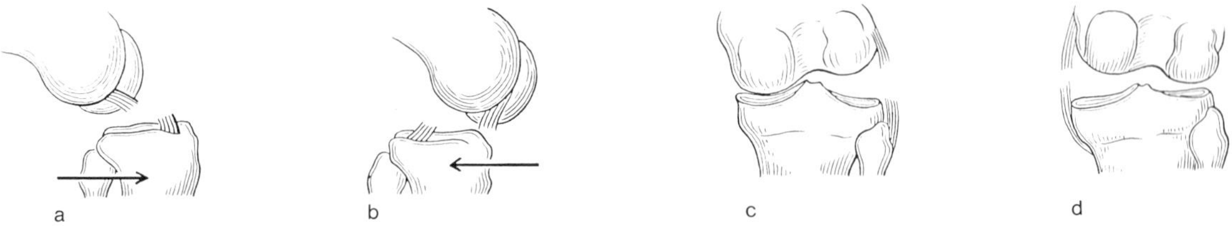

Fig. 6.11a–d. Symptoms due to tearing of ligaments at the knee.

a) Drawer phenomenon in tearing off of the anterior cruciate ligaments.
b) Drawer phenomenon in tearing off of the posterior cruciate ligaments.
c) and d) Opening up of the joint space due to tearing off of the medial or lateral ligament.

(From H. R. Zatzkin:
The Roentgen Diagnosis of Trauma. Chicago, Yearbook Medical Publishers, Inc., 1965. Used by permission.)

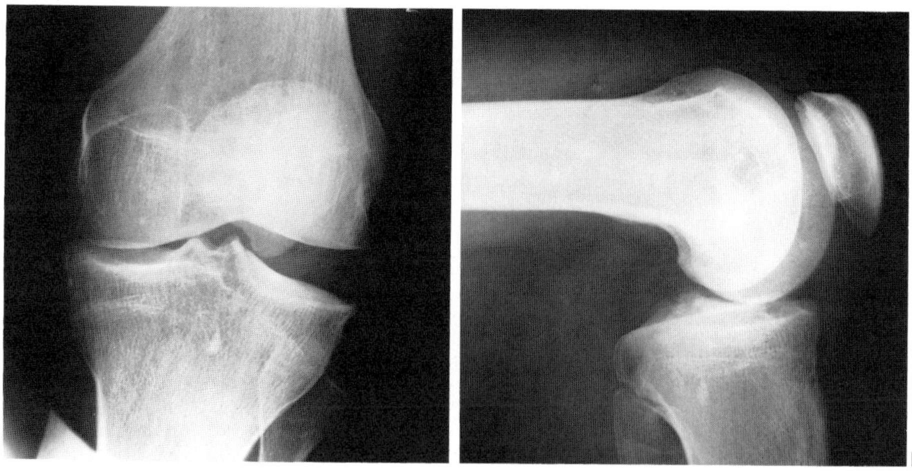

a b

Fig. 6.12a and b. A 29-year-old man. a) Opening up of the joint space laterally when patient's lower leg is held in abduction = complete tear of the lateral collateral ligament. b) Drawer phenomenon after dorsal tear of the posterior cruciate ligament.

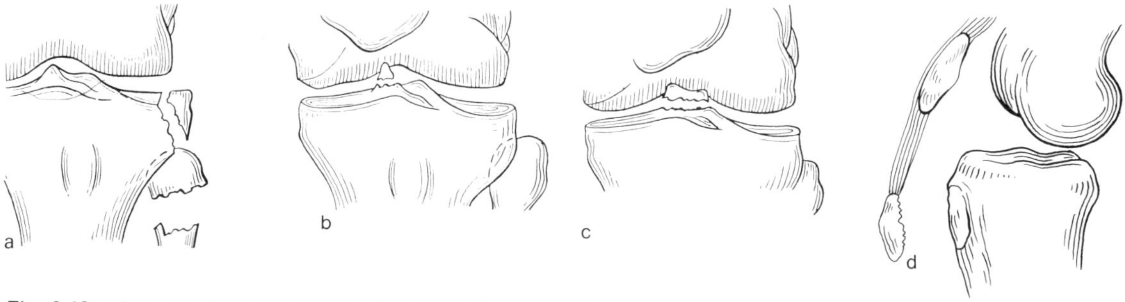

Fig. 6.13a–d. Avulsion fractures at the knee joint.
a) Avulsion fracture at the lateral corner of the tibial plateau and the fibular head.
b) Avulsion of the medial tip of the intercondylar eminence.
c) Avulsion of the intercondylar eminence.
d) Complete avulsion of the tibial tuberosity.

(Fig. a–c from H. R. Zatzkin: The Roentgen Diagnosis of Trauma. Chicago, Yearbook Medical Publishers, Inc., 1965. Used by permission.)

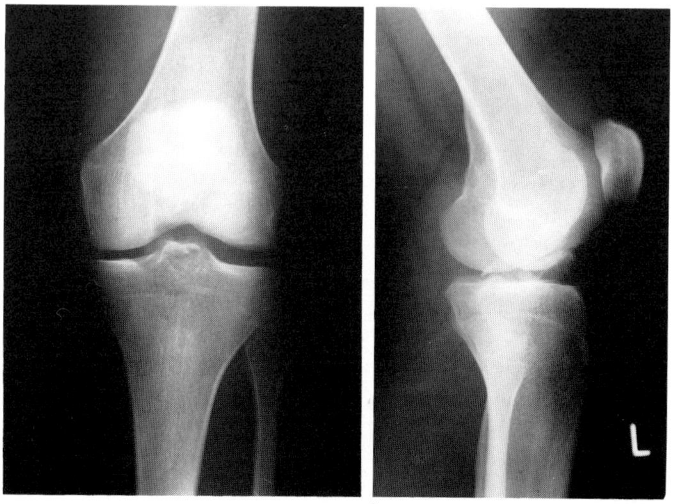

a b

Fig. 6.14a and b. Avulsion fracture of the intercondylar eminence. Hemarthrosis.

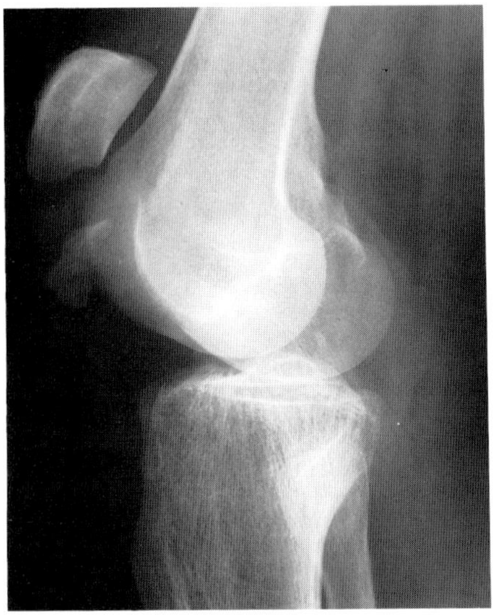

◀ Fig. 6.15. A 73-year-old man after a fall while working in the garden. Tearing off of the patellar ligament at its origin on the tibial tuberosity.

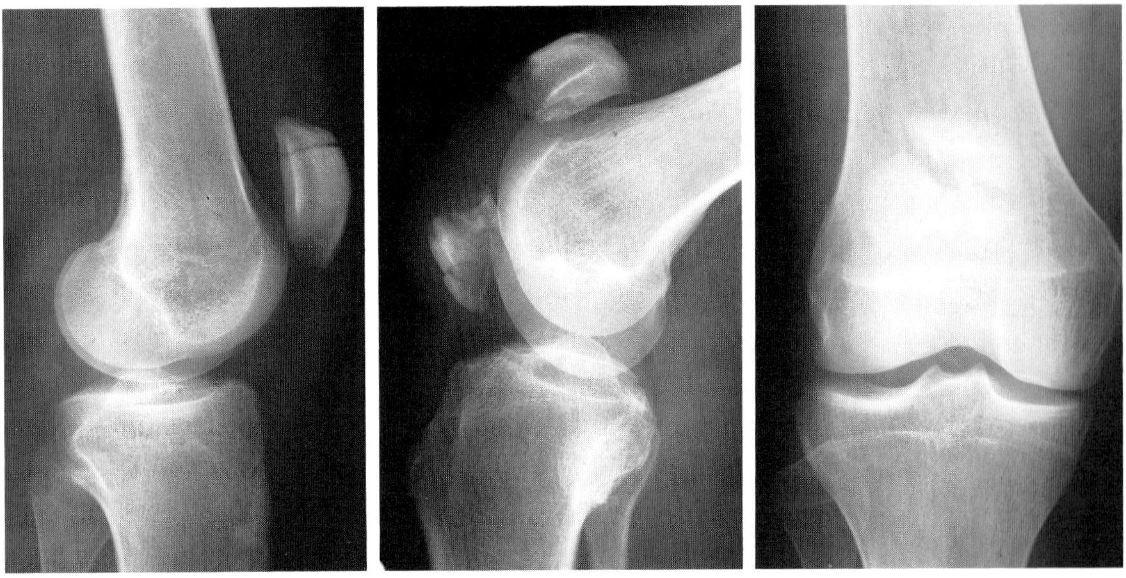

Fig. 6.16a b c

Fig. 6.16a–c. Fractures of the patella.
a) Fissure without significant dislocation.
b) Transverse fracture with marked dislocation.
c) Stellar fracture = comminuted fracture without marked dislocation.

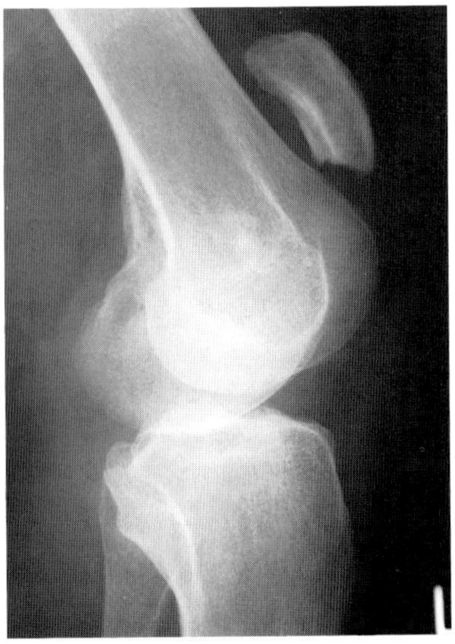

◀ Fig. 6.17. A 57-year-old man with a complete tear of the patellar ligament, with dislocation of the patella superiorly.

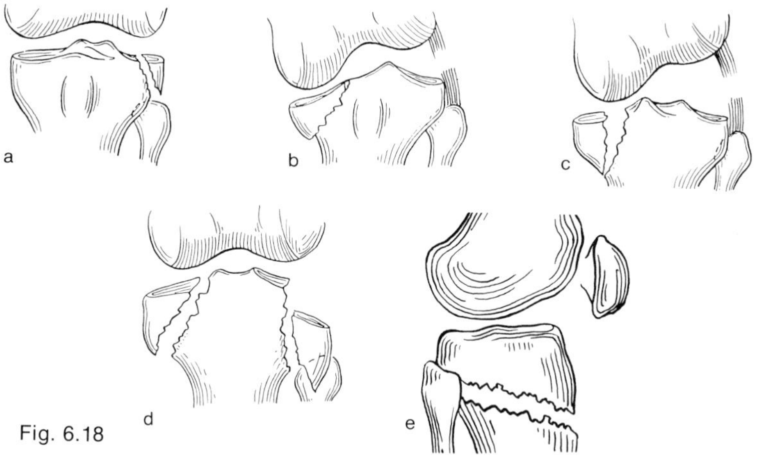

Fig. 6.18

Fig. 6.18a–e. Tibial plateau.

a) Fracture of the lateral corner of tibial plateau.

b) Impression fractures with a tear of the contralateral collateral ligament.

c) Fracture through the medial tibial plateau, with tearing off of the contralateral ligament.

d) Comminuted fracture.

e) Intracondylar fracture of the tibia.

(From H. R. Zatzkin: The Roentgen Diagnosis of Trauma. Chicago, Yearbook Medical Publishers, Inc., 1965. Used by permission.)

Fig. 6.19. A 68-year-old man who suddenly fell on the street when his left knee gave way. Depressed fracture of the lateral tibial plateau, with complete fracture of the fibular head. Rupture of the medial ligament.

Fig. 6.20a and b. Transitional types between the tibial plateau and the subcapitular fracture. (Fracture of the patella and small accumulation of fluid in the joint).

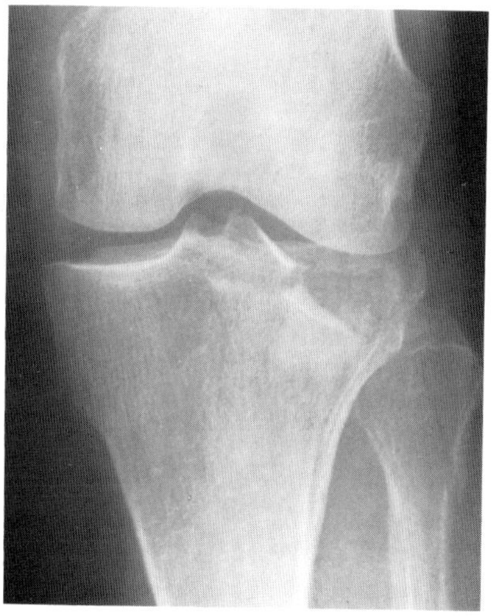

Fig. 6.19

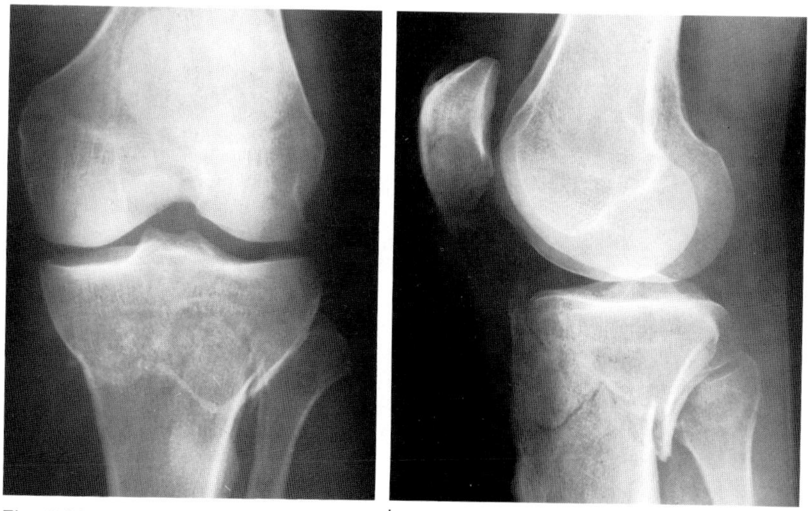

Fig. 6.20a b

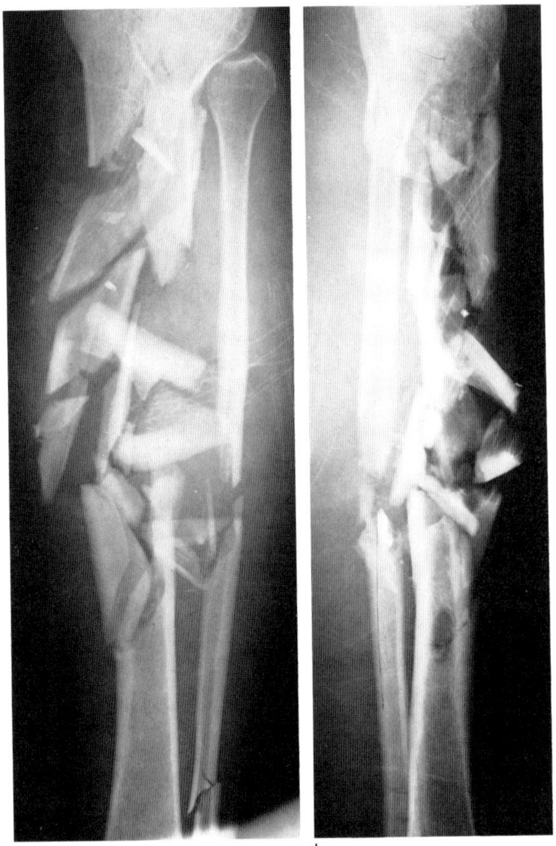

a b

Fig. 6.21a and b. A 39-year-old man who was a passenger in a car in an accident. Massive comminuted fracture of the left shank. Further fractures of the right and left femurs and the pelvis.

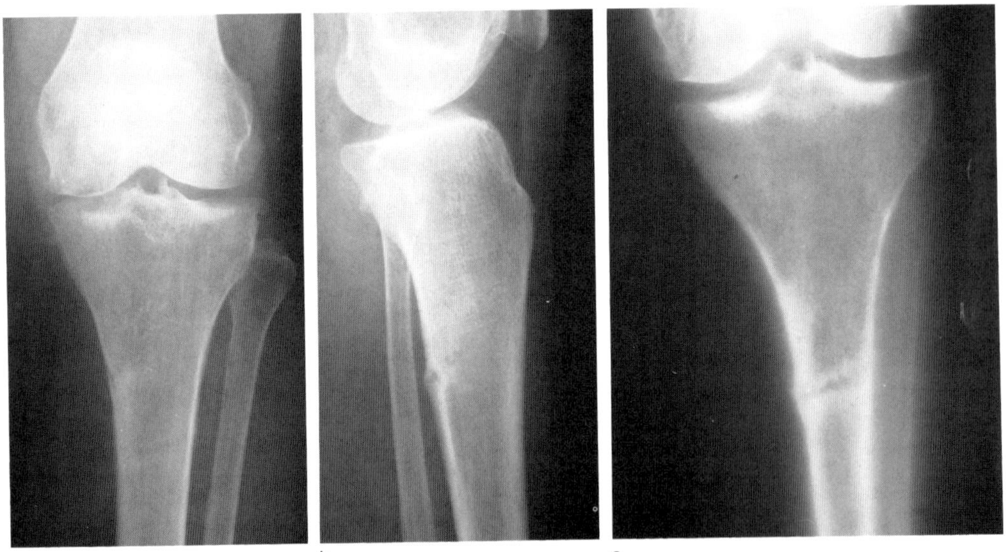

a b c

Fig. 6.22a–c. A 68-year-old woman. Follow-up after 6 weeks. No residual findings. Fatigue fracture of the left tibia. a and b) Routine views; c) tomogram.

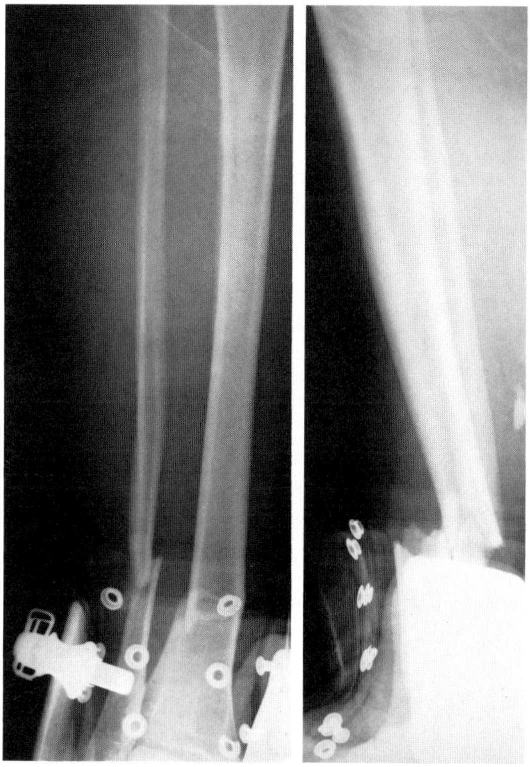

Fig. 6.23a and b. An 18-year-old skier with a fracture above the rim of the ski boot involving the right shank. X-ray obtained with the boot in place.

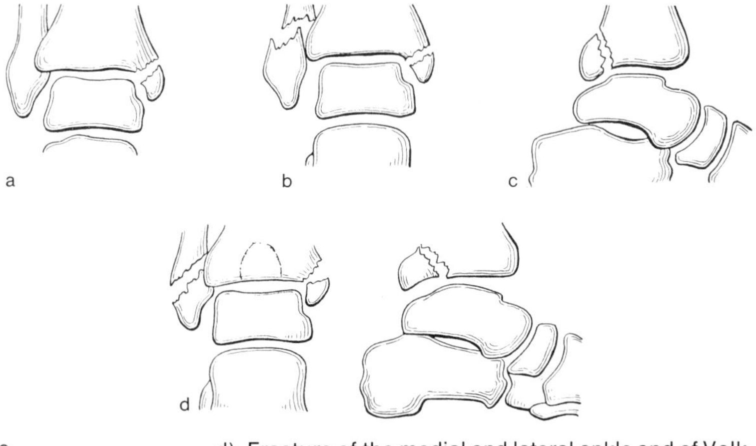

Fig. 6.24a–d. Fractures of the ankle.

a) Isolated fracture of the medial or lateral ankle; displacement of the talus toward the side of the fragment is indication of the tearing of the contralateral ligament.
b) Bimalleolar fracture.
c) Isolated fracture of the posteroinferior corner of the tibia (triangle of Volkmann).
d) Fracture of the medial and lateral ankle and of Volkmann's triangle, also referred to as trimalleolar fracture.

(From H. R. Zatzkin: The Roentgen Diagnosis of Trauma. Chicago, Yearbook Medical Publishers, Inc., 1965. Used by permission.)

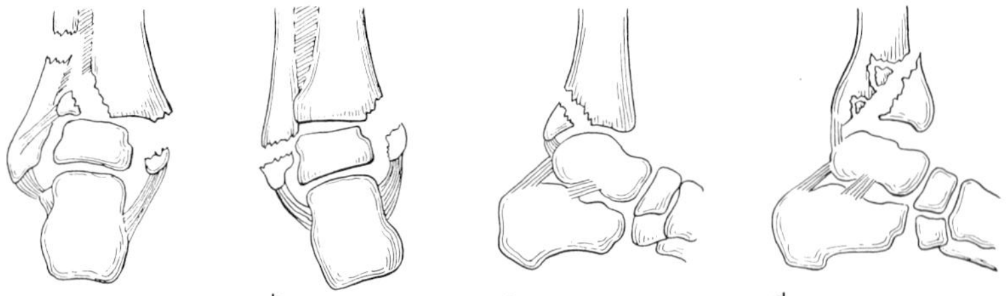

a b c d

Fig. 6.25a–d. Ankle fractures with subluxation and lesions of ligaments.
a) Pronation fracture with subluxation of the talus laterally; high fibular fracture always indicates a rupture of the tibiofibular syndesmosis.
b) Supination fracture with subluxation of the talus medially.
c) Fracture of a posterior portion of the tibia (and both bones of the ankle), with posterior dislocation of the talus.
d) Fracture of an anterior wedge of the distal tibia (and both bones of the ankle), with anterior displacement of the talus.
(From H. R. Zatzkin: The Roentgen Diagnosis of Trauma. Chicago, Yearbook Medical Publishers, Inc., 1965. Used by permission.)

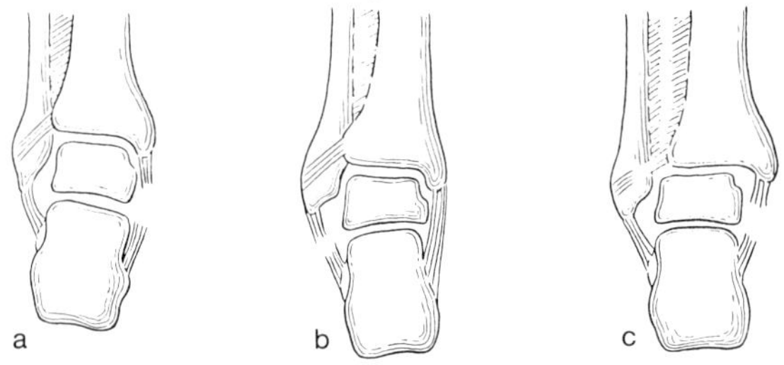

a b c

Fig. 6.26a–c. Tear of ligaments at the ankle joint.
a) Tear of the medial ligament
b) Tear of the lateral ligament.
c) Tear of the medial ligament; rupture of the tibiofibular syndesmosis and the tibiofibular ligament with lateral displacement.
(From H. R. Zatzkin: The Roentgen Diagnosis of Trauma. Chicago, Yearbook Medical Publishers, Inc., 1965. Used by permission.)

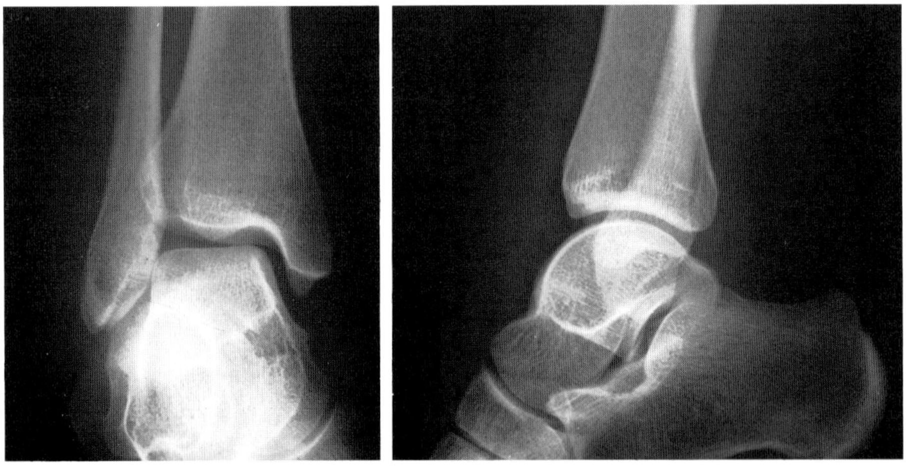

a b

Fig. 6.27a and b. A 15-year-old girl with distortion of the right ankle with a tear of the lateral ligament.

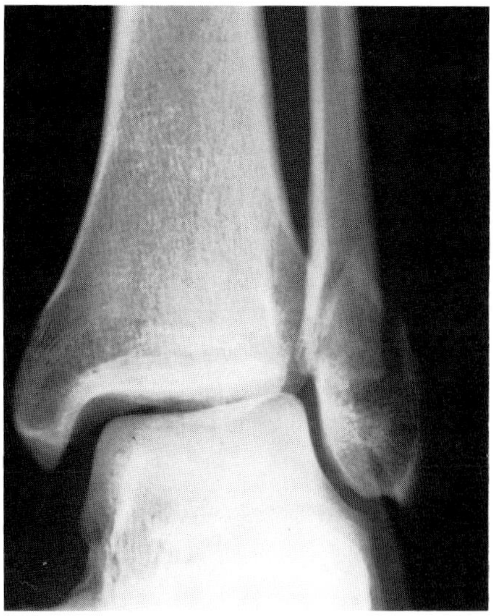

a

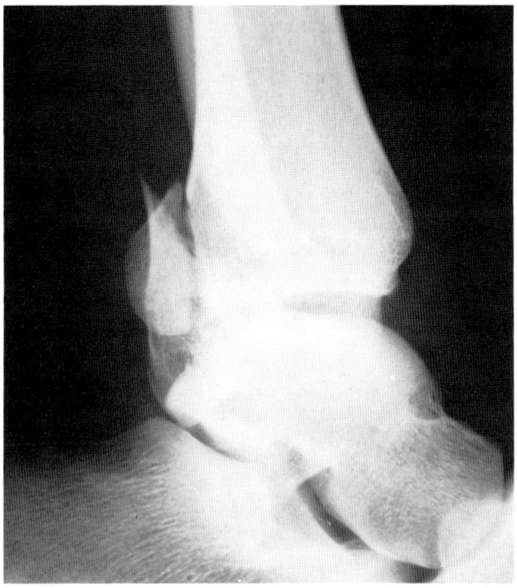

b

Fig. 6.28a and b. Fracture of the distal end of the fibula and of Volkmann's triangle; lesion of the medial ligament (widening of the medial and vertical portions of the joint space and of the tibiofibular syndesmosis in combination with displacement of the talus).

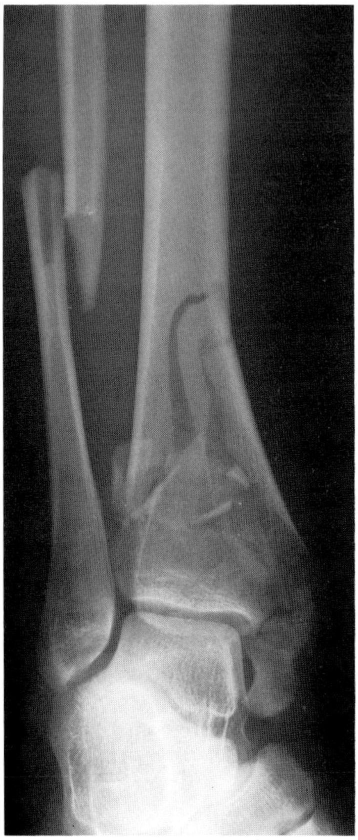

Fig. 6.29. A 37-year-old man after an accident at work. Rupture of the tibiofibular syndesmosis in a comminuted fracture of the distal tibia; fracture of the fibula in its distal 3rd and of the medial portion of the ankle.

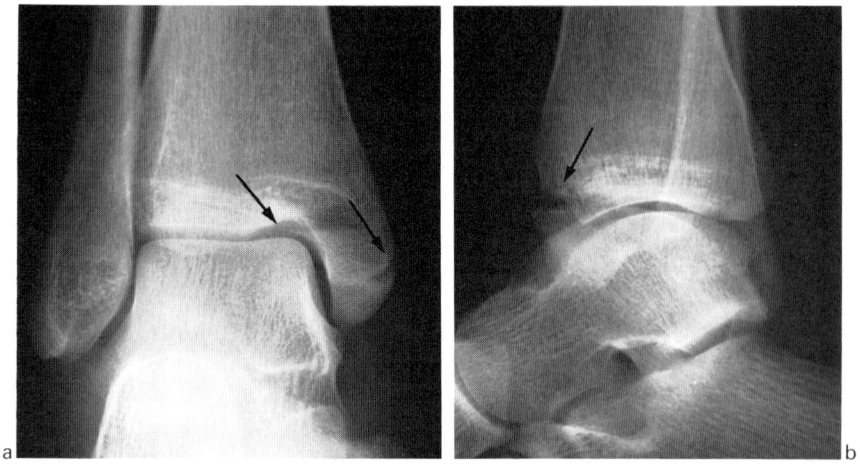

Fig. 6.30a and b. A 22-year-old woman with a fracture of the medial ankle and minimal displacement on both views.

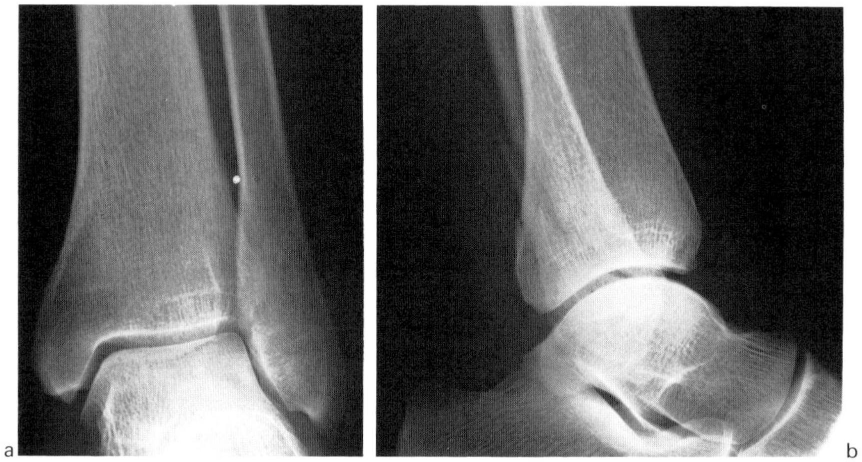

Fig. 6.31a and b. A 37-year-old man with a fracture of the lateral aspect of the ankle, with avulsion of one of Volkmann's triangles; well recognized only on the lateral view.

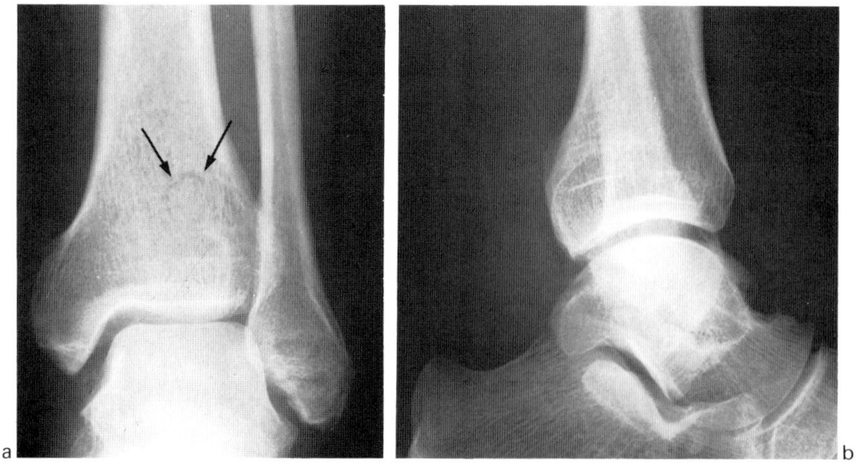

Fig. 6.32a and b. A 65-year-old man with a fracture of the lateral ankle and avulsion of Volkmann's triangle *(arrows)*.

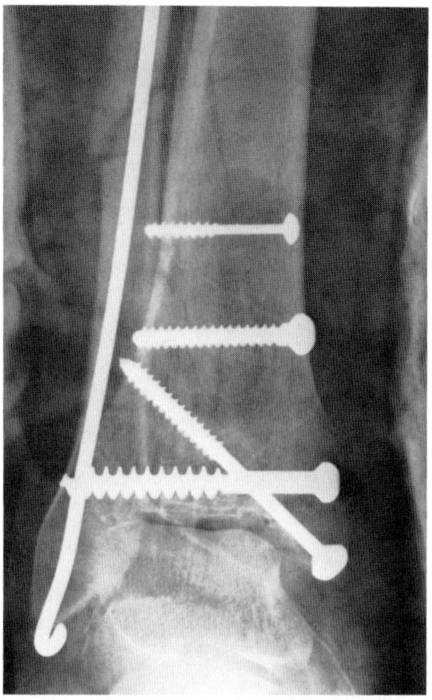

Fig. 6.33. Follow-up examination through a plaster cast after internal fixation of a comminuted fracture of the distal tibia, fracture of the medial ankle, high fibular fracture and rupture of the syndesmosis. Rush pin within the fibula. Screws from above downward. Navicular screw, cortical screw (ankle screw with self-cutting thread) and spongiosa screw for fixation of the syndesmosis.

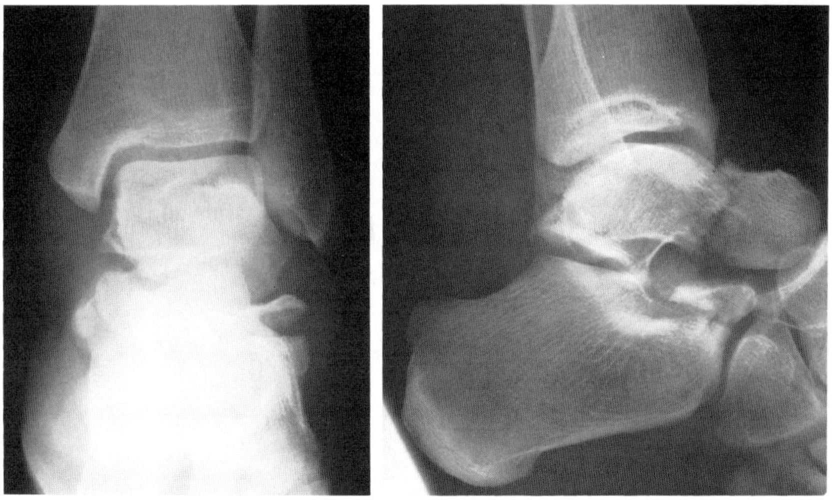

a b

Fig. 6.34a and b. A 21-year-old woman after a car accident. Fracture of the talus and the anterior process of the calcaneus. Dislocation of the lower calcaneal joint.

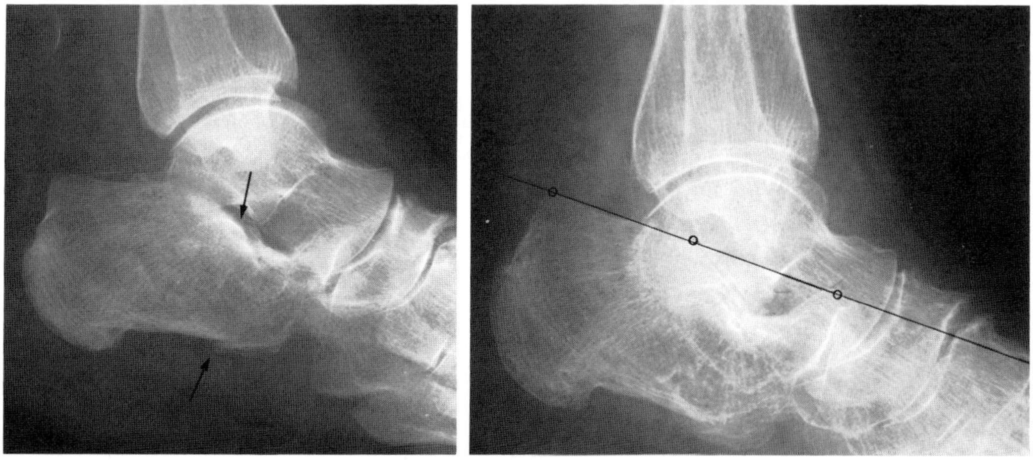

a b

Fig. 6.35. A 58-year-old woman after a fall from a stool while taking down laundry.
a) Compression fracture of the calcaneus, extending into the joint *(arrows)*.
b) Nine months after the fracture, there is good consolidation, the joint space is narrow and the angle between the tuber and joint has disappeared (traumatic flat foot).

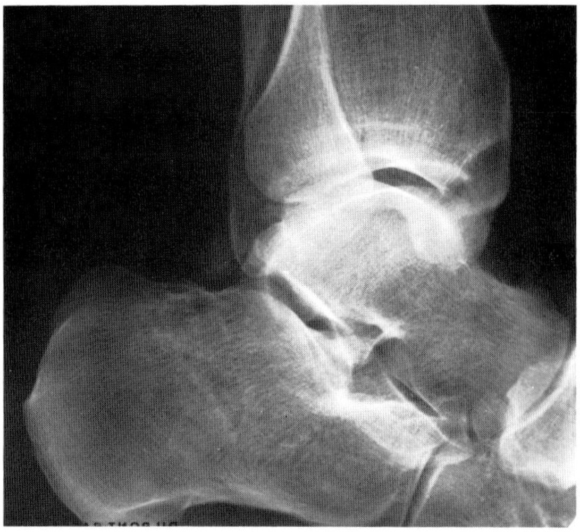

Fig. 6.36. A 60-year-old mason with an extra-articular fracture of the calcaneus.

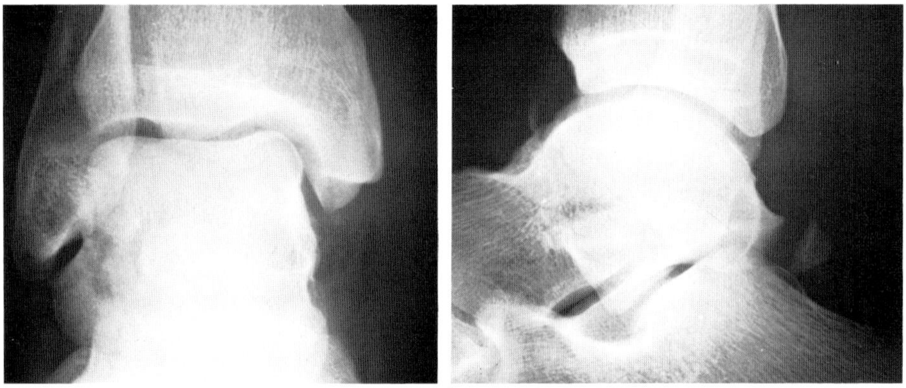

a b

Fig. 6.37a and b. A 23-year-old man who fell from a ladder. Multiple avulsion fractures of the talus; posterior process of the talus; lateral process of the talus as well as the medial and anterior articular rim.

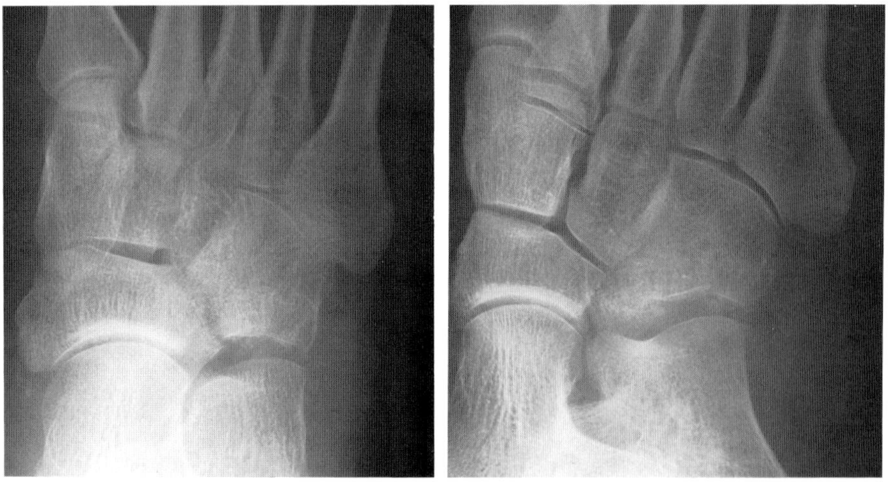

a b

Fig. 6.38a–c. a and b) A 30-year-old woman with a fracture of the cuboid bone. c) A 30-year-old woman with a fracture of the 1st cuneiform bone.

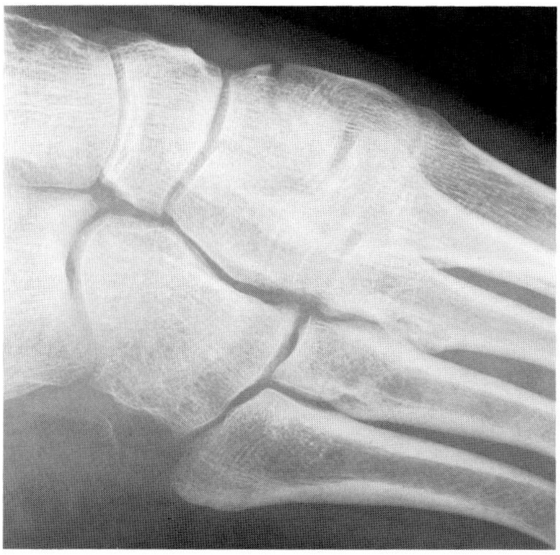

Fig. 6.38c

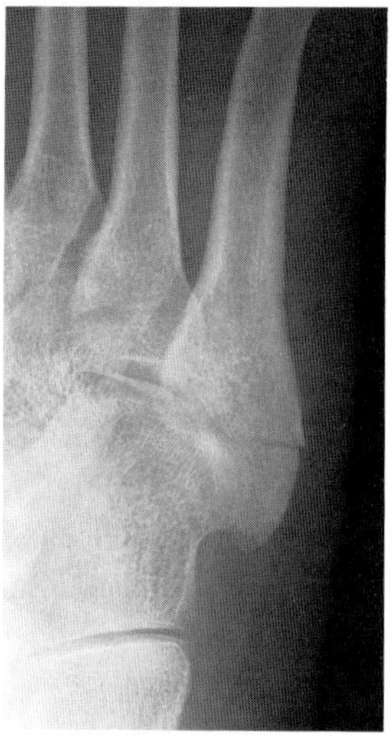

Fig. 6.39a

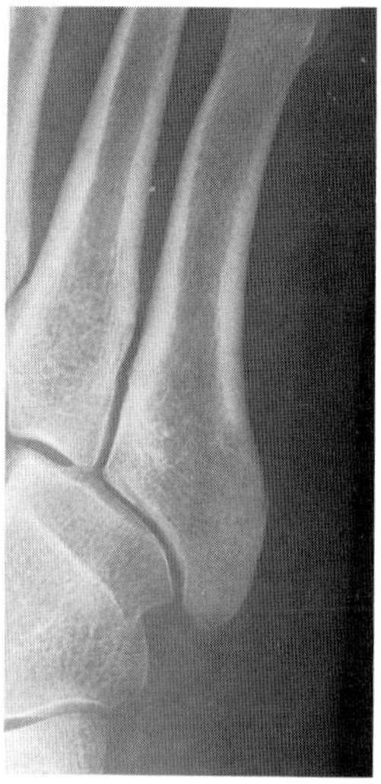

b

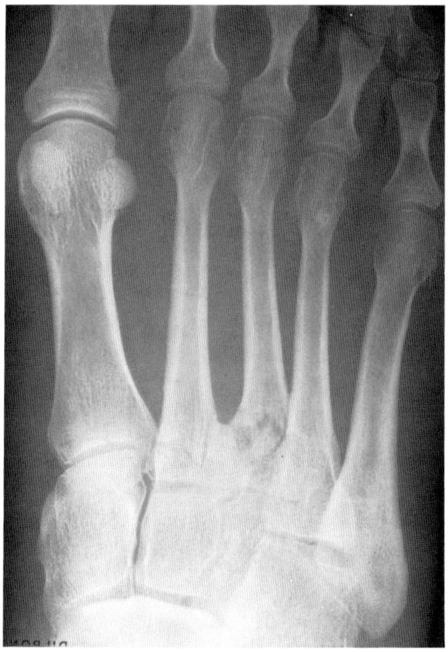

c

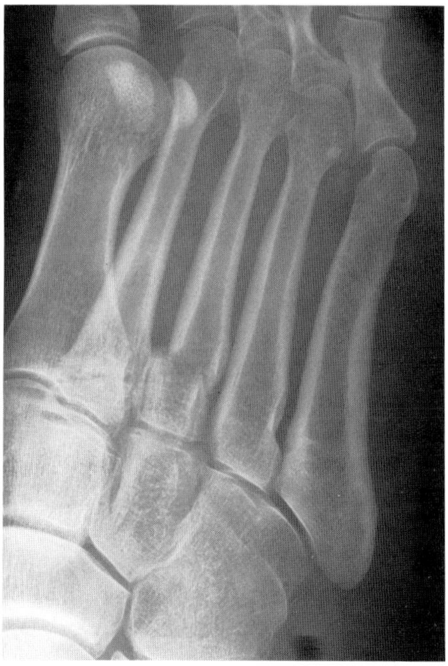

d

Fig. 6.39a–d. a and b) A 22-year-old woman after an accident at home. Fracture at the base of the metatarsal V.
c and d) A 45-year-old woman after an accident at home. Fracture of the metatarsal bones II and III close to the base.

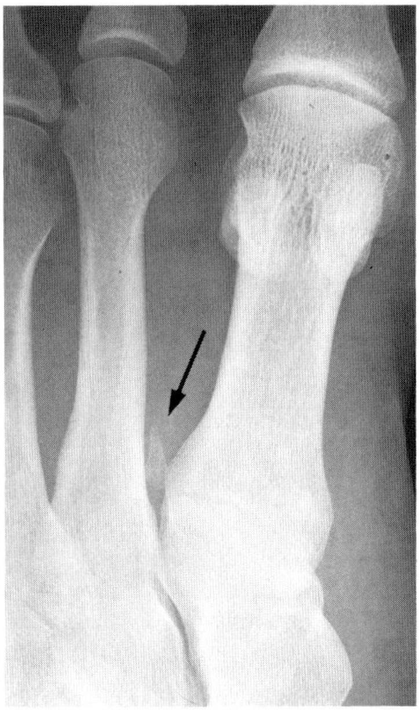

Fig. 6.40. A 23-year-old woman with distortion of the metatarsus. This is an intermetatarsal bone and not an avulsion.

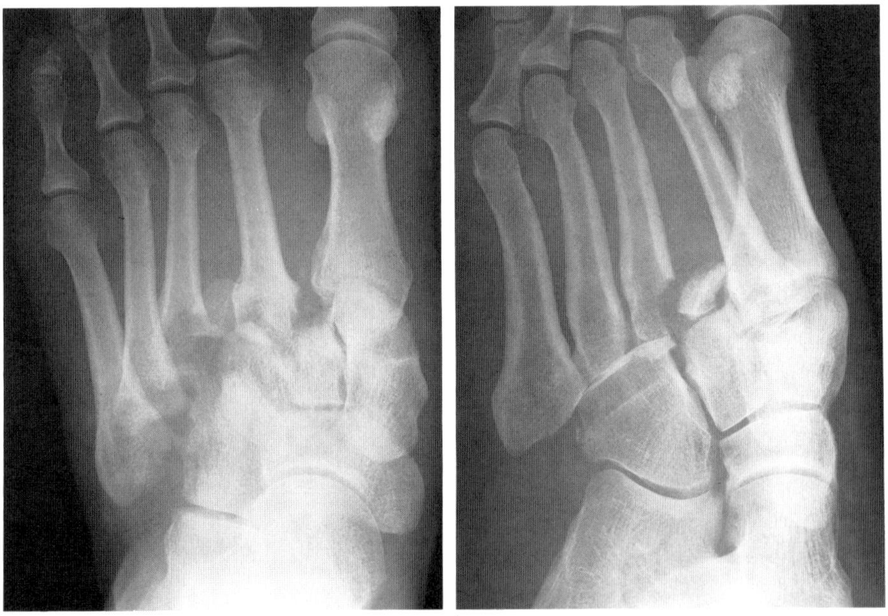

a b

Fig. 6.41a and b. A 41-year-old transport worker with luxation in Lisfranc's joint and multiple avulsion fractures.

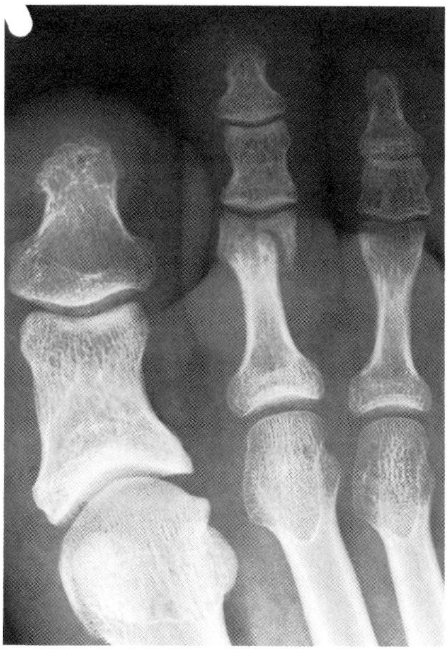

Fig. 6.42. Fracture of the head of the ground phalanx II with extension into the joint.

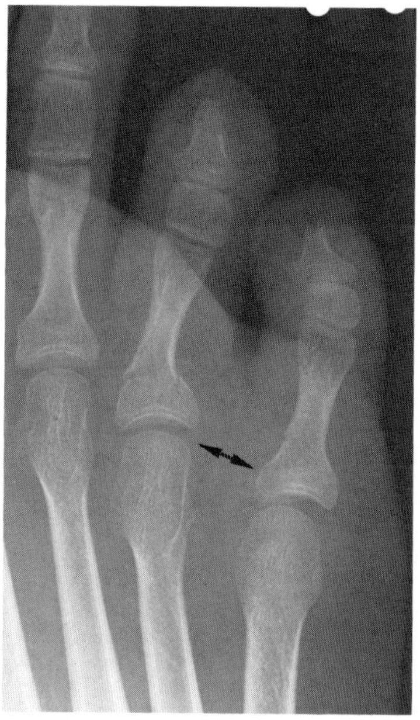

Fig. 6.43. An 18-year-old man who fell with his right foot caught in a banister. Fracture of the ground phalanges IV and V close to the base. Rupture of the deep metatarsal ligament *(arrow)*.

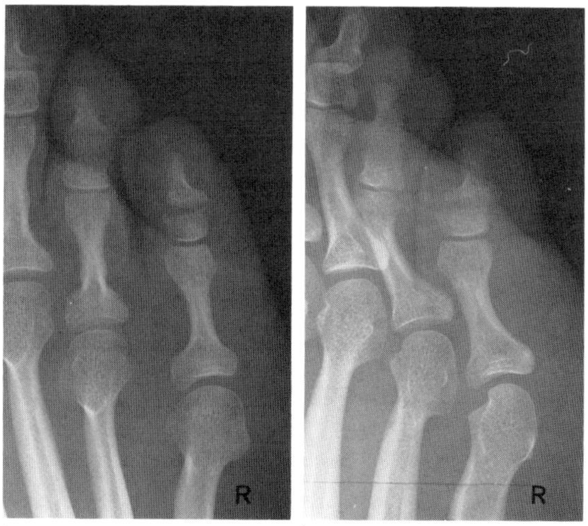

a b

Fig. 6.44a and b. A 26-year-old man with a fracture of a developmentally fused middle and end phalanx of the small toe. Fracture occurred at the level of the missing joint space. The 4th toe also shows a missing distal joint space.

7 Pathologic Fractures

Pathologic fractures may occur as spontaneous fractures. They are defined as fractures resulting from such minimal trauma as normally would never be adequate to cause a fracture. They are thus due to a reduced stability of bone caused by a local or generalized abnormal process. Only the so-called march or fatigue fractures do not occur as a result of a preexisting pathologic local alteration. The most frequent cause of a pathologic fracture during childhood and adolescence is osteogenesis imperfecta. Juvenile bone cysts as well as benign cystic lesions of bone and fibrous dysplasia must also be considered. In adults, however, bony metastases, Paget's disease and osteoporosis are chiefly considered. Furthermore, spontaneous fractures have been seen in all types of tumors, osteomyelitis, Bekhterev's disease, syphilis of bone (gumma), storage diseases and also, on an iatrogenic basis, after intensive x-ray therapy of parts of the skeleton.

The patient's history will often reveal important information as to the basic disorder (such as earlier fractures, metabolic diseases, surgery or x-ray therapy) (Fig. 7.1). Some pathologic fractures show atypical localization such as the march fracture of metatarsal II (Fig. 7.2) or of the tibia, or the fatigue fracture in osteoporosis or osteomalacia (Fig. 7.3).

Pathologic processes of bone are often recognized only after a fracture results from minimal trauma. This refers particularly to cysts and benign tumors of bone (Figs. 7.4 to 7.7). Based on x-ray symptoms and their localization, important information can be derived regarding the diagnosis and differential diagnosis of the underlying pathologic process. Local bony atrophy, posttraumatic or postinfectious processes and advanced generalized osteoporosis are frequently underestimated in their importance as causes of spontaneous fractures (Figs. 7.8 and 7.9). A characteristic picture is usually presented in pathologic fractures with Paget's disease, particularly because of the deformity and abnormal structure of the bones but also because of the abruptness of the fracture (Fig. 7.10). A similar type of fracture results from deformity and destruction of bone in hemophilia (Fig. 7.11). Infectious processes of bone can usually be recognized by the bony defects, reactive sclerosis and periosteal reaction. In the case of marked atrophy of the bone, reactive changes are much less marked or may be totally absent (Fig. 7.12). Among many spontaneous fractures as a result of tumor tissue, metastases of a carcinoma of the breast, a carcinoma of the bronchus and tumors of the kidneys and thyroid must most often be expected. A diagnosis of the exact nature of the underlying tumor, however, is only rarely possible (Figs. 7.13 to 7.15). In the differential diagnosis, Recklinghausen's disease should be considered, especially its tumoral form (Fig. 7.16). Among iatrogenic pathologic fractures, those resulting from radiation, particularly to the femoral neck in patients with gynecologic lesions are best known (Fig. 7.17). In some areas, especially the clavicle and the ends of the ribs, it is difficult to delineate metastatic fractures. Sometimes only a follow-up examination or biopsy will bring an answer (Fig. 7.18). Full knowledge of the fields of radiation, the dose of radiation applied, and whether there were skin changes may provide important clues. Difficult further problems are posed, finally, by neurogenic pathologic fractures such as those resulting from poliomyelitis, tabes, syringomyelia and other neuropathic disorders (Figs. 7.19 and 7.20).

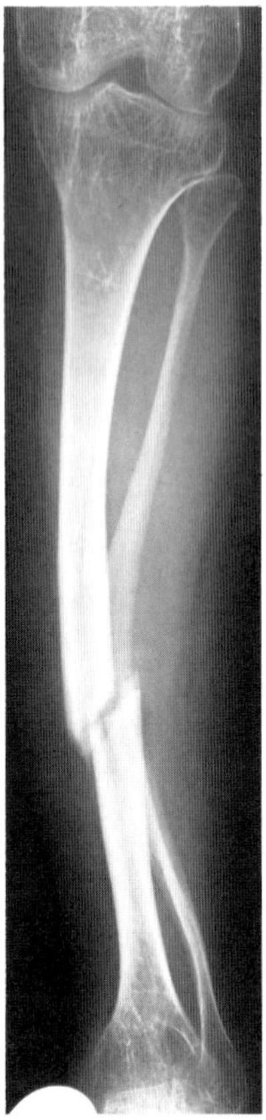

Fig. 7.1. A 17-year-old girl with blue sclerae and a hearing disorder. At 3 years of age, a fracture of the right femur; 1 year ago, a fracture of the right tibia. Pathologic fracture in osteogenesis imperfecta.

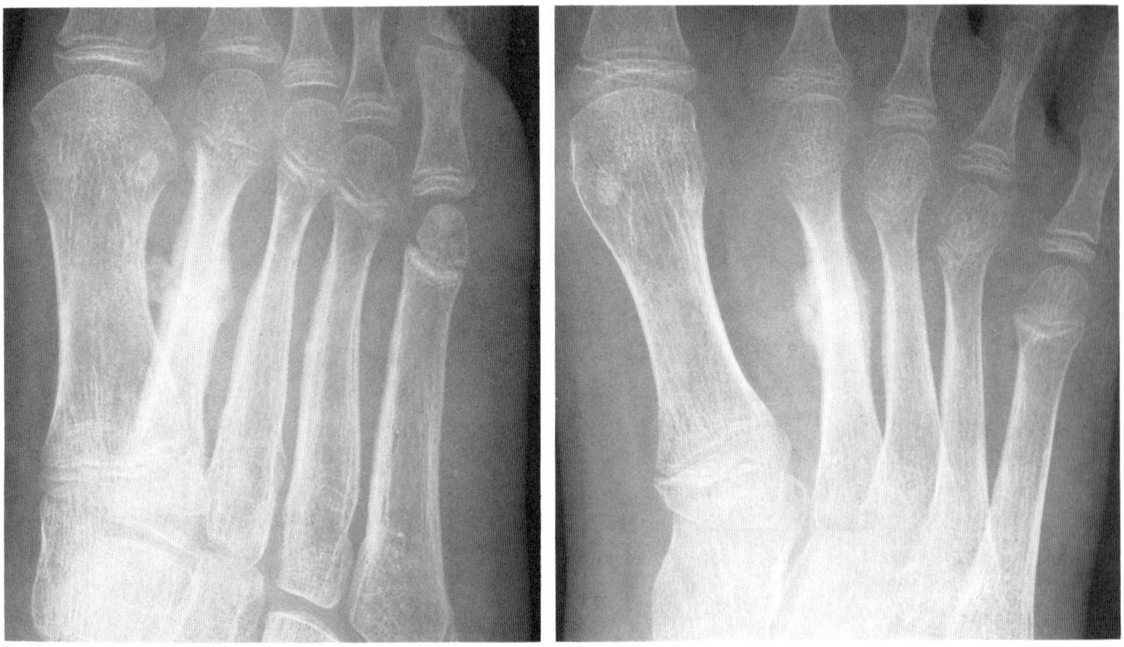

a b

Fig. 7.2a and b. A 10-year-old girl who for weeks had painful swelling of the right midfoot. Fatigue fracture of the 2nd metacarpal bone.

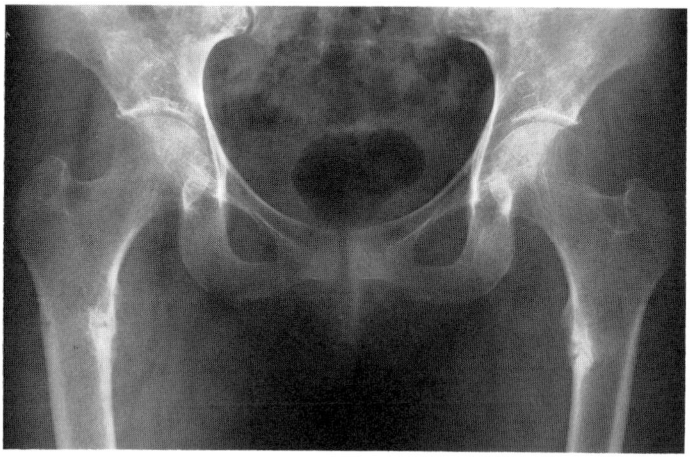

Fig. 7.3. A 57-year-old woman with a symmetrical fracture of both femora below the trochanter due to osteomalacia.

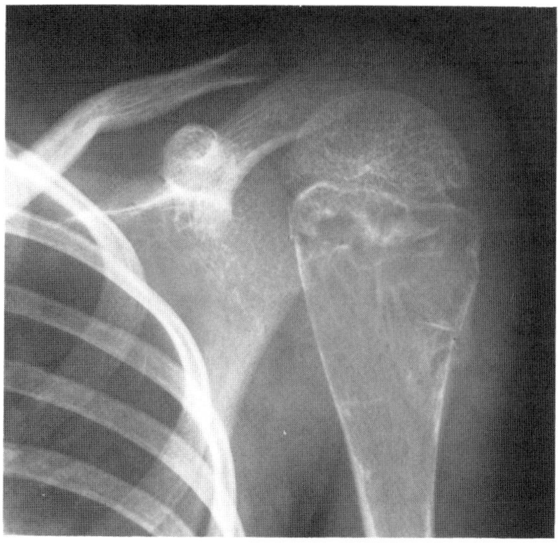

Fig. 7.4. An 8-year-old boy after a fall from a bicycle. Pathologic fracture in the presence of a solitary primary bone cyst. The trauma led to detection of this condition.

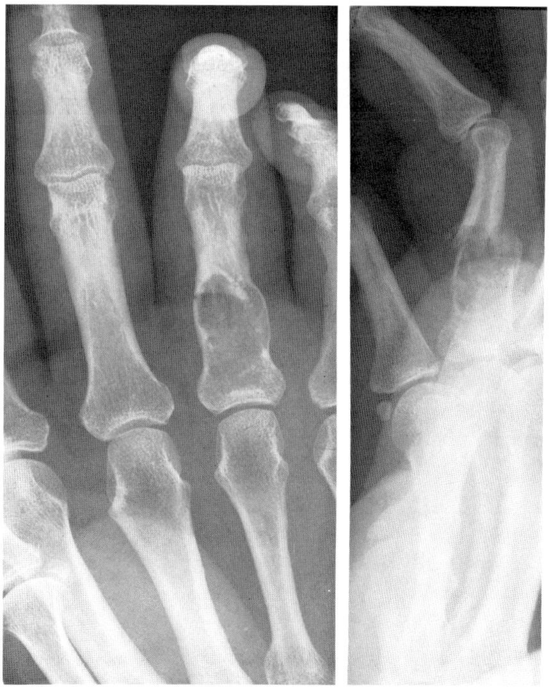

a b

Fig. 7.5a and b. Spontaneous fracture of the ground phalanx of the right ring finger as a result of minimal trauma in the presence of a large enchondroma.

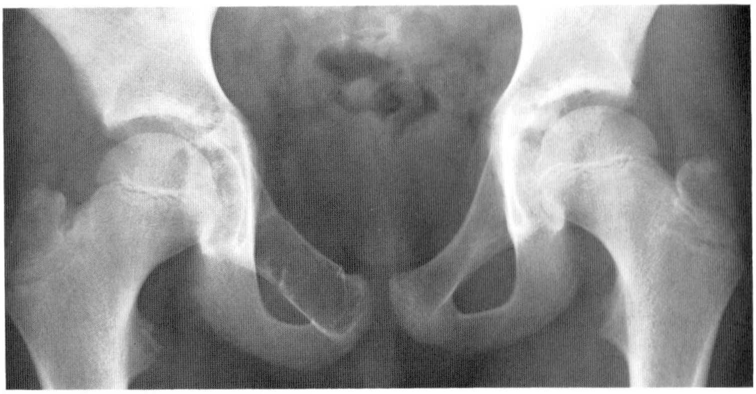

Fig. 7.6. Spontaneous fracture of the right pubic bone due to osteoclastoma.

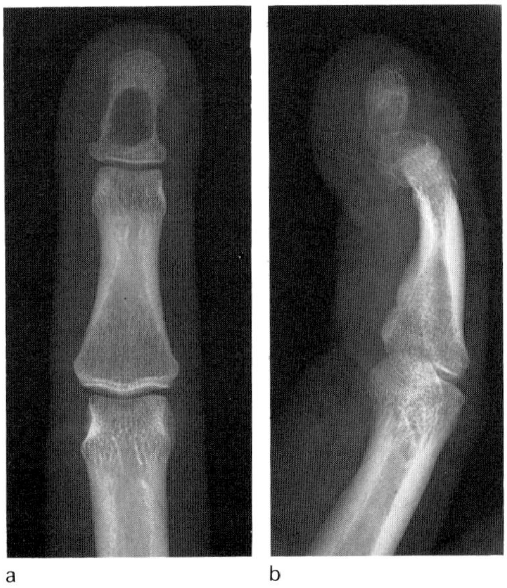

Fig. 7.7a and b. A 32-year-old woman after an accident at work, with marked compression of the midportion of the middle finger. Pathologic fracture in the presence of adequate trauma. Old traumatic epithelioid cyst of the end phalanx of the middle finger.

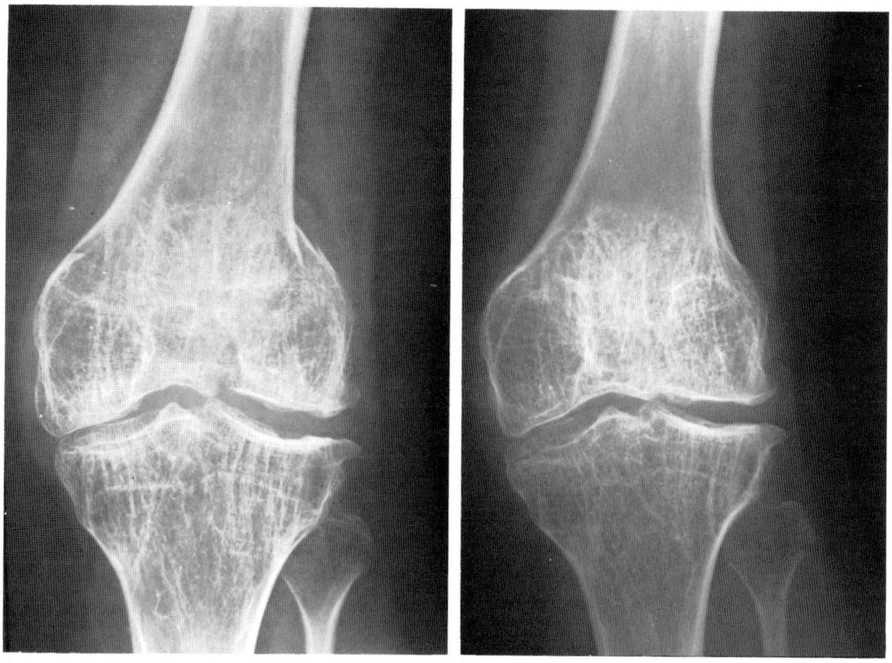

a b

Fig. 7.8a and b. A 25-year-old woman. a) Fracture of the lateral femoral condyle as a result of minimal trauma in severe bony atrophy after coxitis.
b) X-ray follow-up $1\frac{1}{2}$ years later shows good and complete bony consolidation.

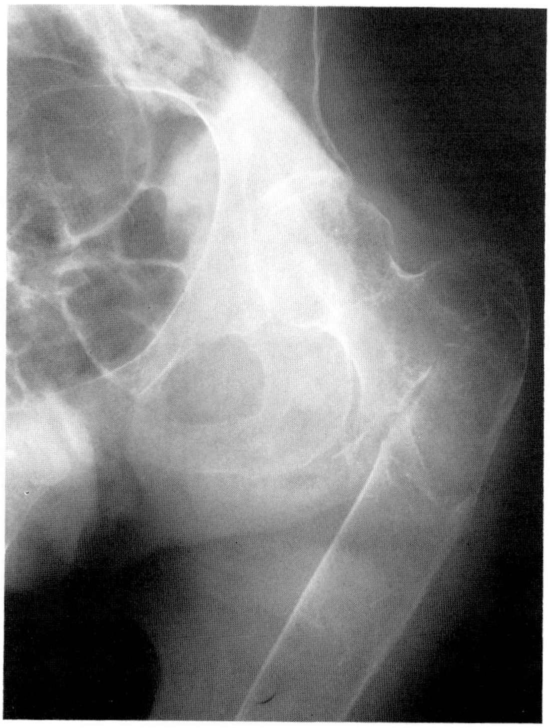

Fig. 7.9. A 63-year-old woman with spontaneous fracture of the hip in bed in the presence of severe osteoporosis after years of immobilization in bed due to multiple sclerosis.

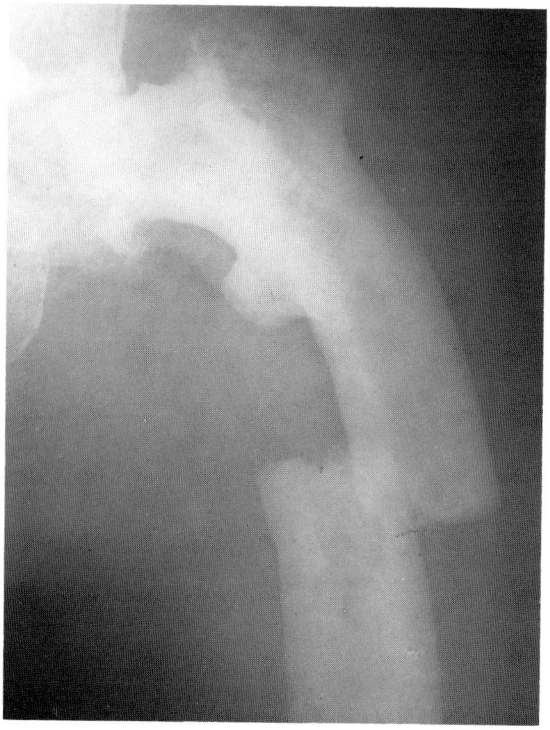

Fig. 7.10. A 73-year-old woman with spontaneous fracture of the femur due to Paget's disease. The deformity and abnormal density of the bone are typical, as is the blunt transverse fracture.

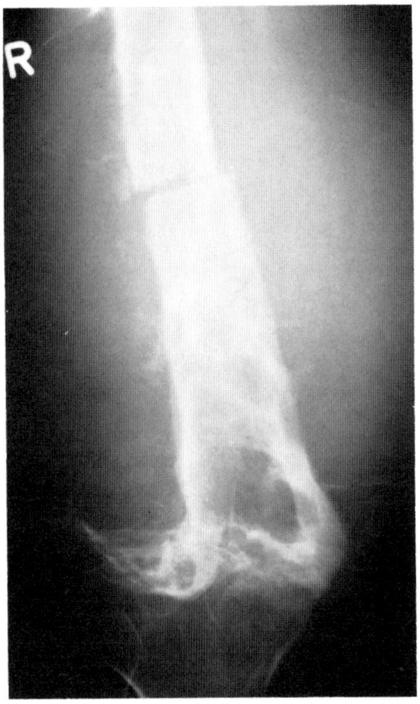

Fig. 7.11. A 33-year-old woman with a pathologic fracture of the right femur due to hemophilia.

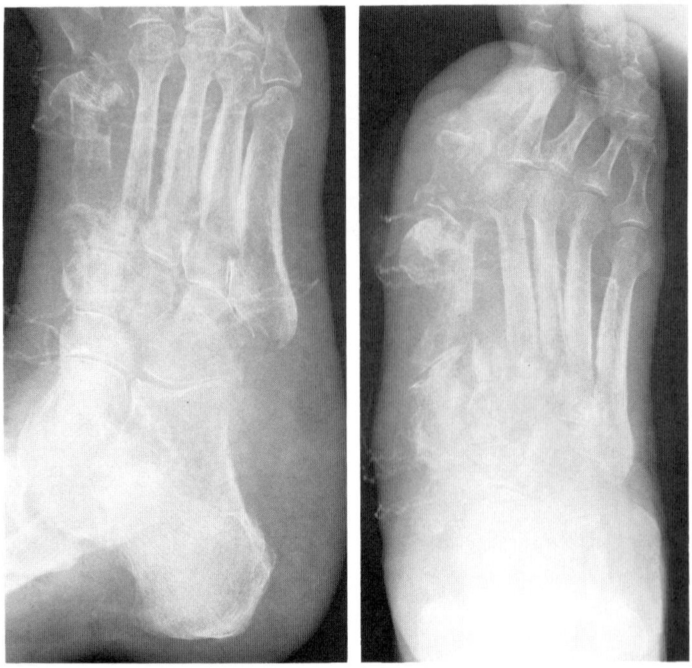

a b

Fig. 7.12a and b. Pathologic fracture of the metatarsal bones I to IV due to severe local infection in a diabetic.

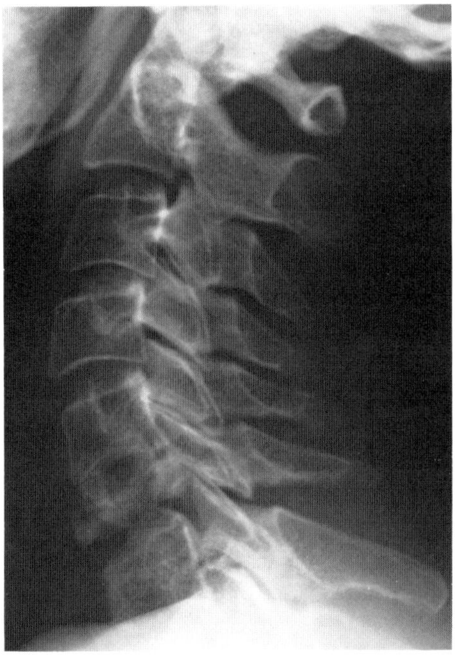

Fig. 7.13. A 59-year-old man with a spontaneous fracture of the 6th cervical vertebral body due to metastasis of a carcinoma of the esophagus.

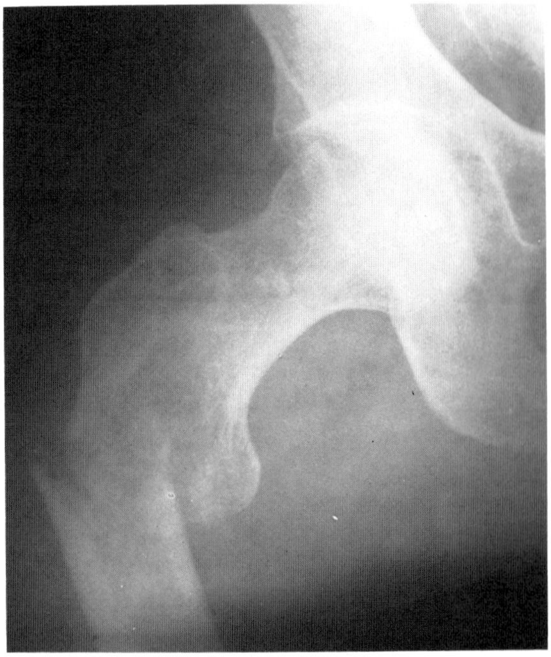

Fig. 7.14. A 46-year-old woman with a pathologic fracture of the right femur due to plasmacytoma.

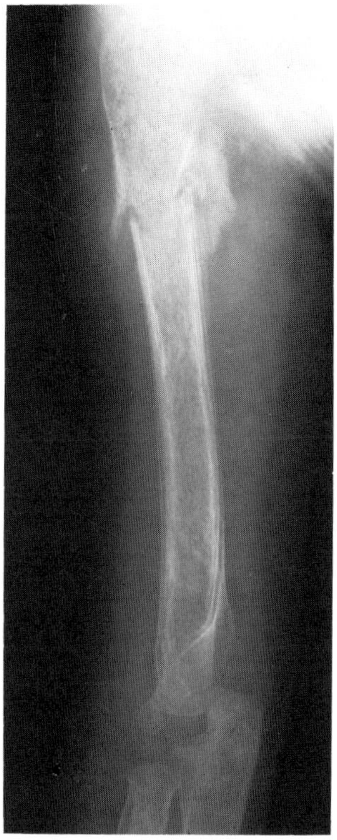

Fig. 7.15. A 3-year-old boy with a pathologic fracture of the right humerus in paramyeloblastic leukemia.

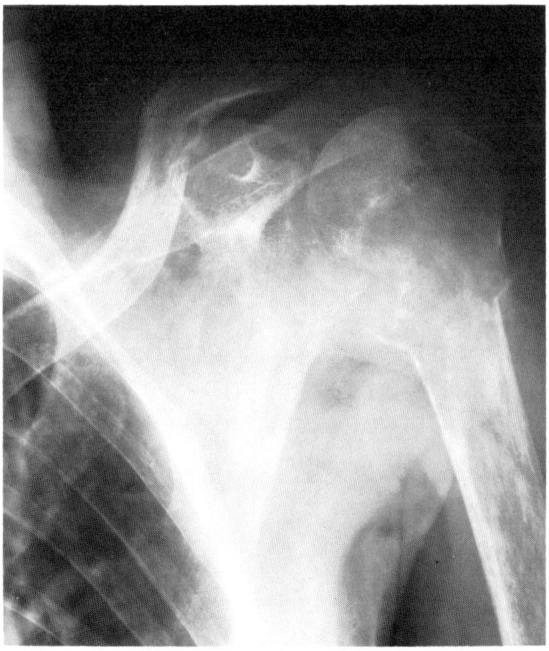

a

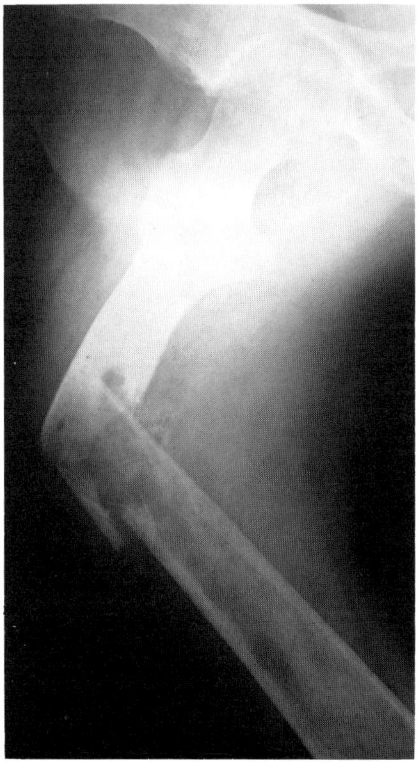

b

Fig. 7.16a and b. A 56-year-old man with a pathologic fracture due to a tumoral form of Recklinghausen's disease.

a) Fracture of the left humeral neck.

b) Fracture of the right femur 2 years later.

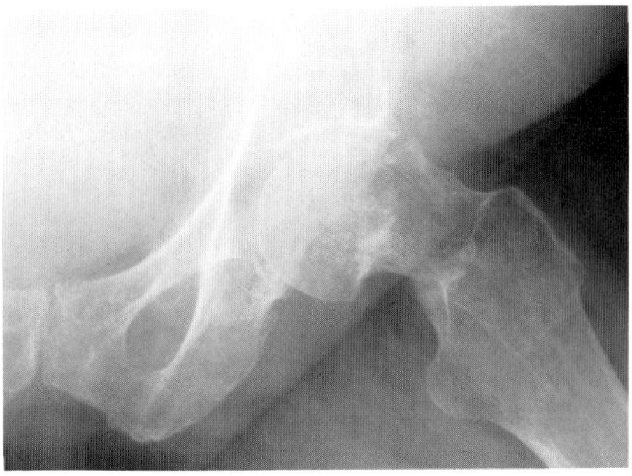

a

Fig. 7.17a and b. A 63-year-old woman with a femoral neck fracture caused by radiation damage 2 years after a local dose of 5500 r in cobalt teletherapy and 2000 mgeh radium implant for a recurrent carcinoma of the neck. For 1$^{1}/_{2}$ years, she had pain in her left hip. X-ray six months prior to this study did not reveal a fracture.

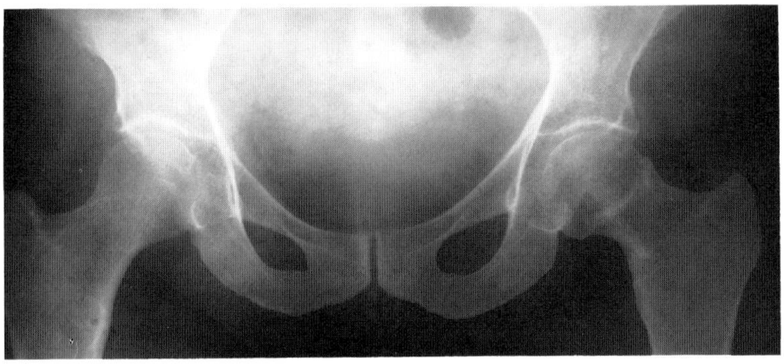

b

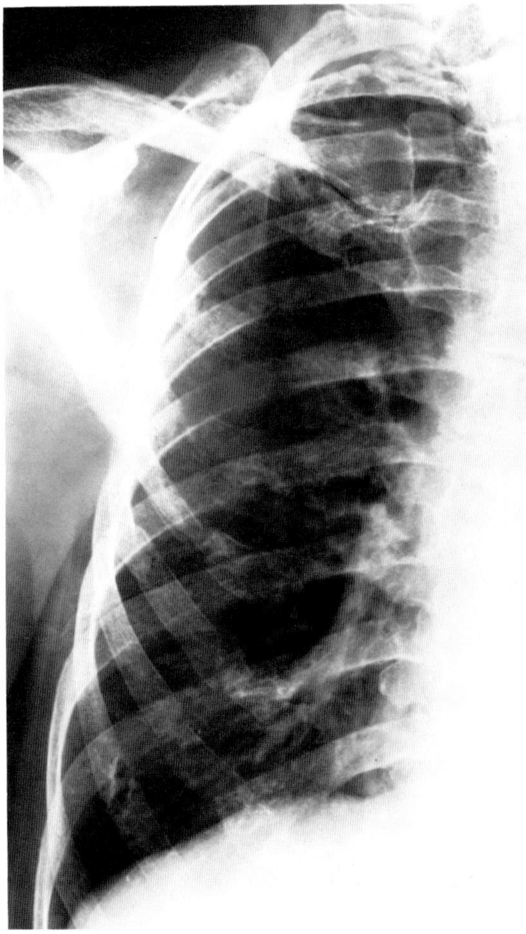

Fig. 7.18. A 52-year-old woman with a fracture of the right clavicle after irradiation. The 2nd to 7th ribs on the right anteriorly also show fractures after intensive postoperative irradiation for carcinoma of the breast. Almost complete lack of periosteal callus formation.

Fig. 7.19a and b. A 47-year-old man with an altered sensitivity due to alcoholic neuropathy.
a) Pathologic avulsion-fracture of the calcaneal tuberosity.
b) Fracture of the metatarsal V.

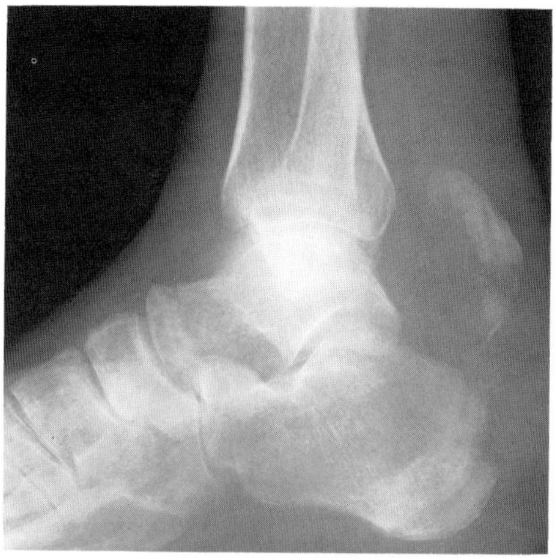

a

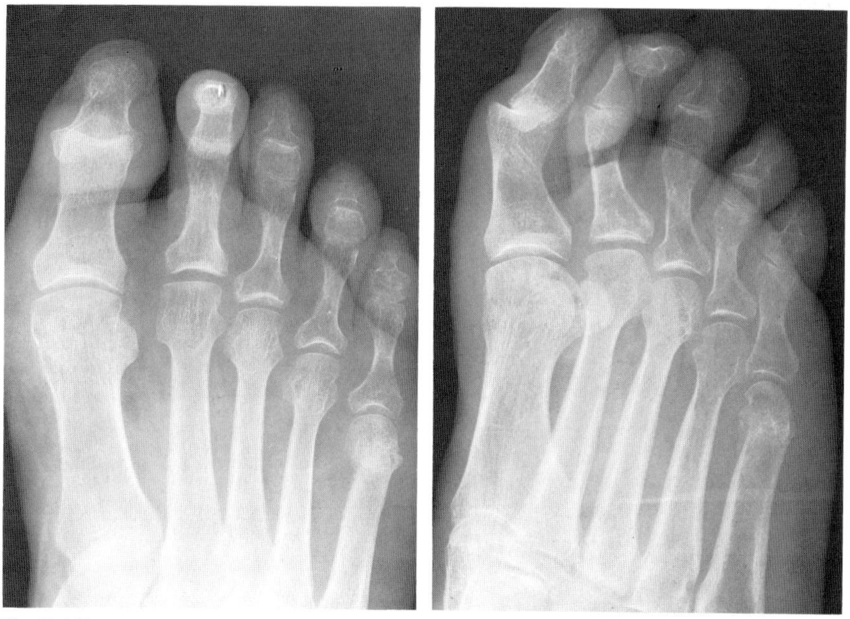

Fig. 7.19b

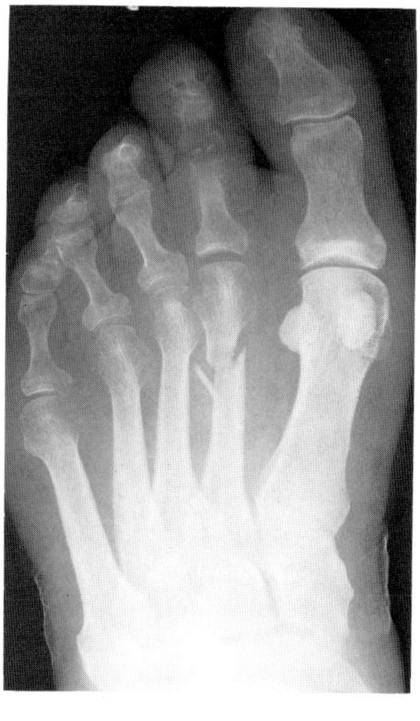

Fig. 7.20. A 57-year-old man with a painless spontaneous fracture of the 2nd metatarsal due to lumbar syringomyelia. Trophic ulcer of the 2nd toe, with involvement of the underlying bone and joint.

8 Thorax

Blunt trauma to the thorax occurs much more frequently than open injuries during peacetime. According to Gremmel and Vieten (1966), 58 per cent of such injuries are the result of traffic accidents, 24 per cent are due to accidents at work and 12 per cent occur during daily activities. The remainder usually occur during sports activities. The major distinctions are: contusion, compression and bruising with or without injury to the thoracic skeleton and to the internal organs of the thorax. About 5 to 6 per cent of injuries to the thorax are open penetrating wounds (Dick, 1900; cited in Lorenz, 1966). Such injuries are usually the result of projectiles, stabbings or thrusting wounds. All injuries of the thorax, with the exception of isolated fractures of the ribs, are particularly serious and have a high mortality. For blunt injuries to the thorax, a mortality of 7 per cent has been quoted by Gremmel and Vieten (1966), and may go as high as 20 per cent according to Keller et al. (1967). Thoracic trauma, also in the absence of fractured ribs, is frequently associated with severe injuries to the internal organs or with traumatic injuries to other parts of the body. A synopsis of the radiologic symptoms in injuries to the thorax is given in Figure 8.1.

The most frequent radiologic finding is traumatic pneumothorax with or without fractured ribs, hematothorax and hematopneumothorax (Figs. 8.2 to 8.4). Single fractures of the ribs without marked dislocation usually do not have a concomitant injury to the pleura or soft tissues (Figs. 8.5 and 8.6), whereas an extensive series of fractures and large fracture areas of the chest wall often do have a simultaneous pneumothorax, a hematothorax and subcutaneous or mediastinal emphysema (Figs. 8.7 and 8.8). Hematothorax and pneumothorax may present only days and sometimes even weeks after the trauma (Fig. 8.9). Markedly dislocated fractures of the ribs may sometimes cause only a minimal pleural reaction without emphysema of the soft tissues, hematothorax or pneumothorax. Fractures of the sternum are localized most frequently within the body. There is a whole spectrum of involvement – from minimal anterior depression of the cortical layer to complete fracture with marked dislocation of a portion into the deeper region of the mediastinum (Figs. 8.10 and 8.11). A concomitant injury of the thoracic organs can, however, also result from minimal dislocation of a fractured sternum. In such situations, we must consider the sternal fracture as only a part of the major thoracic injury. Although the majority of sternal fractures are best seen on a lateral view of the thorax, it is still recommended that one obtain special views of the sternum in the prone position and with the right side elevated. When in doubt, one should either obtain a contact film with the cassette placed right on the sternum and the x-ray tube positioned toward the right side of the spine or get a tomogram. Often it is necessary to expose several films to arrive at a reliable documentation. Tomographic views are particularly useful in demonstrating a dislocation of the sternoclavicular joint (Fig. 8.12).

Contusion of the lung is usually recognized on x-rays because of somewhat marked intrapulmonary hemorrhage; the opacification can be more oval or rounded in shape (Figs. 8.13 and 8.14). During resorption of such pulmonary hematomas, traumatic cysts of the lung may be found. These may be the result of tears of alveolar structures (Fig. 8.15).

Extensive, patchy, usually bilateral opacification of the lung is the result of aspiration of water during drowning. The marginal regions of the lung usually remain free of opacification (Fig. 8.16). In spite of visible improvement in the radiologic findings, there may still be a fatal result. Massive bilateral opacification of the lung fields due to edema of the lungs and hemorrhage may eventually, together with subcutaneous and mediastinal emphysema, be the result of pulmonary injury caused by an explosion (Fig. 8.17). Similar alterations in interstitial infiltration can be seen in chemical intoxication (Fig. 8.18). In the adult, these are usually the result of suicide attempts with sleeping pills or barbiturates; during childhood, they are the inadvertent consequence of swallowing toxic household products such as kerosene, spot removers, furniture polish or turpentine.

Interstitial edema of the lung can also be seen after massive burns. The differential diagnosis, particularly in older patients and regardless of the type of trauma, must include a cardiac cause for the pulmonary edema that is precipitated by the accident.

Pulmonary opacification similar to that caused by edema can be seen in fat embolization (Fig. 8.19). Atelectasis can be recognized by a shift of the mediastinum toward the affected side. There may be an indication of an obstruction, rupture or torsion of one of the major bronchi (Fig. 8.20); small areas of atelectasis usually have an uncharacteristic streaky or ribbon-shaped appearance and may be the sole result of obstruction by secretions.

Rupture within the major airways occasionally involves the trachea and, somewhat more frequently, the main or intermediate bronchi. Radiologic symptoms in order of decreasing frequency are: pneumothorax, subcutaneous emphysema, mediastinal emphysema, hematothorax and chylothorax. In only about $^1/_3$ of all cases is the diagnosis made early. Atelectasis is always a late finding (Fig. 8.21). In every case, an attempt should be made as early as possible to reestablish continuity of the airway. Reconstructions of the bronchus in delayed cases have shown that an atelectatic lung may resume its function even years later (Krauss, 1956).

Rarer than a rupture of the bronchus are injuries of the thoracic duct or of a large vessel leading toward it, with a consequent chylothorax. These changes may be the result of wounds caused by a knife or projectiles, by blunt trauma to the thoracic wall, as well as by a iatrogenic action such as surgery within the thoracic cage. Occasionally such changes result from perforation of the lower third of the esophagus by a foreign body. The main radiologic finding is the presence of free fluid within the pleura, its location being determined by the level of the injury. Distinction between chylothorax and hematothorax is possible only after pleural aspiration. Also, a hematothorax has the tendency to develop much faster.

Traumatic rupture of the esophagus is extremely rare and results only from maximal forces such as an explosion. Other injuries usually accompanying severe blunt trauma to the thorax in or near the abdomen may make a proper diagnosis difficult. Small amounts of fluid and air-fluid levels in the posterior mediastinum should suggest a rupture of the esophagus. In order to confirm the perforation and its exact location, it is necessary to use a water-soluble, sterile contrast agent.

Like iatrogenic perforation during an esophagoscopy or gastroscopy penetrating wounds due to projectiles or a knife are not at all rare (Fig. 8.22).

More and more significance should be attached to incomplete rupture of large blood vessels. It can be the result of traffic accidents, an elevator crash or a fall onto the back, and involves particularly the area of the aortic isthmus, the ascending aorta, the descending aorta and the aortic arch, but also the larger arteries arising from the aorta. As a result of an improperly treated incomplete rupture, a false aneurysm may develop, with the constant danger of a rupture or a dissecting aneurysm.

The hematoma after a rupture will, depending on its location and extent, lead to a widening of the vascular shadow or of the entire mediastinum and can best be recognized on high-kV x-ray technique or on overexposed x-rays (Sanborn et al., 1970). If doubt exists, angiography is indicated (Kümmerle, 1965) (Fig. 8.23).

Traumatic diaphragmatic hernias and ruptures of the diaphragm are frequently seen as additional injuries after contusion of the thorax or abdomen or following combined thoraco-abdominal trauma. They are seen more often on the left, since on the right the liver apparently serves as a barrier that prevents prolapse of abdominal organs into the thoracic cage. The organs most frequently seen to prolapse are the omentum, colon, stomach, small intestine, spleen and liver. This complication typically occurs after a head-on collision in a traffic accident or after a fall from a great height. Blunt diaphragmatic injuries due to blunt trauma are frequently recognized accidentally and much later than the traumatic event. A proper radiologic approach will include fluoroscopy in different views, survey films on two planes, contrast investigation of the gastrointestinal tract and finally, as the frequently decisive study, a diagnostic pneumoperitoneum. The x-ray investigation should confirm or rule out conclusively the presence of a ruptured diaphragm, as well as the location and type of rupture and whether the abdominal organs have prolapsed. One should always remember the danger of incarceration (e. g., of the stomach or colon) within the hernia, with the risk of perforation due to an ulcer affecting the prolapsed part of the gastrointestinal tract (Figs. 8.24 to 8.26).

In a penetrating injury of the thorax, the involvement of certain organs and structures can be only suspected radiologically, particularly when the penetrating foreign body has already been removed, such as in a stabbing. The presence of pleural and abdominal symptoms may indicate a lesion of the diaphragm.

Injuries caused by radiologically recognizable foreign bodies are reviewed in Chapter 10.

Blunt trauma affecting the heart may lead to a concussion or a contusion of the heart. A clinical and roentgenologic distinction between these conditions is not possible. Concussion must be recognized as a functional alteration with coronary spasm, whereas contusion is defined as damage to the heart muscle itself. Frequently, the ECG will be diagnostically more informative than an x-ray. According to de Muth et al. (1967), the following electrocardiographic signs and clinical findings will help in the diagnosis: pericarditis and subendocardial infarction, T-wave changes in V_4, right bundle branch block, infarct in the septum, RST-alterations as usually seen in myocardial damage, reversal of T-wave in the chest wall lead, intermittent bundle branch block and ST-alterations as seen in ischemia.

Severe chest pain and tachycardia unexplained on the basis of the traumatic history should alert one to the distinct possibility of traumatic damage to the heart. Radiologic symptoms of a concussion or a contusion of the heart are: cardiac dilatation with pulmonary congestion, enlargement and change in contour of the cardiac silhouette due to small rents in the myocardium or on the valves or damage to coronary arteries, possibly with tamponade after bleeding into the pericardial sac. Larger rents in the pericardium result in a possible displacement of the heart, with a corresponding change in the contour of the heart.

Open heart injuries are seen relatively rarely during peacetime. They are mostly the result of stabbings. In surviving patients there is accumulation of blood in the pericardium, with tamponade or a pneumopericardium (Fig. 8.27). The same symptoms, with and without hemothorax, have been described after rupture of the heart following blunt trauma (Noon et al., 1971).

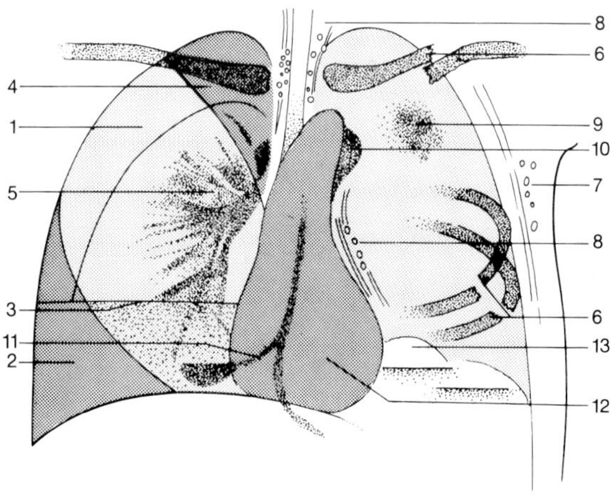

Fig. 8.1. Synopsis of x-ray findings in an injury to the thorax:
1 Pneumothorax, tension pneumothorax
2 Hematothorax
3 Hematopneumothorax
4 Atelectasis
5 Edema or edemalike changes, cardiac pulmonary edema
6 Fractures (ribs, clavicle, sternum)
7 Emphysema of chest wall
8 Emphysema of mediastinum
9 Infiltration (contusion, aspiration)
10 Rupture of large vessels
11 Rupture of esophagus
12 Contusion of heart (ECG)
13 Diaphragmatic hernia or rupture

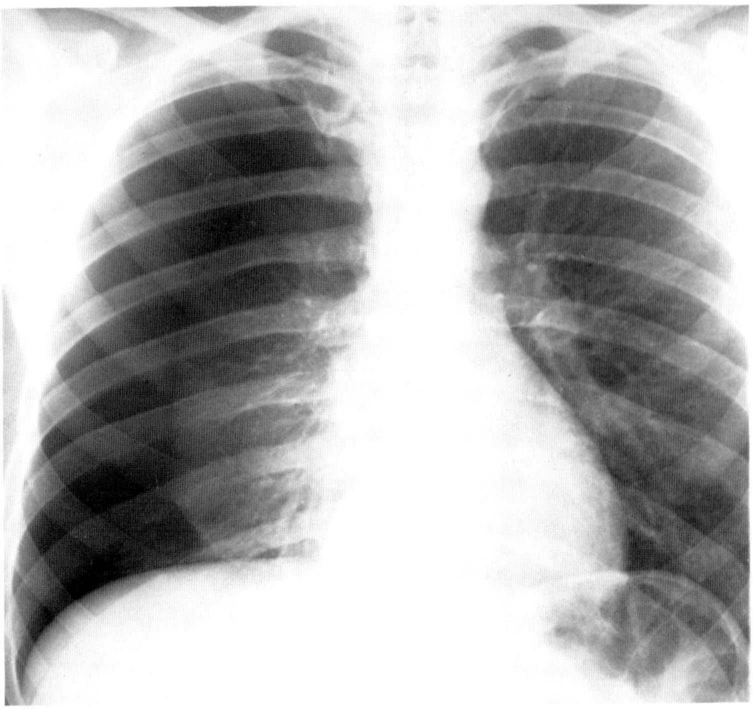

Fig. 8.2a

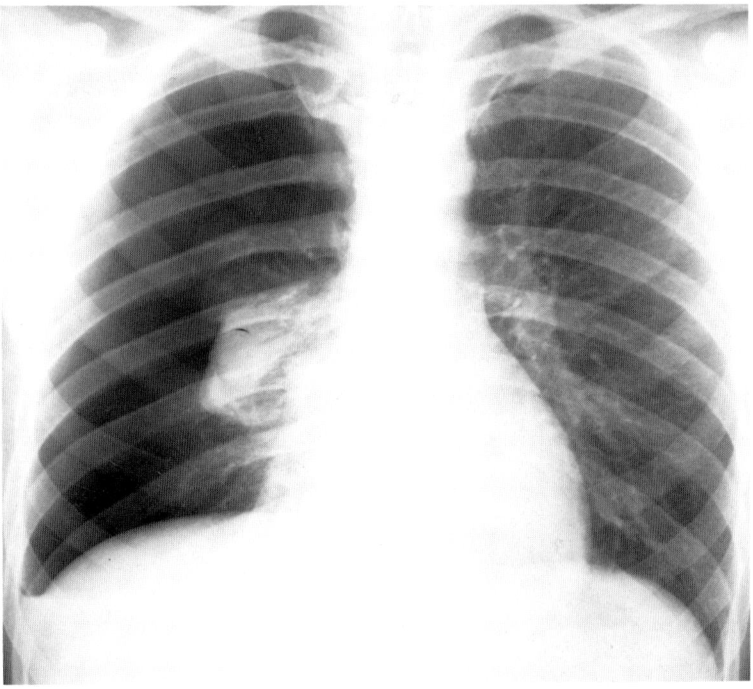

b

Fig. 8.2a and b. A 22-year-old man after a sports accident, a) Pneumothorax on the right; no visible fracture of the ribs.
b) Follow-up one week later: increase in pathology on the right; tension pneumothorax and secondary fluid accumulation.

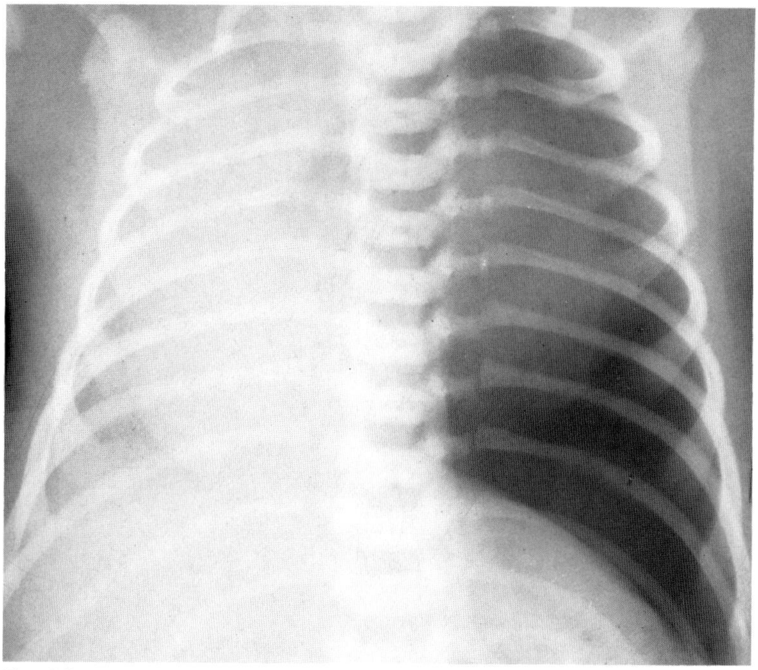

Fig. 8.3a

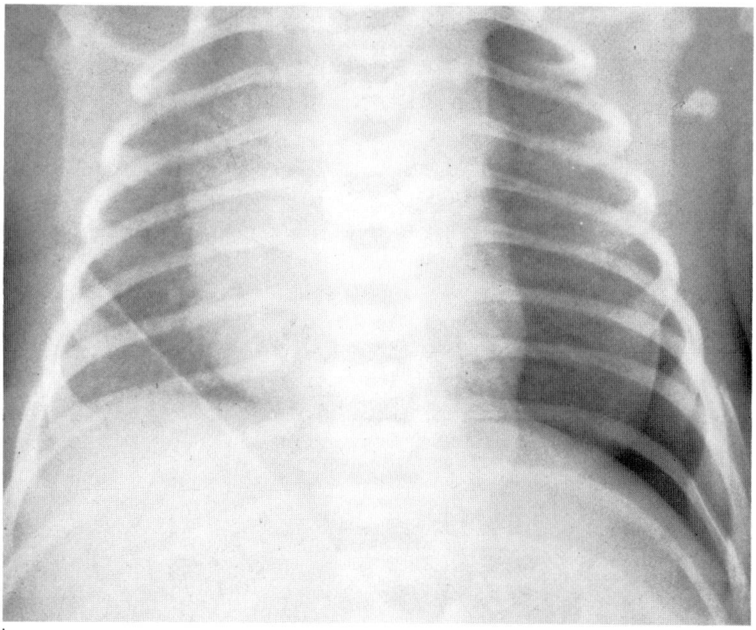

b

Fig. 8.3a–c. a) Tension pneumothorax due to birth trauma.
b) Rapid expansion of the left lung after aspiration of pneumothorax.
c) Further improvement after 3 days. Mediastinum again in midline; small remaining air accumulation at the left base.

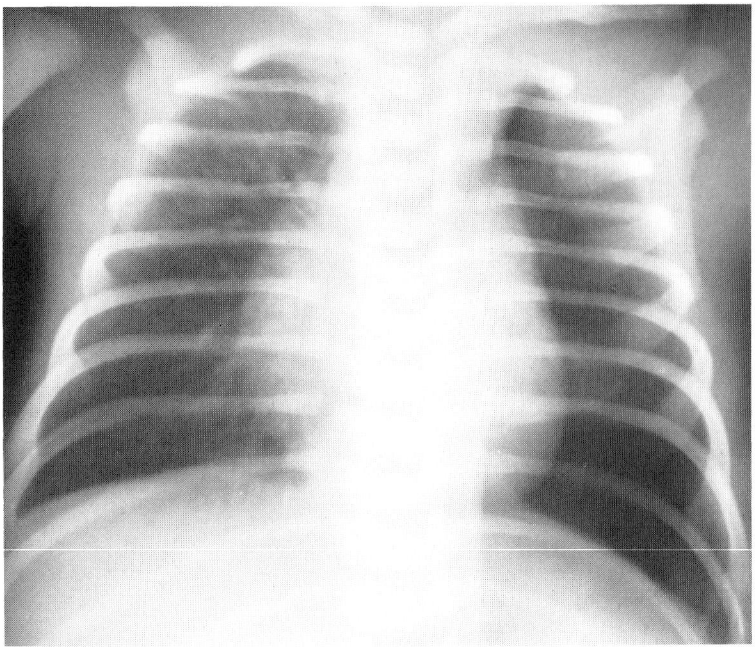

Fig. 8.3c

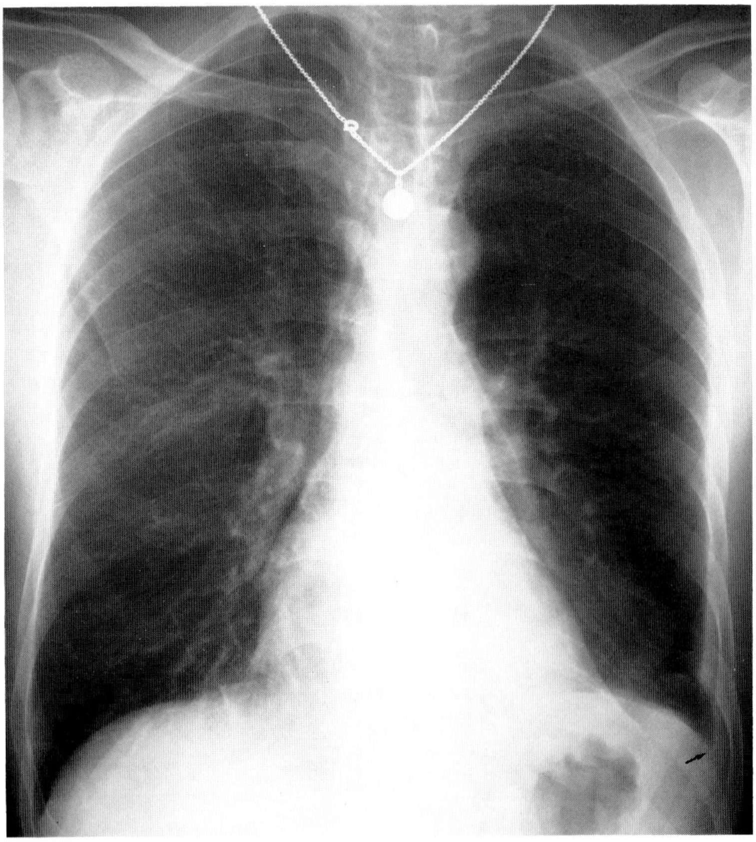

Fig. 8.4. A 47-year-old man after a collision while playing soccer. Small hematothorax on the left (*arrow*). No visible fracture of the ribs.

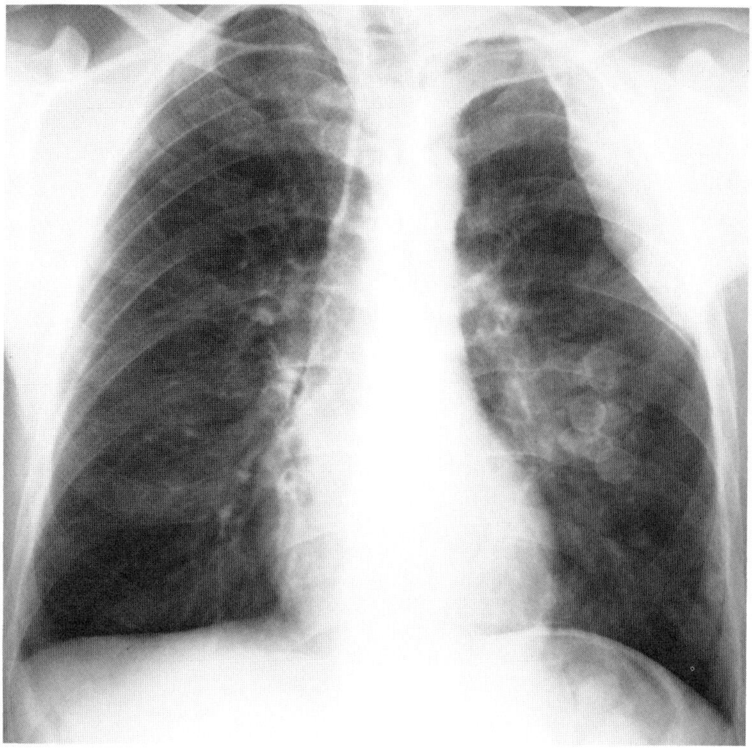

Fig. 8.5. A 34-year-old man with a single fracture of the 4th left rib in the anterior axillary line; old oleothorax with small individual droplets of oil that have descended into the pleural space.

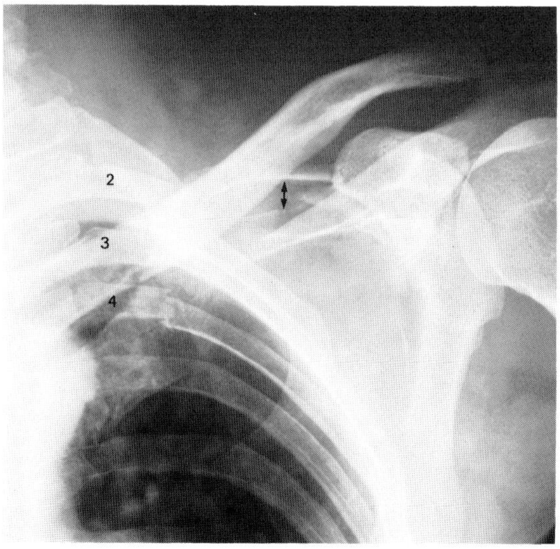

Fig. 8.6. A 67-year-old man after an accident on a farm. Series of fractures on the left 2nd to 4th dorsal ribs, together with a fracture of the scapula (*arrow*). Minimal reaction of the pleura below the dislocated 2nd rib.

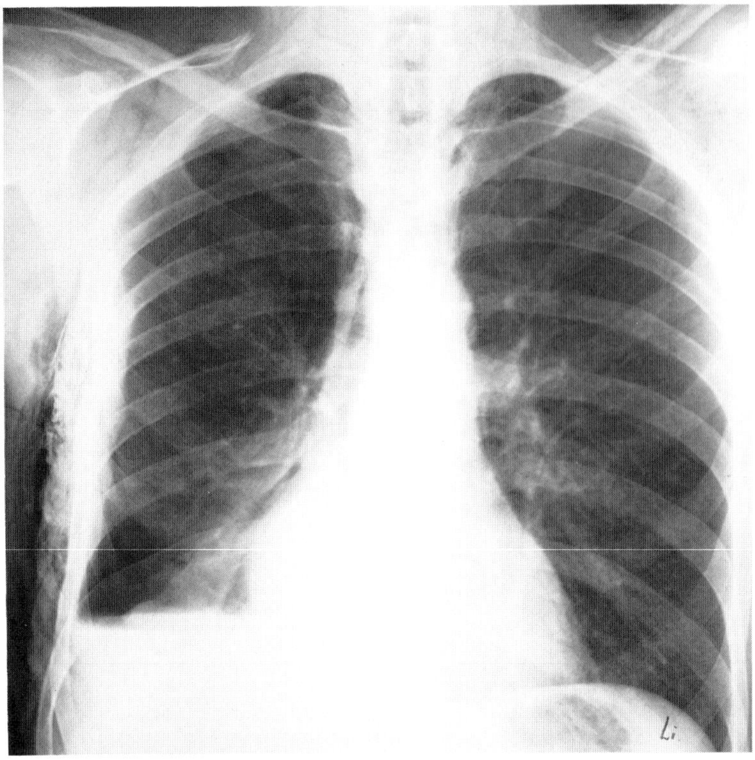

Fig. 8.7. A 39-year-old man who was a passenger in a car in an accident. Series of fractured ribs on the right; hematopneumothorax, emphysema of the skin laterally and emphysema of the mediastinum.

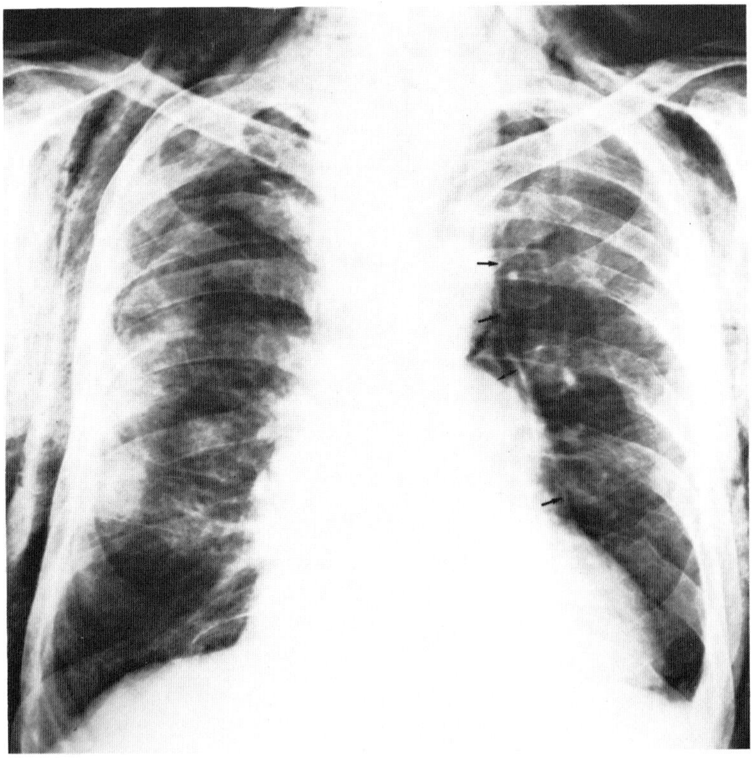

Fig. 8.8. A 52-year-old man after a fall from a car in a vineyard. Extensive series of fractures of the ribs on the right, with marked dislocation. Fresh and old fractures of the ribs on the left. Life-threatening emphysema in the subcutaneous and mediastinal areas *(horizontal arrows)*. Pneumothorax on the right.

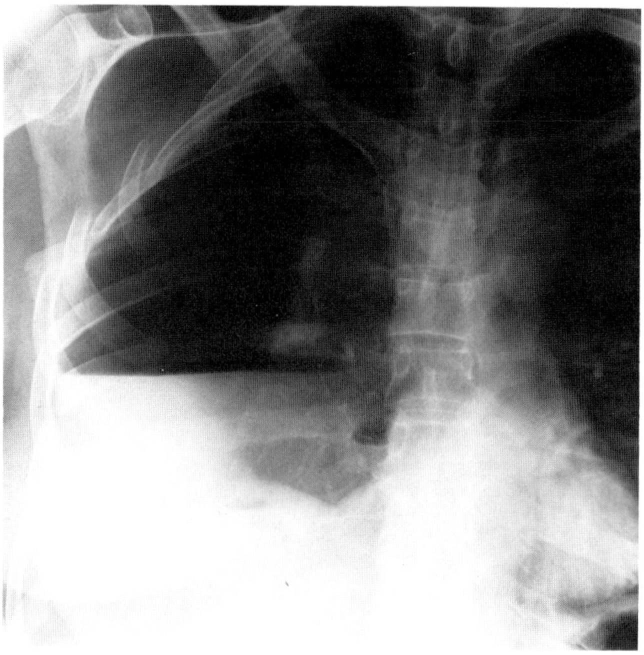

Fig. 8.9. A 48-year-old woman after being catapulted from a car. Series of rib fractures 1-10 on the right; chest wall fractures, 3–5; fracture of the right clavicle, fractures of the 1st to the 4th ribs on the left. Small degree of subcutaneous emphysema on the right. 4 weeks after the accident, sudden appearance of an extensive hematopneumothorax and marked dislocation of the ruptured ribs on the right.

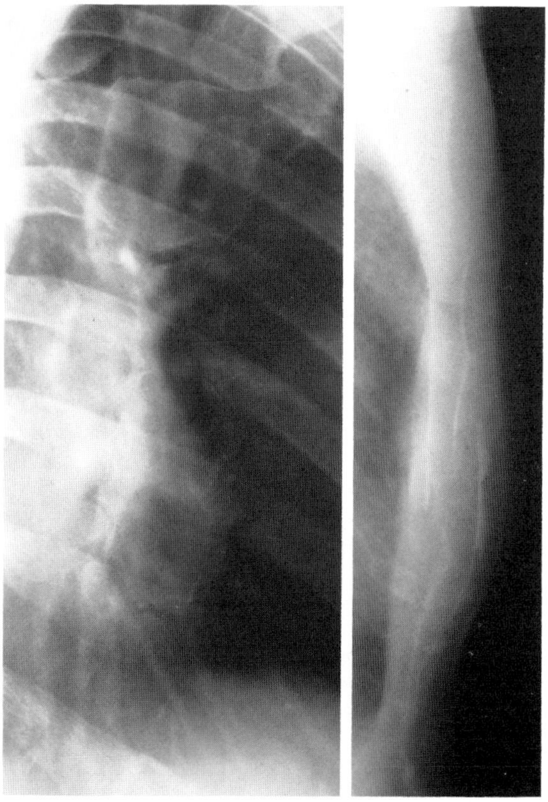

a b

Fig. 8.10a and b. A 46-year-old man after a fall from a scaffold. Complete fracture of the body of the sternum, with dislocation by the thickness of the bone. Even with a special oblique view of the sternum and the good quality of the films, this fracture cannot be confirmed.

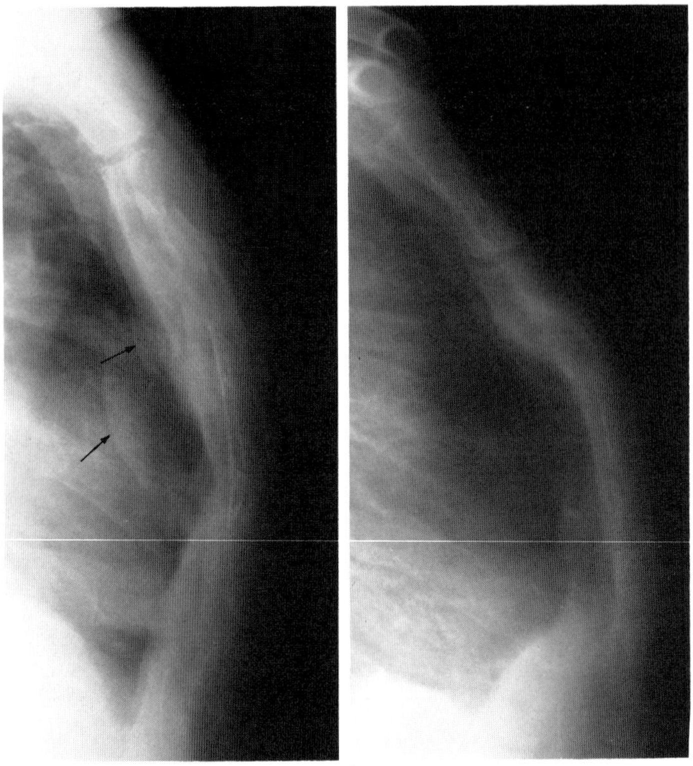

Fig. 8.11a and b. A 63-year-old man after an accident on a farm. Fracture of the body of the sternum, with well-demonstrable dislocation internally. Retrosternal hematoma. Follow-up after 5 months shows bony consolidation.

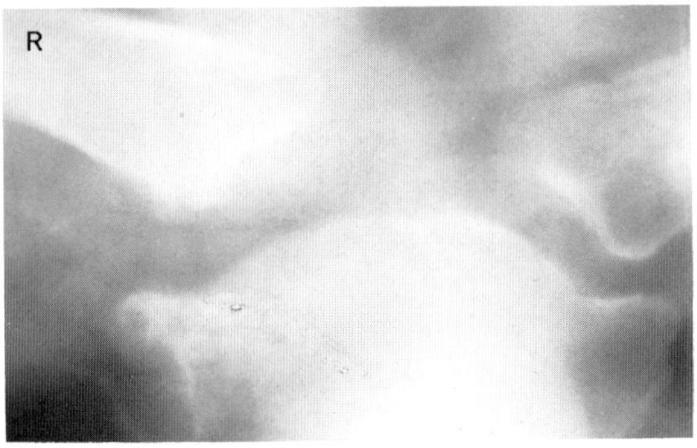

Fig. 8.12. A 38-year-old man after a car accident; subluxation of the right sternoclavicular joint. Tomogram.

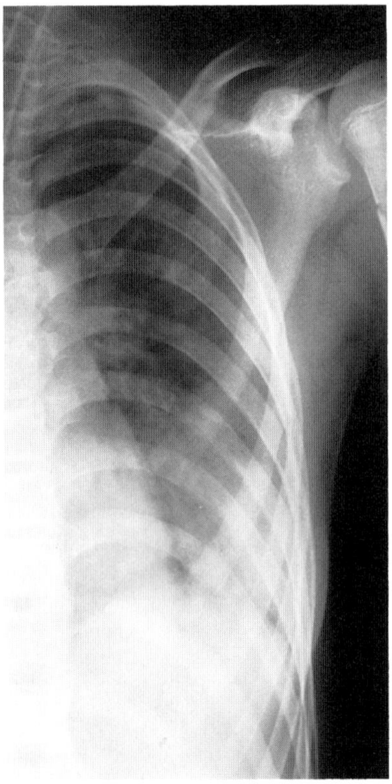

Fig. 8.13. A 12-year-old girl who was hit by a car while on a bicycle. Contusion of the left lung. Extensive patchy opacification of the left lower lung area. Fracture of the clavicle, the humerus on the left and the 12th rib on the left posteriorly.

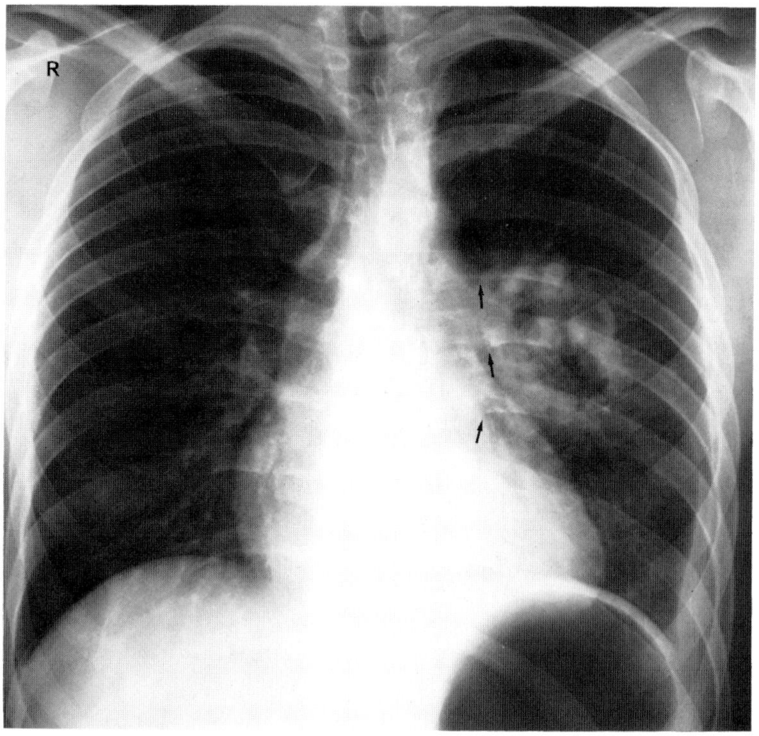

Fig. 8.14. A 22-year-old man after a traffic accident. Contusion of the lung on the left, with hematoma of the lung in its midregion. Hematothorax. Paravertebral fractures of ribs 5 to 8 on the left.

Fig. 8.15. Traumatic cyst of the lung, with an air-fluid level in the right middle lung field four hours after bilateral chest trauma. (From C. J. Fagan: Am. J. Roentgenol. *97:* 186, 1966.)

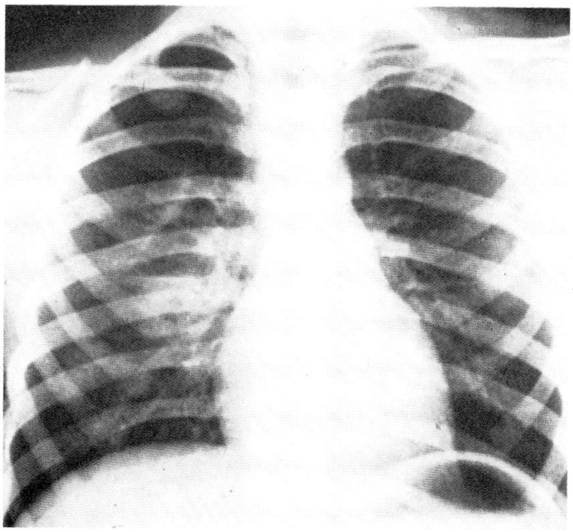

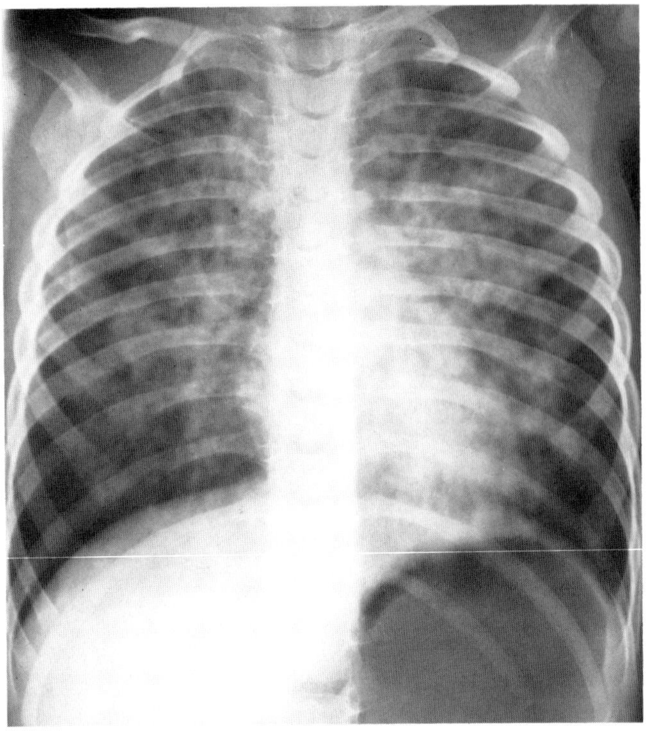

Fig. 8.16. A 2½-year-old child after a fall into a rainwater container. Eventually good outcome. Extensive patchy areas of densities bilaterally as a result of water aspiration. Enormous air accumulation in the stomach.

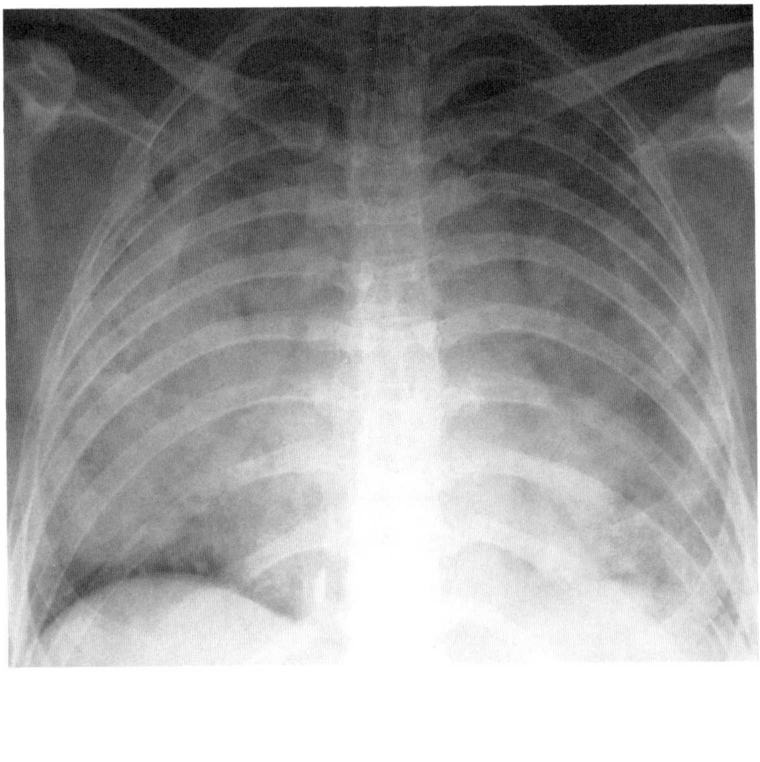

Fig. 8.17. A 51-year-old woman who died as a result of severe edema of the lungs after an explosion of gas which caused first-, second- and third-degree burns over the entire body.

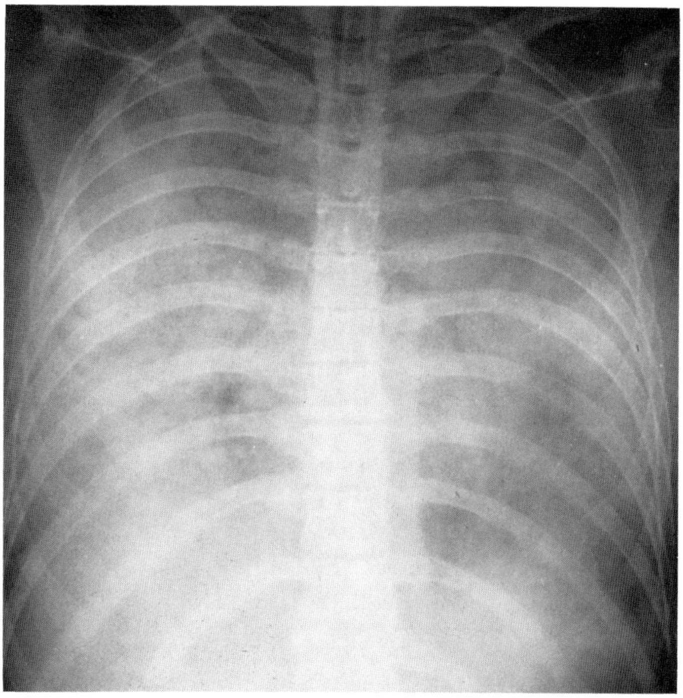

Fig. 8.18. A 25-year-old woman who died as a result of interstitial edema of the lungs after intoxication with sleeping pills (carbamide).

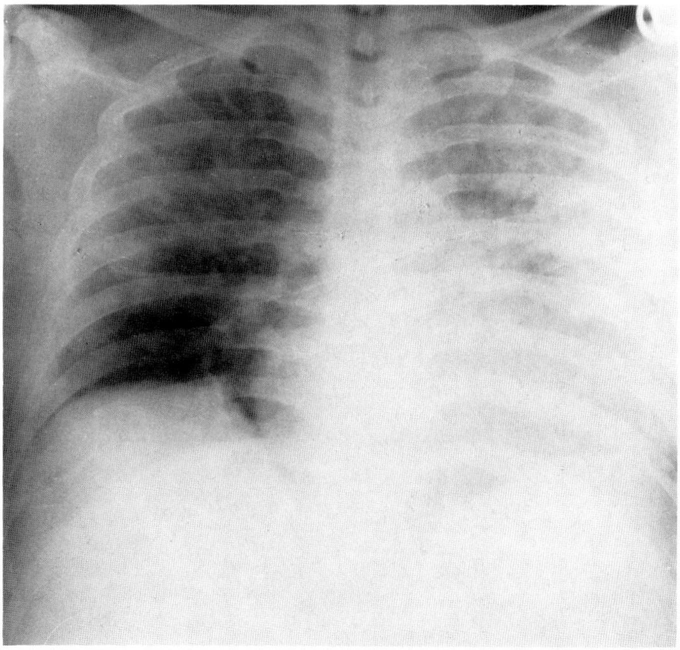

Fig. 8.19. A 30-year-old man with fractures of the femur and shank. Edemalike opacification of the lung, in this case due to fat embolism.

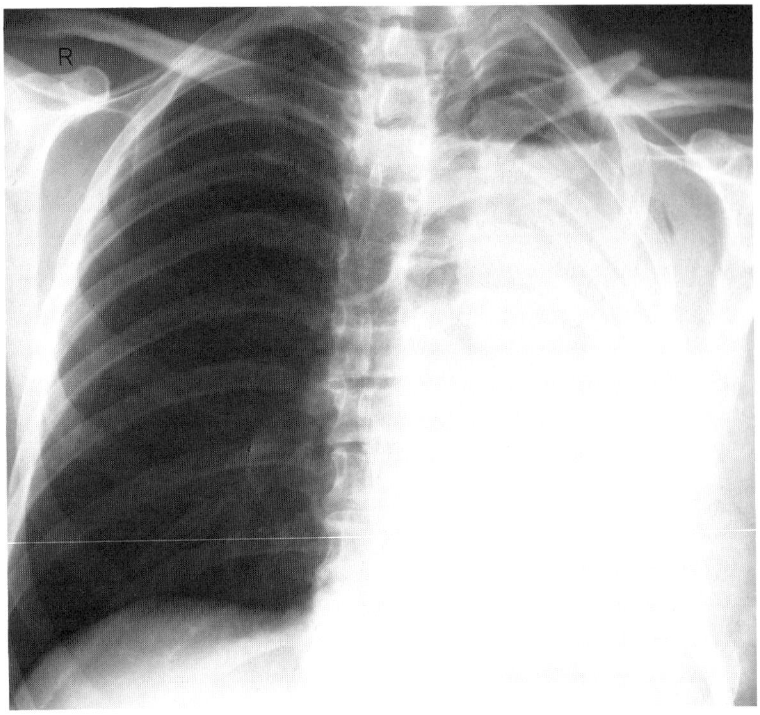

Fig. 8.20. A 45-year-old man after a motorcycle collision with a car. Torsion of the left lower lobe of the lung. Marked displacement toward the left of the mediastinum as a result of atelectasis. Massive hemato-pneumothorax. Fracture of the thoracic wall and clavicle on the left.

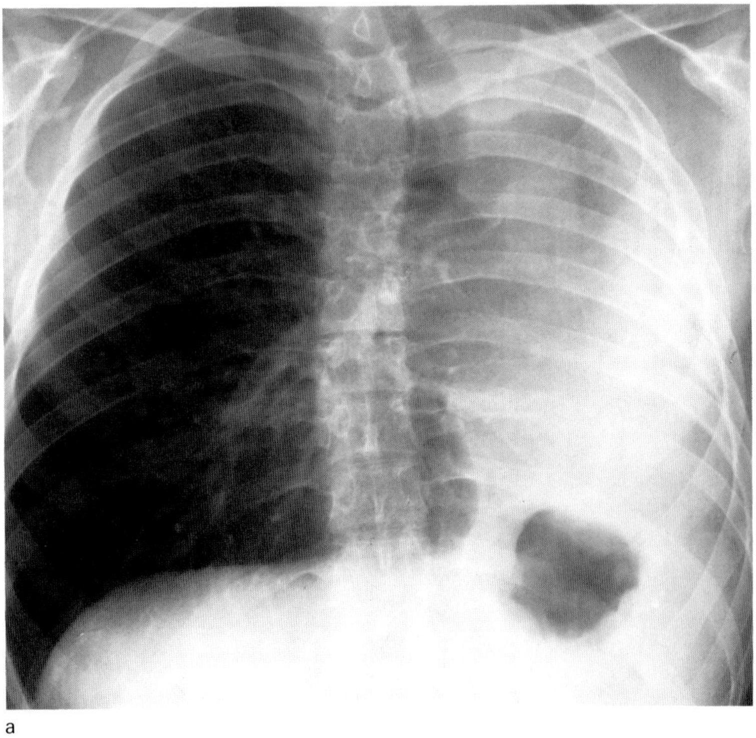

a

Fig. 8.21a–c. A 21-year-old man with a rupture of the left main-stem bronchus. Diagnosis delayed. Atelectasis of the left lung and thickening of the pleura.

a) A. p. survey film.
b) Tomogram.
c) Bronchogram.

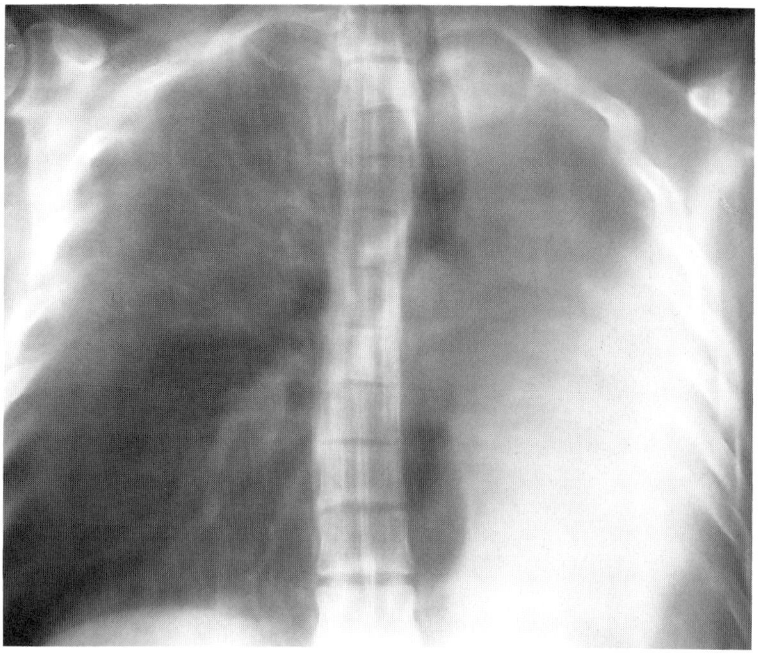

Fig. 8.21b

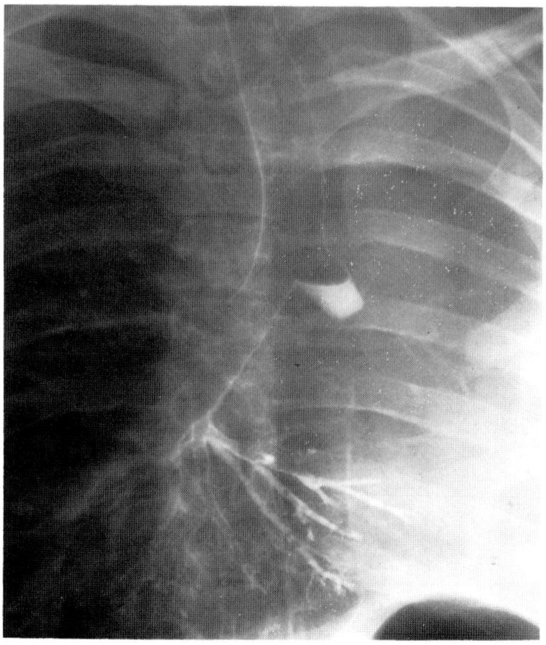

Fig. 8.21c

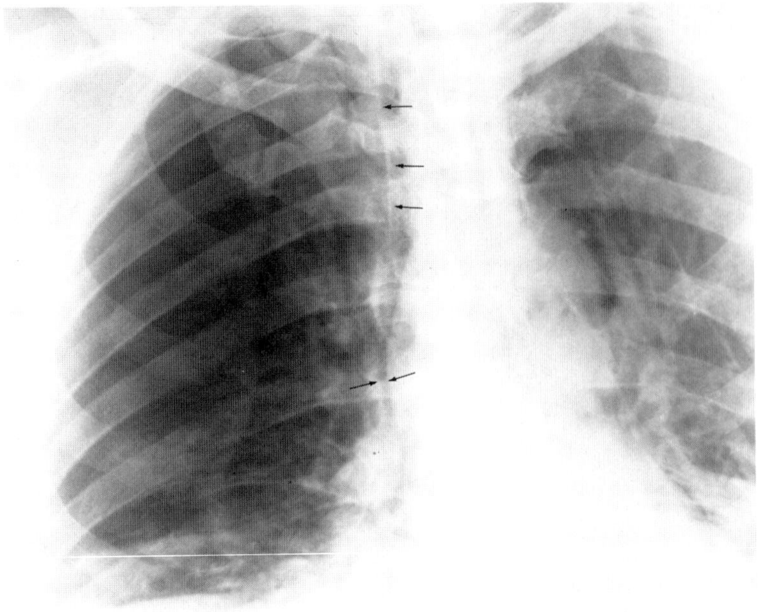

Fig. 8.22a

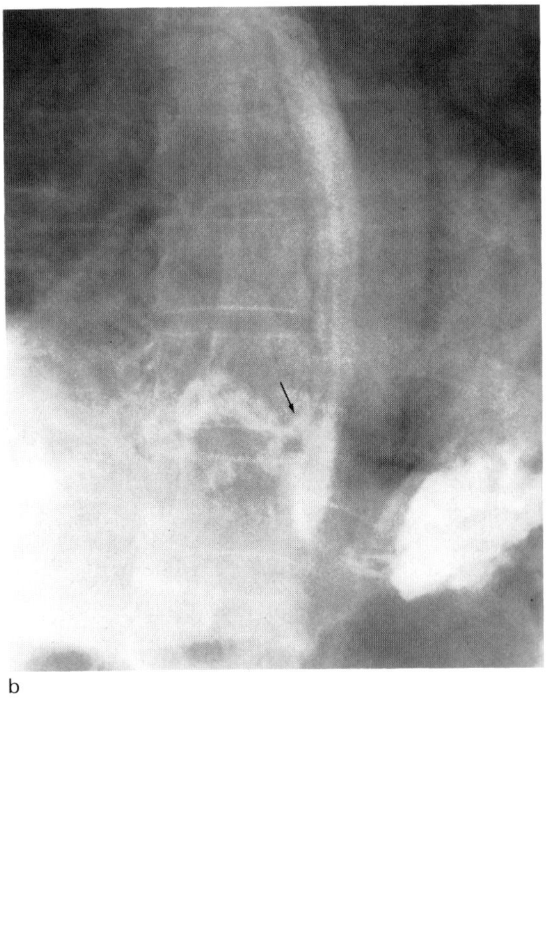

b

Fig. 8.22a and b. A 58-year-old man after gastroscopy. Operation and subsequent healing. Perforation of the esophagus in its lower 3rd on the right. The survey film shows a pneumomediastinum and pneumothorax on the right. Investigation with Gastrografin reveals the area of perforation and accumulation of the contrast agent in the pleural space.

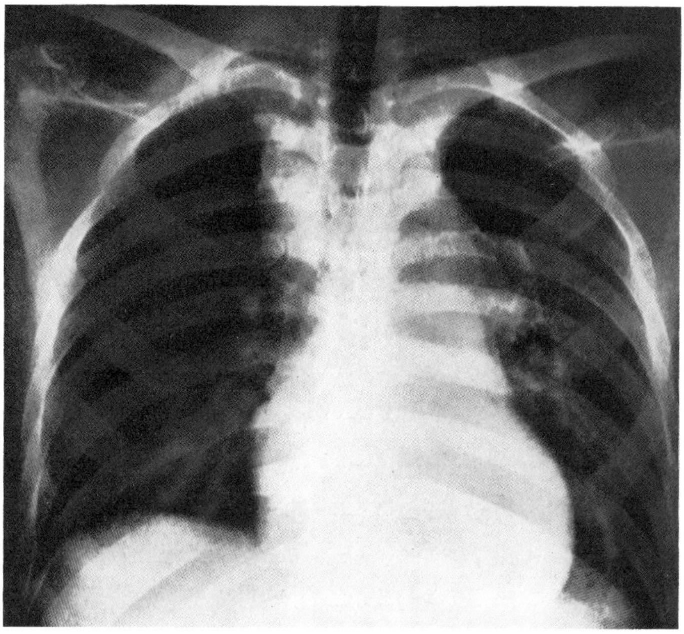

Fig. 8.23a

Fig. 8.23a and b. a) Incomplete rupture of the aorta. A.p. film of the thorax 24 hours after the accident; widening of the mediastinum toward the left.
b) Angiogram; spindlelike widening and dissection of the descending aorta. (From F. Kümmerle: Hefte zur Unfallheilkunde, H. 81: 21, 1965.)

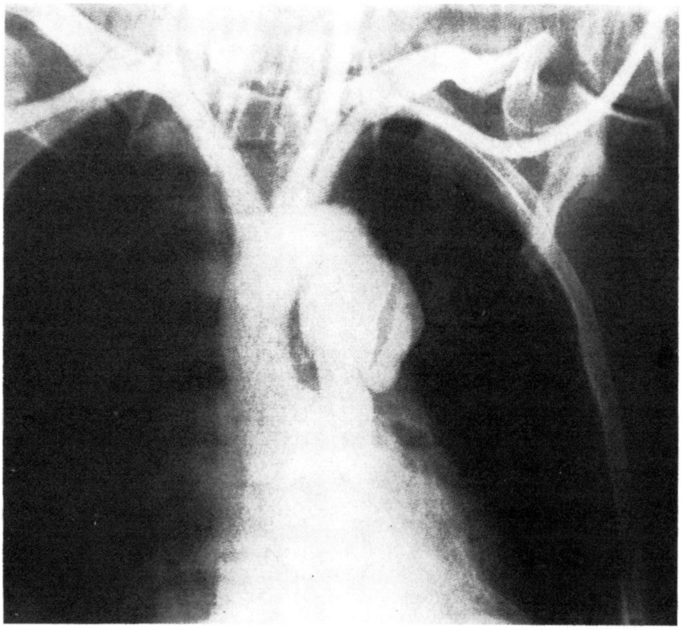

b

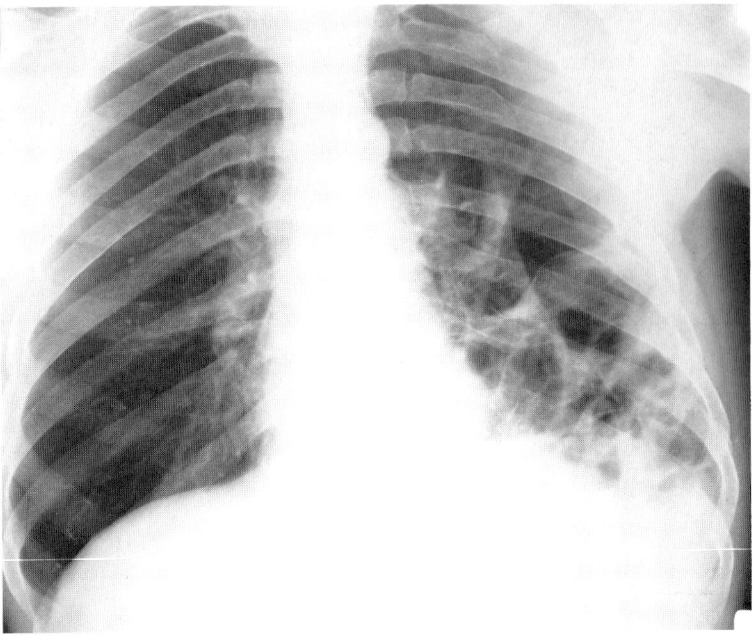

Fig. 8.24a

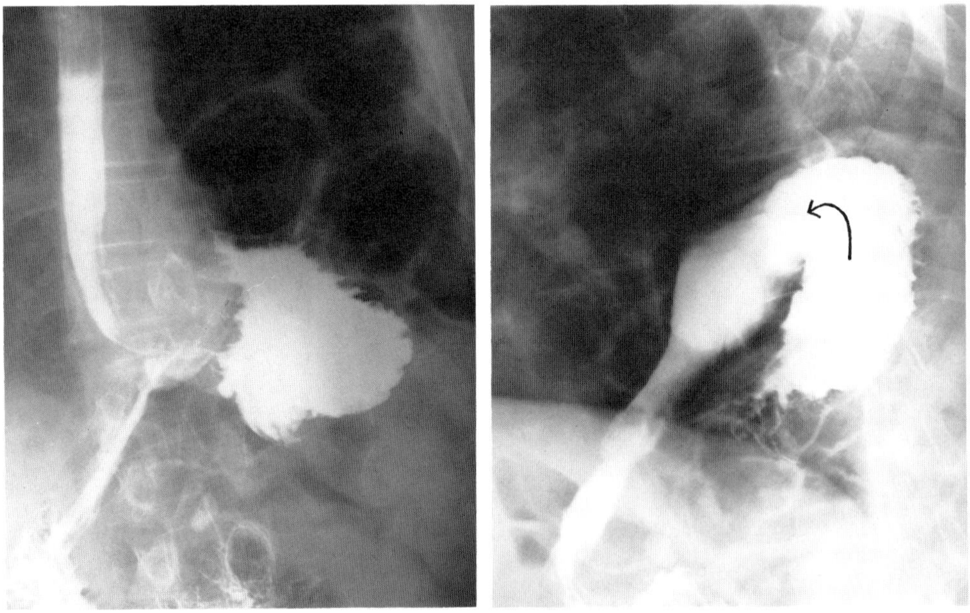

Fig. 8.24b c

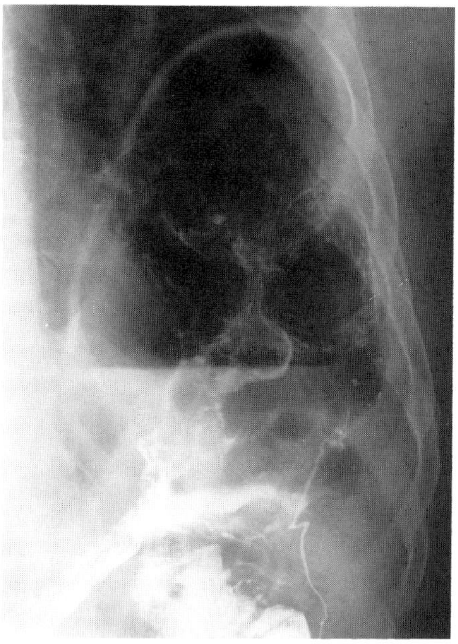
Fig. 8.24d

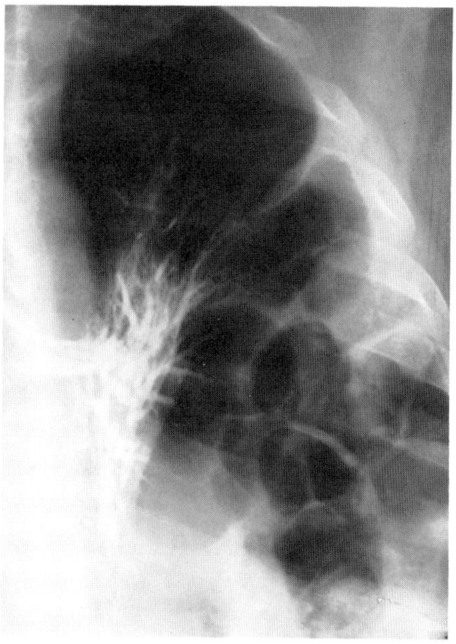
e

Fig. 8.24a–f. A 49-year-old man with a rupture of the left diaphragm after a fall from a poplar tree, about 4 meters high, one year ago.

◀ a) Thoracic survey film. Rupture of the left diaphragm, with prolapse of the abdominal organs. Fully consolidated fractures of the 3rd to 5th ribs in the scapular line and the 5th to 8th ribs in the posterior axillary line.

◀ b and c) Investigation with a contrast agent showing the displaced stomach; typical curving of the stomach cranially and displacement of the gastric body.

d) Contrast within the colon.

e) Bronchogram to demonstrate the compression of the lung and bronchi, particularly in the lower lobe area.

f) Chest films 7 months after corrective surgery. There is now only minimal scarring of the pleura on the left base laterally.

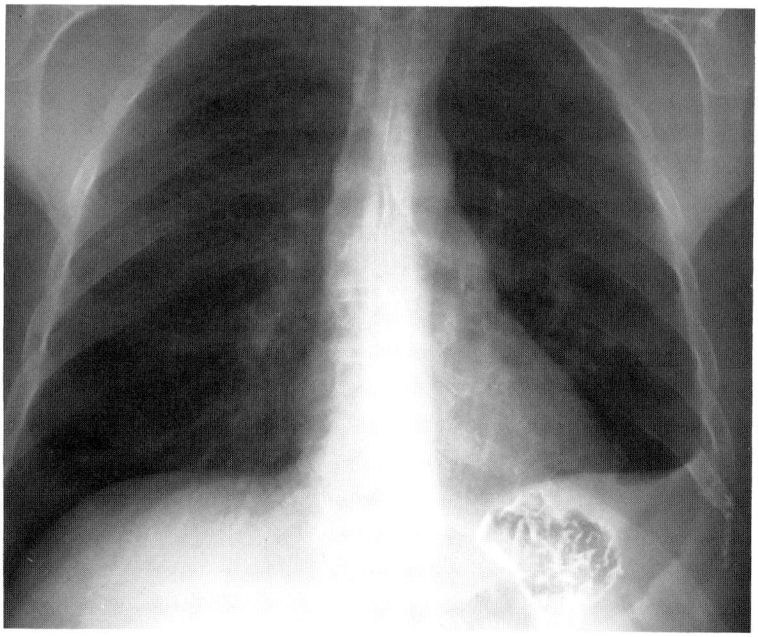
Fig. 8.24f

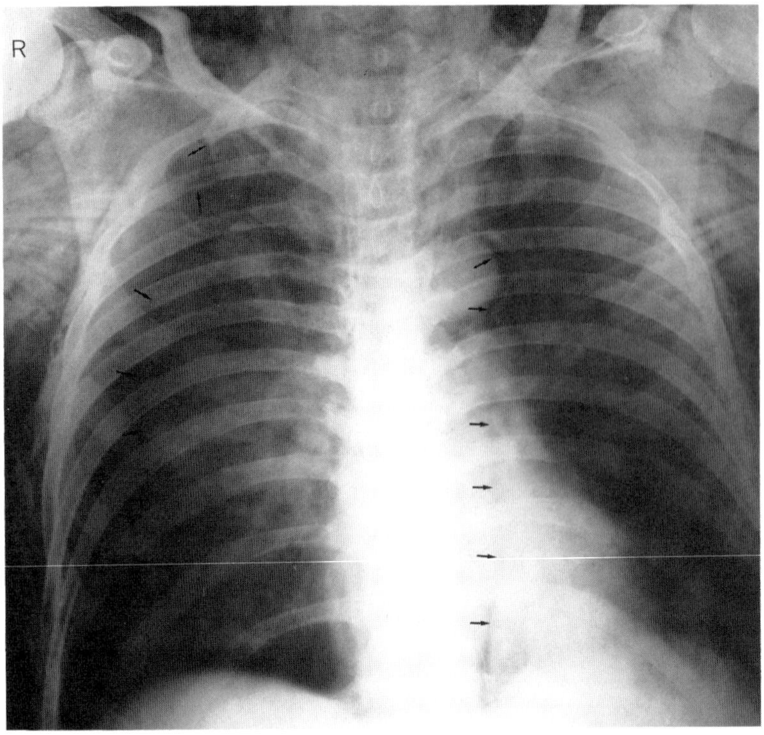

Fig. 8.25a

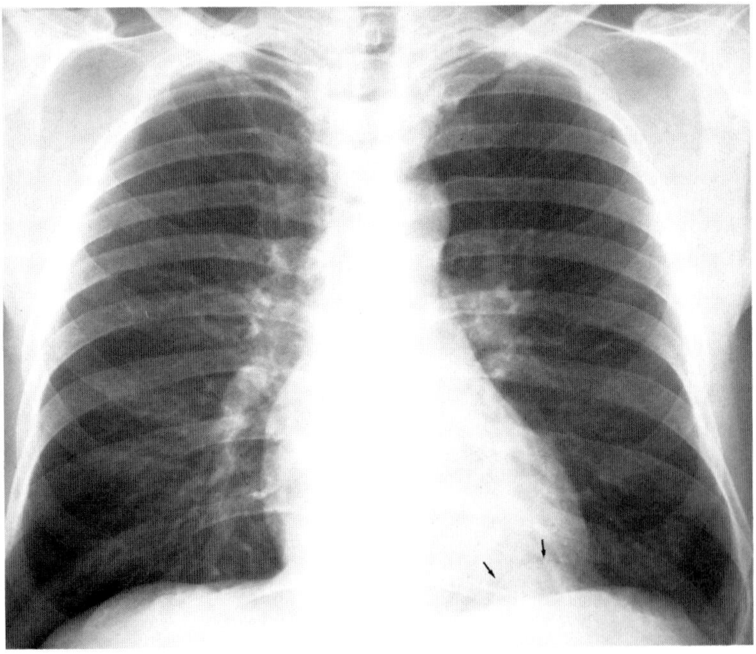

Fig. 8.25b

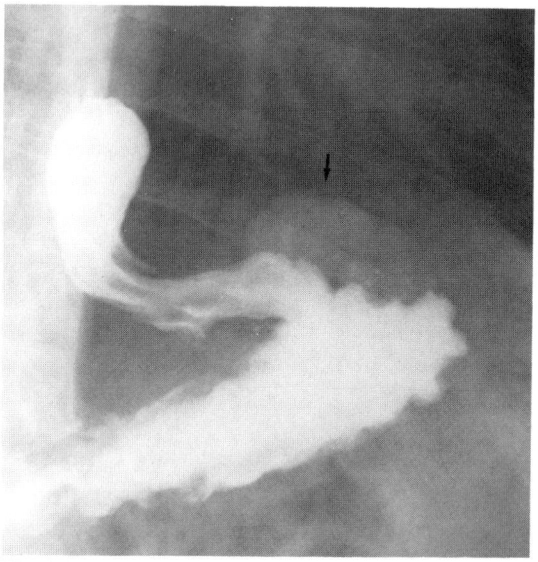

Fig. 8.25c

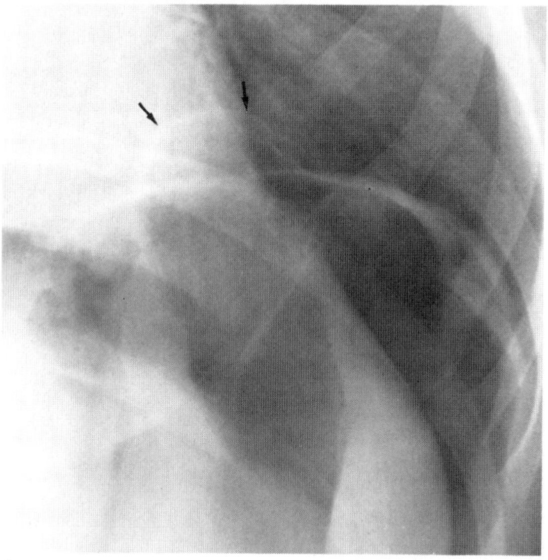

d

Fig. 8.25a–d. A 32-year-old man who sustained a steering-wheel injury to the chest cage in a collision. Traumatic herniation of the diaphragm on the left.
a) Immediately after the accident: pneumothorax on the right; pneumomediastinum; air around the aorta. Massive subcutaneous emphysema, with feathering in the area of the pectoral muscle. Fracture of the 1st and 3rd ribs on the right and the 2nd rib on the left.
b) At investigation prior to discharge 4 weeks after the accident: rounded opacification above the left diaphragm.
c) Contrast investigation of the stomach reveals signs of a diaphragmatic hernia with a prolapsed stomach.
d) Proof of the diagnosis after pneumoperitoneum. The gas (N_2O) migrates into the peritoneal sac.

Fig. 8.26. A 60-year-old woman after being hit by a car on the street. Cerebral concussion; contusion of the thorax; combined pelvic fracture, with extraperitoneal rupture of the bladder. Fracture of the shank. Diaphragmatic rupture on the left, with prolapse of the abdominal organs into the pleural and pericardial spaces. Delayed incarceration. Eight months after the accident, sudden clinical signs and symptoms of an acute abdomen. Radiologically there is incarceration of the colon, with ileus. Surgical intervention. Intrapleural fixation of about 30 cm. of colon; prolapse of parts of the colon, the fundus of the stomach and the left lobe of the liver into the pericardial sac.

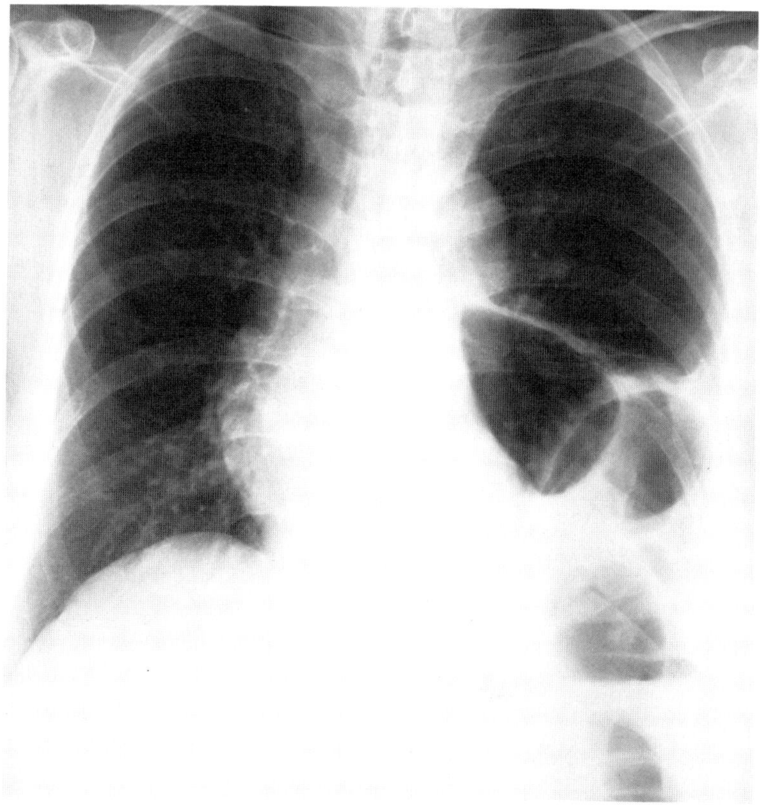

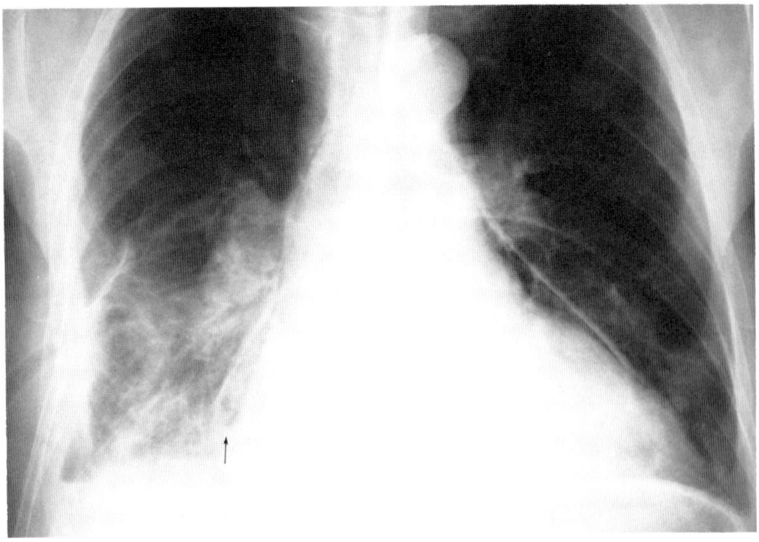

Fig. 8.27. A 60-year-old man with pneumopericardium after a stabbing injury to the pericardial sac. Hemorrhage into the lung and pleura and, to a lesser degree, into the pericardium (*arrow*).

9 Abdomen

Blunt trauma to the abdomen, forces hitting the abdomen broadly and penetrating abdominal injuries are particularly dangerous because of possible internal hemorrhage or peritonitis. An exact history or visible external marks may be very helpful if there is a limited direct effect of forces such as a fist blow, a kick or other type of blow. Often it is impossible to decide immediately if there is a simple contusion of the abdomen or if there are internal injuries. Only the later clinical course and observation of the patient will tell. Hemorrhage from natural orifices or from a catheter placed in the stomach or bladder always is a direct sign of an internal injury. Because the unclear clinical symptoms are often somewhat misleading in the presence of coexisting injuries, it is particularly important to conduct a thorough radiologic investigation. This should immediately follow the clinical examination. The radiologist must pay special attention to lifethreatening conditions such as disturbed respiration and circulation. The x-ray investigation may have to await improvement of the patient's general condition.

Accidents usually associated with abdominal injury are, in the order of decreasing incidence: traffic accidents; injury due to a direct kick; a blow, push or fall from a great height; a fall during sports or everyday activities; getting crushed; and being buried alive. Obviously, gunshot or stabbing accidents do carry a very high risk of injury to internal organs. According to Vielberg and Schnepper (1966); the incidence of injury to individual organs after blunt abdominal trauma is: spleen, 30 per cent; liver, 25 per cent; kidney, 20 per cent, gut, 10 per cent; omentum, 7 per cent; bladder, 3 per cent; stomach, 2 per cent; pancreas, uterus and gallbladder, 1 per cent. Concomitant injury, according to Klieber (1958), occurs in the following percentage distribution: thorax, 28 per cent; skull, 12 per cent; extremities, 10 per cent; spine, 5 per cent; pelvis, 4 per cent.

Figure 9.1 is a schematic survey of the radiologic symptoms of abdominal injuries. Injuries to the diaphragm have already been discussed in detail in Chapter 8.

Considering the danger to the patient's life with injuries accompanied by shock, one must attempt to arrive at as reliable a diagnosis as possible from simple survey films. If, however, this is not possible with the clinical findings, contrast examination and visualization of parenchymatous organs, hollow organs and the vasculature must be performed.

As a nonspecific symptom, one frequently sees, even with simple contusion of the abdomen, dilatation and meteorism within the area of the gastrointestinal tract as an expression of local loss of tonicity (Fig. 9.2).

Hematoma of the abdominal wall, with bleeding into the musculature or into the extraperitoneal fatty tissue, can be recognized radiologically by soft tissue opacification. This finding must be distinguished from intraperitoneal hemorrhage and is important for the simple reason that it marks the immediate area of impact. As a result of pain and as a positional response to it, there is usually skoliosis, with the concavity directed toward the affected side, particularly with muscular involvement.

Accumulation of free fluid within the peritoneal cavity (such as in hemorrhage) depending on its localization, can result in a somewhat circumscribed or diffuse opacification that is visible especially in the lateral and marginal areas of the abdomen and the inner pelvic region. If there are doubts about the presence of a hematoperitoneum, a diagnostic pneumoperitoneum will fully clarify the situation. If there is free blood, there will be an air-fluid level. Due to fibrinous changes, the peritoneal surface may not always be completely flat; occasionally one finds deposits of fibrin on the parietal or visceral peritoneum (Fig. 9.3). A massive hematoperitoneum, with displacement of the colon from the lateral abdominal wall (Fig. 9.4) or displacement of gas-containing bowel loops, is the result (Fig. 9.5); in the absence of gas within the bowel, the exact course of the colon can readily be visualized by rectal air insufflation.

Retroperitoneal hemorrhages will result in the disappearance of the psoas shadow and possibly also the renal shadow on the involved side and, within the pelvis, an opacification extending from the bladder to the os pubis, frequently in association with displacement of the bladder to the contralateral side (Figs. 9.6 and 9.7). Abdominal hemorrhage always raises the suspicion of an organ injury. The intraperitoneal or retroperitoneal location of the hematoma will indicate the organs actually affected. Intraparenchymatous or subcapsular hemorrhage will always result in an increase in size of the organ. A complete rupture will result in the disappearance of the normally visible borders of a given organ.

The most common injury to an internal organ after blunt abdominal trauma is rupture of the spleen. We distinguish primary and secondary or delayed rupture of the spleen. The latter will develop from an initially intracapsular hemorrhage, with rupture of the capsule hours, days and even several weeks after the actual trauma as the result of constantly increasing pressure within the organ. Such delayed rupture also has been seen to affect the liver, gut, kidney and diaphragm but occurs with the highest incidence within the spleen. The mortality of rupture of the spleen, if there is no surgical intervention, is 90 per cent; after surgical intervention for simple rupture of the spleen, 0 to 20 per cent; and for complicated injuries of the spleen (rupture and severe concomitant injuries, particularly within the abdominal area), 40 to 80 per cent (Lorenz, 1966).

The radiologic findings in rupture of the spleen are: opacification of the left upper quadrant; hematoperitoneum located between the descending colon and the parietal peritoneum; displacement of the stomach (possibly reduced air or contrast filling) toward the right and inferiorly; displacement of the left splenic flexure of the colon inferiorly; elevation of the left diaphragm; loss of detail of the left psoas shadow and of the renal outline; and displacement or compression of the left kidney (Fig. 9.8). Schorr and Danon (1967) have described a valuable symptom visible on a.p. views in the left lateral decubitus position. In order to obtain this information, it is important to have a slight degree of contrast filling of the stomach. As the result of enlargement of the spleen and the perisplenic hematoma, there is a mildly concave impression on the greater curvature of the stomach, its location remaining at some distance from the lateral abdominal wall. The direct angiographic confirmation of a ruptured spleen is technically much more demanding. Premature venous filling and small contrast extravasation, filling defects during the parenchymatous phase and interruptions of the contour of the organ, as well as displacement and deformity of the vessels, are proof of direct injury to the organ (Fig. 9.9). Despite the possibility of direct angiographic documentation it is recommended that the x-ray diagnosis of rupture of the spleen be based on the simpler noninvasive methods with the smallest risks. With good and reliable technique and a careful approach to interpretation based on sound experience, it is often possible to arrive at a reliable diagnosis. After the spleen, the liver has the next highest incidence of organ injury due to blunt abdominal trauma. Differentiation should be made between subcapsular hematoma and central and open rupture. The danger of injury to the liver is twofold: internal hemorrhage and bile peritonitis. Formerly, there was a lethality of over 60 per cent (Reifferscheidt, quoted from Lorenz, 1966). Only in the past 20 years have advances in surgery and the possibility of properly managing the very high incidence of postoperative complications improved this situation considerably. Subcapsular hemorrhage and central rupture may be very difficult to diagnose; it is entirely possible that they sometimes remain unrecognized and healing occurs with the possibility of formation of a pseudocyst. Hematobilia as a result of parenchymatous lesions of ruptured vessels or bile ducts may remain hidden for some time.

Radiologically the intracapsular injury of the liver is noticeable because of an increase in size of the liver shadow and the elevation and reduced excursions of the right diaphragm. Air bubbles within the liver are a highly reliable sign of central rupture. For further diagnostic clarification, one can resort to intravenous and intraoperative cholangiography and celiacography. Intraoperative cholangiography will demonstrate lesions of the bile ducts; arteriography will show vascular lesions, directly or by the displacement and abnormal appearance of the vessels (Fig. 9.10). In the case of rupture of the liver and its capsule, there may be massive bleeding into the peritoneal cavity. The roentgenogram will show a dense opacification of the upper abdominal region prominently on the right; elevation of the right diaphragm; a lack in contours of the liver, the kidney and the psoas shadow; and displacement of the transverse colon and the hepatic flexure (Fig. 9.11). Occasionally rupture will occur in liver with a preexisting abnormal local condition; this was described by Hodel (1968) as a "pathologic rupture" of the liver.

Types of injury to the gastrointestinal canal are: contusion, rupture, perforation (such as by projectile, stabbing or foreign-body injury) and complete avulsion. Contusions are usually the result of localized forces; rupture and avulsion are often due to large objects hitting the abdomen or a fall from a great height. About 80 per cent of blunt abdominal trauma and 25 to 40 per cent of perforating abdominal injuries will involve the small bowel (Lorenz, 1966; Kümmerle, 1959). The outcome of injury to gastrointestinal structures will depend largely on an early surgical intervention (Kümmerle, 1959). Even in the absence of radiologic findings, surgery is indicated if, within 6 hours after the trauma, the presenting abdominal pain and tenderness do not decrease (Boosworth, quoted after Lorenz,1966). After a simple contusion, there may be, as a reflex, loss of tonicity. This will be demonstrated on a roentgenogram as a dilatation of the affected portion of the gastrointestinal canal. Hematoma of the bowel wall, most frequently localized within the duodenum, may lead to a local stenosis. This finding may be documented by contrast agent visualizing the stomach and duodenum only (Fig. 9.12). In injuries of the gastrointestinal tract (especially of the stomach) with direct perforation (rupture or avulsion), there will be a subphrenic half-moon as a result of free gas within the abdominal cavity; this is the same sign seen after perforation of an ulcer. In order to fully appreciate this finding, however, x-rays are needed with the patient in the standing or sitting posture. Perforation or rupture of the gut will not show this finding as frequently and there may be only minimal free air. It should be possible to demonstrate free air within the abdominal cavity in about 80 per cent of all traumatic perforations. The absence of free air never completely excludes the possibility of a perforation. If, because of loss of consciousness or other major symptoms, it is not possible to obtain views with the upper part of the body in the vertical position, one should at least obtain an a.p.view with the patient supine and one additional view in the left lateral decubitus position. Often free intraperitoneal air will then be visible as a rounded "half-moon" within the upper abdomen or as a sickle at the lower rim of the liver; if the x-ray is taken in the left lateral decubitus position there will be a greater accumulation of free air between the liver and the right inner abdominal wall (Figs. 9.13 and 9.14). If air escapes from a perforation by way of an abdominal wall rupture, there will be soft-tissue emphysema of the thorax and abdomen; free air then may not be visible below the diaphragm (Fig. 9.15).

Perforation of those parts of the gut localized retroperitoneally will result in a characteristic x-ray appearance. There will be free gas in the retroperitoneal space, particularly in the perirenal region (Fig. 9.16).

In some geographic areas, perforating projectile or knife injuries are the chief cause of perforating abdominal trauma involving the gut. Thus Morton and Jordan (1968) report that in Houston, Texas, among 131 open duodenal injuries, there were 14 blunt abdominal traumas but 15 projectile and 22 stabbing injuries. Obviously the number of additional penetrating injuries to other abdominal organs is particularly high in this group: liver, 38 per cent; transverse colon, 30 per cent; small bowel, 29 per cent; pancreas, 28 per cent; stomach, 24 per cent; kidney, 21 per cent; vena cava, 17 per cent; gallbladder, 9 per cent; ureter, 8 per cent; superior mesenteric artery, 7 per cent; aorta, renal arteries and choledochal duct, 5 per cent. If the connection of a penetrating injury to the peritoneal cavity and internal organs cannot be fully determined, Cornell et al. (1967) recommend inserting a catheter into the wound and injecting contrast agent. The water-soluble, sterile contrast agent can be mixed with 1 ml. methylene blue in order to mark the course of the perforation which may be helpful during subsequent surgery. The x-rays obtained on two planes and possible additional views (often spot films obtained during fluoroscopy) will allow great accuracy in answering the question of whether there is a communication with the peritoneal cavity (Figs. 9.17 and 9.18).

Isolated injury of the pancreas occurs relatively rarely. During blunt abdominal trauma, the most frequent mechanism is a jolt by the steering wheel in the upper abdominal region during a car accident. The head of the pancreas is most frequently affected but the adjacent organs (duodenum, choledochus, vessels and transverse colon) are quite often also involved. With 53 per cent of steering-wheel injuries being fatal, mortality is very high compared with other blunt injuries of the pancreas (29 per cent) (Wilson et al., 1967). There are concomitant injuries due to blunt abdominal trauma, with pancreatic involvement in 77 per cent and penetrating trauma in 89 per cent. However, based on a larger number, mortality due to penetrating pancreatic injury is with 27 per cent lower than that due to blunt abdominal trauma (38 per cent) (Wilson et al., 1967).

The different types of pancreatic injury – contusion with hemorrhage, rupture, complete avulsion, and fragmentation – cannot be differentiated radiologically. X-ray symptoms strongly indicating an injury to the pancreas are: opacification of the abdominal region; displacement of the body of the stomach and the antrum to the right; displacement of the transverse colon downward, and the so-called pressure symptoms in the area of the left half of the transverse colon and the left kidney (Fig. 9.19). Contrast study of the stomach with water-soluble contrast agent will allow a simultaneous comment on a possible concomitant injury of the stomach or upper small bowel. As a result of contusion of the pancreas, a pseudocyst can develop within days; this occurs most frequently in children. Radiologically, the diagnosis can be made reliably based on an impression upon and displacement of the stomach from behind and displacement of the duodenojejunal flexure downward (Fig. 9.20).

Isolated injury of the gallbladder and bile ducts, the mesentery or omentum and the serosa is rare and hardly ever reason for special radiologic investigations. Rents in the omentum or the mesentery will present with signs and symptoms of intraperitoneal hemorrhage; avulsion of larger mesenteric vessels may lead to a gangrenous bowel, with radiologically demonstrable emphysema of the bowel wall (Fig. 9.21). Including simple contusions, the kidney is the most frequently injured organ in abdominal trauma. Slight contusions may result in hematuria. Thus, kidney injuries can be detected much more readily than those involving other internal organs. Because of its location, the kidney is exposed to direct forces from in front, from behind and from the sides. Rapid deceleration during traffic accidents or a fall from a great height will result in forces pulling at the renal pedicle. Less frequently than simple contusion, we see rupture with subcapsular hematoma, rupture with involvement of the capsule and perirenal hematoma, fragmentation and avulsion of the renal pedicle. Projectile injury of the kidney is among the most severe, with a mortality of over 50 per cent (Heim, according to Lorenz, 1966). Indirect signs of traumatic renal involvement may be fractures of the lower ribs and of the transverse processes or vertebral bodies. In the presence of a right-sided renal injury, there is often also involvement of the liver; if the left side is affected, the spleen. The abdominal survey film with soft technique reveals a vague opacification on the side affected by the retroperitoneal hematoma, with loss of the psoas contour and an increase in size and poor delineation of the kidney itself. Further information may be obtained by intravenous urography which may show a whole series of radiologic findings. There may be a mild degree of caliceal deformity or of difference in contrast delineation when comparing both sides in simple contusion, whereas contrast agent may accumulate the vicinity of the kidney (Fig. 9.22) in rupture of the kidney or in a nonfunctioning kidney. In unilaterally reduced or absent excretion of contrast agent, retrograde pyelography may offer some information on the actual damage (Fig. 9.23). If intravenous or retrograde urography cannot clarify the existing pathology, renal angiography is indicated. This can be performed using the catheter technique or high translumbar direct puncture. Traumatic alterations can be demonstrated directly by this method (Figs. 9.24 and 9.25). It certainly is most unusual to encounter the formation of a collateral circulation in a delayed traumatic occlusion of a renal artery (Fig. 9.26). Occasionally traumatic changes may occur within a kidney already abnormal by some pathologic process. Reiss (1967) reports on the rupture of a renal cyst, and Houston et al. (1968), on the traumatic rupture of a horseshoe kidney.

Besides demonstrating the type and degree of renal trauma, one of the key tasks of the x-ray investigation is to ascertain the presence of a second fully functional kidney. Important radiologic information will determine whether it may be possible to preserve part of the traumatized kidney injuries can be detected much more readily than those involving other internal organs. Because of its location, kidney is exposed to certain the sequelae of trauma, renal angiography will be used with increasing frequency (Bergmann, 1965; Buschmann and Kerk, 1965).

Rupture or avulsion of the ureter is a rare event. The most frequently involved site is the upper portion of the ureter. Because of the other severe injuries accompanying the rupture, the diagnosis may be markedly delayed if one does not attach the proper significance to retroperitoneal fluid accumulation. A retroperitoneal hematoma may cause temporarily, or later result in, stenosis of the ureter (Fig. 9.27). Iatrogenic injuries to the ureter or the renal pelvis luckily are almost always without ill effect (Fig. 9.28).

Injuries to the bladder and the urethra frequently accompany pelvic fractures and have already been discussed. Here they are of interest insofar as contusion of the bladder and rupture and injury of the urethra may occur in the course of blunt or penetrating abdominal trauma without fractures of the pelvis. The radiologic investigation will include sequentially: intravenous urography, cystography, transurethral or suprapubic catheterization and urethrocystography. With respect to rupture of the bladder, one should differentiate between its intraperitoneal and its extraperitoneal location (compare Fig. 4.15). In perineal perforating injuries, there is particular danger to the urethra (Fig. 9.29).

Involvement of the uterus, tubes and ovaries is rare. Radiologically, there will be only mild signs of intraperitoneal hemorrhage. The pregnant uterus is more susceptible to trauma and there may be massive intraperitoneal hemorrhage. Rupture can be recognized by the extrauterine position of the fetus and a large accumulation of free intraperitoneal fluid. The extremely rare rupture of the chylous cisterna will result in the accumulation of chylous ascites.

Traumatic rupture of large arterial or venous structures within the abdominal cavity usually will lead to rapid death. Thus, measures to salvage the patient will usually be to no avail. Vascular occlusion or stenosis due to contusion, however, may be radiologically recognized immediately after trauma or at some later time (Fig. 9.30).

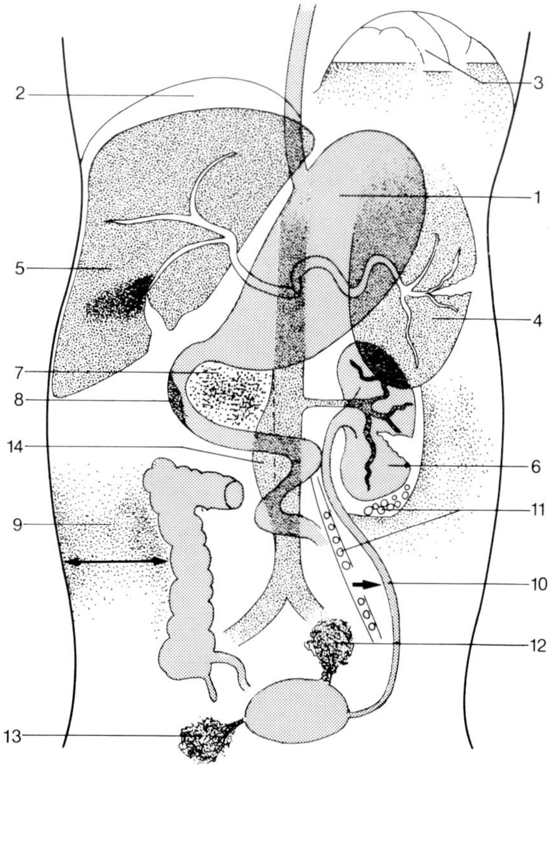

Fig. 9.1. Synopsis of the roentgen findings in abdominal injuries:
1 Reactive dilatation of the stomach
2 Free air in the abdominal cavity (perforation)
3 Ruptured diaphragm
4 Ruptured spleen
5 Ruptured liver
6 Ruptured kidney
7 Ruptured pancreas
8 Intramural hematoma of the gut
9 Intraperitoneal hemorrhage
10 Retroperitoneal hemorrhage
11 Retroperitoneal perforation (gas accumulation beside the psoas and around the kidney)
12 Intraperitoneal rupture of the bladder
13 Extraperitoneal rupture of the bladder
14 Rupture of the abdominal aorta or other blood vessels

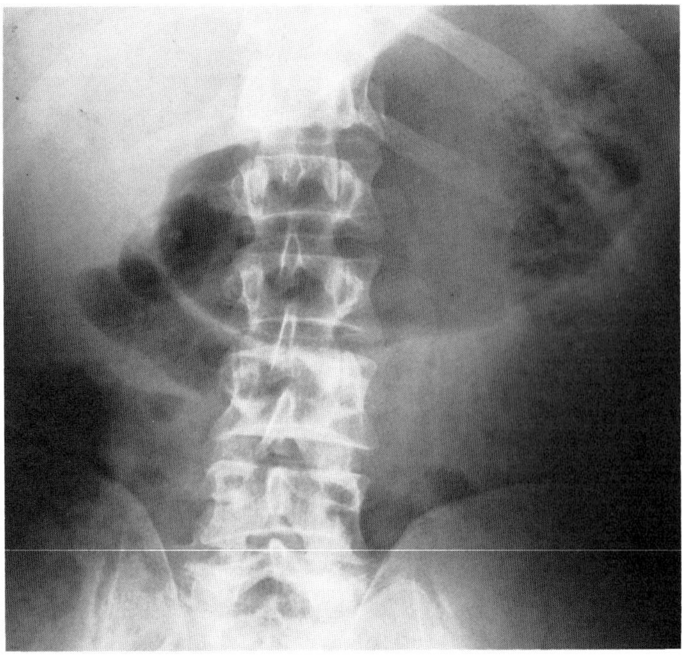

Fig. 9.2. A 26-year-old man after blunt trauma to the abdomen. Traumatic atony with dilatation of the stomach.

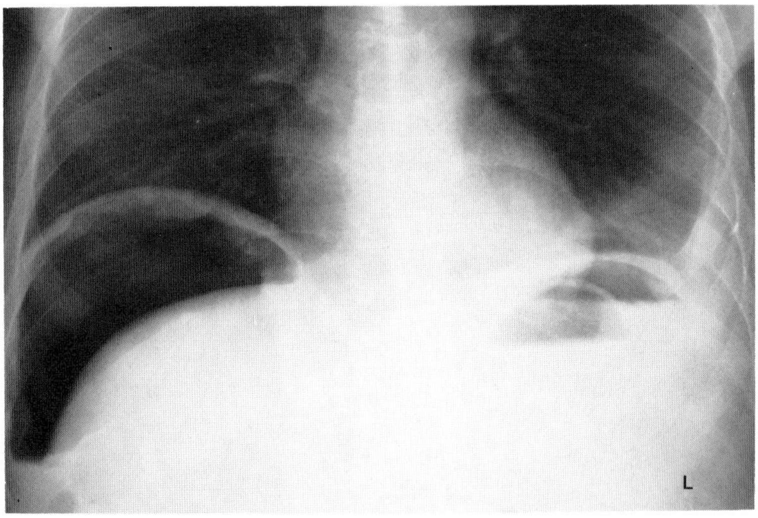

Fig. 9.3. A 21-year-old man after combined blunt trauma to the chest and abdomen. Proof of a hemoperitoneum by diagnostic pneumoperitoneum. Fibrinous alterations in the area of air-fluid level below the gas sickle (N_2O) and between the liver and diaphragm. Deposits of fibrin on the parietal peritoneum.

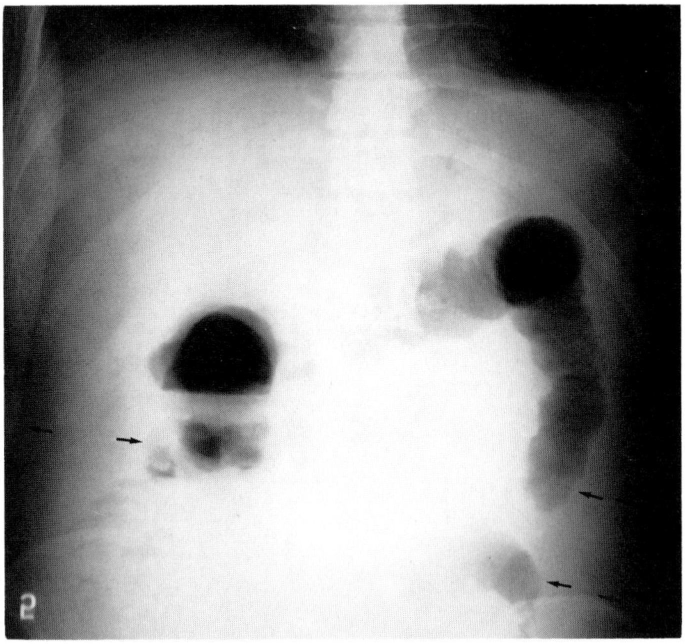

Fig. 9.4. A 30-year-old man after a traffic accident. Massive bleeding into the peritoneal cavity. Fluid accumulation between the parietal peritoneum and the descending colon, with marked displacement of the colon from the lateral abdominal wall (*horizontal arrows*).

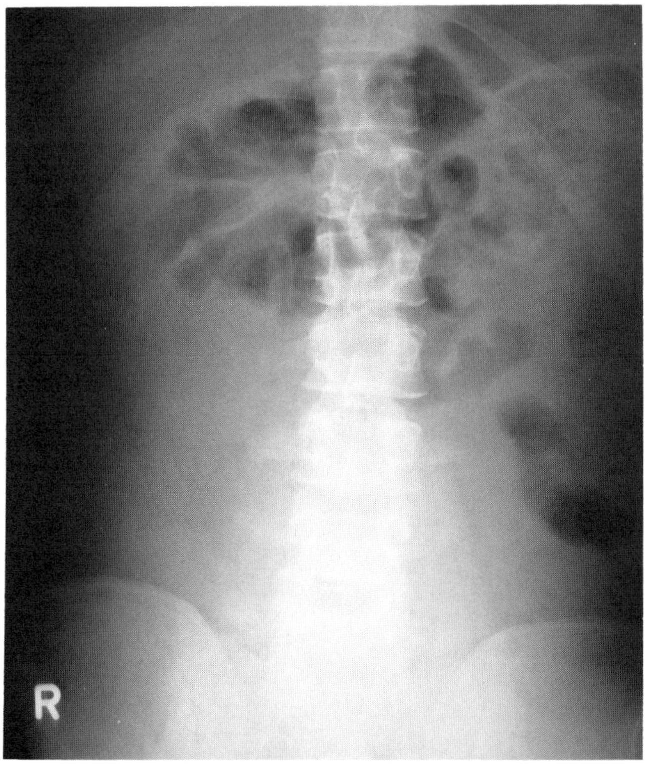

Fig. 9.5. Same case as Fig. 9.3. Massive bleeding into the peritoneal cavity, with displacement of the gas-containing cecum and ascending colon.

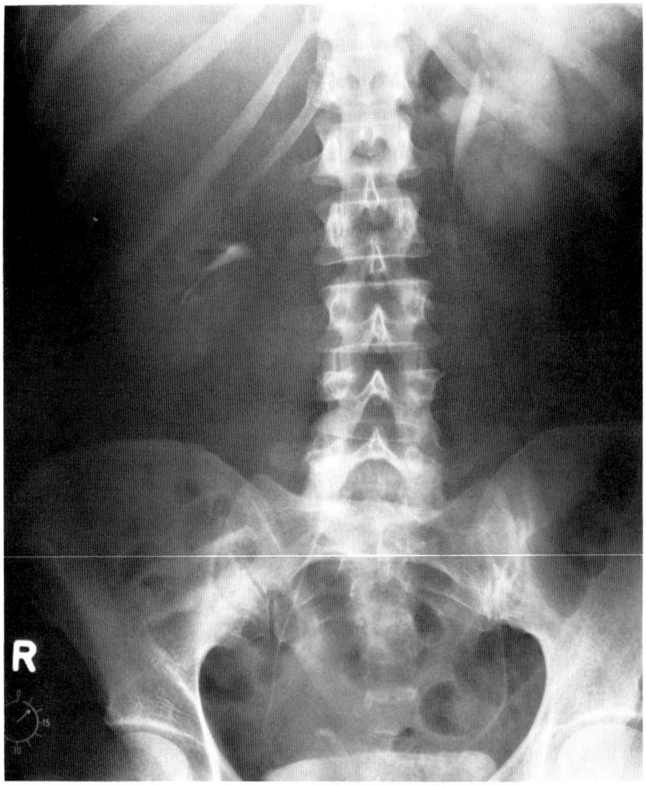

Fig. 9.6. Retroperitoneal hemorrhage and contusion of the right kidney. No psoas delineation on the right. No contrast agent in the right upper pole area. Concavity of the scoliotic posture toward the injured side. Displacement of the right ureter toward the left.

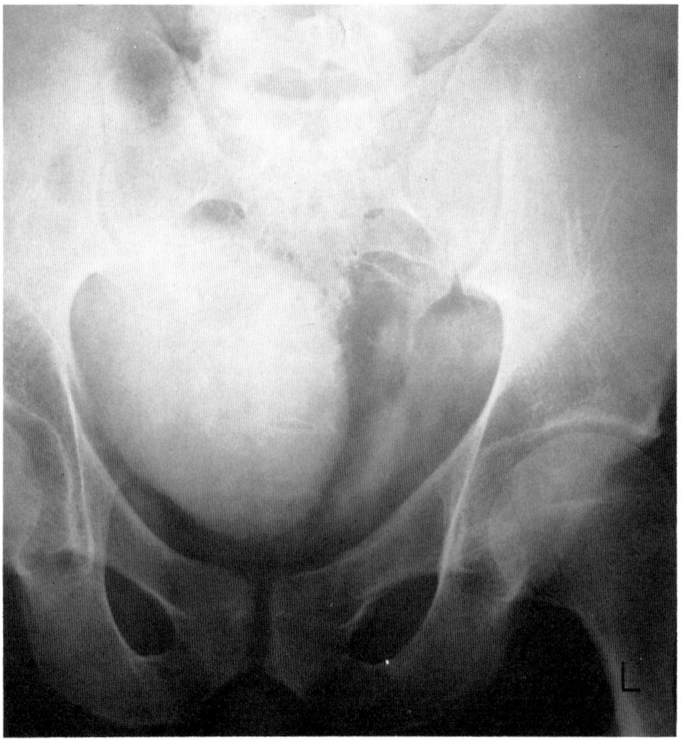

Fig. 9.7. A 34-year-old man who, while drunk and with a plaster cast on one leg, drove his car into a gasoline pump. Deep retroperitoneal hemorrhage on the left, with a fracture of the left pubic bone. Opacification of the inner pelvic area on the left beside the bladder which is displaced toward the right.

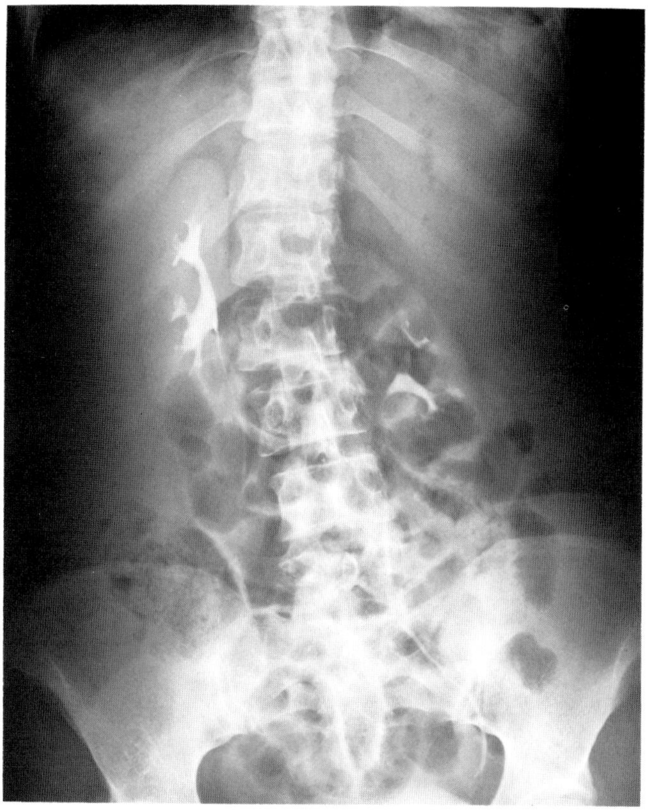

Fig. 9.8. A 49-year-old woman with a ruptured spleen. Abdomen at intravenous urography: opacification of the left upper quadrant; displacement of the left splenic flexure downward; and a compression effect of the left kidney.

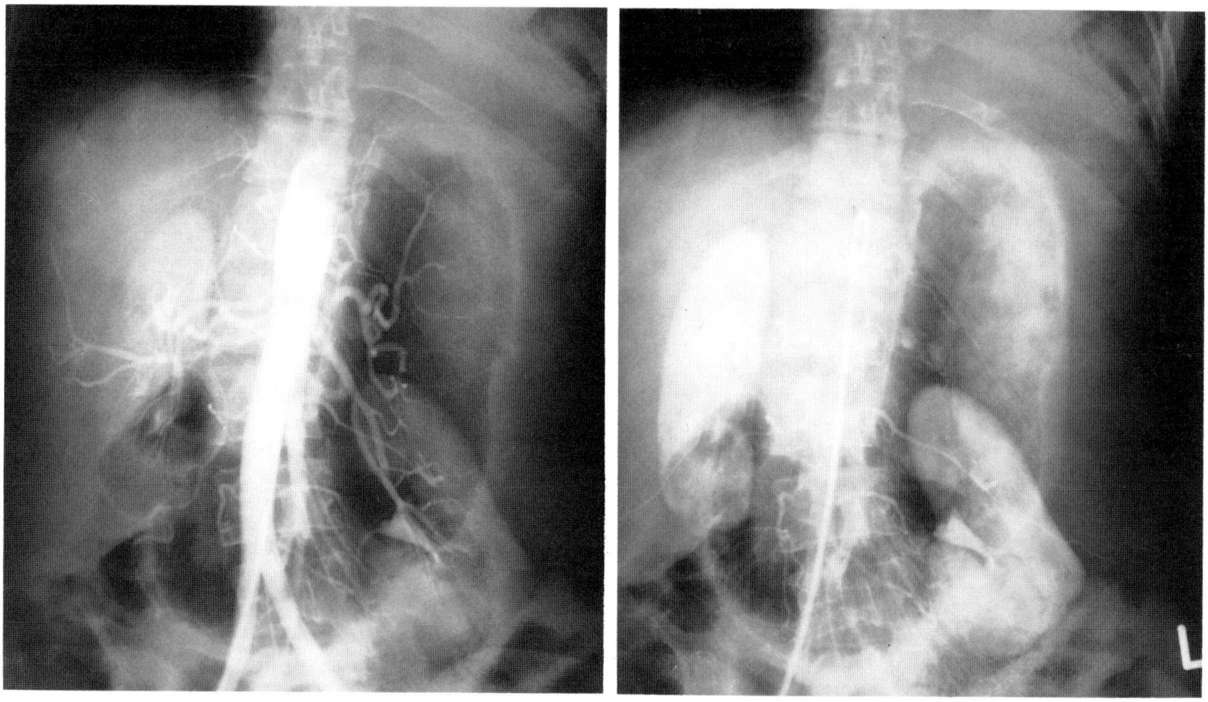

a b

Fig. 9.9a and b. Same case as Fig. 9.8. Midstream angiography in a rupture of the spleen. a) Arterial phase: splenic artery pushed toward the aorta. Arching and deformity of the small vessels. b) Parenchymatous phase: displacement of the abnormally formed and enlarged cortex medially due to the hematoma.

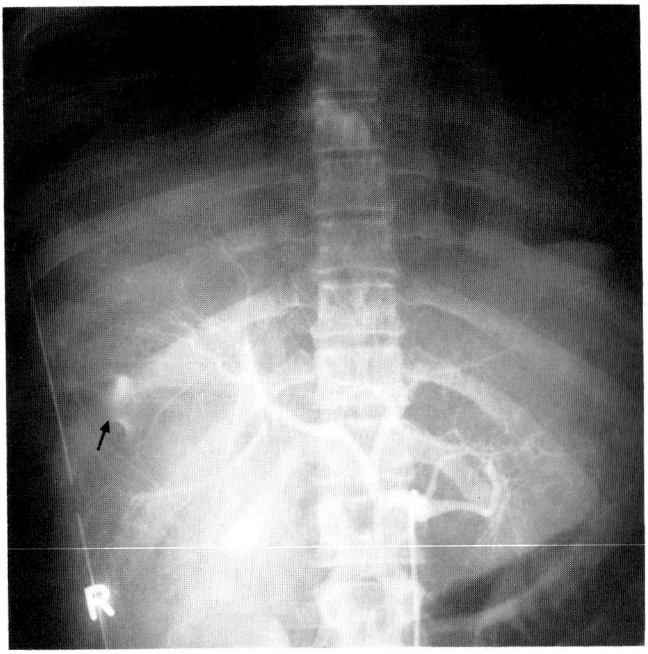

Fig. 9.10. A 22-year-old man after a ski accident. Central rupture of the liver. His condition after removal of the spleen because of rupture and surgical repair of a superficial rupture of the liver. Because of continued bleeding (hematobilia), selective angiography was employed and revealed: displaced large vessels within the right lobe of the liver; abnormal shape of the small vessels; and extravasation of the contrast agent (*arrow*). Note the increased size of the liver without proper delineation toward the right kidney and the elevation of the right diaphragm.

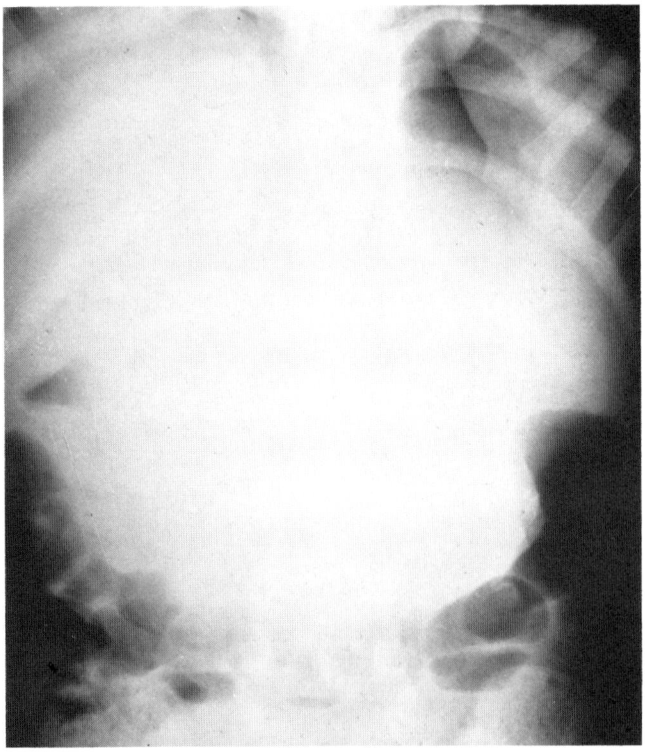

Fig. 9.11. Rupture of the liver, with a tear in the liver capsule; massive bleeding into the peritoneal cavity, marked opacification by the hematoma. Elevation of the right diaphragm. Contours of the liver, kidney and psoas cannot be recognized. Trasverse colon displaced downward. (From H. Vielberg and E. Schnepper: Röntgenblätter *19:* 405, 1966.)

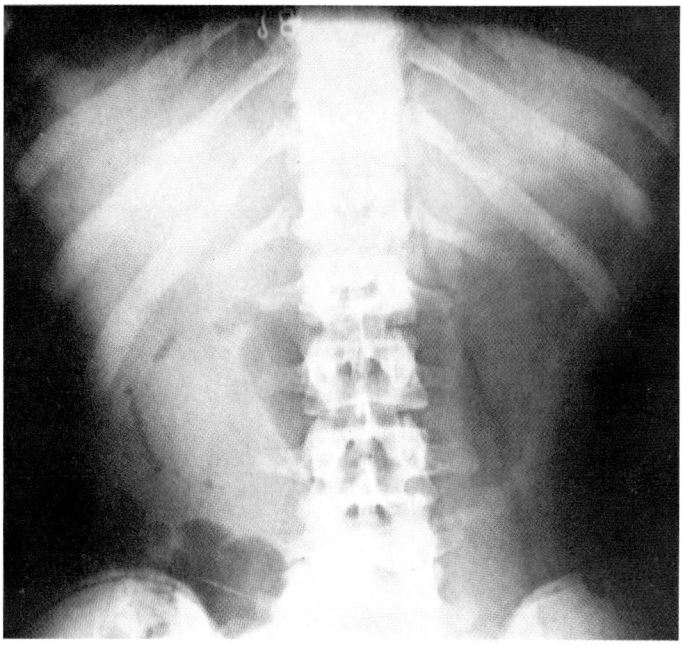

Fig. 9.12a

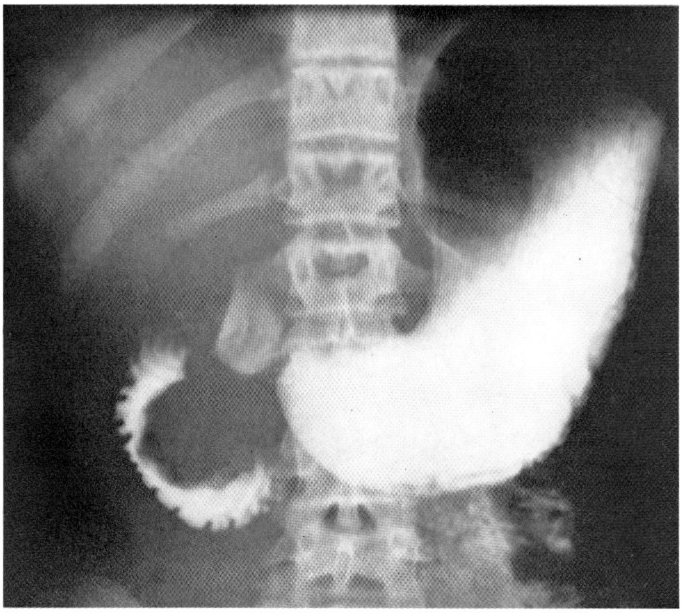

Fig. 9.12b

Fig. 9.12a and b. A 15-year-old girl after a kick by a horse in the midabdominal region. Conservative management. X-ray follow-up after 3 months was normal. Intramural hematoma of the duodenum. Obstruction by the filling defect arising from the wall with smooth and flat characteristics.
a) Abdominal survey film.
b) Contrast agent in the stomach and duodenum. (From J. J. McCort: Radiographic Examination in Blunt Abdominal Trauma. Philadelphia, W. B. Saunders Co., 1966.)

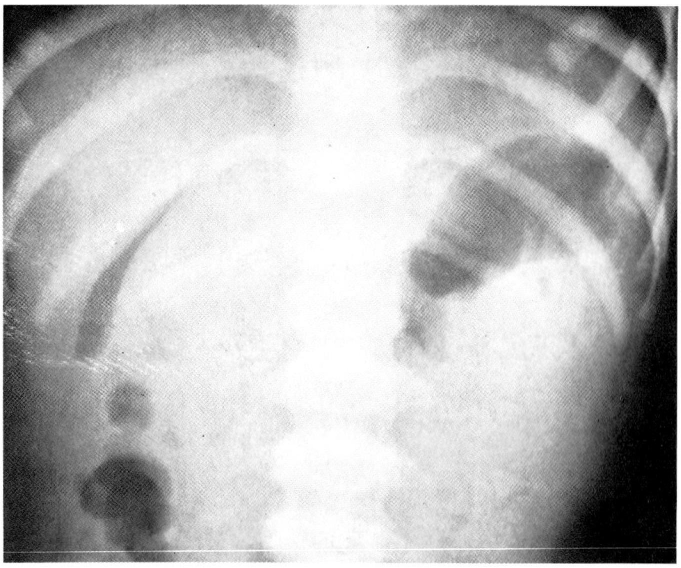

Fig. 9.13. Free air below the right lobe of the liver; intraperitoneal rupture of the duodenum. (From J. J. McCort: Radiographic Examination in Blunt Abdominal Trauma. Philadelphia, W. B. Saunders Co., 1966.)

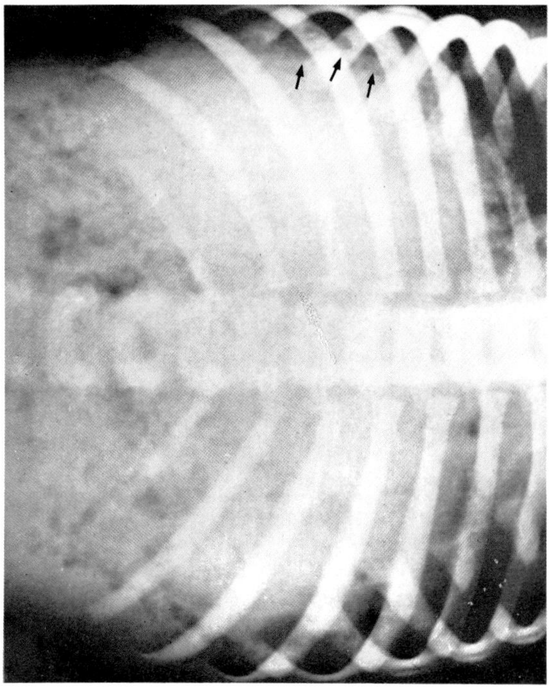

Fig. 9.14. Rupture of the jejunum during a car accident. A. p. view in the left lateral decubitus position. Free air between the liver and the right border of the parietal peritoneum.

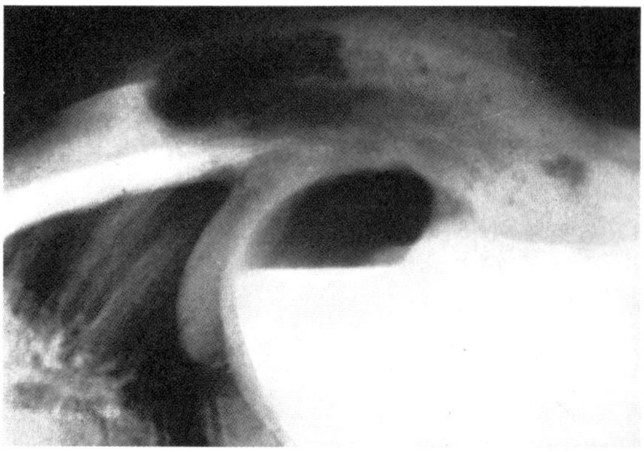

Fig. 9.15. A 16-year-old girl after a traffic accident. Air has escaped into the anterior abdominal and the thoracic wall from a traumatic perforation in the small bowel, with a coexisting rupture of the abdominal wall. (From J. Kaude: Br. J. Radiol. *39:* 950, 1966.)

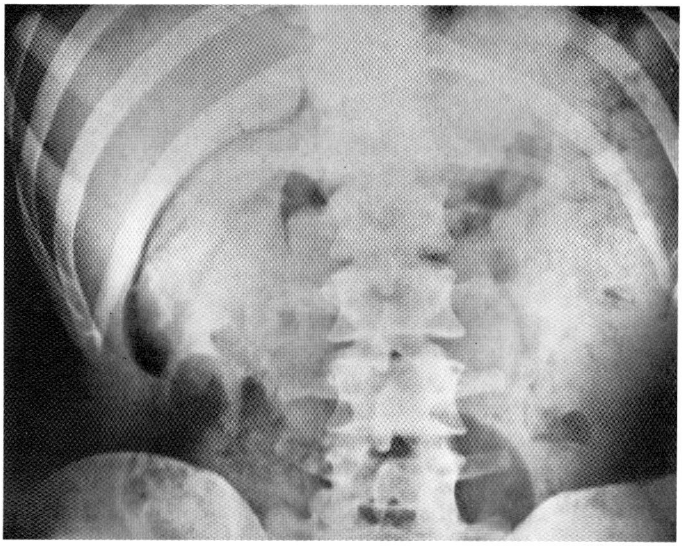

Fig. 9.16. Patient was hit in the abdomen during a brawl. Perirenal gas collection. Apparently gas has migrated from a perforation in the duodenum into the retroperitoneal region. (From J. J. McCort: Radiographic Examination in Blunt Abdominal Trauma. Philadelphia, W. B. Saunders Co., 1966.)

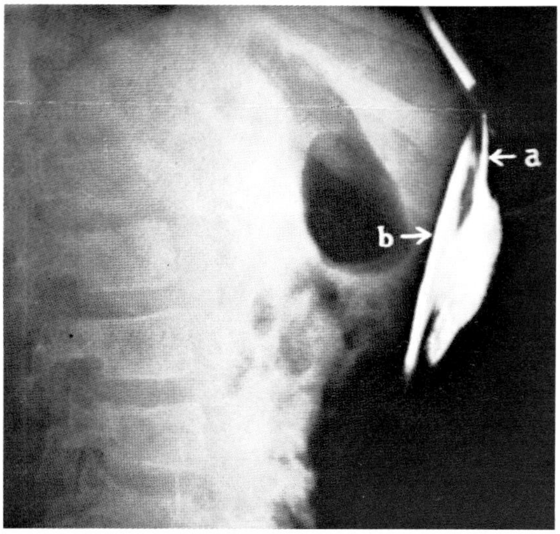

Fig. 9.17. Stabbing injury of the upper abdomen. Contrast instillation (*a* and *b*) shows no communication with the abdominal cavity. (From W. P. Cornell, P. A. Ebert and G. D. Zuidema: J. Surg. Res. *5:* 142, 1965.)

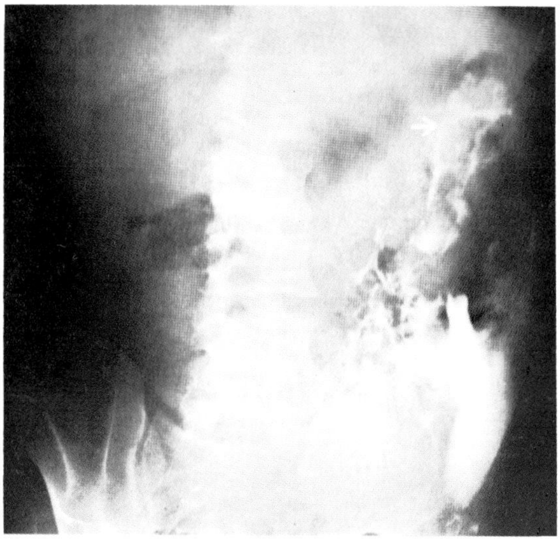

Fig. 9.18. Penetrating injury of the abdomen, with communication to the peritoneal cavity. Contrast agent has coated the liver and peritoneal surface of the gut, as well as the dependent parts of the abdominal cavity. (From W. P. Cornell, P. A. Ebert and G. D. Zuidema: J. Surg. Res. *5:* 142, 1965.)

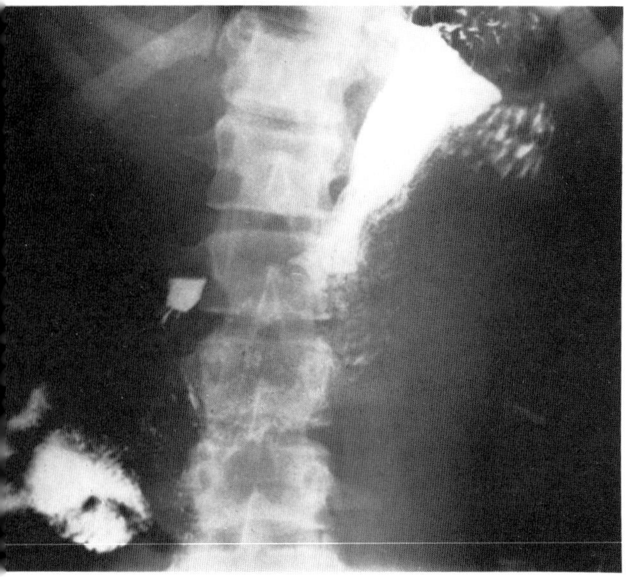
a

Fig. 9.19a–c. a) Opacification of the midabdomen and displacement of the stomach toward the right in rupture of the pancreas.
b) Displacement of the transverse colon downward and pressure symptoms in the area of the left half of the transverse colon in rupture of the pancreas.
c) Pressure symptoms of the left kidney in rupture of the pancreas.
(From H. Vielberg and E. Schnepper: Röntgenblätter *19:* 405, 1966.)

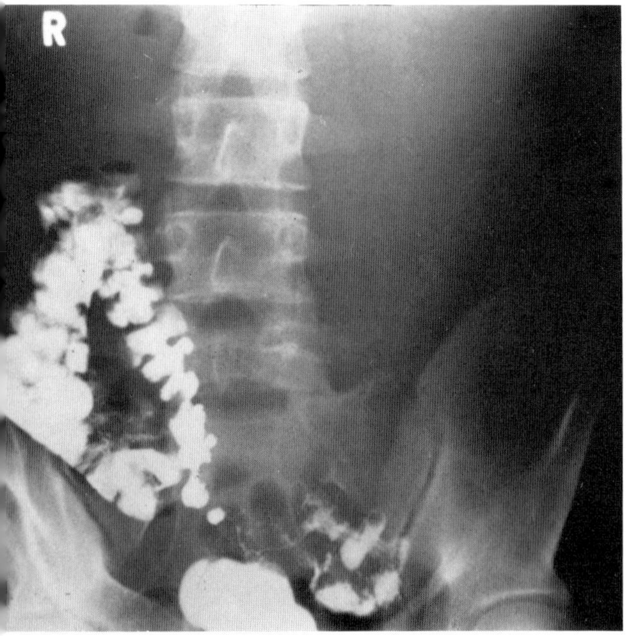

Fig. 9.19b

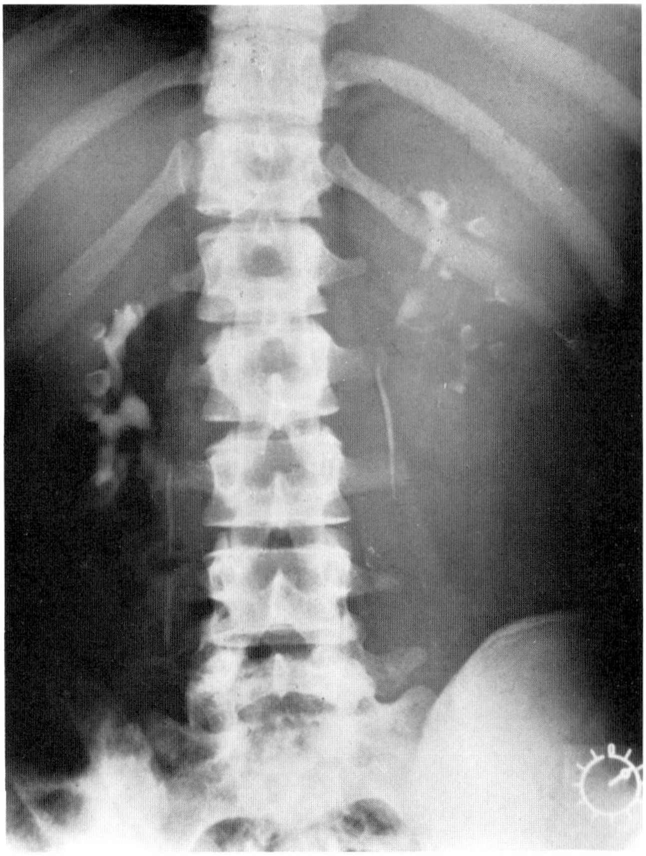
c

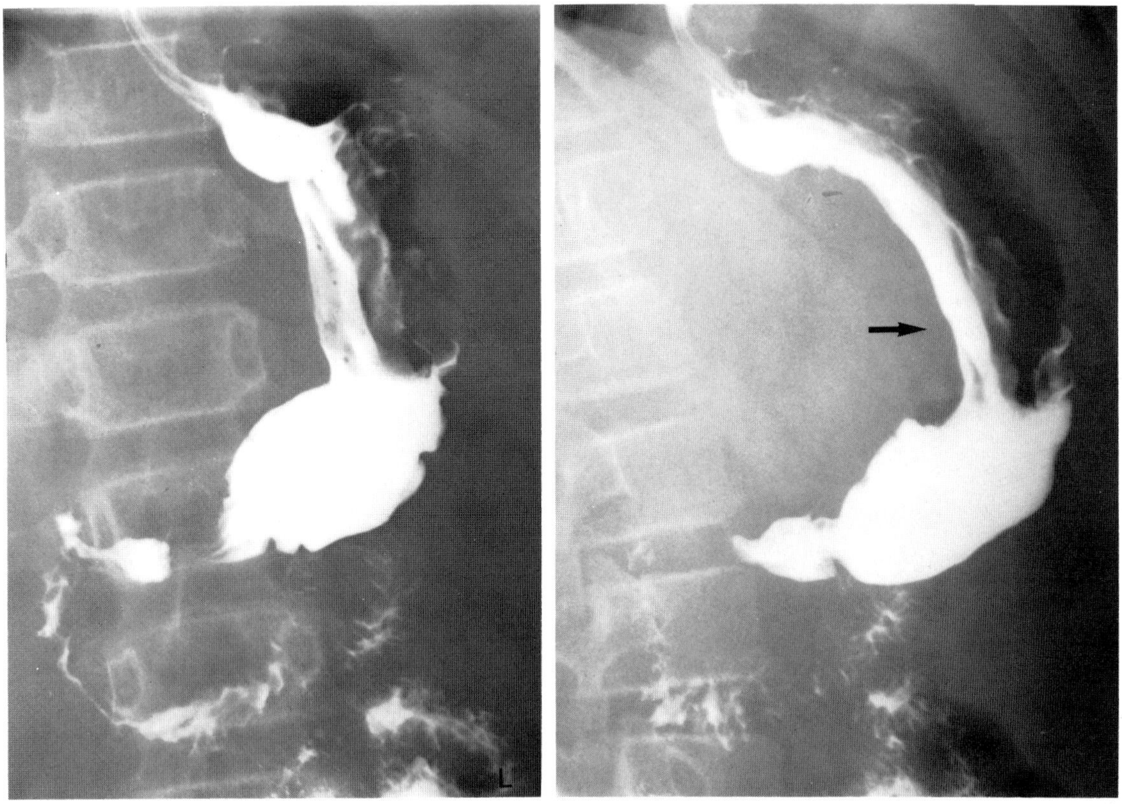

Fig. 9.20a b

▲

Fig. 9.20a and b. A 9-year-old girl who, three weeks ago, fell from a bicycle; trauma to the left upper quadrant when she hit the handle bar. Traumatic cyst of the pancreas. Impression of the stomach from behind with anterior displacement; downward displacement of the duodenojejunal flexure.

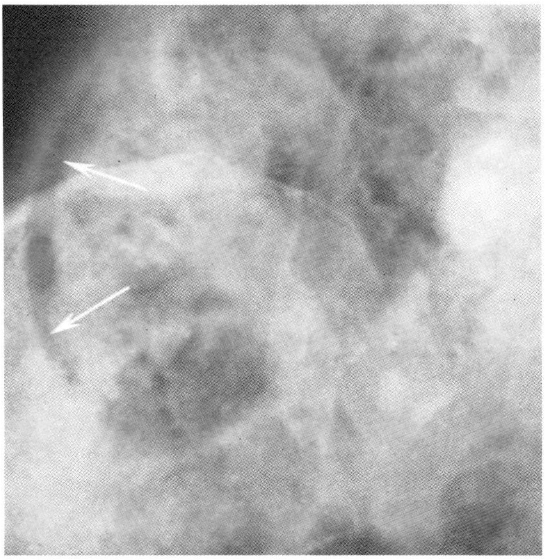

Fig. 9.21. Emphysema of the bowel wall in necrosis of the cecum as the result of blunt abdominal trauma. (From J. J. McCort: Radiographic Examination in Blunt Abdominal Trauma. Philadelphia, W. B. Saunders Co., 1966.)

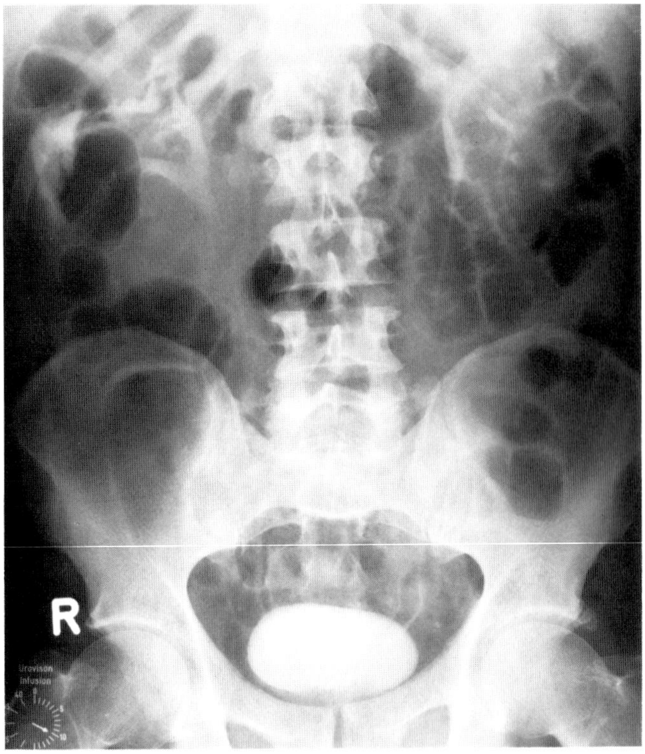

Fig. 9.22. Intravenous urography in rupture of the kidney on the right. Free contrast agent in the perirenal area.

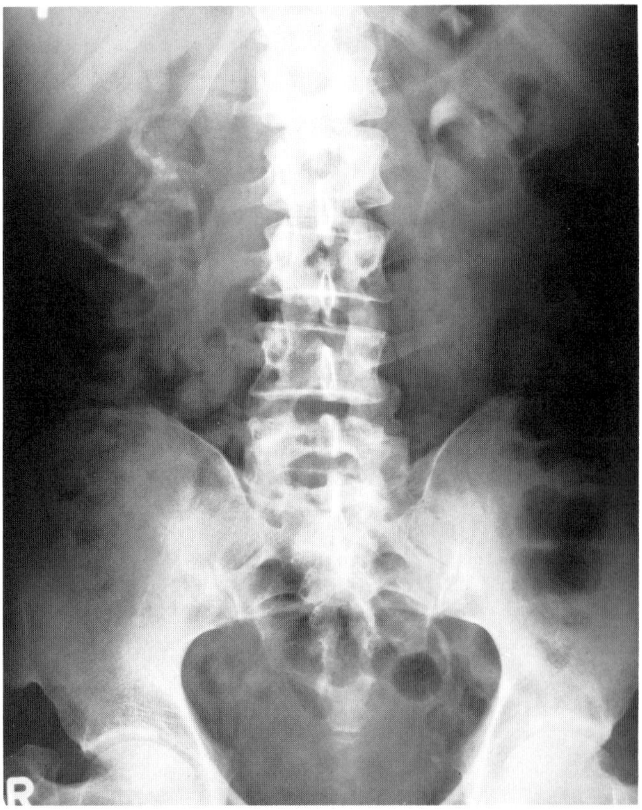

Fig. 9.23a

Fig. 9.23a–c. A 51-year-old man after a fall from a scaffold. Nephrectomy on the right.

a) Reduced excretion of the contrast agent on the right after contusion of the kidney.

b) Retrograde filling: multiple areas of rupture.

c) X-ray follow-up 6 months later; scarring of the upper pole (no excretion on the right during intravenous urography and hypertension).

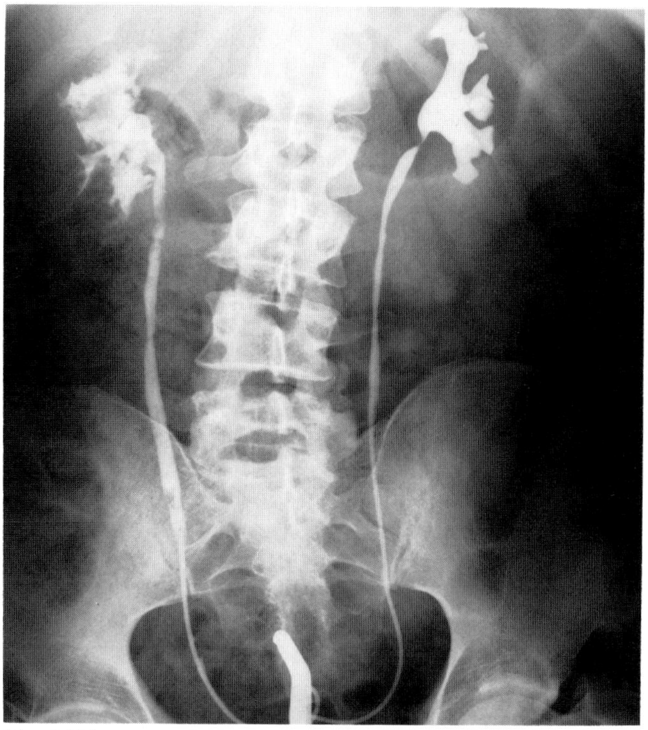

Fig. 9.23b

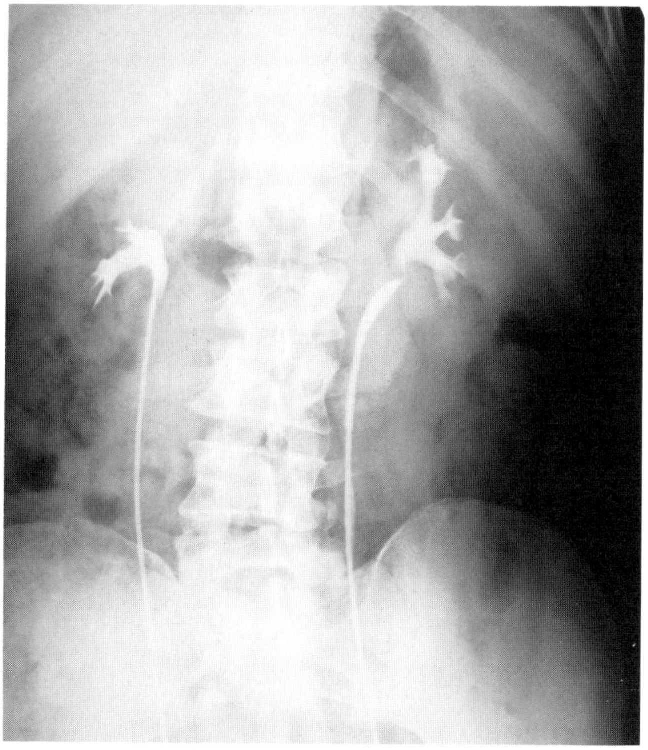

Fig. 9.23c

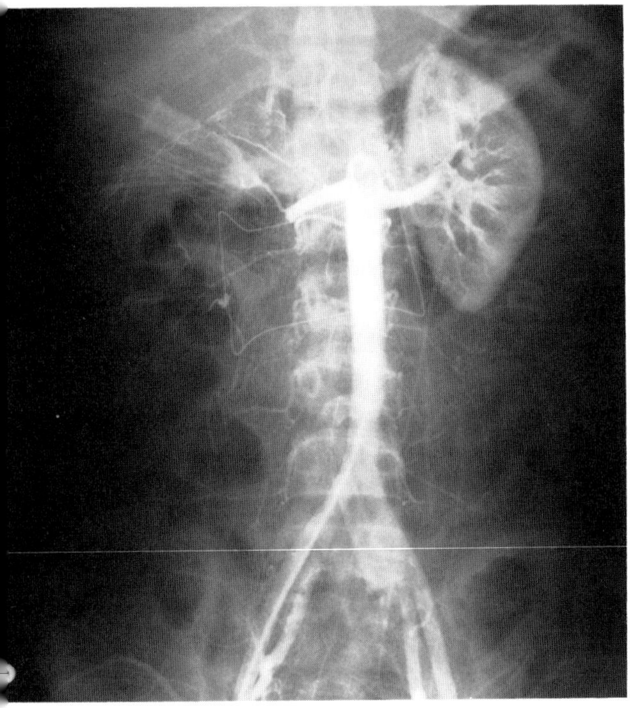

Fig. 9.24

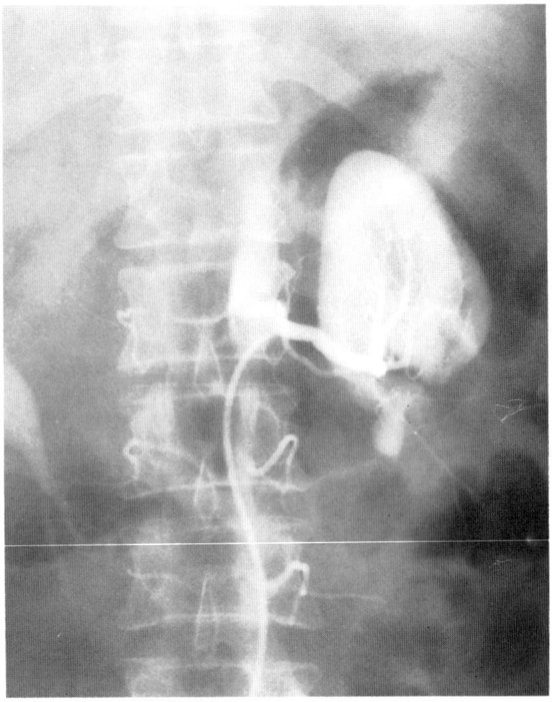

Fig. 9.25

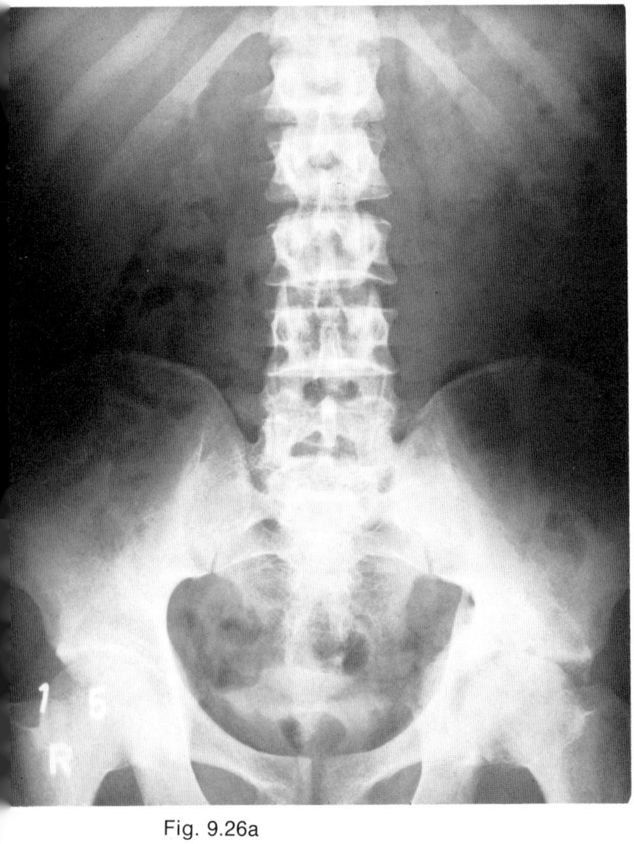

Fig. 9.26a

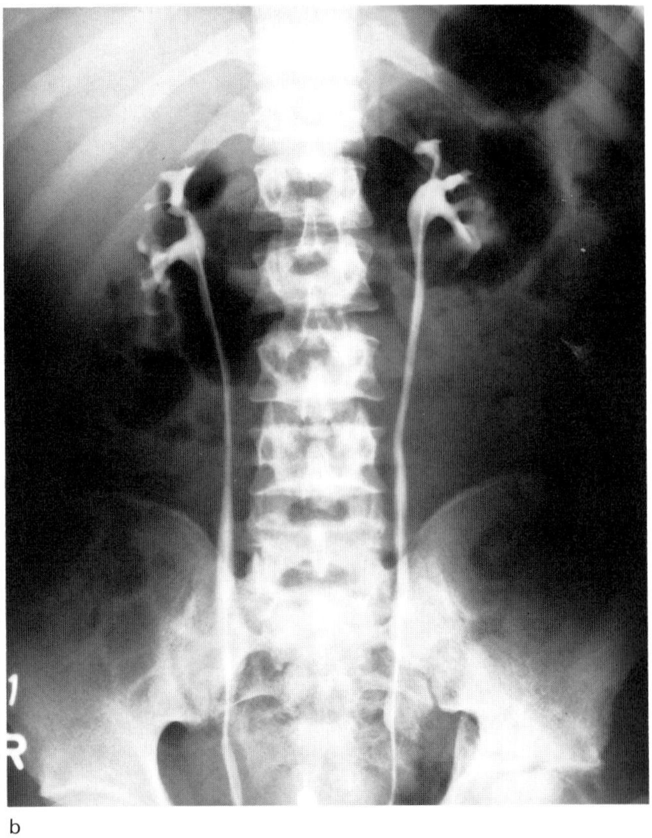

b

◀ Fig. 9.24. A 15-year-old boy. Laparotomy performed because of initial suspicion of a ruptured liver. Renal angiography; avulsion of the right renal artery after a fall from a bicycle.

◀ Fig. 9.25. Rupture of the left kidney during selective angiography.

Fig. 9.26a–d. A 22-year-old man after an accident with a motorcycle. Multiple fractures and contusion of both kidneys. Anuric for 16 days; dialysis performed five times. Because of hypertension, nephrectomy was performed on the left. Secondary gout is a consequence of insufficient arterial blood supply to the remaining right kidney by a capsular artery. Delayed traumatic occlusion of the right renal artery.

a) Intravenous urography: only minimal excretion of the contrast agent.

b) Retrograde urography: slight deformation of the calyces.

c) Translumbar aortogram: filling of the right renal artery by way of a hypertrophic capsular artery. No visualization of the left renal artery.

d) Parenchymatous phase of aortography: massive infarct of the right kidney. No significant concentration of dye within the left kidney.

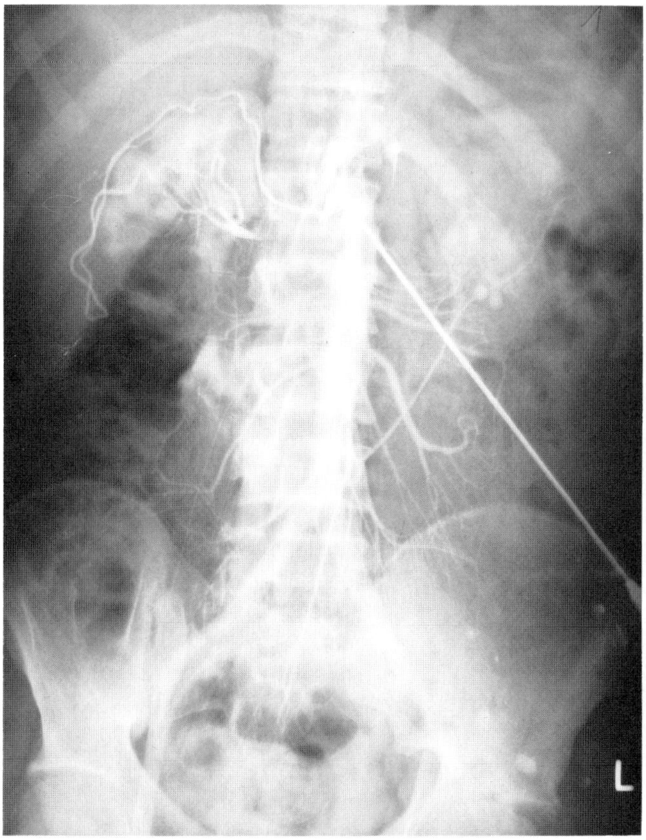

Fig. 9.26c

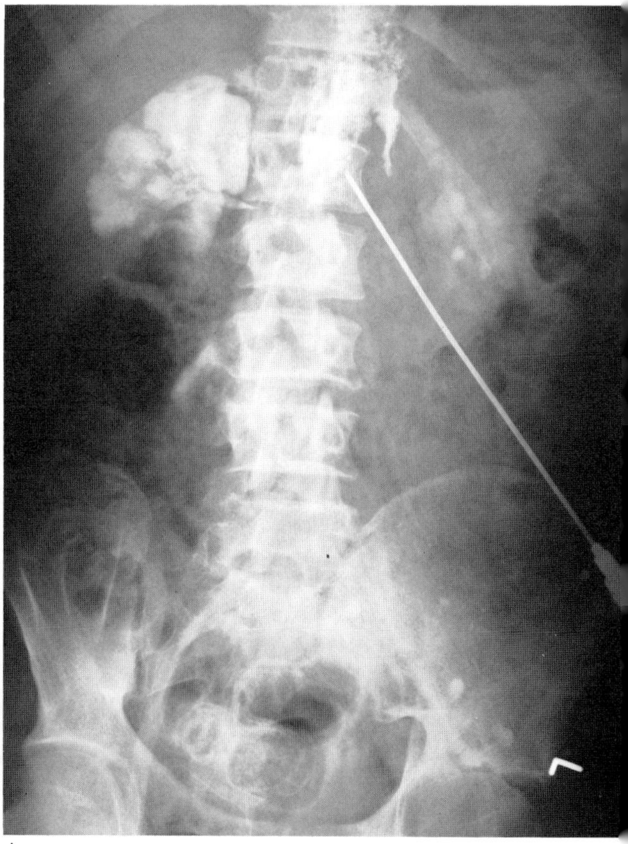

d

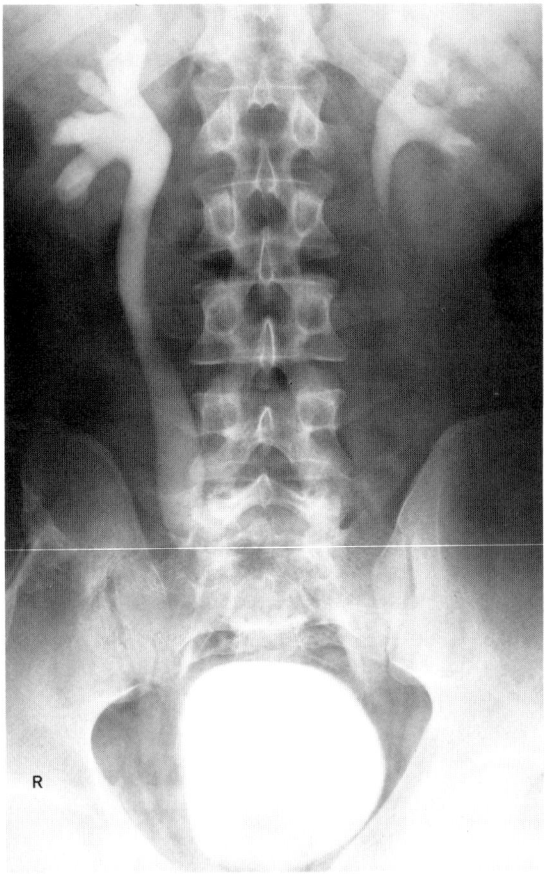

Fig. 9.27. Fibrous stenosis of the right ureter after a retroperitoneal hematoma.

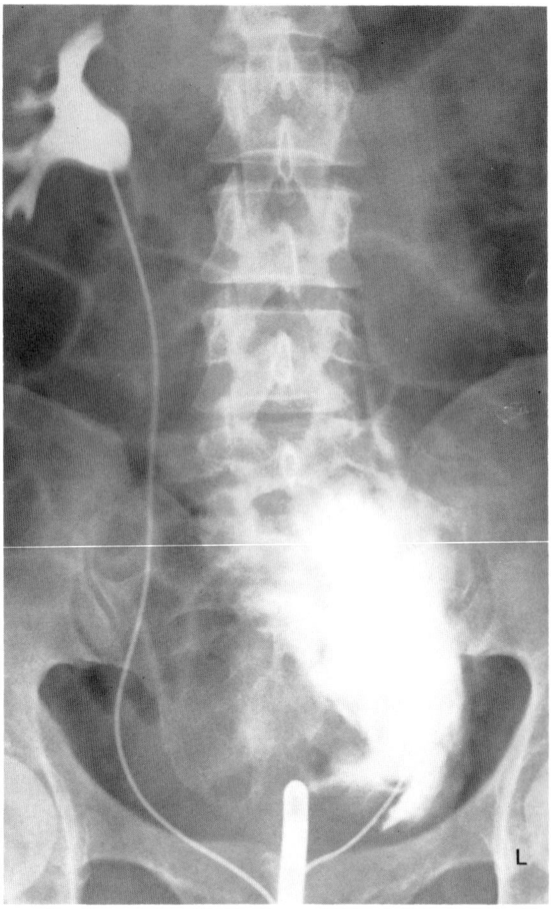

Fig. 9.28. Perforation of the left ureter at retrograde pyelography. Retroperitoneal accumulation of contrast agent.

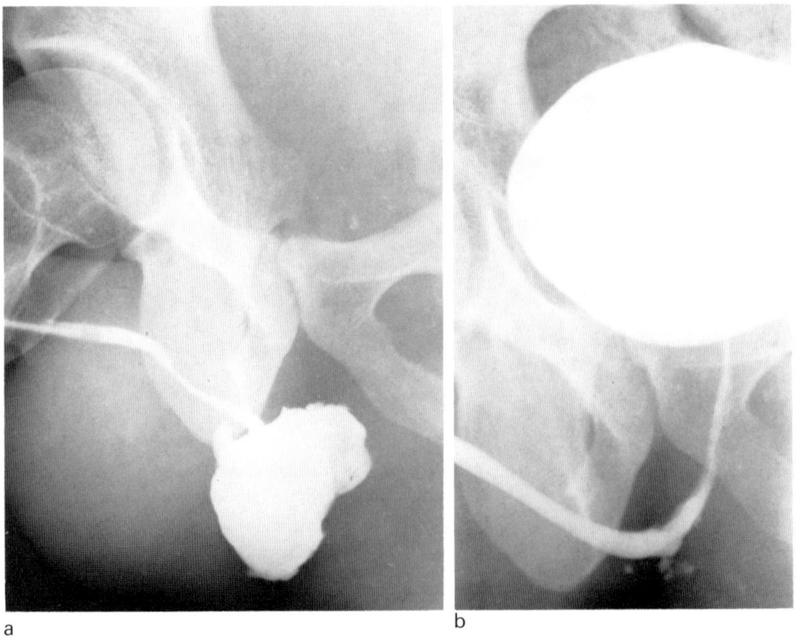

Fig. 9.29a and b. Rupture of the urethra as a result of a perforating perineal injury.
a) Urethrocystogram: disruption of the urethra; extravasation of dye.
b) Follow-up after surgical correction.

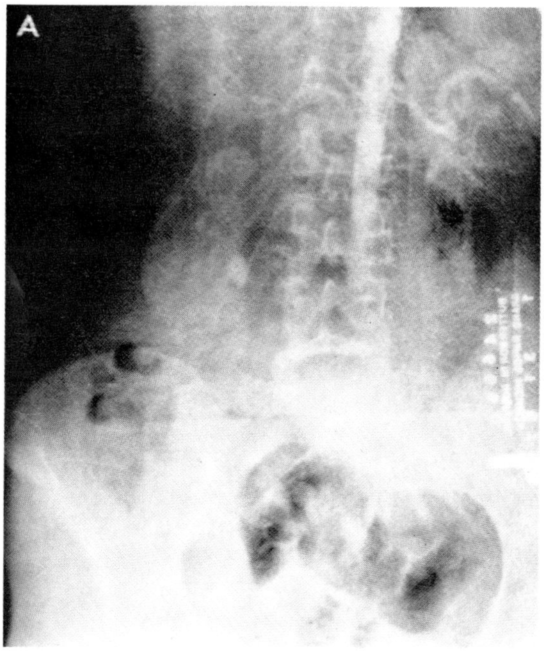

Fig. 9.30a

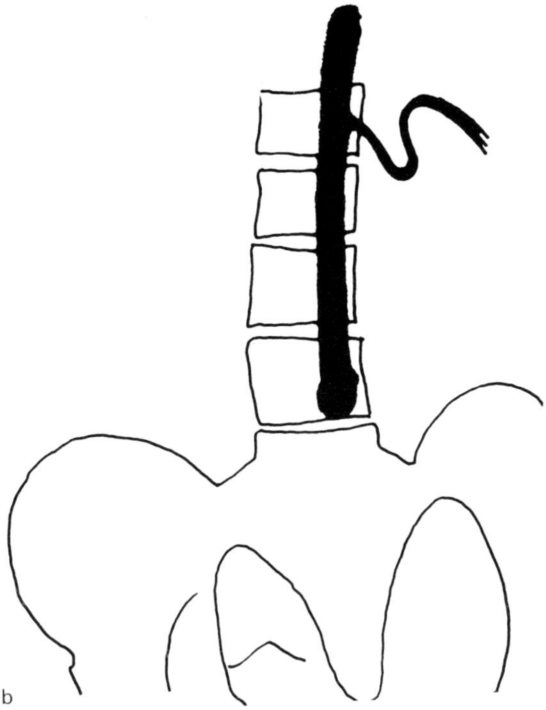

b

Fig. 9.30a–c. A 27-year-old woman after a car accident in which she fell against the steering wheel. Traumatic occlusion of the abdominal aorta by a subintimal hematoma.
a) Aortogram (Seldinger method from the left cubital artery): stop somewhat above the bifurcation of the aorta.
b) Schematic drawing of the aortic occlusion.
c) Local finding at operation.
(From L. A. Tomatis, F. A. Doorndos and J. A. Beard: J. Trauma *8:* 1095, 1968.)

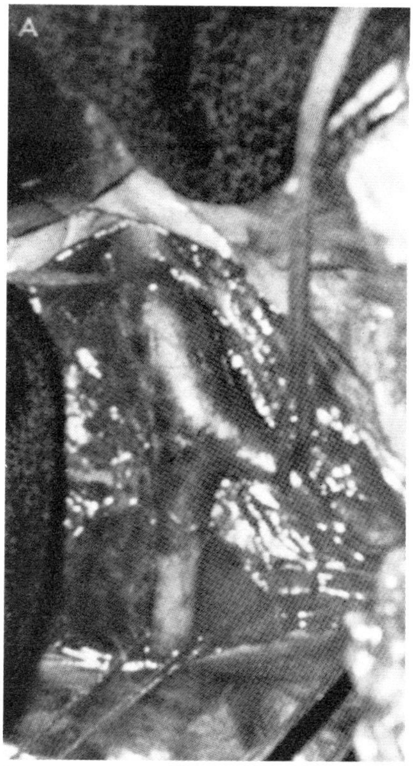

c

10 Foreign Bodies

The demonstration of the presence, type and localization of foreign bodies is one of the most interesting and satisfying tasks of x-ray diagnosis. Foreign bodies that enter by ingestion through the natural openings or by forcible percutaneous means reach several areas within the human body. Sometimes foreign bodies, such as metallic splinters from war injuries or broken tips of needles, are discovered accidentally. Usually, however, they are the object of a search on the basis of a known history.

The material and structure of a foreign body are the key factors in its radiologic recognition. Metallic foreign bodies are usually easy to find. However, it is possible that splinters, even entire projectiles, may evade detection if they are hidden within the organ shadows of dense parenchymatous structures or the spinal column. This will be the case if the films are somewhat underexposed or if the patient moved when they were taken. Even relatively large sewing needles may not be recognized if they are close to the spinal column and if the patient is examined by only fluoroscopy. There are not only diagnostic reasons for always obtaining x-rays on two or more views. Small metallic particles, particularly of light metal, can be recognized only on films of excellent quality with soft penetration. In order to avoid confusion of a metallic foreign body with dirt in the cassette, it is recommended that a second film be obtained with another cassette with the same exposure data. When investigating soft-tissue areas, it is best not to use screen films. Small particles of regular glass usually can be recognized as very fine areas of shadow. Where they are very small and overlap with the bone, it is easy to overlook them. Glass containing lead or other metals, such as crystal, will cast a dense shadow.

Larger wooden splinters can be recognized only if they are within soft tissues and project outside of skeletal parts. Small thin wooden and glass splinters within the soft tissues can be visualized better with the new mammography technique (Fischer, 1973). Dirt and tiny stones are visible by a contrast of almost the same density as bone. The most difficult problem is to recognize foreign bodies made of plastic. If in doubt, it is best to take an x-ray of a similar plastic object if it can be obtained. This should determine whether it is possible to recognize the object in question radiologically.

Many foreign bodies have a tendency to change their location, and this must be kept in mind. Within the gastrointestinal tract, there is a change in position due to peristalsis; within the tracheobronchial tree, due to coughing and gravity; within the vascular system, by the blood stream; and within soft tissues, because of muscular activity. A follow-up radiographic investigation immediately prior to an attempt at surgical removal is always indicated. Nonopaque foreign bodies may be recognized by using contrast agents, resulting in an area of radiolucency within the contrast due to the presence of the foreign body within the esophagus, gastrointestinal canal, urethra or bladder.

Every foreign body should be primarily pinpointed as to its accurate topographic or anatomic location. However, foreign bodies within the eye or within the thicker soft tissues can be approached using geometric methods of exact localization. Well-known methods are those of Comberg and Pfeiffer to determine the location of intraocular foreign bodies (Fig. 10.1). With respect to other geometric methods, the literature should be consulted (Büchner, 1965). They have been superseded by improved methods of topographic-anatomic localization and by improved investigative methods of detecting metallic foreign bodies (electromagnetic devices and image intensifier combined with television). The value of a careful x-ray investigation cannot be overemphasized. Finally, one should always remember the great importance of stereoscopic roentgenograms. With this very simple technique, valuable diagnostic information can be obtained (Fig. 10.2). With this method, for instance, the exact location of a multitude of small shotgun pellets and their relation to bones, joints and internal organs can be determined rapidly. As a result of radiologic determination of type and location of a foreign body, there may well be important conclusions in view of the urgency and type of operation necessary. Besides x-ray evidence of internal hemorrhage or perforation, the demonstration of dangerous metallic tips or parts of knives and the recognition of chemical or potentially toxic hazards may significantly influence the surgical approach.

The ingestion of foreign bodies is generally harmless and even large foreign bodies will leave the human body by natural avenues. Within the esophagus, there may be a problem in that relatively small foreign bodies may get stuck, because they can cause local spasm, which will retain them. In the adult this is most frequently the result of poorly chewed food particles – pieces of ham, small bones or fish bones – and possibly also parts of an artificial denture (Fig. 10.3). It may be very difficult to accurately recognize small bones, fish bones and glass splinters. The best approach is to check for their presence in the upper esophagus by using a soft-tissue technique on the lateral neck (Fig. 10.4).

The true size, location and form of a foreign body are sometimes impossible to determine properly, such as when there is a local obstruction. If in doubt, endoscopy without delay is always indicated (Fig. 10.5).

Besides coins, bobby pins, glass marbles, needles, buttons and parts of toys, thumbtacks are the most frequently swallowed foreign bodies during early childhood (Figs. 10.6 and 10.7).

If a perforation of the esophagus by a foreign body is suspected, clarification using one mouthful of aqueous contrast agent can be attempted. Such an approach is equally important in demonstrating the integrity of the esophagus after successful extraction of the foreign body, particularly after a difficult technical procedure.

Most swallowed foreign bodies will pass through the esophagus and reach the stomach and beyond. Wadolowski (1965), in a careful analysis of 1014 cases, has determined that all swallowed foreign bodies of up to 14 cm. in length were spontaneously evacuated. Normal anatomic and functional conditions within the gastrointestinal canal must, however, be present. The numbers and types of swallowed foreign bodies are enormous, as is the variety of reasons and motives for their ingestion (Figs. 10.8 to 10.10). Unless there is immediate reason for surgery because of an obvious obstruction or imminent danger, radiologic follow-up is indicated. Metallic mercury is almost nontoxic to the gastrointestinal tract (Fig. 10.11). Within tissues and if present in a very fine dispersion, there may be resorption and intoxication (Fühner 1947). Nonopaque foreign bodies such as wooden or plastic toothpicks (used with party snacks) or glass splinters may escape observation even during the passage of contrast material. Bezoars which rarely form within the stomach, such as phytobezoars, trichobezoars and shellac bezoars, are usually detected radiologically; often, however, they are initially considered to be local tumors (Fig. 10.12). As a result of pathologic local conditions, otherwise harmless foreign bodies may be the cause of a local obstacle, forming an occlusion (Fig. 10.13).

Besides obstruction, there is also the danger of perforation intraperitoneally, with subsequent subdiaphragmatic accumulation of free air, as well as retroperitoneally, with collection of gas in the perirenal space. The possibility of perforation or penetration by gastric or intestinal catheters should be kept in mind, along with the concomitant serious foreign-body effect of barium if introduced into the peritoneal cavity (Fig. 10.14).

There are many exceptional cases of foreign-body ingestion. Only one such example should be mentioned here: Because of a bet, a young man swallowed 30 intact frogs, whereupon he developed intestinal obstruction because of the undigested bones (Kern et al., 1964).

Aspiration of foreign bodies occurs less frequently than ingestion. The key symptom is a sudden attack of severe coughing or suffocation. This cannot go unnoticed, except for patients with an abnormal state of consciousness. After an initial coughing episode, there is usually a somewhat symptom-free phase until the development of secondary mechanical or infectious local responses. Particularly in children with bronchopulmonary pathology resistant to therapy, the possibility of aspiration of a foreign body must be seriously considered. About $^3/_4$ of all foreign body aspirations are observed among children under 6 years of age. At the end of the 19th century, the mortality rate for foreign-body aspiration was about 50 per cent (Maurer and Hoefer-Janker, 1966); today this is less than 1 per cent. This improvement certainly is in large part due to the effectiveness of x-ray diagnosis, advances in anesthesia and also the improved endoscopic techniques of extracting foreign bodies. In all cases of foreign-body aspiration or ingestion, endoscopy should be attempted early (Minnigerode, 1972). The majority of small foreign bodies will rapidly pass through the trachea and reach the right main-stem bronchus or the right lower lobe as the result of its steeper and downward slope. In emergency cases, immediate bronchoscopy and occasionally even tracheotomy may be indicated. In general, however, it should be possible to perform a thorough radiologic investigation. This approach should always include careful fluoroscopy, with excellent preparation and adaptation of the viewer using image intensification and television to obtain multiple views in different directions, some with higher and some with lower kV technique. Subsequent tomography or bronchography may be useful. In the presence of dense foreign bodies, it is usually possible to prove not only the existence but also the exact location within the tracheobronchial tree. Metallic foreign bodies are easily visible during fluoroscopy (Figs. 10.15 and 10.16). Mediastinal shift during the respiratory phases or atelectasis is an indication of stenosis or complete occlusion of a bronchus (Fig. 10.17). Similar importance should be attached to the so-called Hitzenberger's sniff test: during forceful inspiratory sniffing, there is elevation instead of depression of the diaphragm on the involved side. Both of these fluoroscopic signs are especially valuable if one is dealing with nonopaque foreign bodies. Further indirect signs of foreign-body aspiration are atelectatic or bronchopneumonic shadows (Figs. 10.18 and 10.19). The complication of perforation of a bronchus by a foreign body after entering percutaneously can be localized within a bronchus. Pulsation of the foreign body and pulmonary hemorrhage are strong indications of a very close relationship between the foreign body and the larger vessels.

Foreign bodies may change their position if the patient assumes a different position or coughs. This is a strong argument for radiologic control during bronchoscopy (Fig. 10.20). Also, after successful extraction of the foreign body, x-ray follow-up can be very important in ascertaining the complete removal of, or in determining the location and type of, remaining particles (Fig. 10.21).

Foreign-body injuries within the urethra, bladder and rectum are frequently concealed when these are the result of self-inflicted mishaps. If the foreign body is opaque, it will be recognized readily on roentgenograms (Figs. 10.22 to 10.25). Only rarely will there be another way in which foreign bodies can reach the bladder or urethra. Projectiles or splinters may enter after perforation (Fig. 10.26), whereas catheters or parts thereof are iatrogenic in origin (Fig. 10.27).

Nonopaque foreign bodies will be made visible as a defect within the contrast-filled organ. Foreign bodies within the rectum occur rarely and are self-inserted; sometimes they are iatrogenically derived (Figs. 10.28 and 10.29). Complications may be the result of perforation or penetration but also of local formation of concrements (Figs. 10.30 and 10.31). Within the urethra, the danger of a local stricture is significant.

The largest number of open, perforating and serious foreign-body injuries occurs as a result of shooting accidents even during peacetime, if the smaller superficial foreign-body injuries occurring during daily activities are not counted. The type and severity of gunshot wounds are the result of many different factors. The distance of the shot and the velocity and weight of the projectile will determine the force of the blast, the winding or straight course of the projectile, the barrel of the weapon, the stability of the axis of the projectile and the type of projectile (lead or lead mixture, the cover of the projectile, and whether a small shot). All of these are decisive factors for the type of splintering and distribution within the body. Fine metal splinters may mark the trajectory of the projectile within the body. The point of entrance of the projectile is usually smaller than the actual caliber and the exit is larger (as in the area of the skull). Sometimes there may be several exit wounds due to splintering of the projectile. In general, one can distinguish between grazing shots, buffer shots, a shot lodging within the body and a shot passing through it. In a situation when the projectile is stuck and occasionally fragments into many pieces it simulates the presence of several projectiles. Occasionally, a projectile is deflected in the body, thus taking an oblique course (Fig. 10.32).

In all cases of injury by projectiles, there should be a careful extensive radiologic investigation, especially if the cause of the patient's death is strongly suspected to be by shooting (Neiss, 1968). The roentgenogram is of great importance as a medical record, but possibly more so as a medicolegal document. In many cases, it will be possible to determine exactly the type of projectile in question. A prerequisite, however, is a good knowledge of the various guns used today, and being able to identify properly the most important projectiles (Figs. 10.33 to 10.35). The task of the radiologist is primarily to define the type and localization of the foreign body and possibly also the course taken by the projectile (Figs. 10.36 to 10.43). In addition, there should always be a search for symptoms of injury to internal organs, intrathoracic as well as abdominal hemorrhage (Figs.10.44 and 10.45), pneumothorax (Fig. 10.46), infectious reactions (Fig. 10.47) and perforations affecting the gastrointestinal tract, among others (Figs. 10.48 and 10.49). Despite the presence of threatening injuries, the radiologic symptoms may be minimal. The type and extent of damage must always be evaluated on the basis of the clinical symptoms and within the context of the course the projectile has taken within the body. Suspected injury to bones will usually be visible on the roentgenogram (Fig. 10.50).

In all gunshot wounds, one must consider that the point of penetration into the body and the actual location of the projectile may be widely separated. Besides taking a normally direct course, projectiles may migrate within the body to the bronchial system, the pleura, the gastrointestinal tract and the vasculature (compare Fig. 10.46). Any x-ray investigation must, therefore, consider all the possible suspected areas of the body where a projectile may have migrated. In the case of shooting from very close range and also with gas or warning-shot ammunition, gases of the exploding charge may enter the tissues. The extent of accumulation of gas within subcutaneous tissues is easily recognized on roentgenograms (Fig. 10.51).

Stabbing injuries always require careful radiologic work-up. One must always consider the possibility of concomitant bony injuries, injury of parenchymatous tissue or other internal organs (pneumothorax, hemorrhage, perforation) or a foreign body being lodged somewhere within the body (Figs. 10.52 and 10.53).

In the case of a murder or suspected suicide, the help of the radiologist is frequently sought. According to Zatzkin (1965), one must consider the following important points:

1. Postmortem roentgenograms should be utilized to discover so far unknown but possibly malignant diseases.
2. Besides the search for projectiles, the skeleton should be carefully scrutinized for possible traumatic alterations. Multiple injuries to bones, bone-related symptoms due to the battering of a child or fractures within facial structures or the skull may be significant findings.
3. X-rays must be taken if at all possible prior to autopsy in order to determine whether there was pneumothorax or rupture of a hollow organ such as would be caused by stabbing.
4. Air embolization, as seen after criminal abortion, will require x-rays with the body in an upright position and in a lateral decubitus position. The most important sign to be sought is an air-fluid level within the right ventricle or pulmonary artery. The veins of the trunk, head and neck should also be investigated for the possible presence of air. Interstitial emphysema may be present within the pelvis and the abdomen.
5. Recently one has to consider the possibility of injury by projectiles from bolting devices used in manufacturing and propelled by gunpowder. The projectiles from these devices are capable of perforating heavy plates of plaster and still enter deep into the human body (compare Fig. 10.56).
6. In cases when projectiles or splinters are suspected in the body, qualitatively good roentgenograms must be obtained of the entire body so that fragments embedded in bone can be recognized. In an evaluation of the number of projectiles present, it must always be considered that the splintering of projectiles made of soft lead may cause erroneous impressions. An evaluation can also be difficult because of the presence of metallic foreign bodies from earlier injuries.

Accidents at work caused by metallic or glass foreign bodies are today seen regularly. The most endangered parts of the body are the hands and face, and particularly the eyes. If there are opaque splinters within the region of the orbit, the localization, according to Comberg or Pfeiffer, should again be emphasized. In every case, it is necessary to obtain at least two views on two planes for localization (Fig. 10.54). Metal splinters or parts from machines can spring loose and enter the body at great velocity, leading to life-threatening injuries (Figs. 10.55 and 10.56) similar to those due to metal or glass splinters resulting from explosions (Fig. 10.57).

In injuries due to splinters in traffic accidents or in those occurring during daily activities, glass particles are usually involved. Nonbreakable patented glass from car windshields is often implicated in injuries resulting from traffic accidents. Such particles may enter the body deeply and may then be overlooked owing to overlap with bone of about similar density (Fig. 10.58). Sand and gravel, depending on their particle size and quantity, can be recognized quite accurately because of their irregular but typically shaped shadow (Fig. 10.59). Injuries due to glass particles in accidents of daily life are by no means always minor. An externally small and insignificant wound sometimes belies a serious internal injury (Fig. 10.60). Foreign bodies may also enter the body as the result of a physician's intervention. Pieces of cotton or compresses, clamps and fragments of broken tips of needles have all been seen within a surgical field. Cotton or compresses currently can be recognized on x-rays because they are marked by opaque threads (Fig. 10.61). Great care should be exercised in evaluating every dubious radiologic finding, shadow or calcification of tissue in order not to mistake them as calcified cotton left behind at surgery or to misinterpret a metal marker of the Holzknecht palpation instrument as a broken surgical needle (Fig. 10.62); furthermore, the patient should be informed immediately of such "incontestable findings". The search for broken dislocated catheters or objects within the vascular system or the heart can be very difficult (Fig. 10.63). An extensive description and discussion of these problems, presently of increasing significance, can be found in the report by Trede and Encke (1970).

Less dramatic is the search for foreign bodies known to be located somewhat superficially within the soft tissues on the basis of a known history. Regular needles or fragments are probably the most frequently seen foreign body of this type (Figs. 10.64 and 10.65). Nails, pieces of wire, fishing hooks and other objects entering the soles of feet when walking without shoes are hardly ever located so far under the skin that they cannot be recognized from the surface. Still, a roentgenologic investigation may be necessary to determine a possible injury to the bone or the type and extent of the hidden part of the foreign body.

Dramatic pictures are sometimes the result of failures or accidents during investigations with contrast agents. Luckily most of these are survived by the patient without permanent damage (Fig. 10.66). Nonsoluble, nonresorbable contrast agents may be the cause of extensive foreign-body reaction (Fig. 10.67). Coincidentally, one occasionally sees today small splashlike residual deposits of metallic salts in the soft tissues of the gluteal muscle following antisyphilitic therapy (Fig. 10.68).

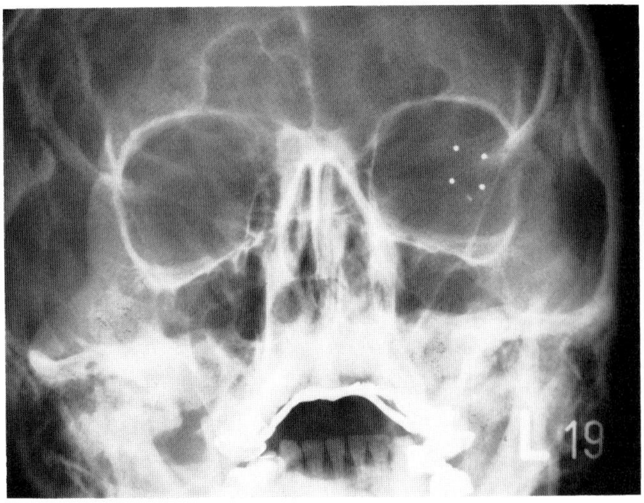

Fig. 10.1a

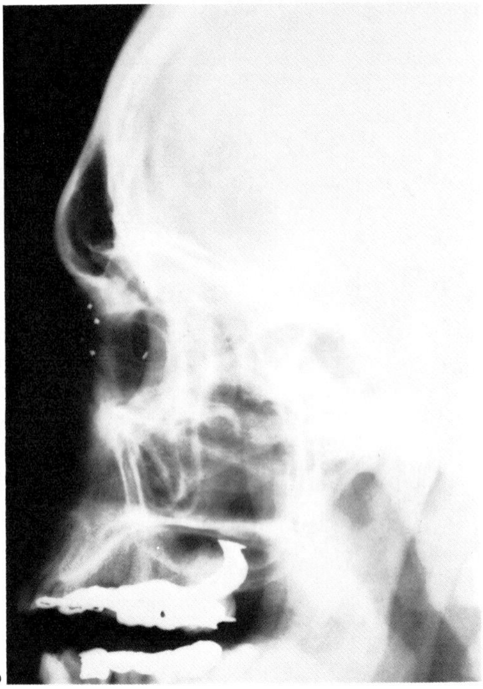

b

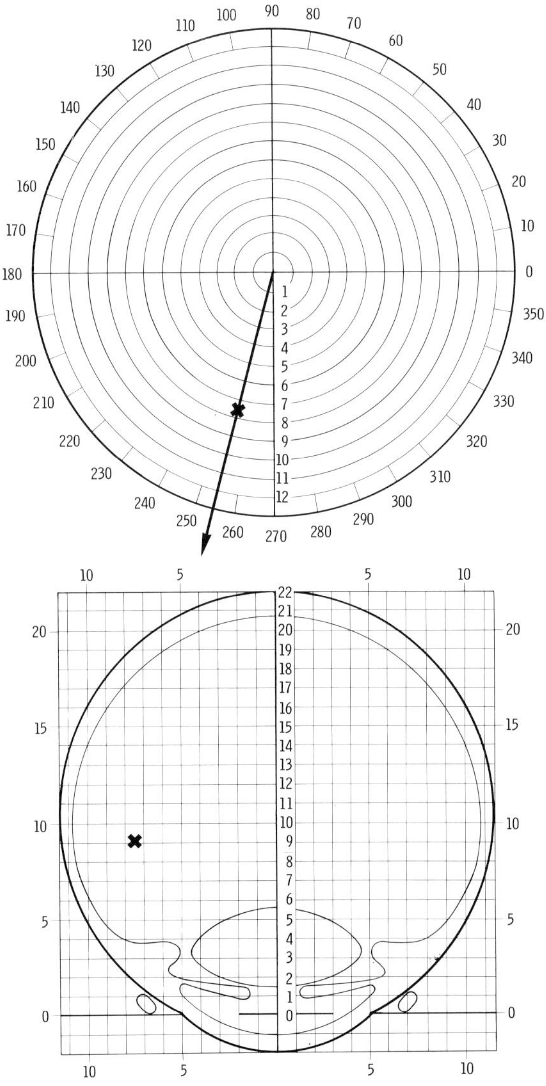

c

Fig. 10.1a–c. Localization of radiopaque foreign bodies in the eye according to Comberg (1927) (see also Pfeiffer, 1940).

a) A line is drawn through the zygomaticofrontal suture on either side (anatomic horizontal). The point of intersection of the lines through the lead points of Comberg's shell will determine the anatomic axis. The line drawn through the foreign body and the anatomic axis will form an angle with the anatomic horizontal, determining the arc value of the foreign-body meridian.

b) On the lateral view, a vertical is constructed through the upper and lower lead points. To this, at right angles, a vertical is connected and runs through the foreign body. Thus, the distance of the foreign body from the plane of the marker can be measured.

c) Schematic drawing with a marked foreign body (*x*). To fully account for the magnification factor, it generally will be sufficient to reduce the measured value on an a. p. view by 10 per cent and, on a lateral view, by 5 per cent (according to R. Thiel).

Fig. 10.2a and b. Stereoscopic x-rays.
a) Stereoscopic exposure technique: with the patient in an absolutely controlled, relaxed position without moving and with the film and cassettes also in a fixed position. Two subsequent exposures are obtained with the x-ray tube moved from a midposition 3.5 cm. toward one side (F_1) for the first exposure, and 3.5 cm. toward the other side (F_2) for the second exposure. If the film focus distance is more than 1 meter, lateral displacement by 5 cm. gives the best results. If one uses grids, one must pay attention to their arrangement (possibly they should be moved parallel to the grid). The film exposed by moving the tube toward the left should be marked with a L (or vice versa, but both films should never be marked, because this will disturb the stereoscopic effect or nullify it completely). The differing projections (P_1, P_2) of the foreign body (x) on both films will result in a stereoscopic image to the viewer, allowing him to localize the depth of the position of the foreign body.
b) Method of viewing stereoscopic images: course of beam in the formation of an image with the stereobinocular according to Stumpf (from Büchner).

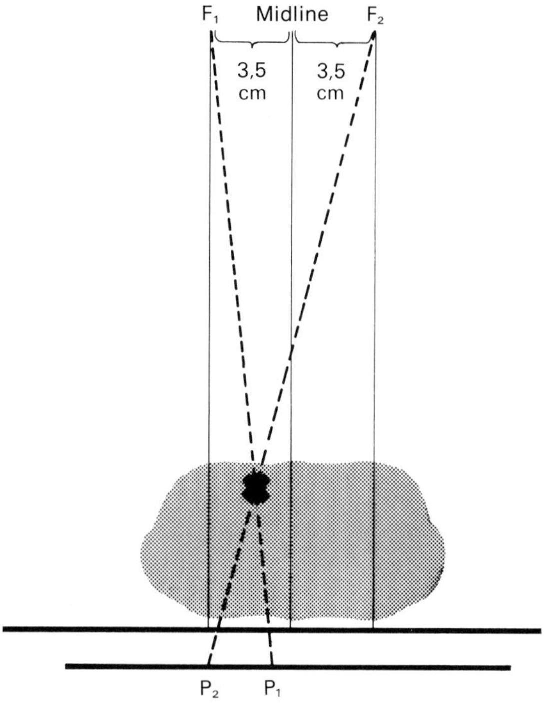

Fig. 10.2a

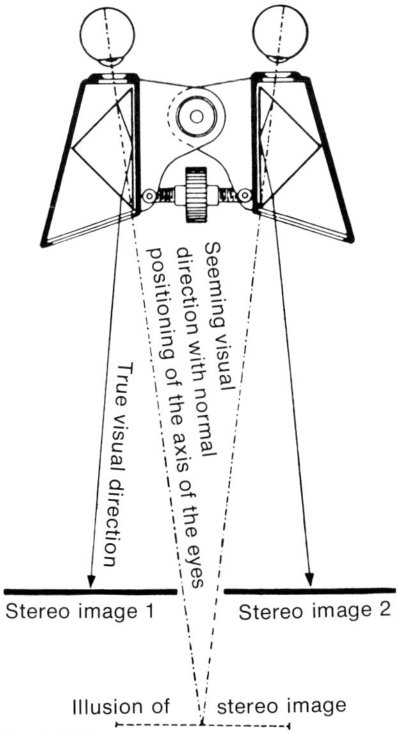

Fig. 10.2b

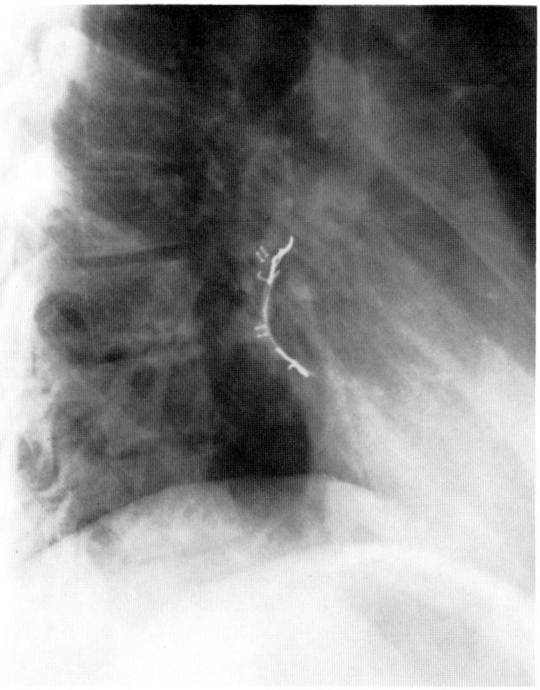

Fig. 10.3. A 21-year-old man who swallowed a dental prosthesis which is shown in the esophagus.

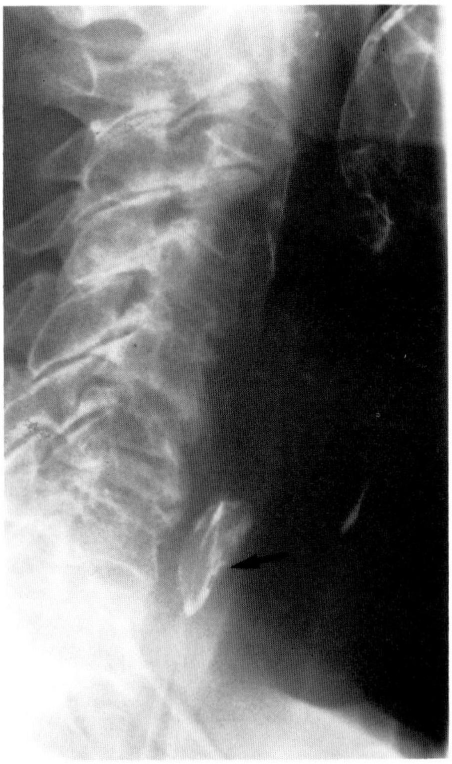

◀ Fig. 10.4. A 68-year-old woman with a glass splinter stuck in the cervical esophagus. Demonstration of a foreign body with Gastrografin.

Fig. 10.5a and b. A 53-year-old woman with a chicken bone stuck in the esophagus.
a) Roentgenogram: negative effect in a barium-filled esophagus due to an oblong nonopaque foreign body. Protrusion of the anterior wall of the esophagus.
b) The endoscopically removed chicken bone (operation by Professor Wiemers).

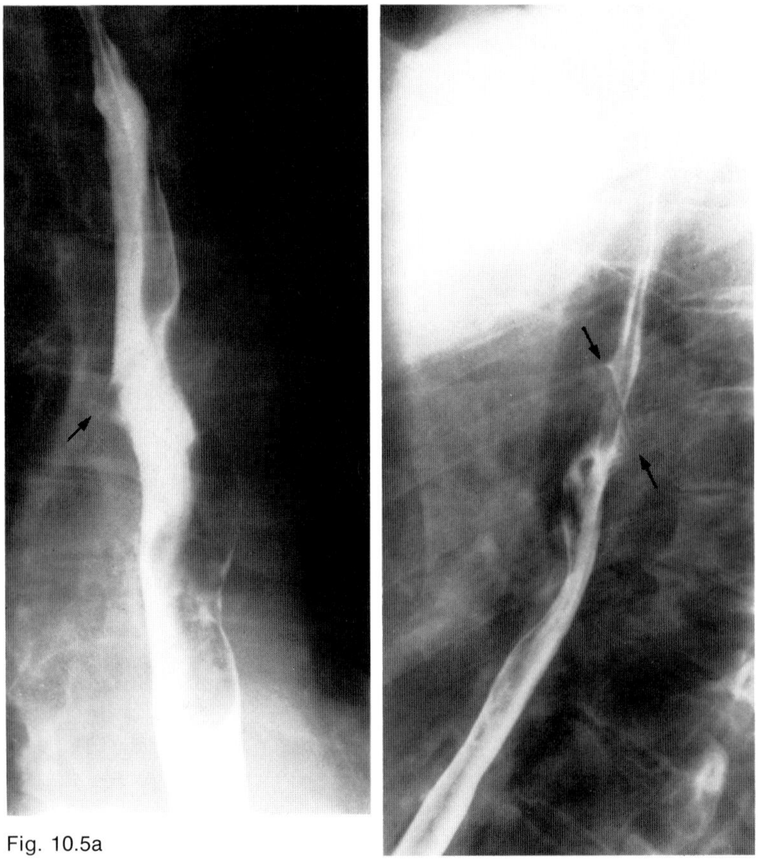

Fig. 10.5a

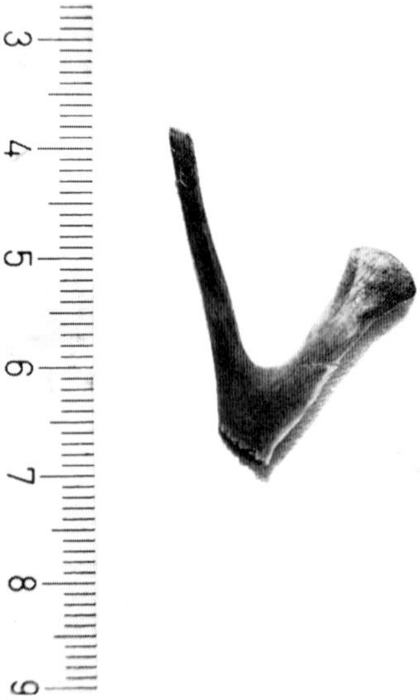

Fig. 10.5b

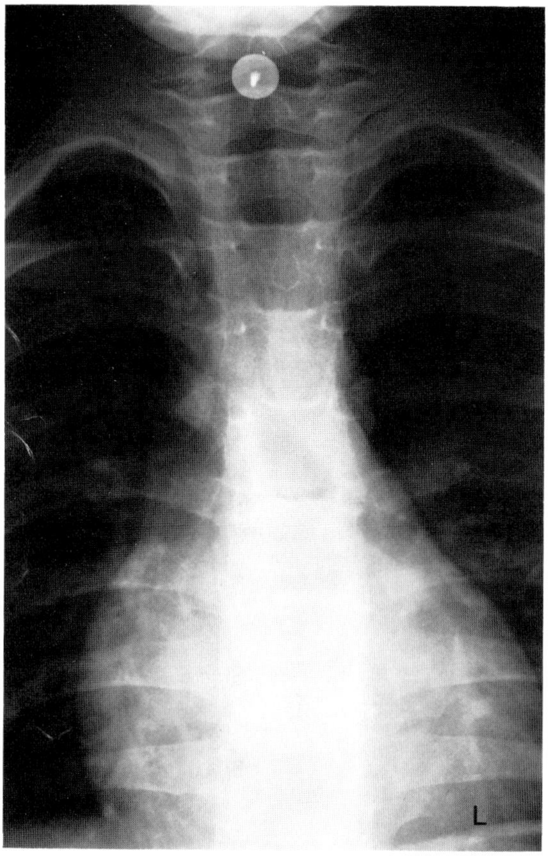

a

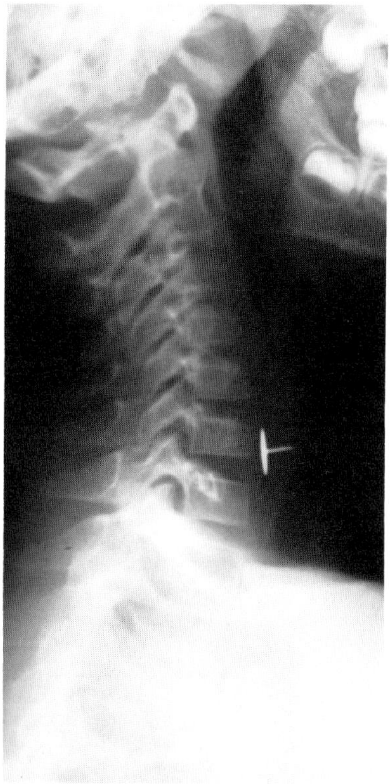

b

Fig. 10.6a and b. A 7-year-old child with a thumbtack in the upper esophagus. Extraction using an esophagoscope.

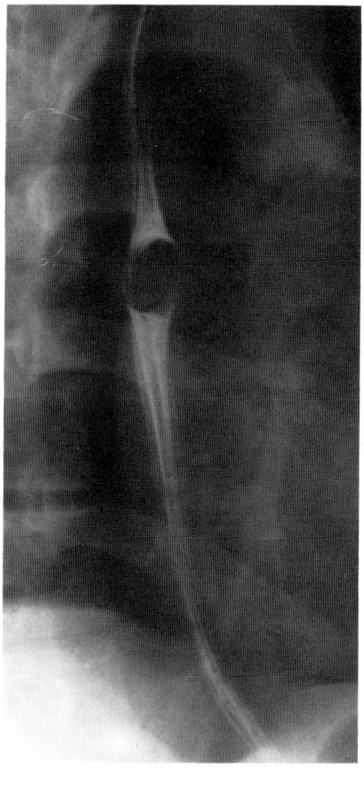

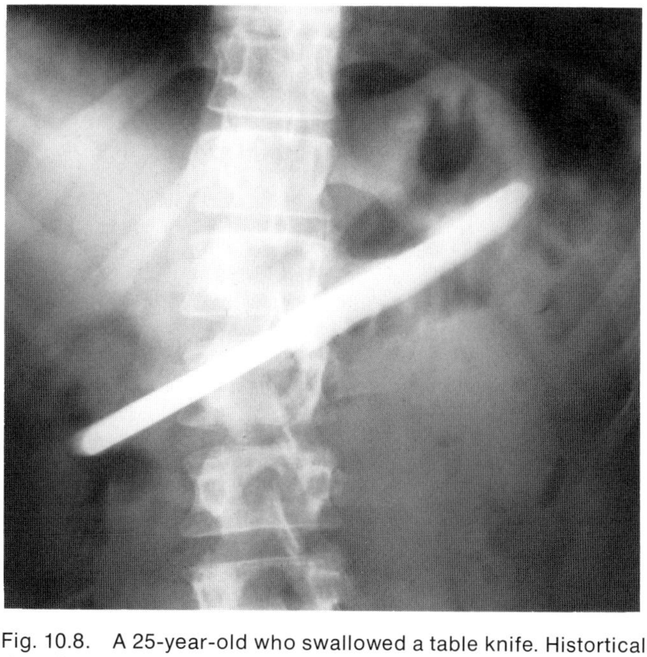

Fig. 10.8. A 25-year-old who swallowed a table knife. Histortical data. Surgical removal from stomach.

◀ Fig. 10.7. Plastic capsule in the esophagus, which, only after barium swallow, is recognizable as a negative effect in the esophagus. Extraction using an esophagoscope.

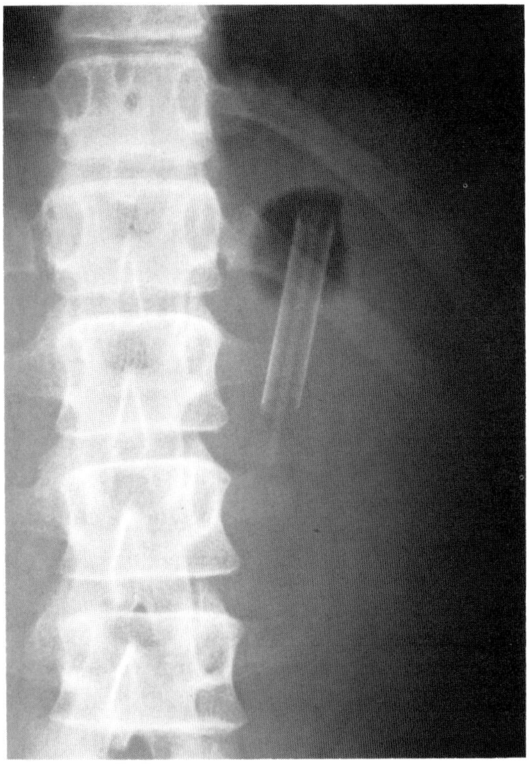

Fig. 10.9. A 10-year-old girl who swallowed a pencil which is pointing downward in the stomach.

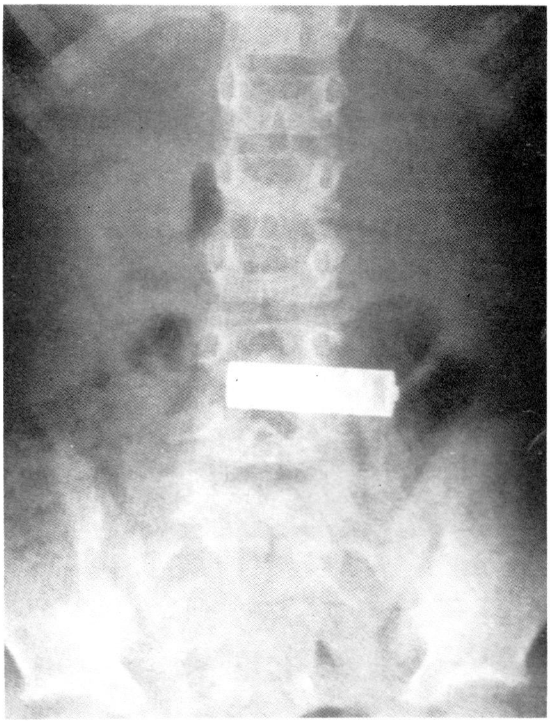

Fig. 10.10. A 5-year-old boy who swallowed a battery which is shown in the stomach. Operative removal because of the danger of chemical injury. (From E. Kern, J. Klöss and A. Bremer: Verschluckte Fremdkörper und Bezoare im Gastrointestinaltrakt. Dtsch. med. Wschr. *89:* 480, 1964.)

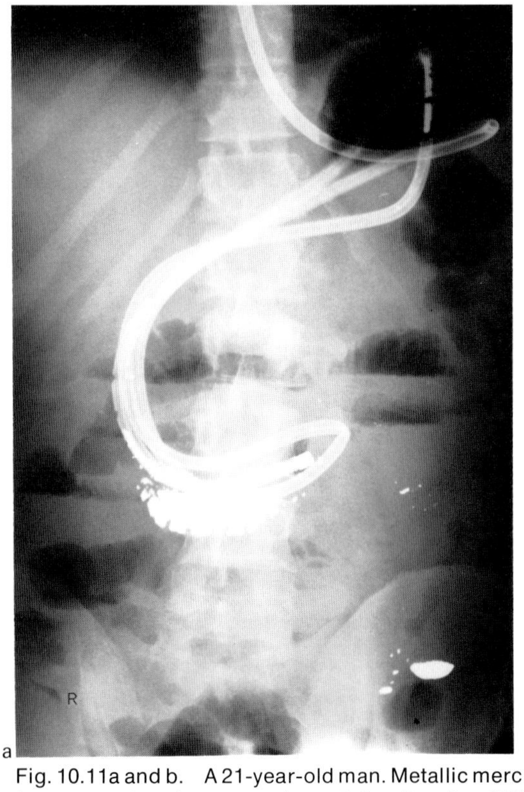

a

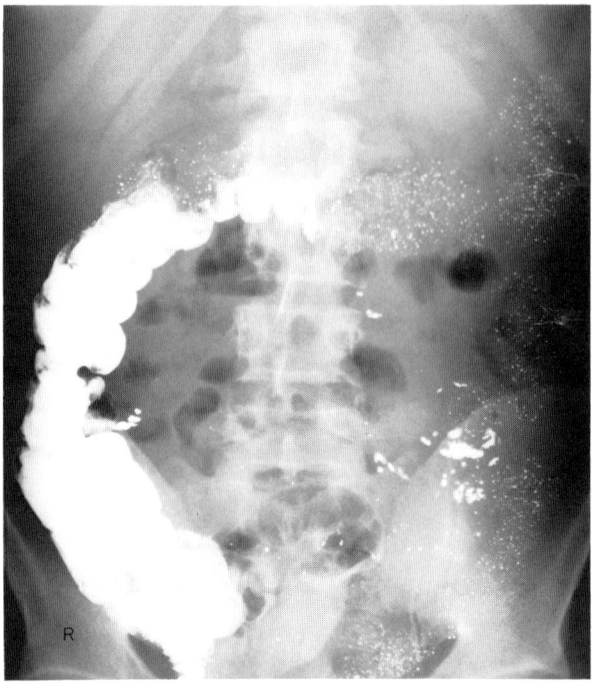

b

Fig. 10.11a and b. A 21-year-old man. Metallic mercury from a ruptured mercury bag at the tip of a Miller-Abbott-Tube:

a) Within the small bowel.

b) Five weeks later, finely dispersed within the large intestine.

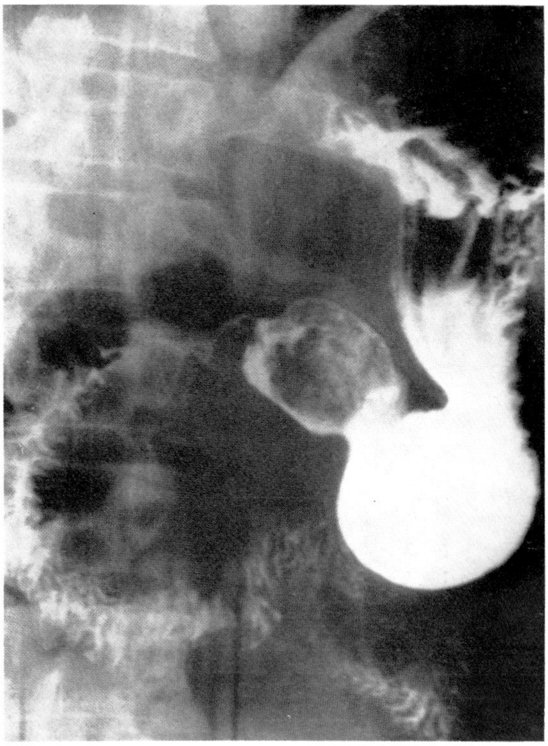

Fig. 10.12. A 48-year-old man who frequently ingested raw herb roots. Bezoar in the gastric antrum which was at first thought to represent a polypoid carcinoma (operation by Professor Dr. E. Kern).

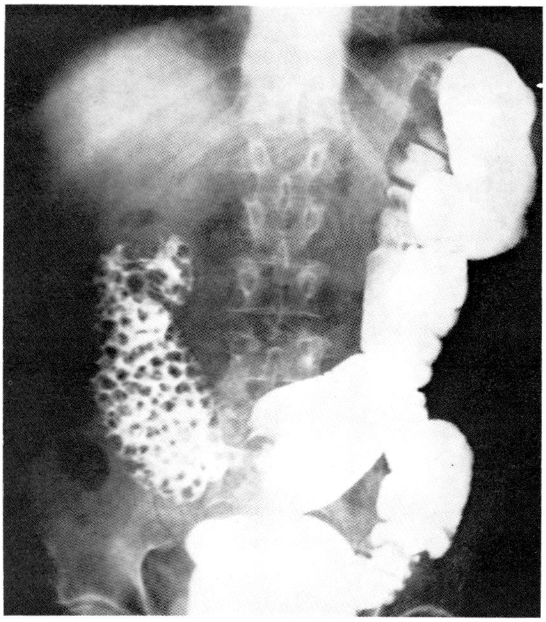

Fig. 10.13. A 61-year-old man with an obstructing accumulation of intentionally swallowed cherry stones, whose aim was to clean the bowels. The stones were localized at the level of a carcinoma of the transverse colon. (From H. Birzle and R. Zix: Kontrasteinlauf mit seltenem Nebenbefund. Fortschr. Röntgenstr. *110:* 574, 1969.)

Fig. 10.14. Remaining barium sulfate in the peritoneal cavity 6 months after perforation of the rectum during barium enema.

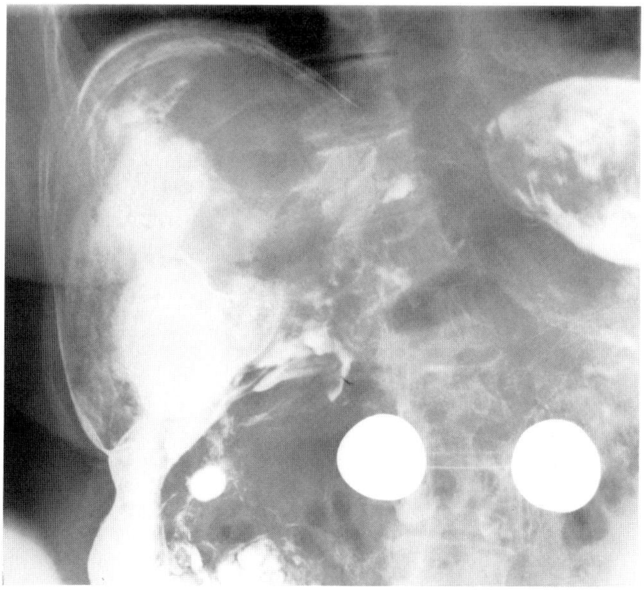

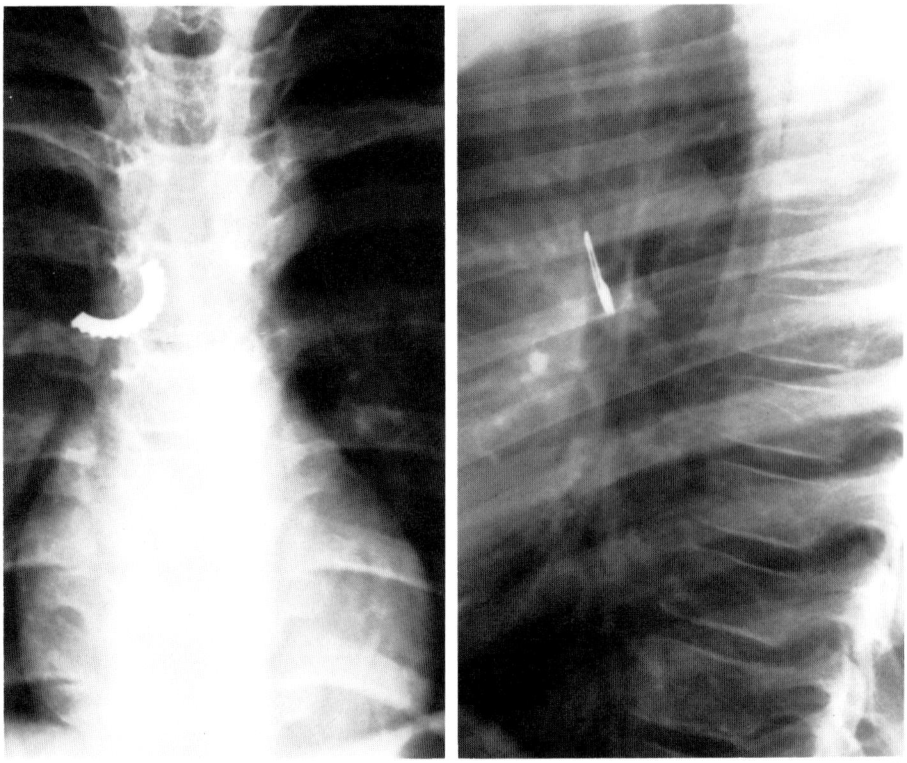

a b

Fig. 10.15a and b. A 12-year-old boy with a metallic foreign body (cogwheel part) in the right mainstem bronchus.

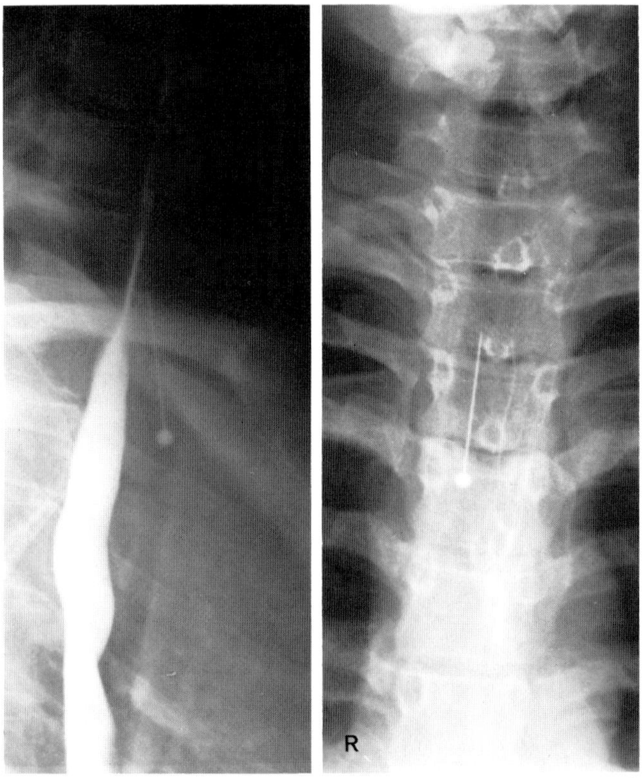

a b

Fig. 10.16a and b. A 25-year-old seamstress with a glass-headed pin in the trachea, the tip pointing superiorly and the cork inferiorly.

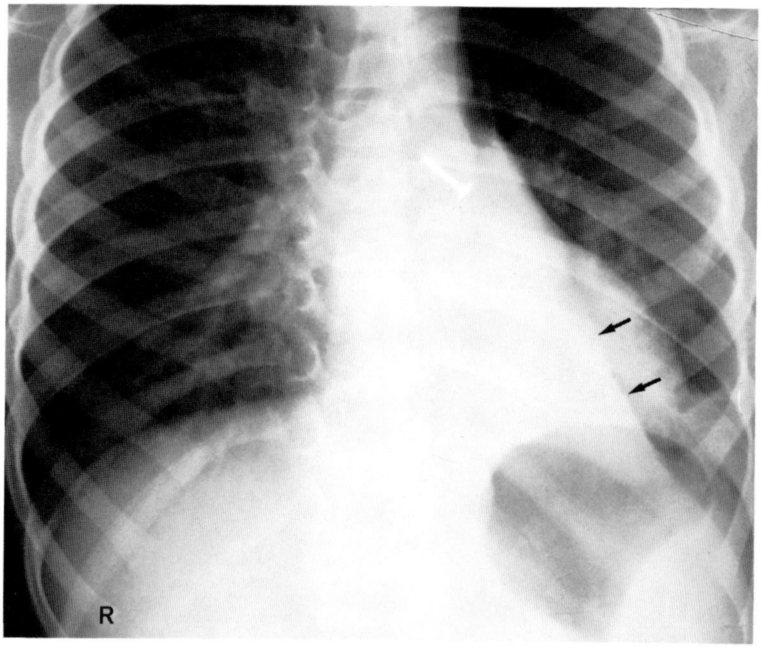

Fig. 10.17a

Fig. 10.17a and b. A 3½-year old boy with an upholstery tack in the left main-stem bronchus, the head of the nail occluding the lower lobe bronchus. Atelectasis of the left lower lobe (*arrows*).

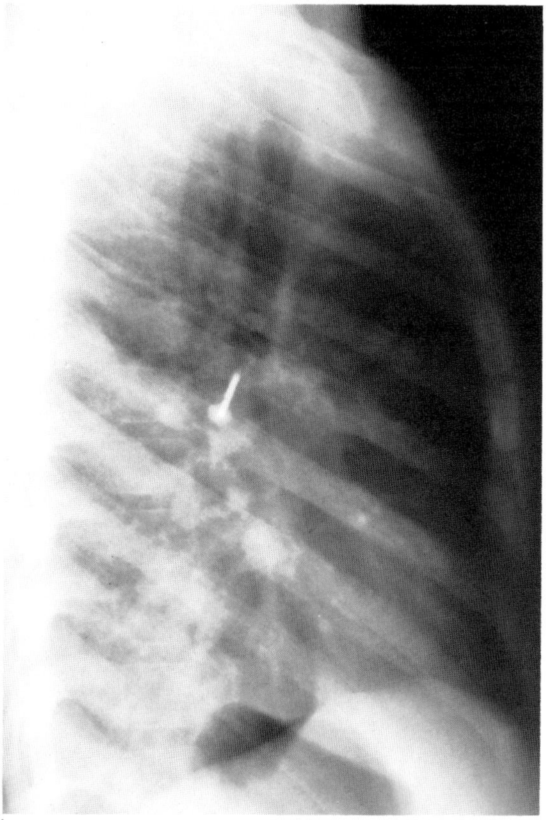

b

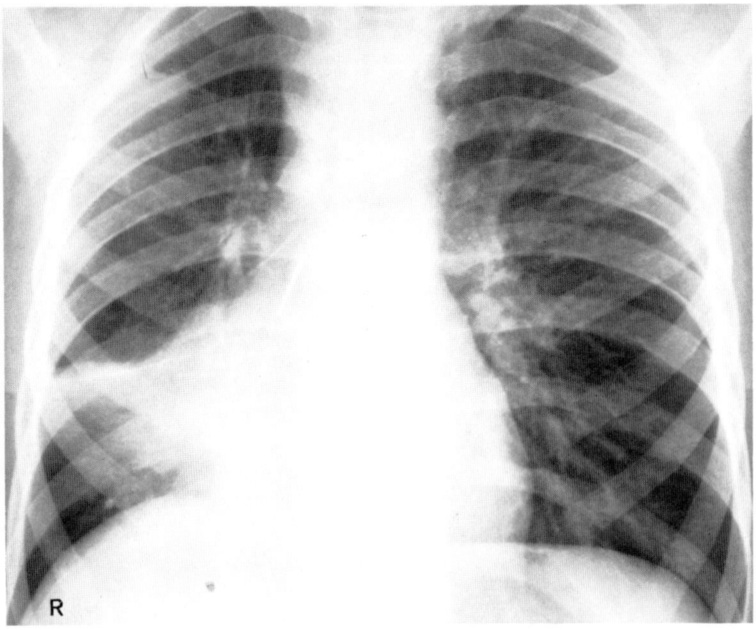

Fig. 10.18a

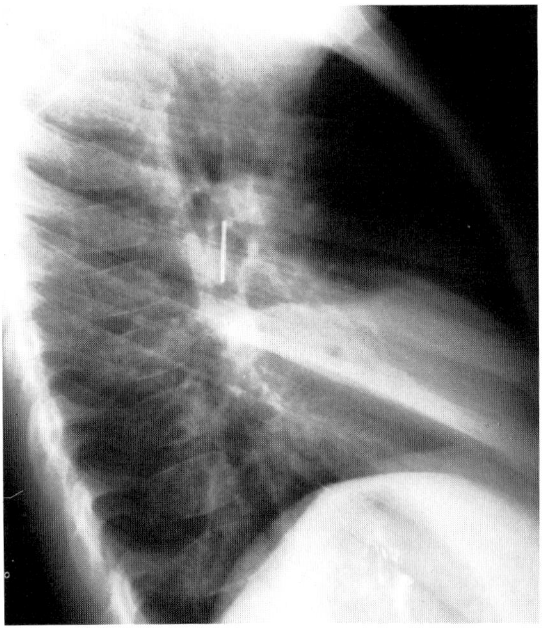

b

Fig. 10.18a and b. A 6-year-old boy with the axle of a toy car lodged in the intermediate bronchus. The atelectasis of the middle lobe indicates that the foreign body must be larger than its visible metallic parts. The invisible plastic wheel occludes the origin of the middle lobe bronchus.

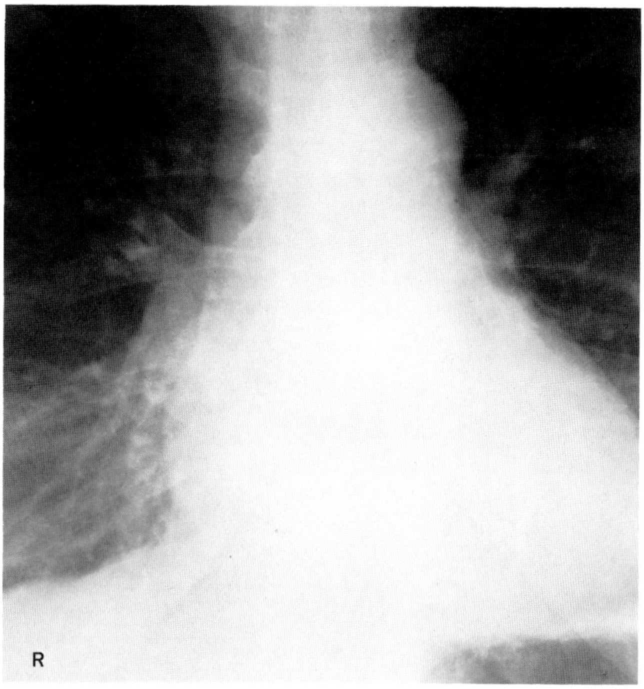

Fig. 10.19a

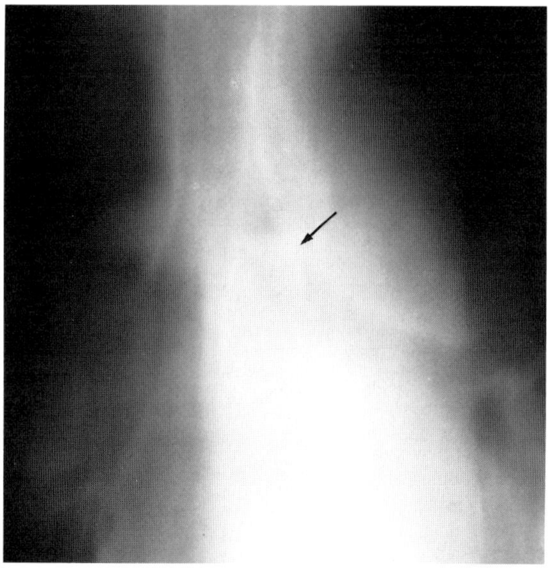

b

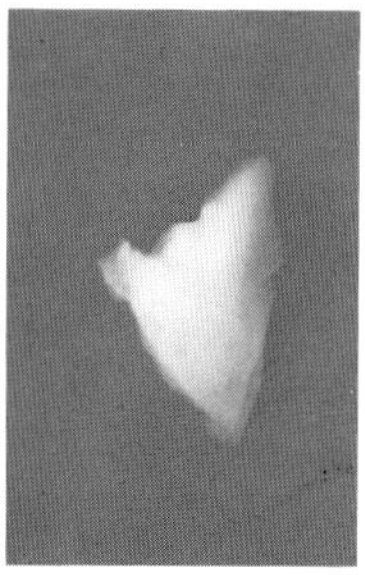

c

Fig. 10.19a–c. A 52-year-old woman.
a) Aspiration of a bone splinter which is not visible on this frame. Slight bronchopneumonic alterations at the lower right, which is the original location of the splinter.
b) After several subsequent coughing attacks, the localization of the splinter by tomography is within the left main-stem bronchus.
c) X-ray of the splinter after extraction using a bronchoscope.

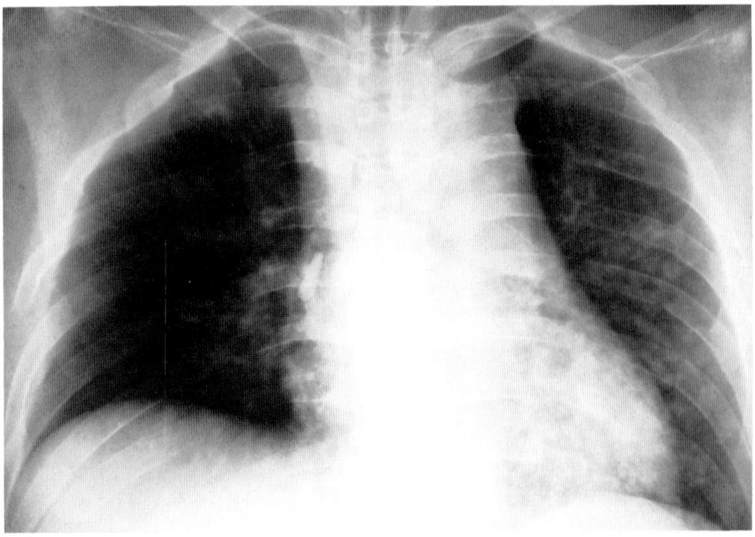

Fig. 10.20a

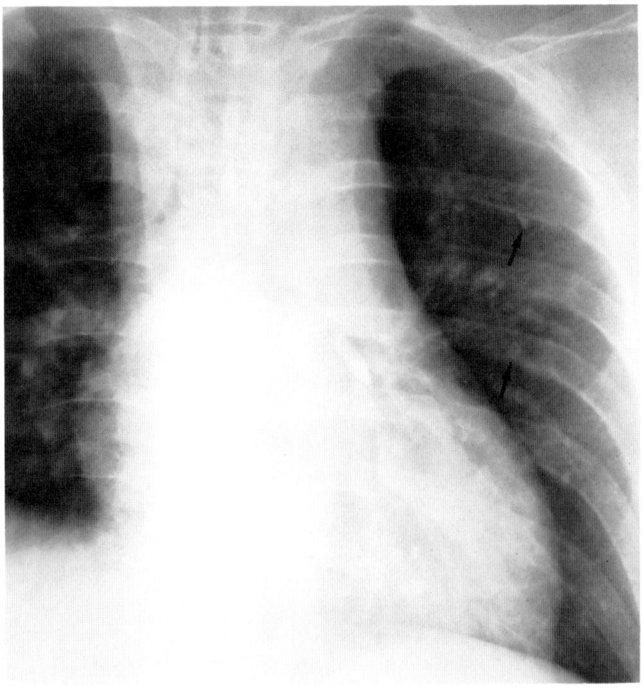

b

Fig. 10.20. A 29-year-old man who, under alcoholic influence, hit the car preceding him.
a) Aspirated tooth in the right main-stem bronchus. Massive aspiration on the left.
b) Follow-up roentgenogram on the same day shows the location of the tooth in the left main bronchus. Glass from the windshield is seen in the left thoracic wall (*arrow*). A series of rib fractures bilaterally.

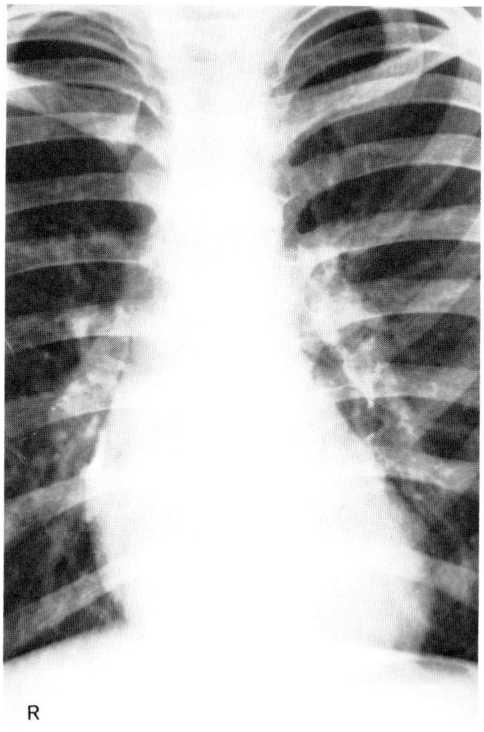

Fig. 10.21a

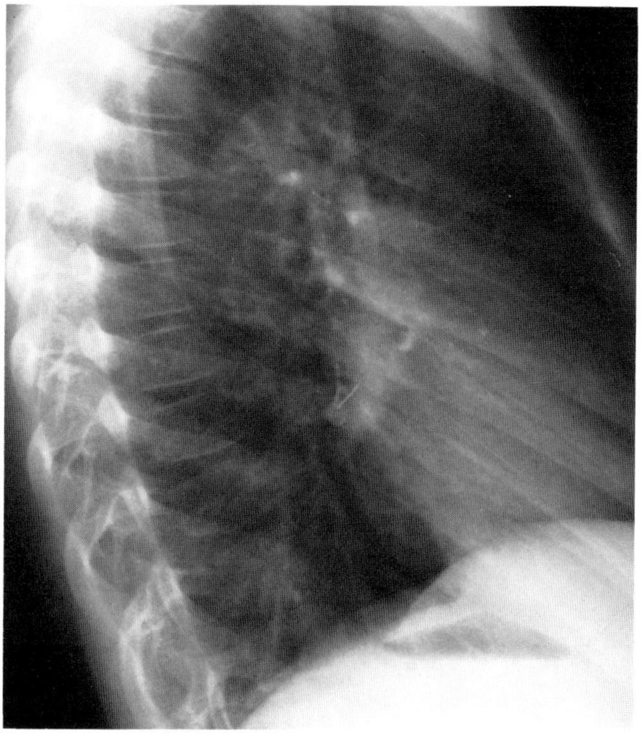

b

Fig. 10.21a–c. A 9-year-old boy.
a and b) Metallic clip in the main bronchus.
c) After extraction using a bronchoscope, a fragment of the clip remains in the right lower lobe brochus.

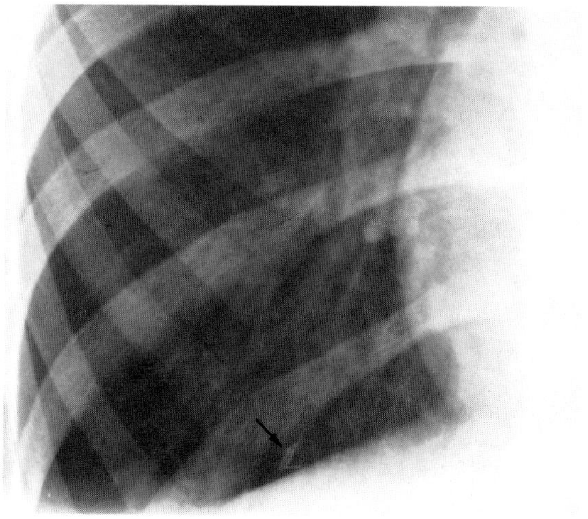

c

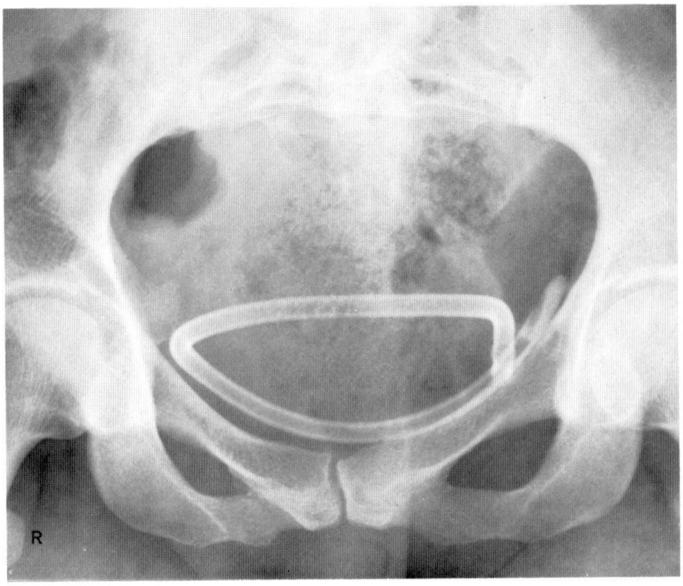

Fig. 10.22. A 35-year-old woman with a catheter that disappeared in the bladder.

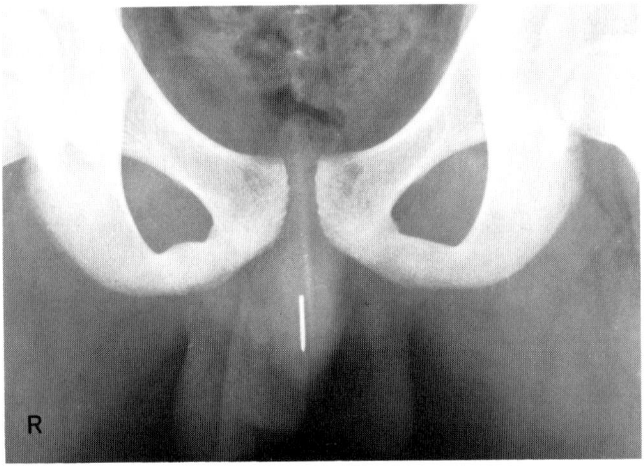

Fig. 10.23. An 11-year-old boy with a sewing needle in the urethra.

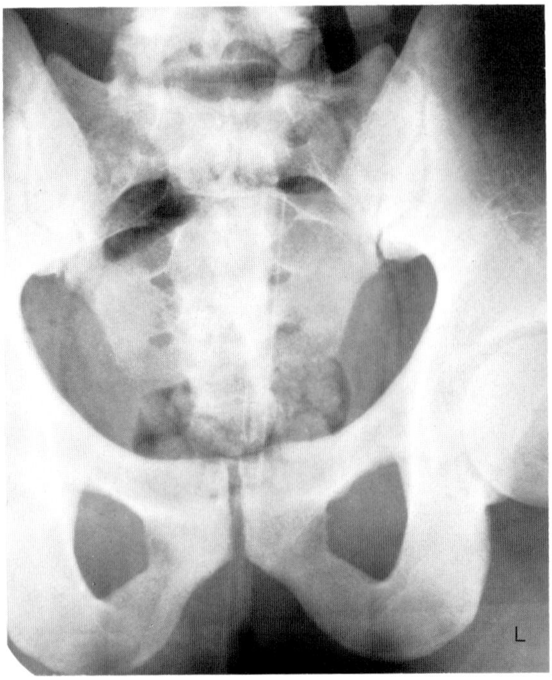

Fig. 10.24. A 22-year-old student with a pencil located in the urethra and bladder.

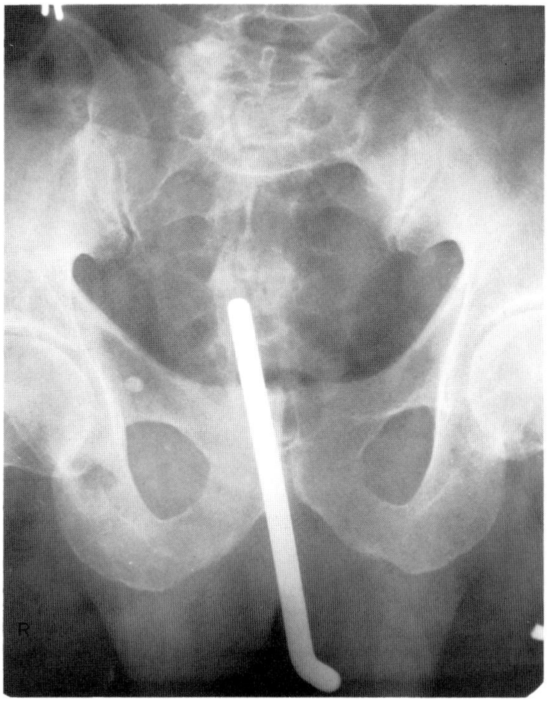

a

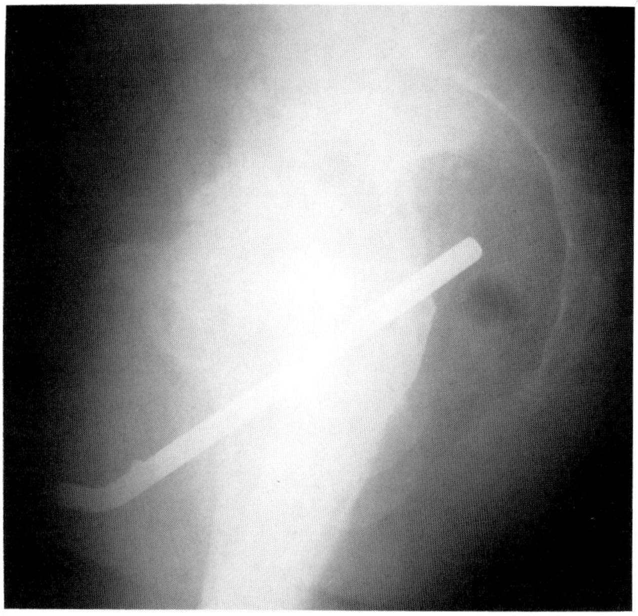

b

Fig. 10.25a and b. A 77-year-old mechanic with a metal bolt situated in the urethra and bladder.

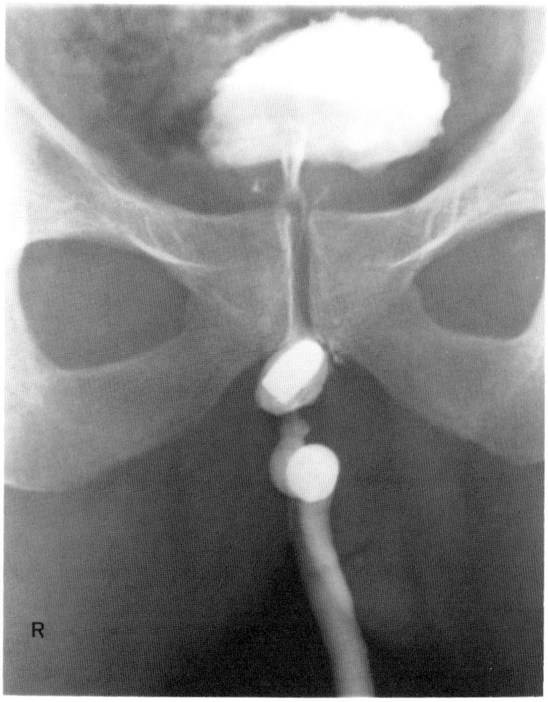

Fig. 10.26. A 41-year-old man seven years after being shot in the groin. At that time, he experienced a short bout of hematuria. Repeatedly had disturbance and difficulty in micturition. In 1951, he suddenly felt pain and resistance during voiding. A bullet from a pistol was located in the urethra.

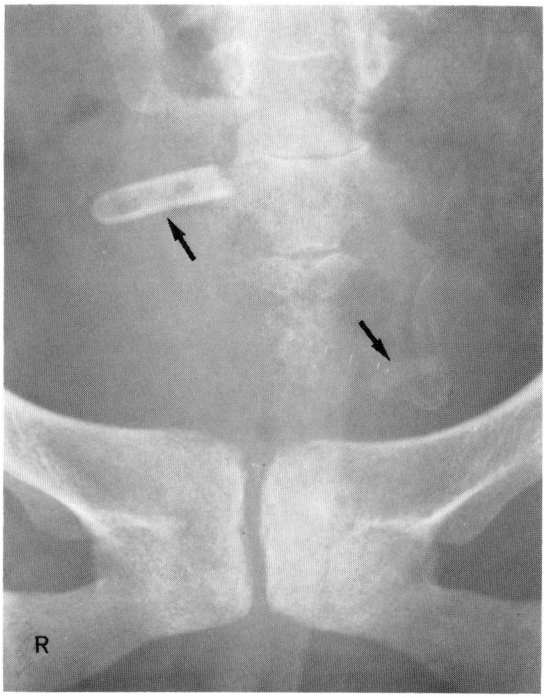

Fig. 10.27. A 25-year-old woman with a broken tip of a glass catheter in the bladder.

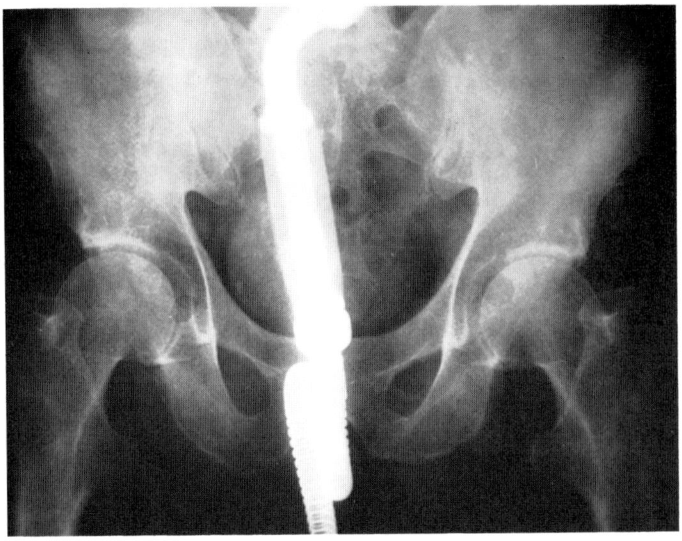

Fig. 10.28. A hand shower in the rectum.

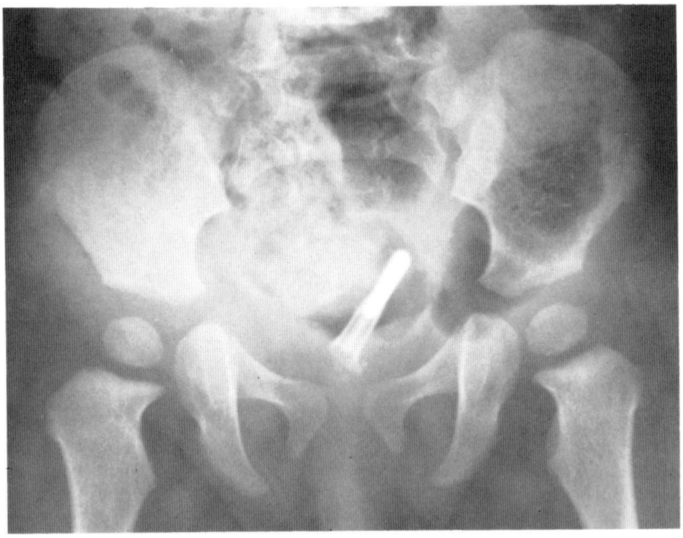

Fig. 10.29. A 10-month-old girl with the broken tip of a thermometer in the rectum.

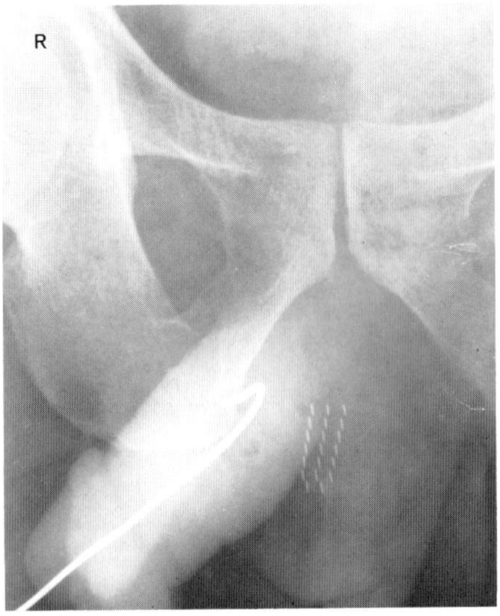

Fig. 10.30. A 57-year-old man with the broken tip of a tooth brush in the posterior portion of the urethra. Wire with a formed hook at the tip (attempt at extraction?) in the anterior urethra. Perforation of the urethra with rapid abscess formation.

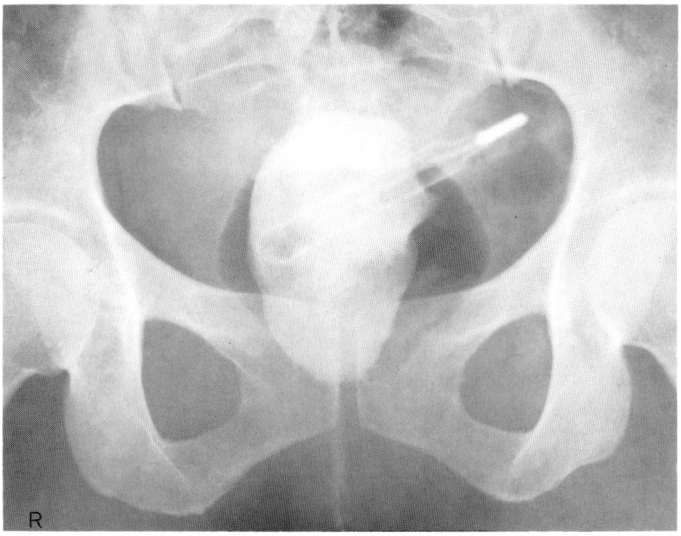

Fig. 10.31. A 29-year-old woman with a thermometer in the bladder. Massive formation of concrement around this foreign body. The tip of the thermometer has penetrated through the anterior abdominal wall.

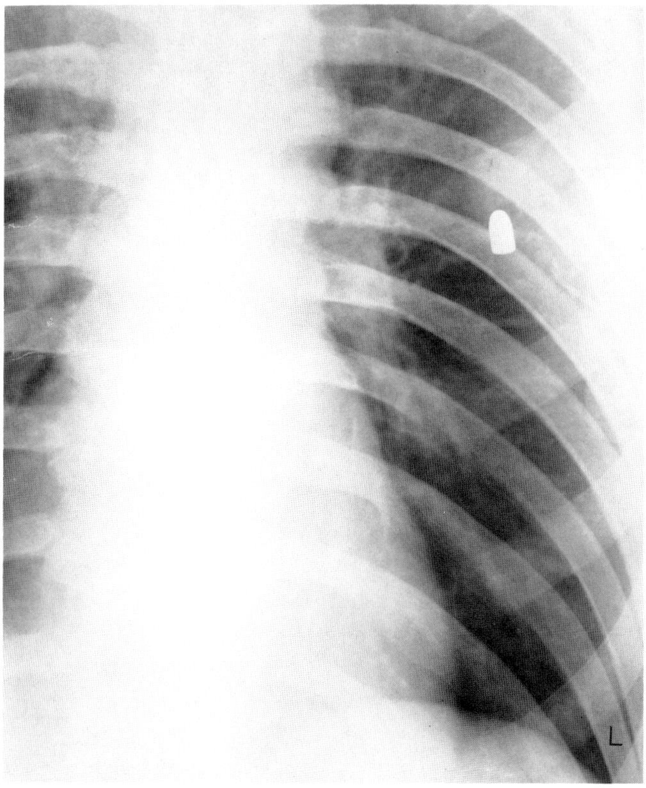

a

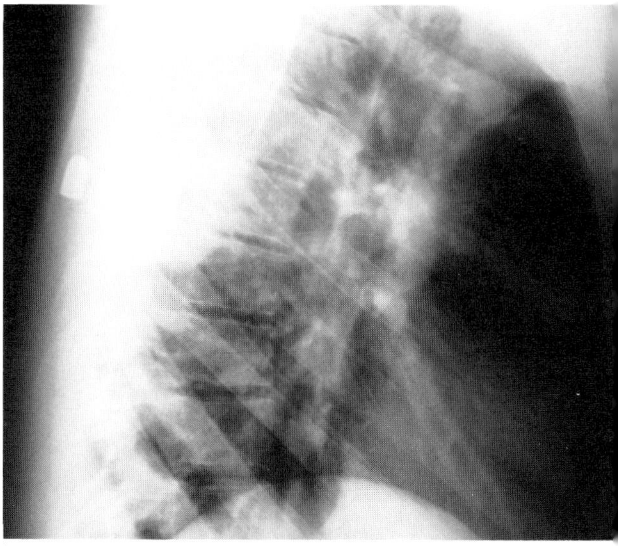

b

Fig. 10.32a and b. A 25-year-old man who attempted suicide with a 6.35 caliber pistol. Deflection of a projectile along the inner thoracic wall. Entrance of the projectile at the level of the left border, splintering the 5th rib. Removal of the foreign body from a subcutaneous location in the back.

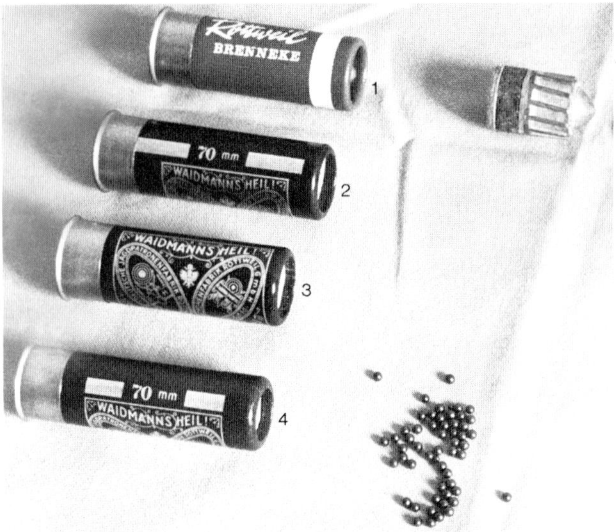

a

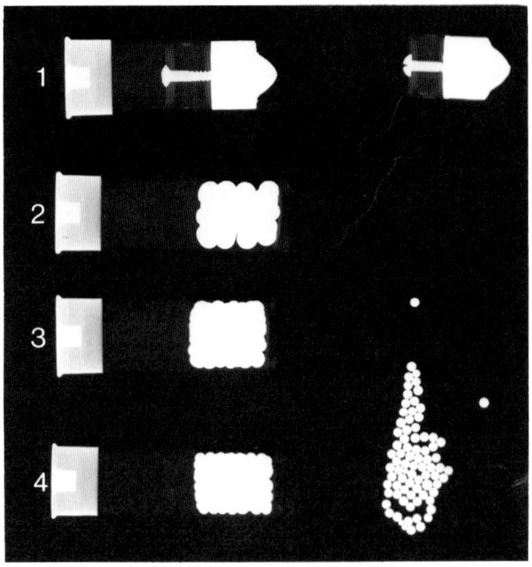

b

Fig. 10.33a and b. Buckshot cartridges for hunting: a) Direct photography. b) X-ray appearance. 1 = Brenneke (rifle ammunition); 2 = lead particles (size 5.6 mm.); 3 = grapeshot (size 4 mm.); 4 = grapeshot (3 mm.). Other commonly used sizes: grapeshot (2.5 mm. and 3.5 mm.).

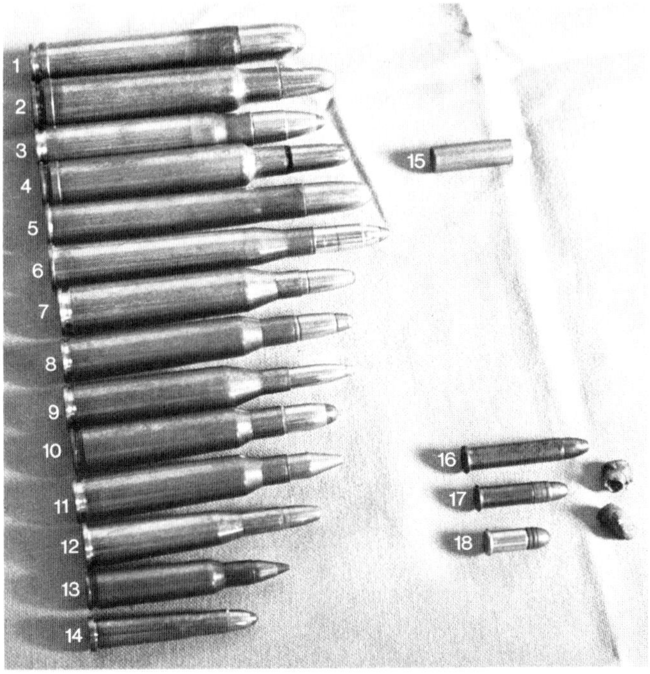

a

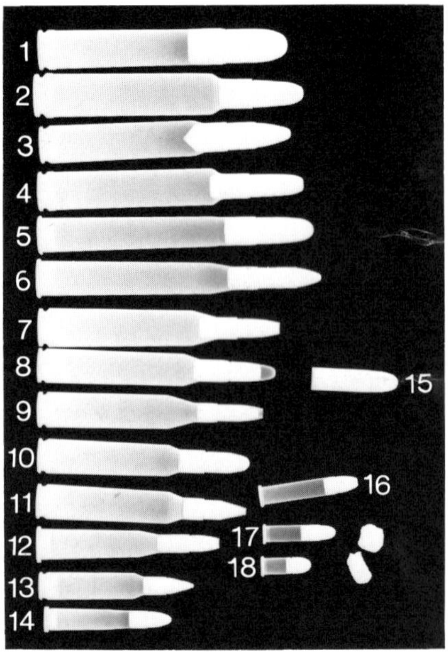

b

Fig. 10.34a and b. Cartridges for hunting rifles: a) Photography. b) Roentgen appearance. 1 = Winchester 458 magnum; 2 = Weatherby 378 magnum; 3 = Brenneke 9.3 x 64; 4 = Weatherby 300 magnum; 5 = RWS 9.3 x 74 R; 6 = Gehmann 7 x 75 R Sup. Expr.; 7 = RWS 6.5 x 68; 8 = 270 Winchester; 9 = vom Hofe 5.6 Sup. Expr.; 10 = RWS 7 x 57; 11 = RWS 6.5 x 57; 12 = RWS 5.6 x 52 R; 13 = 222 Rem.; 14 = 22 Hornet; 15 = 8.57 J partially covered cartridge; 16 = 22 magnum; 17 = 22 long; 18 = 22 short (16 to 18 = cartridges for handguns, caliber 5.62).

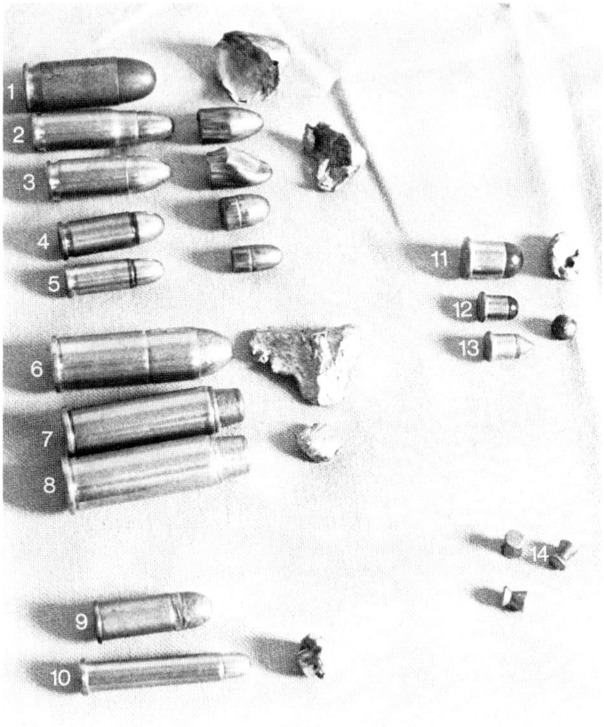

a

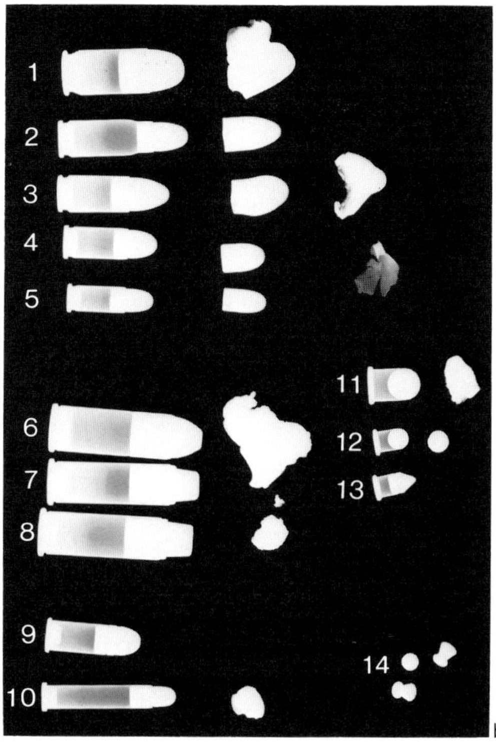

b

Fig. 10.35a and b. Cartridges for pistol and revolver; ammunition for Flobert pistol and air compression rifle: a) Photography. b) Roentgen appearance. Cartridges for pistols: 1 = caliber 45 ACP (11.5 mm.); 2 = Mauser 7.63 mm.; 3 = 9 mm. Parabellum; 4 = 7.65 mm.; 5 = 6.35 mm. Revolvers: 6 = caliber 45 Colt mm.; 7 = caliber 41 magnum; 8 = caliber 44 Rem. magnum; 9 = caliber 320; 10 = caliber 5.7 Velo Dog. Flobert pistols: 11 = 9 mm. round; 12 = 6 mm. round; 13 = 6 mm. pointed; 14 = Diabolo air-compression rifle.

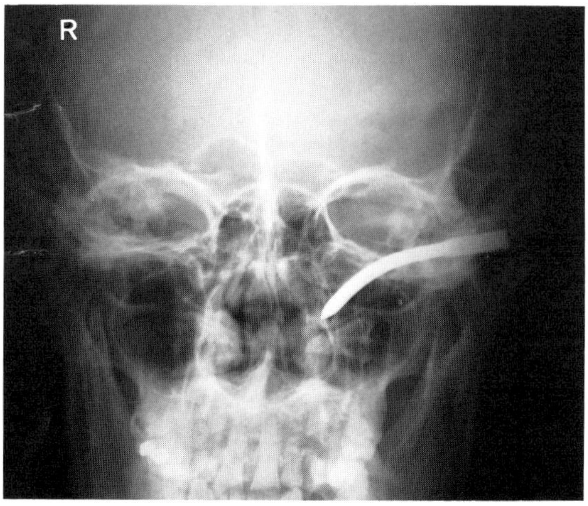

a

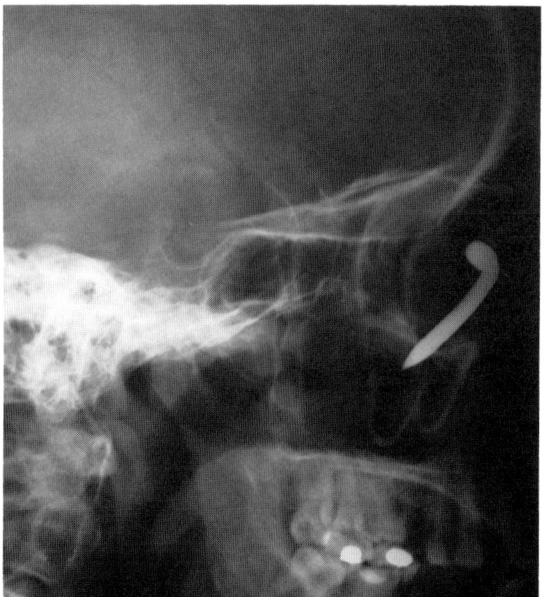

b

Fig. 10.36a and b. 37-year-old man who attempted suicide. Bolt injury of the left orbit and maxillary sinus. Double perforation of the eyeball. Surgical removal of the bolt; the eye was saved. Visual acuity reduced to recognizing light.

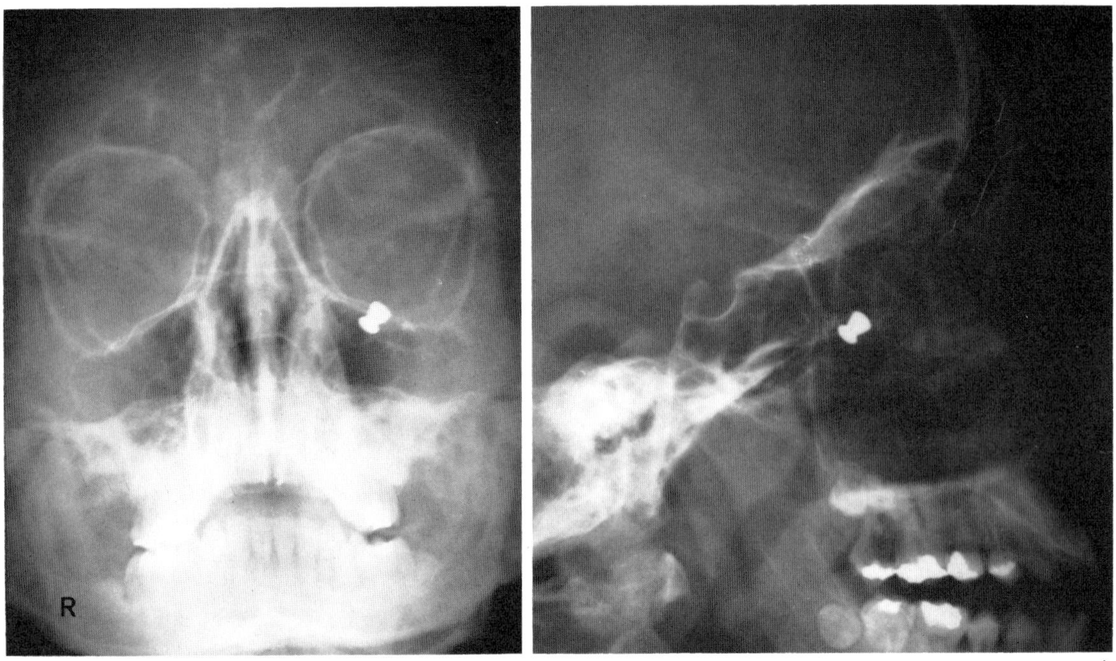

a b

Fig. 10.37a and b. A 14-year-old boy who was hit by a projectile from a Diabolo air-compression rifle. Left dorsobasal area of the orbit. Double perforation of the eyeball due to prolapse of the vitreous body and the uvea. Enucleation.

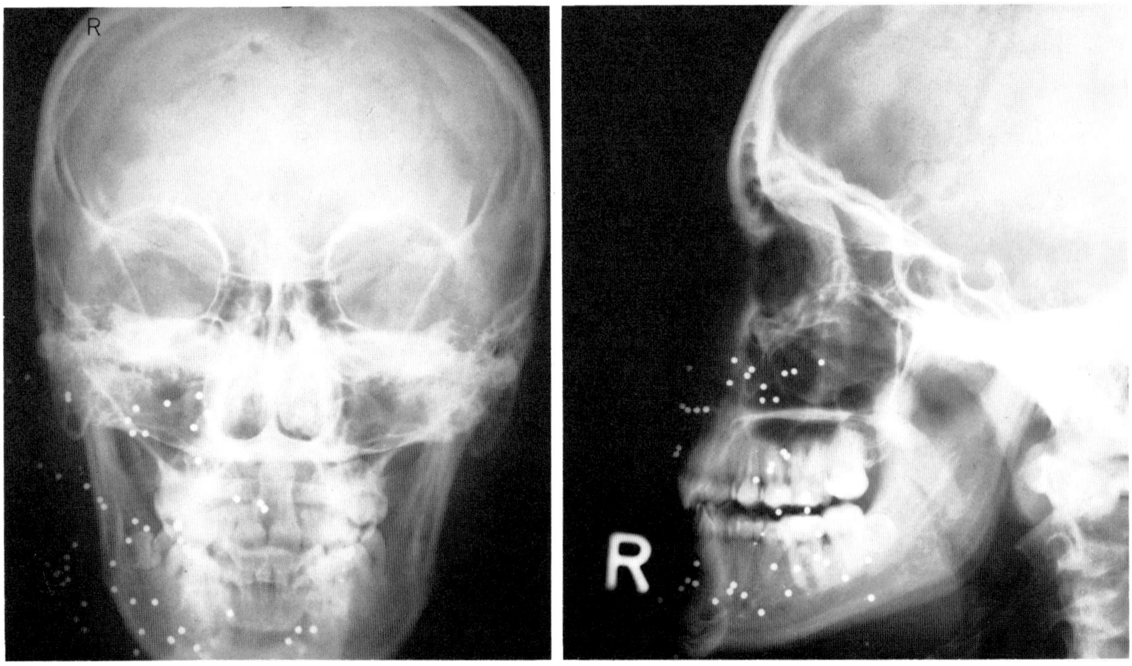

a b

Fig. 10.38a–d. A 16-year-old girl after an accidental grapeshot injury to the face and neck by so-called bird-haze.

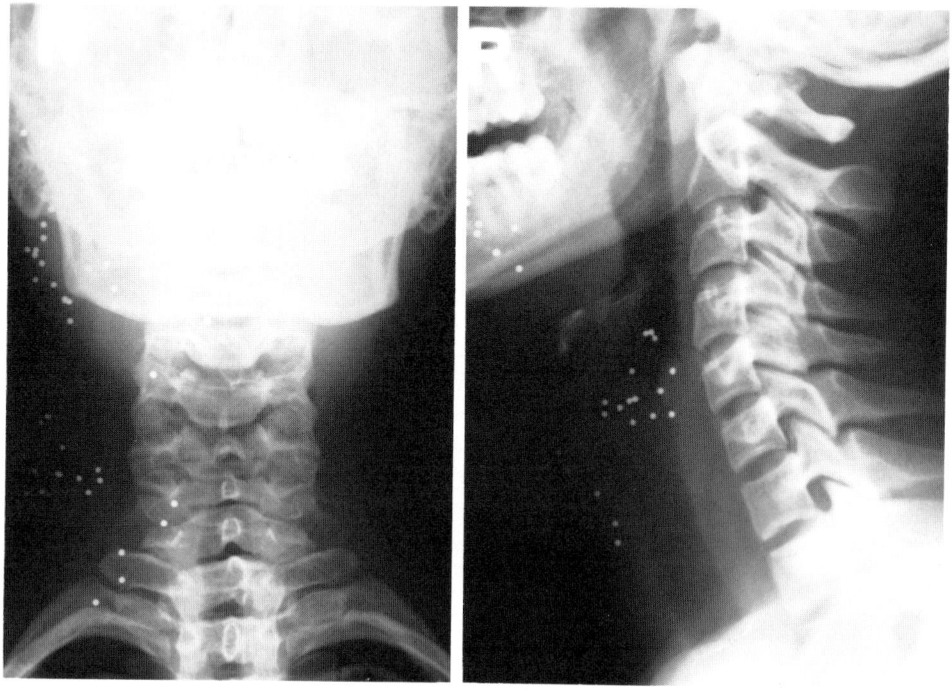

Fig. 10.38c d

Fig. 10.39a and b. A 13-year-old boy who, while helping as a driver, was shot by a hunter. Hunting grapeshot injury of the right thigh. Whether any of the shots actually entered the joint will best be determined by stereoscopic views, possibly with additional air insufflation into the knee joint.

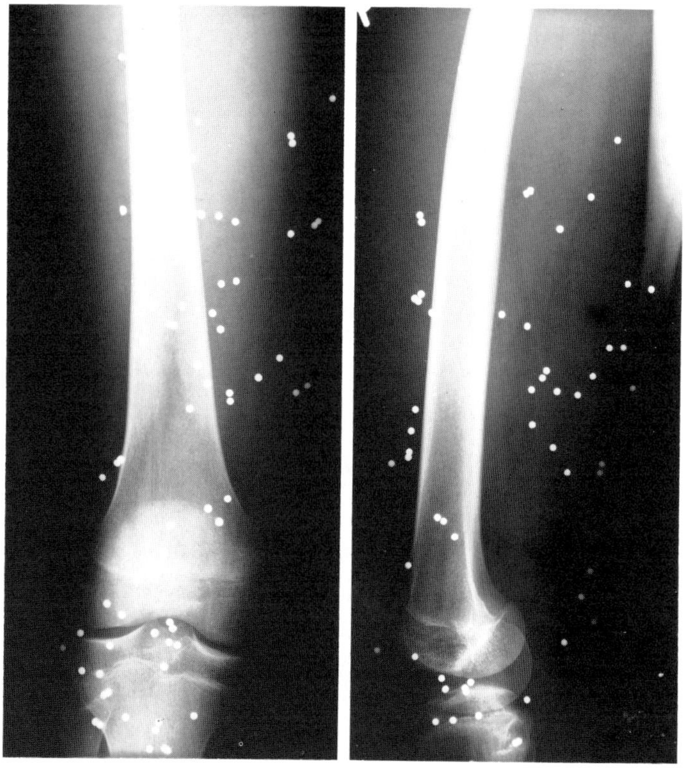

Fig. 10.39a b

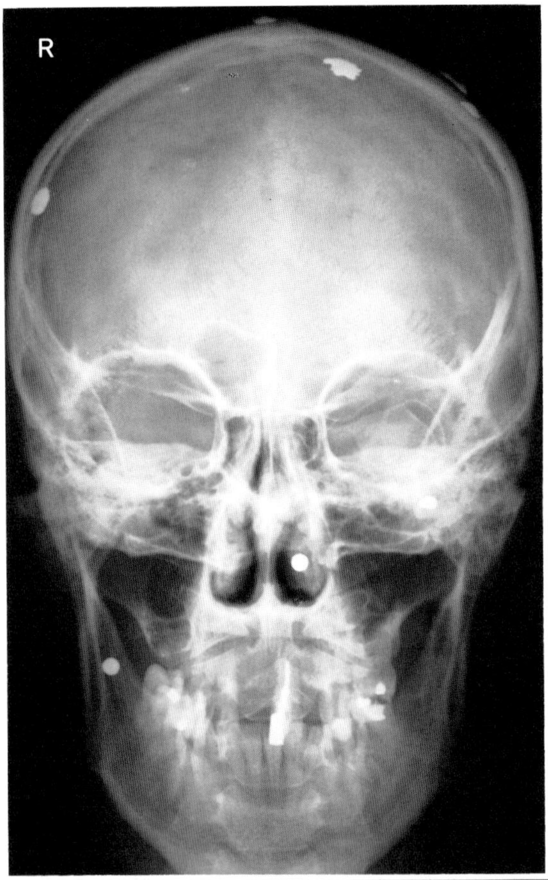

Fig. 10.40a

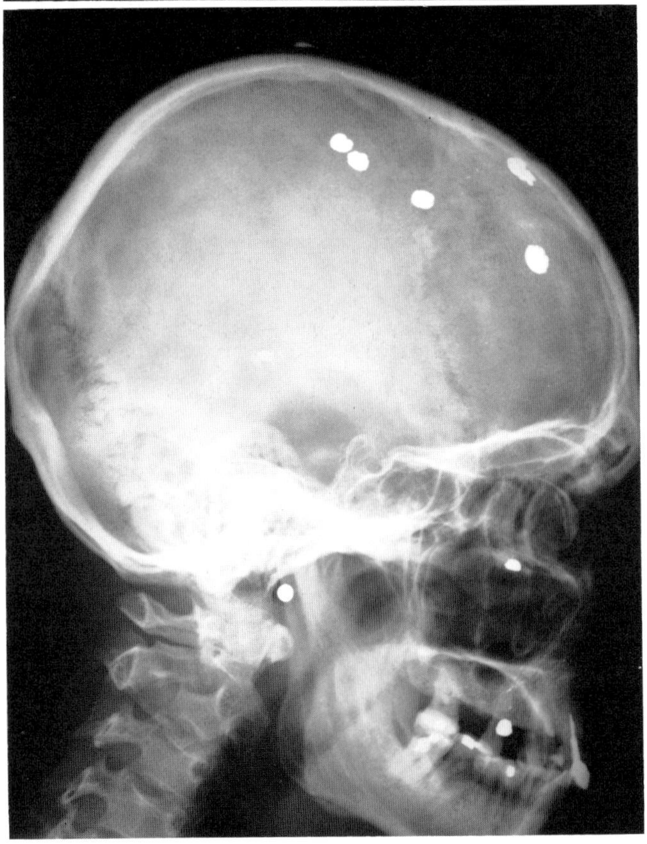

Fig. 10.40b

Fig. 10.40a and b. Grapeshots flattened out when hitting the skull. Additional finding: prosthesis in the left orbit.

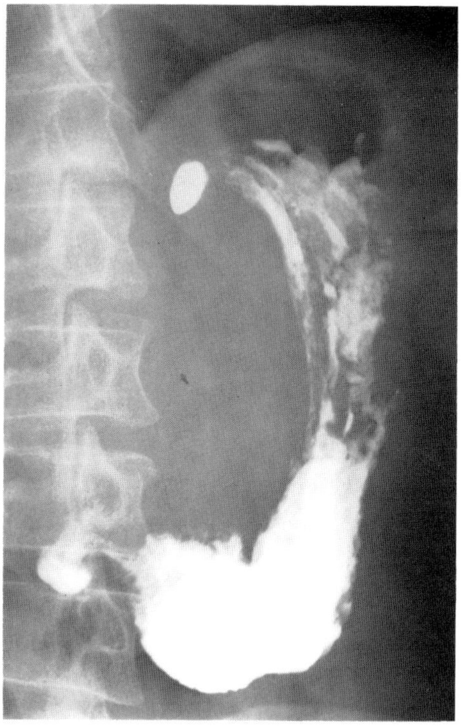

a

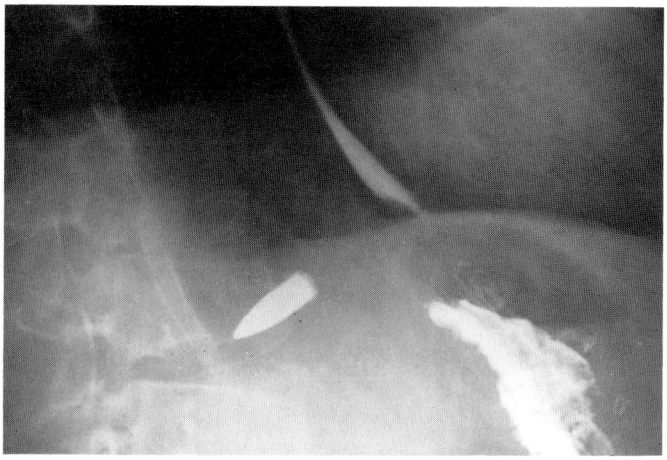

b

Fig. 10.41a and b. A 43-year-old man who was injured during the war when he was 18 years old. Projectile lodged in the left dorsal and paravertebral area of the diaphragm. No pulsation of the projectile.

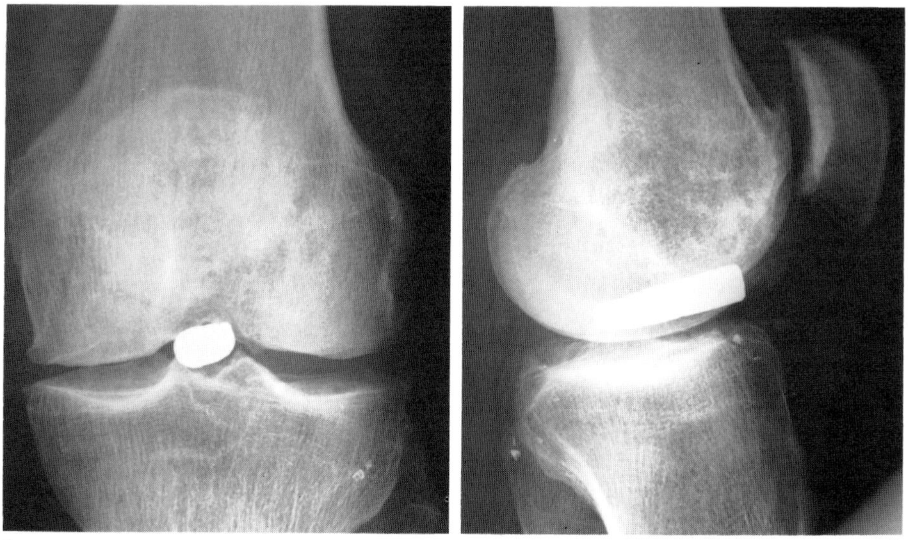

a b

Fig. 10.42a and b. A 62-year-old man with an old war injury. Projectile from a rifle is located in the middle of the knee joint.

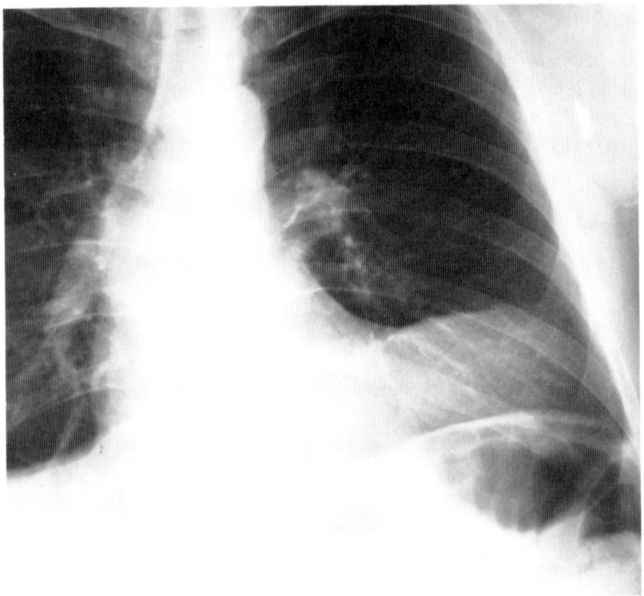

Fig. 10.43a

Fig. 10.43a–c. A 42-year-old man with a war injury. Splinter is stuck at the tip of the heart. This splinter is not visible at all on the a. p. survey film because of the pulsating marginal haze and overlapping with the shadow formed by the heart and diaphragm. On the tomogram, there is an artifact recognized as two seemingly different splinters. This is the result of pulsations. Marked scarring along the course of the canal created by the projectile.

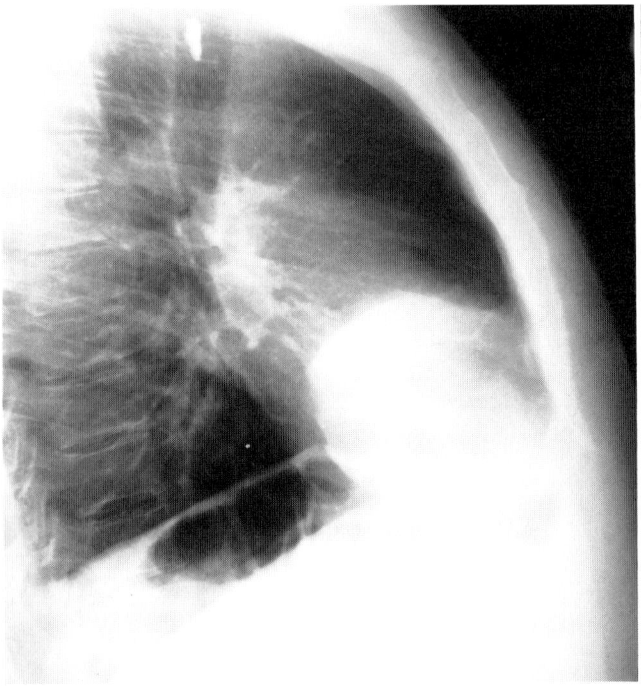

b

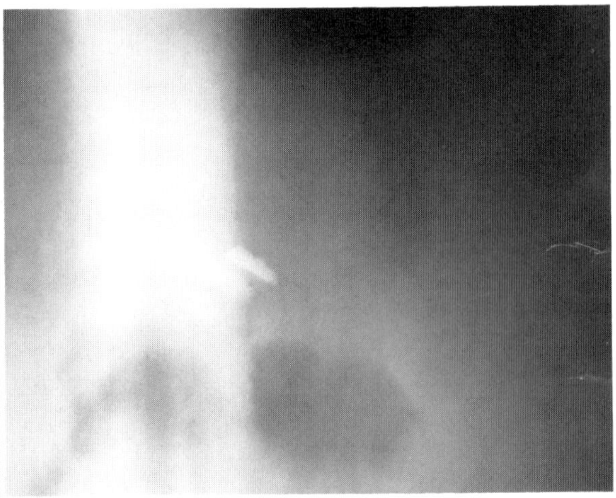

c

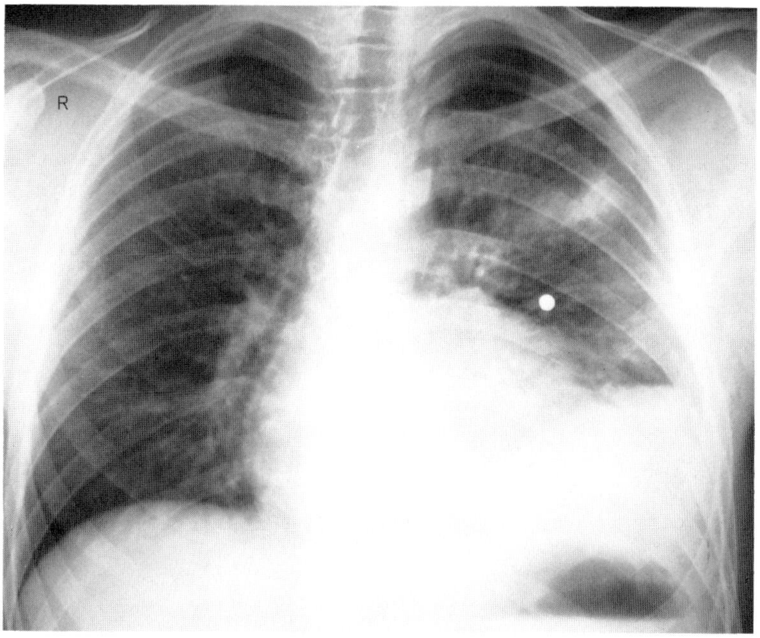

Fig. 10.44a

Fig. 10.44a and b. A 19-year-old man who attempted suicide with an adapted air-compression pistol. Perforating shot through the lung, with hemorrhage in the lung and hematothorax. Entrance of the projectile anteriorly; position of the projectile in the back subcutaneously.

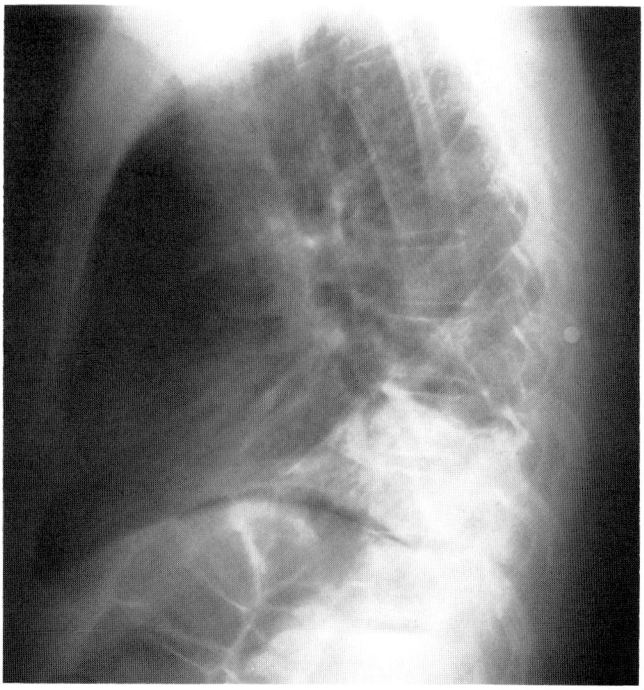

b

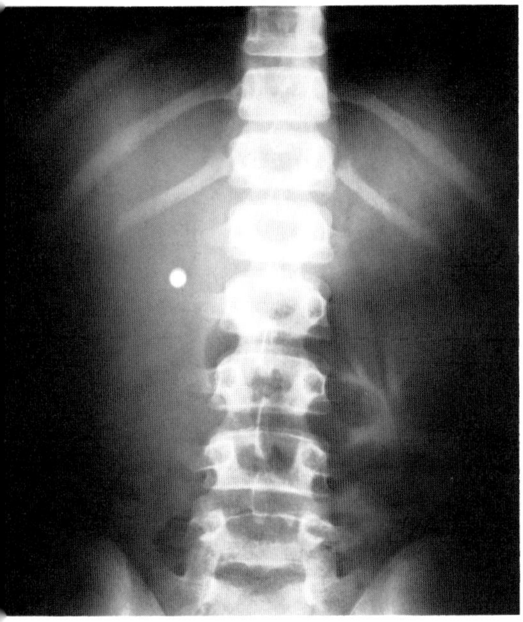

Fig. 10.45. An 11-year-old boy who, while playing with his father's gun, shot himself in the abdomen. Peritoneal and retroperitoneal hemorrhage. Entrance of the projectile into the anterior abdominal wall through the liver, bile ducts and adrenal gland. Removal of the projectile from the subcutaneous area in the back.

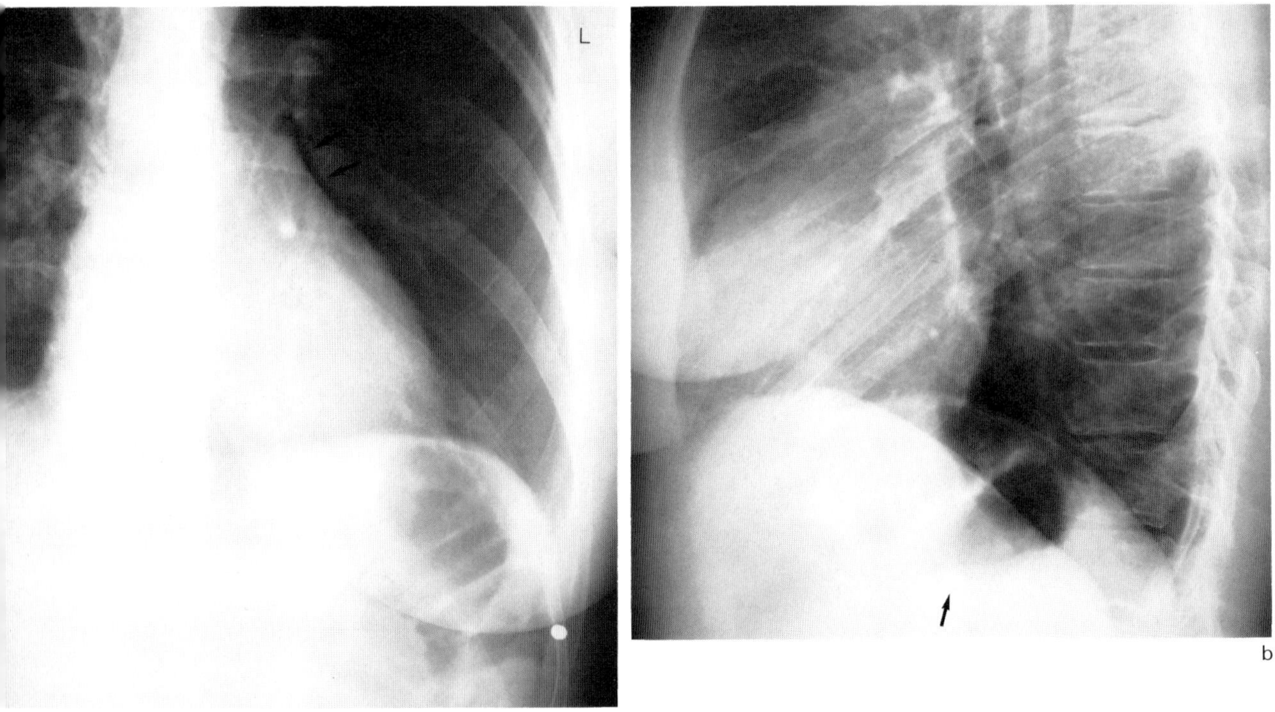

a b

Fig. 10.46a and b. A 43-year-old woman who was injured by a shot from a Diabolo air-compression rifle. Entrance of the projectile in the left supraclavicular region. During the night, pain was felt in the region of the heart. X-ray the following day revealed: projectile in the left pleural sinus; minimal accumulation of free air in the mediastinum; fluid in the diaphragmatic angle.

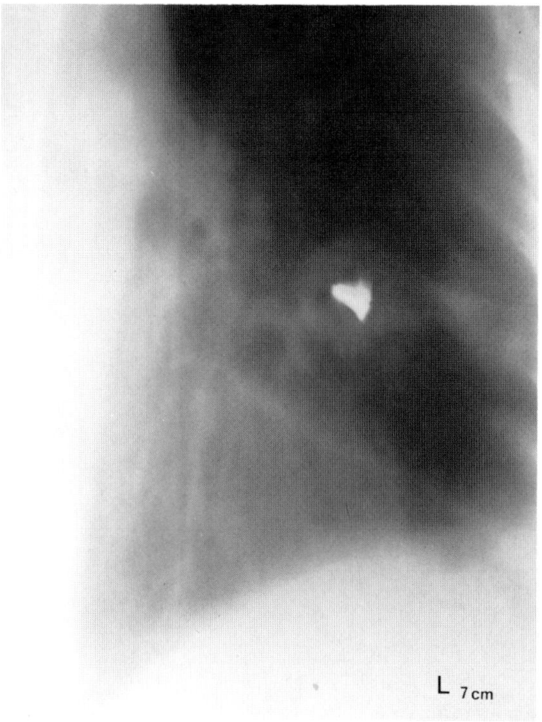

Fig. 10.47. A 33-year-old man with abscess formation around a splinter stuck in the left lower lobe of the lung.

Fig. 10.48. A 15-year-old boy who, while playing with a pistol, accidentally shot himself in the abdomen anteriorly. Perforation of the duodenal bulb; hematoma of the transverse colon. Free air in the abdominal cavity (*arrow*); diffuse shadow from the hematoma in the midabdomen and on the right retroperitoneally. The projectile was palpable in the subcutaneous area of the back and could be removed.

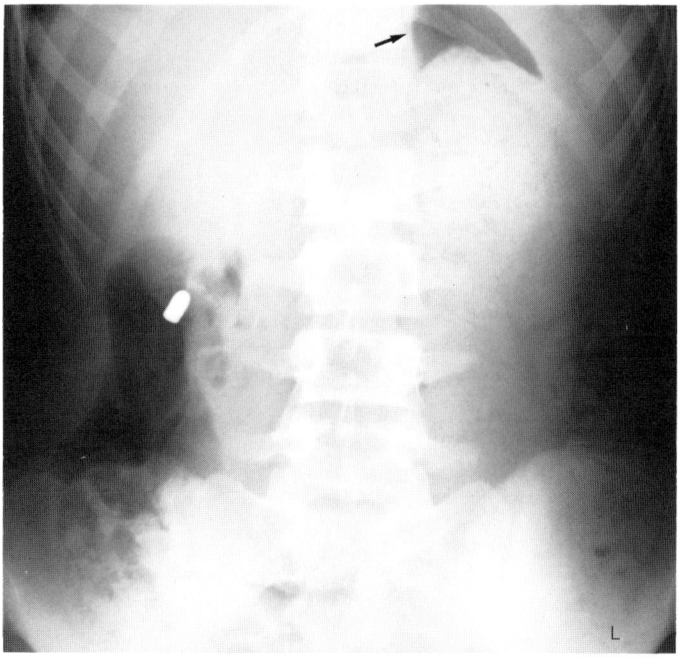

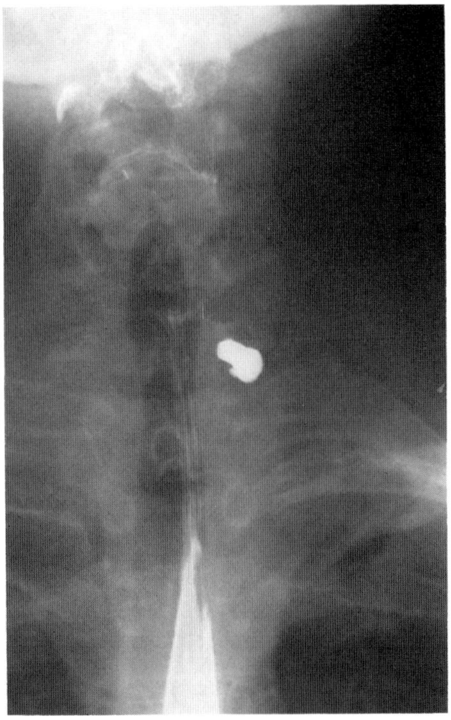

Fig. 10.49a

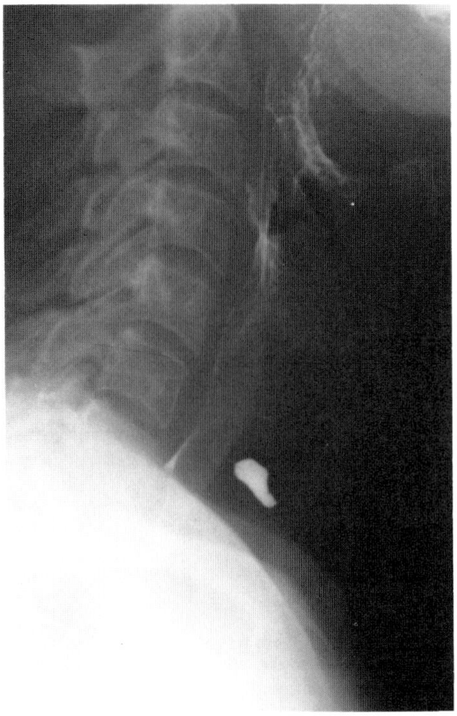

b

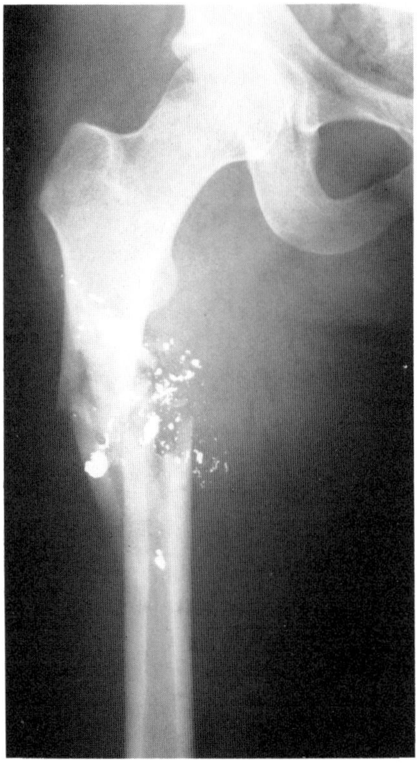

Fig. 10.50

▲ Fig. 10.49a and b. A 32-year-old man who was shot during a holdup. (In such cases, it is very important to find and secure the projectile for the investigating police agency.) Injury to the left lobe of the thyroid. Entrance of the projectile laterally, with injury to the nerve plexus and temporary paralysis of the left arm. Surgical removal of the projectile from the left lobe of the thyroid.

◀ Fig. 10.50. A 28-year-old woman who was injured as a result of careless manipulation of a loaded gun in a car. Gunshot fracture of the right femur; caliber 22 long.

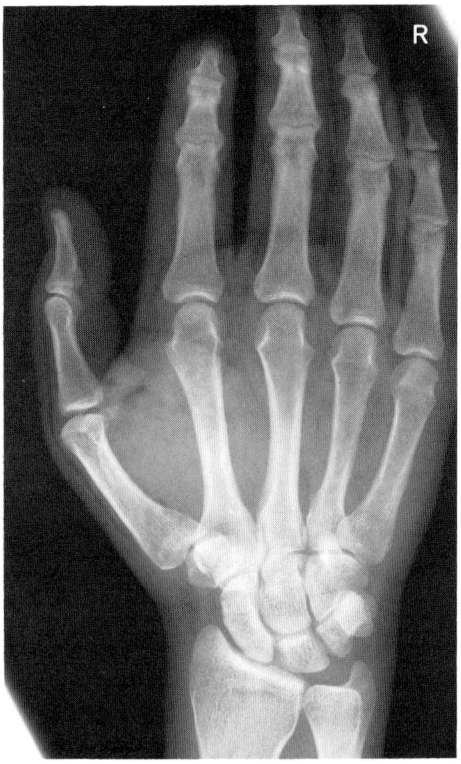

Fig. 10.51. A 32-year-old man who was shot in the hand at close range with a gas pistol. Free gas with extensions along the tendon sheath, particularly on the volar surface of the thumb.

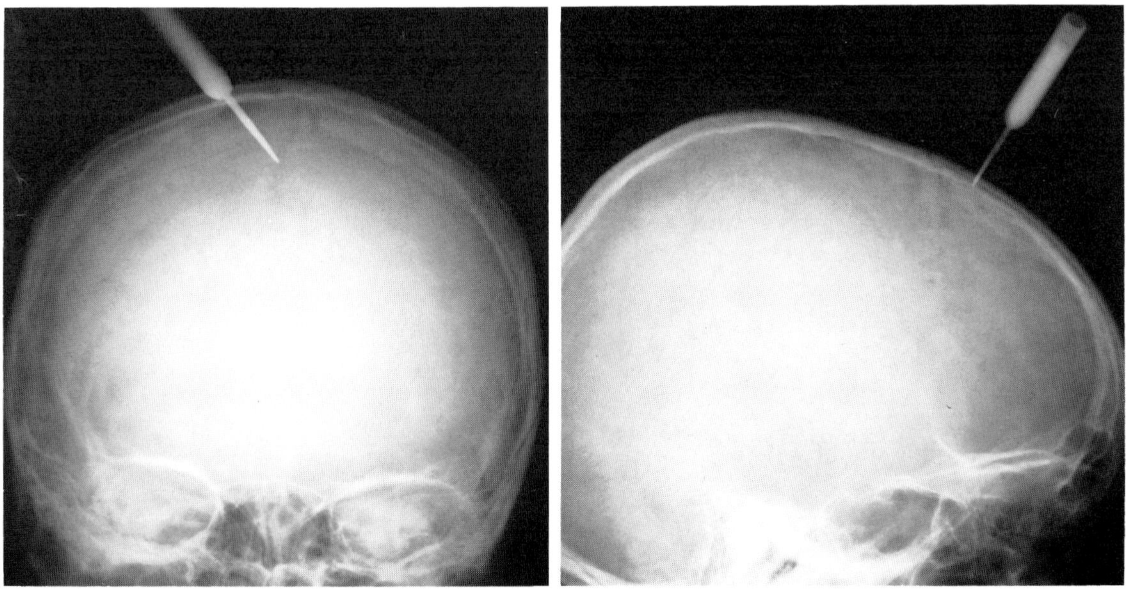

a b

Fig. 10.52. A 13-year-old boy who, while playing Indians, was hit in the head by an arrow. The tip of the arrow entered the superficial tissues of the head. Radiologically and during surgery, no bony injury was observed.

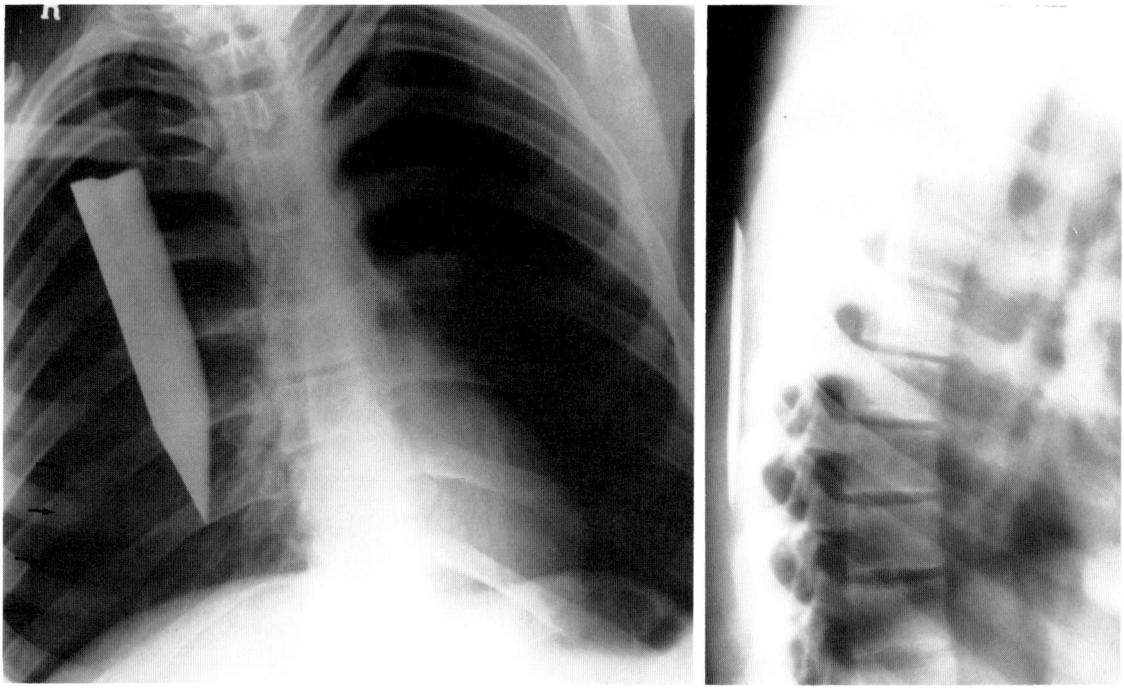

Fig. 10.53a b

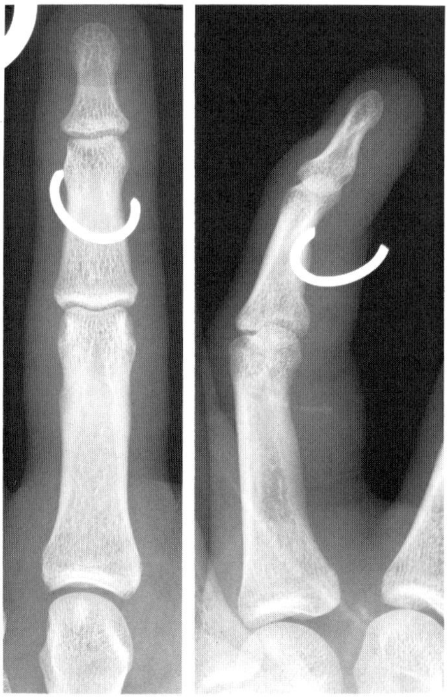

Fig. 10.54a b

▲ Fig. 10.53a and b. A 28-year-old man with a stab wound. Broken tip of knife is lodged in the soft tissue of the posterior thoracic wall on the right. Pneumothorax; slight degree of emphysema in the right supraclavicular soft tissues.

◀ Fig. 10.54a and b. A 19-year-old man after an accident at work. Broken blast ring in the volar soft tissues of the left middle finger. Only documentation on two planes can give adequate information on possible further involvement of bone and about the parts of the foreign bodies that are totally invisible from the outside; this will frequently give important hints as to the most successful and least traumatic removal of the foreign body.

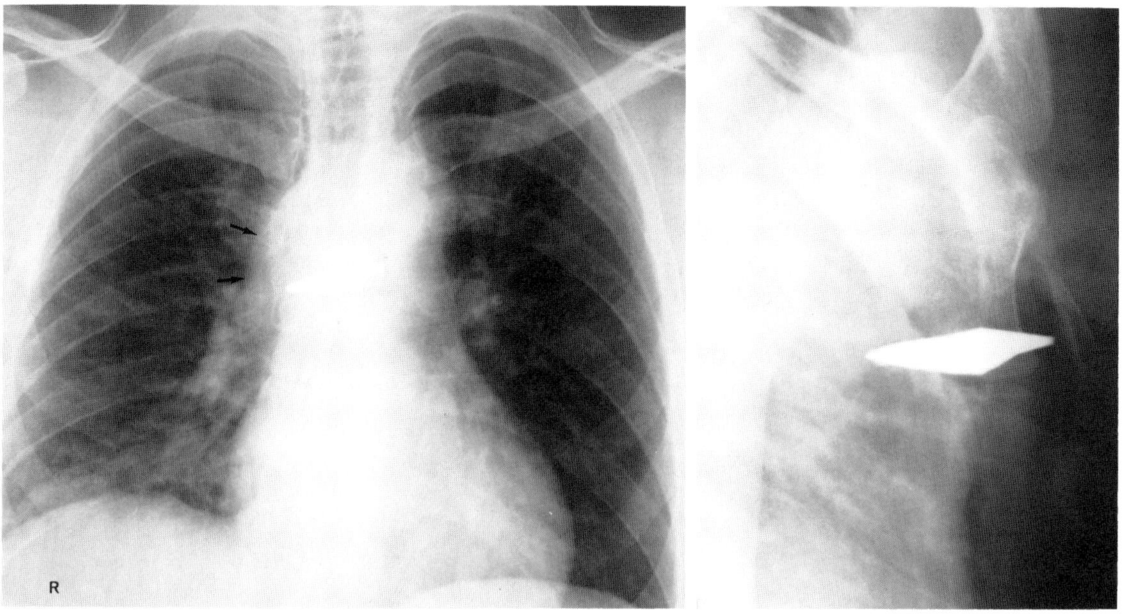

a b

Fig. 10.55a and b. A 49-year-old man after an accident at work. A piece of metal was thrown from a machine, entering the body through the sternum. Radiologic suspicion of a paraaortic hematoma in the area of the ascending aorta. Removal of the fragment by transsternal thoracotomy. The splinter stuck in the ascending aorta. This case should serve as an example of how important it is not to simply remove or pull out splinters at the place of accident. (Operation by Professor Dr. Overbeck.)

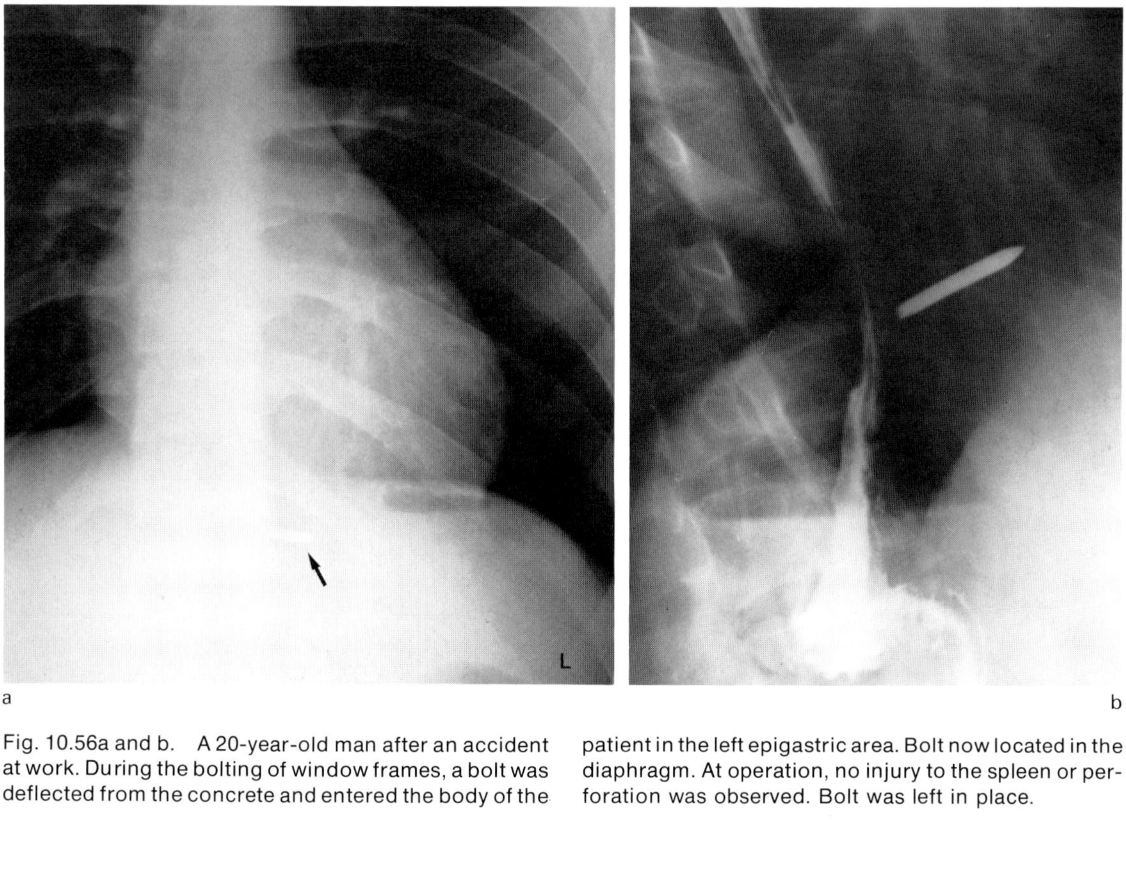

a b

Fig. 10.56a and b. A 20-year-old man after an accident at work. During the bolting of window frames, a bolt was deflected from the concrete and entered the body of the patient in the left epigastric area. Bolt now located in the diaphragm. At operation, no injury to the spleen or perforation was observed. Bolt was left in place.

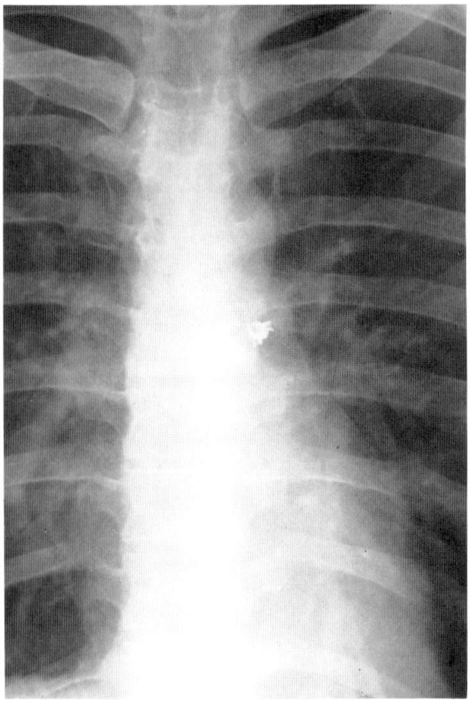

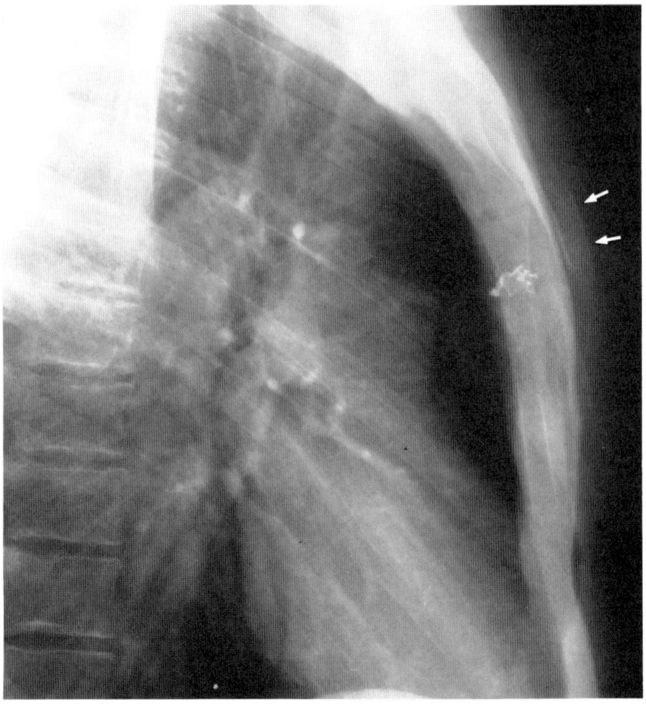

Fig. 10.57a and b. A 31-year-old man who was injured by a metal splinter during an explosion in a chemical factory. The splinter was left in the parasternal area, with gas distributed under the fascia. There are several other splinters in different locations.

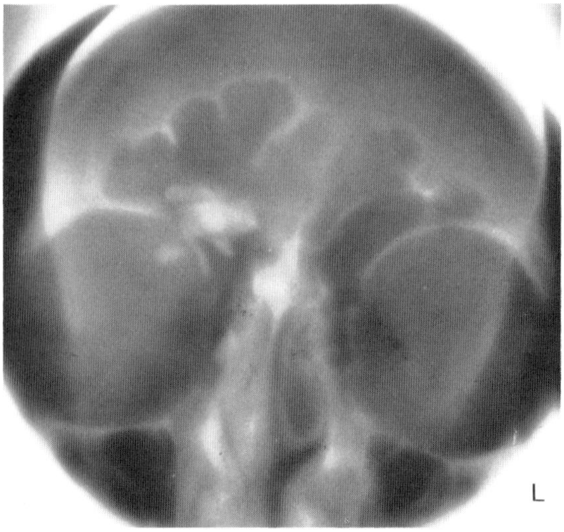

Fig. 10.58. A 21-year-old man with several unknown splinters that entered their present location as a result of a traffic accident five years previously. Glass splinters from the windshield are seen in the frontal sinus and orbit. Tomography.

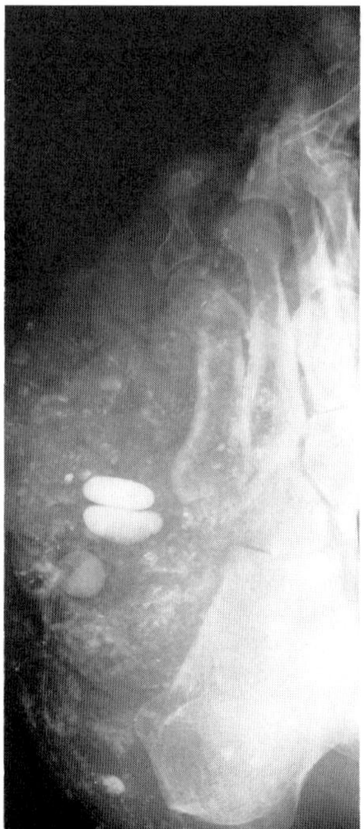

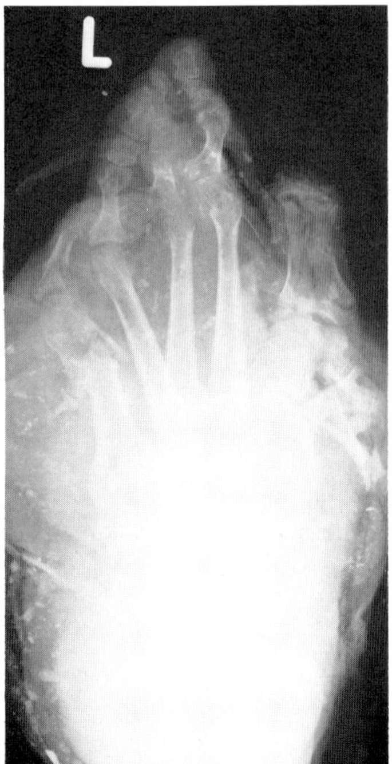

Fig. 10.59a b

Fig. 10.59a and b. A 48-year-old letter carrier who was hit by a railcar while walking between the rails. Amputation of the forefoot. Massive entry of sand and gravel into the soft tissues of the foot. Several open fractures of the forefoot and amputation of the big toe.

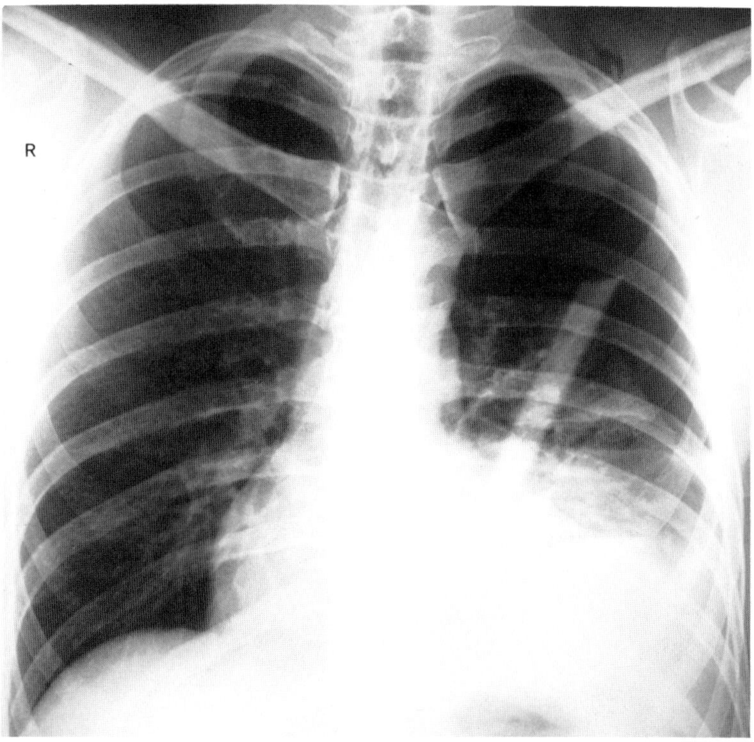

Fig. 10.60a

Fig. 10.60a and b. A 28-year-old man who, after having donated blood, lost consciousness and fell against a glass door. Initially, among other measures taken, a cut in the left supraclavicular area was sutured. Shortly before he was to be released, an x-ray obtained to exclude the possible presence of a pneumothorax revealed a most unexpected finding. Immediate admission to a hospital; thoracotomy was performed and the large glass splinter was removed. Large glass splinter almost shaped like a knife in the left hemithorax. Pneumothorax and hematothorax.

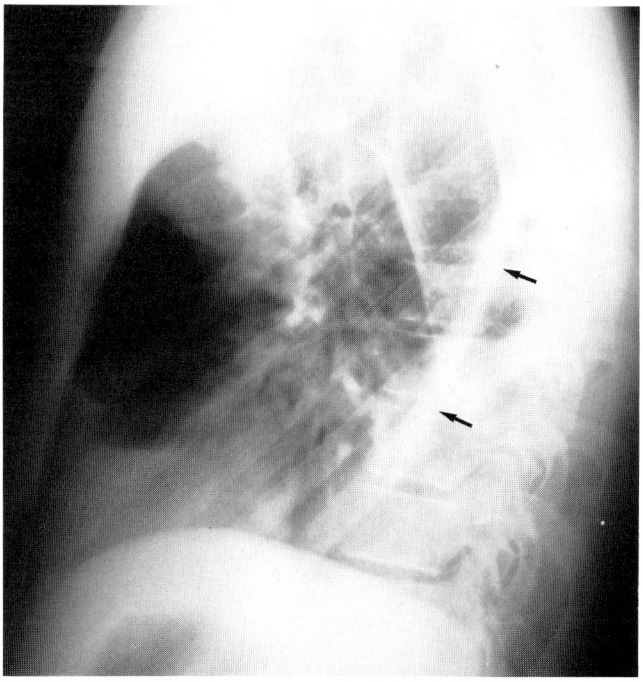

b

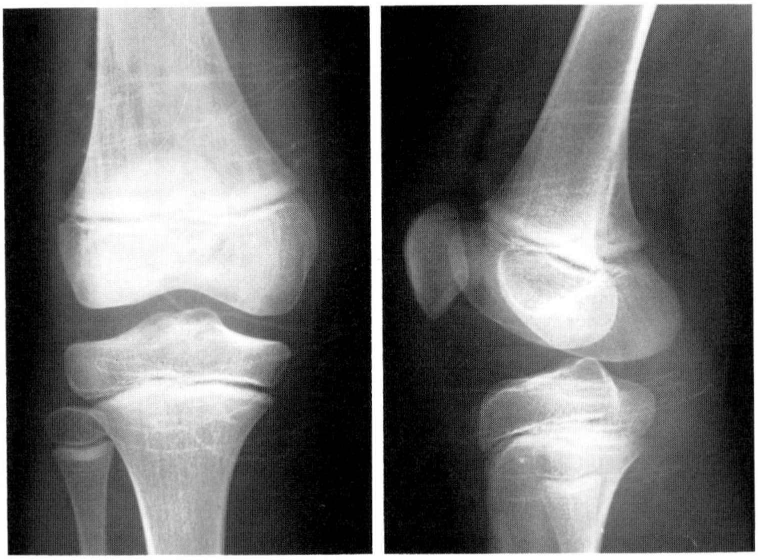

a b

Fig. 10.61a and b. An 8-year-old girl with an open injury of the left knee. Air in the retropatellar and superior recesses. Radiopaque markers in the compresses.

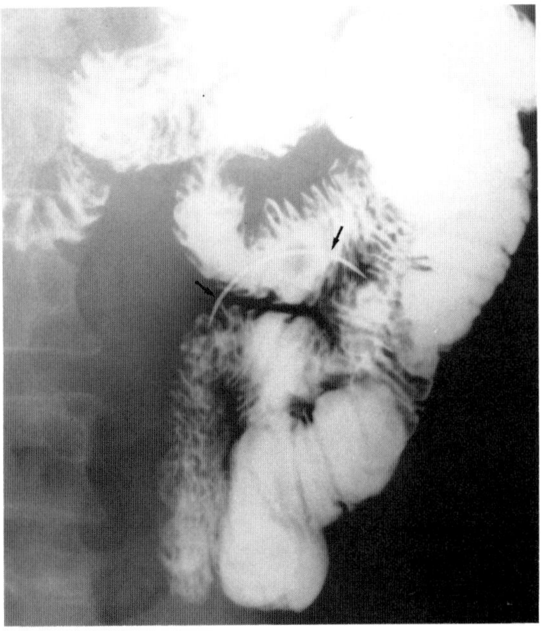

Fig. 10.62. Metal marker of Holzknecht's palpation instrument. This is not a fragment of a broken surgical needle left behind in the abdomen!

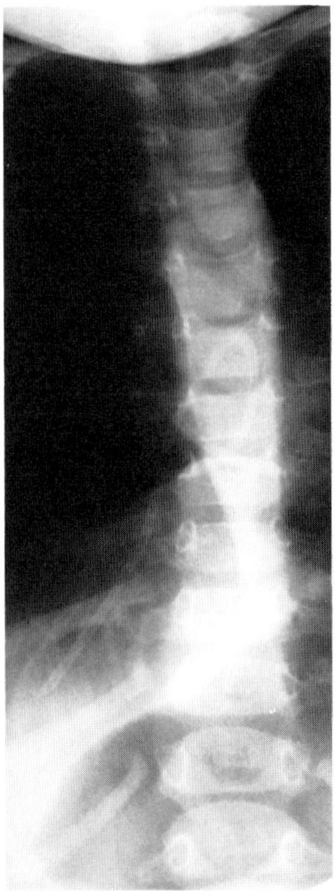

Fig. 10.63

Fig. 10.63. A 2-year-old girl. During revision of a shunt for hydrocephalus, a catheter was displaced and entered the right atrium. Surgical removal. Piece of catheter in the right heart. (Kindly supplied by H. Reinwein, Freiburg.)

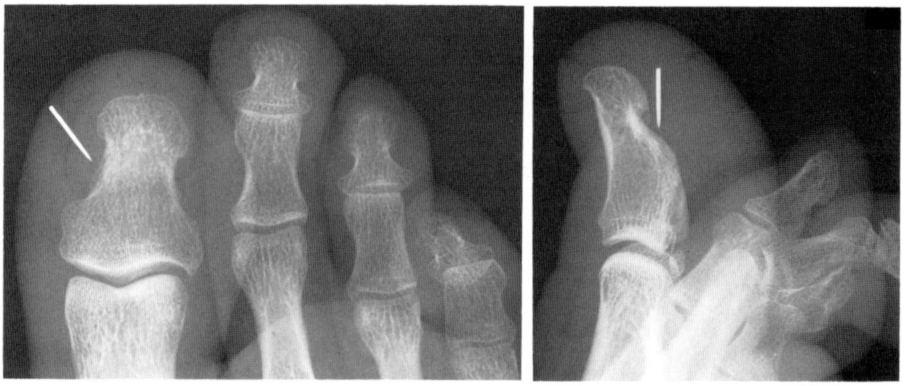

a b

Fig. 10.64a and b. A 25-year-old woman with a fragment of a sewing needle in the soft tissues of the big toe.

Fig. 10.65. A 30-year-old psychopathic woman. Several needles and fragments in the subcutaneous tissues of the anterior abdominal wall and the left breast.

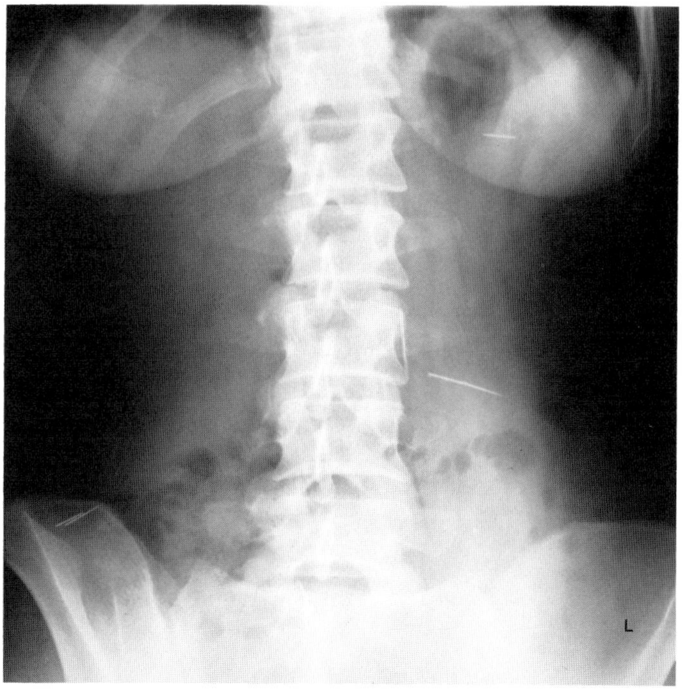

Fig. 10.65

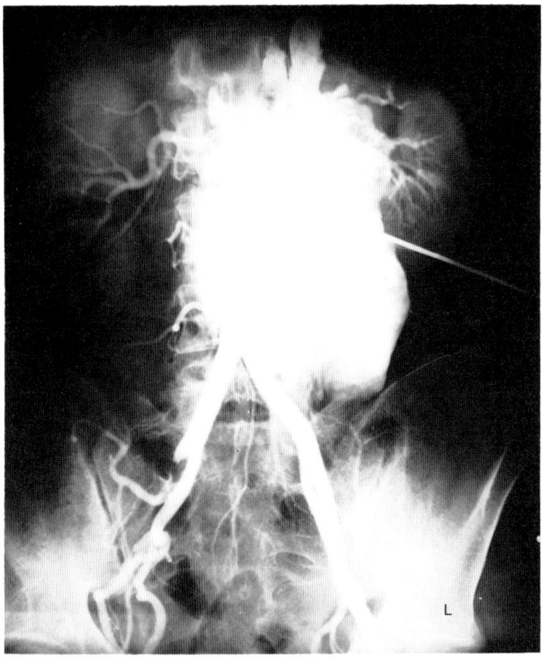

Fig. 10.66. A 47-year-old man after a paraaortic injection of a water-soluble, resorbable contrast agent. For two days, moderately severe lower back pain; otherwise no sequelae. Three months later at follow-up angiography and after disobliteration, normal conditions were observed in the area of the aorta and its large vessels.

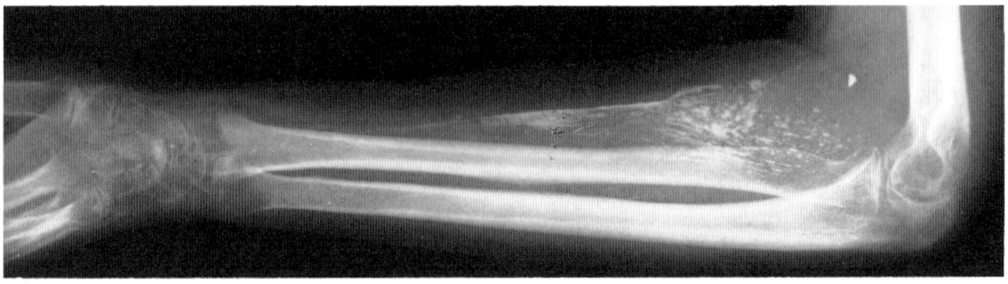

Fig. 10.67. A 39-year-old man whose arm was eventually amputated. Distribution of contrast agent during an unsuccessful attempt at filling an old fistula demonstrates a deep-seated injury. Contrast agent was not resorbable. Necrotizing foreign-body reaction. Severe bony atrophy.

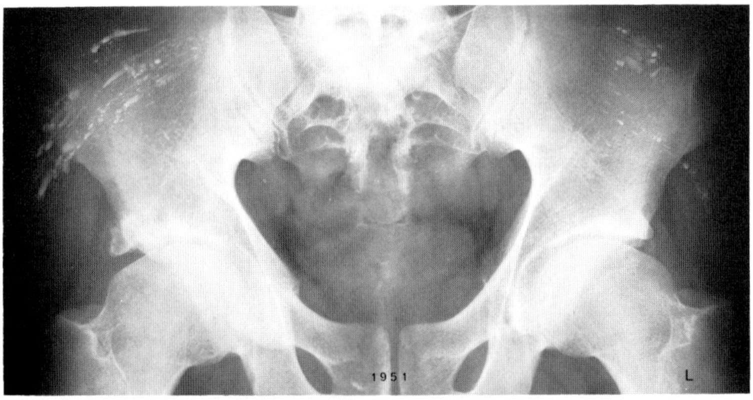

Fig. 10.68. A 24-year-old man with calciumlike dense deposits of metal salts (most likely used in an oily suspension) in the gluteal muscles.

11 Soft Tissues and Peripheral Vessels

After a blunt or penetrating soft-tissue injury of smaller or larger extent, an x-ray investigation is indicated for several reasons. The purpose is not to determine the exact injury or its extent per se, but primarily to exclude the possibility of a deep-seated injury that foils external recognition. In minor soft-tissue injuries so frequently seen, the usual question is that of involvement of bones and joints. In addition, the x-ray can identify the possible admixture of foreign bodies (Fig. 11.1). Particularly in the case of severe and extensive soft-tissue injuries, it is not always possible to reliably exclude radiologically the involvement of bones and joints. Follow-up x-ray examination after several weeks to months will show whether there has been complete healing (Fig. 11.2) or whether reactive bony alterations offering retrospective evidence of bony involvement can be recognized. Also, as a result of unrecognized bony injury such as by extension of an infectious local process, there may be involvement of the periosteal bones or joints; this can usually be recognized on brief radiologic investigation anf follow-up. Traumatic opening of a joint, a frequent injury in severe soft-tissue trauma, is recognized by the presence of air within the joint or its recesses (Fig. 11.3). After small injuries, usually stabbing injuries, there may be in soft tissues and rarely also in bone so-called traumatic epithelioids. These can occasionally be recognized on a roentgenogram (Fig. 11.4; compare Fig. 7.7). Posttraumatic infection of soft tissues and the presence of gas-forming microorganisms will produce a characteristic x-ray appearance, with cystic localized formation of gas (Fig. 11.5). In the case of a severe clostridial infection – gas gangrene – with its very extensive migration of gas along the muscles, there is a typical feathery appearance that may be recognized early on roentgenograms (Fig. 11.6).

Among traumatic injuries to blood vessels, undoubtedly the most important is an acute injury of the arteries. Surgical reconstruction as the method of choice has been developed only within the last 20 years. Even during World War II, injuries to vessels were treated with ligatures, with a resulting amputation rate of 26 per cent for the region of the brachial artery and 72 per cent for the popliteal artery (de Bakey and Simeone, 1946). According to the latest statistics on arterial injuries, during the Vietnam war, the former total amputation rate of 40 per cent has fallen to about 8 per cent (Fisher, 1967).

Nowadays injuries to arteries during peacetime have a relatively high incidence as a result of severe traffic accidents, work-related mishaps, violent crime and personal brawls (mechanism of injury: projectiles, stabs or cuts). Less frequently seen are attempts at suicide, injuries during sports and in the home. According to the literature (Maurer and Scherer, 1969), the following distribution of main arterial injuries can be expected: 60 per cent, upper extremity; 30 per cent, lower extremity; the rest, arteries of the neck and the large vessels in the thorax, abdomen or pelvis. During war time, there is a preponderance of injuries to the arteries of the lower extremity (Fisher, 1967).

If an arterial injury is suspected and the condition of the patient permits, selective arteriography should be performed. To do this procedure prior to surgical correction of a fracture will be to the advantage of the patient and the surgeon.

One should never overlook the technical and time requirements for the performance of arteriography. This procedure is usually much more difficult than in an uninjured patient undergoing angiography, despite the fact that occasionally contrast studies of an extremity can be conducted successfully with the simplest technique (Fig. 11.7). Demonstration of a traumatic disturbance of perfusion and its exact localization can be achieved only with seriography (Fig. 11.8; compare Fig. 11.10); also, this procedure can determine whether there is organic or functional stenosis or complete obstruction of a vessel. Organic stenoses show irregularities in caliber, in the contour of the inner wall and in filling. Functionally narrowed vessels show a smooth inner surface and are completely filled (Fig. 11.9).

If indicated, arteriography can be performed with a plaster cast in place (Fig. 11.10).

Besides occlusion of great arteries, there will also be marked abnormality of circulation, in which there is interruption of flow through smaller vessels in unusual areas normally having a large blood supply (Fig. 11.11).

As a consequence of arterial injury, there may be formation of false aneurysms (Figs. 11.12 and 11.13) or arteriovenous fistulas (Fig. 11.14; compare Fig. 3.8). This is seen most frequently in the area of the femoral and popliteal arteries and veins. In the differential diagnosis, one must consider the possibility of a congenital arteriovenous fistula (Tice et al., 1963). Traumatic arteriovenous fistulas of unusual localization have been described between superficial temporal veins and arteries, the superior gluteal artery and vein, the hepatic artery and the portal vein, the brachiocephalic truncus and the superior vena cava, the coronary artery and the coronary sinus, and between the vertebral artery and vein (Creech et al., 1965). If an arterial pathology is demonstrated after a lengthy interval subsequent to a trauma it is quite difficult to judge the cause-and-effect relationship. The area of localization and the lack of other vascular pathology are good indications of a traumatic origin. Arterial stenosis or occlusion can also be the result of extensive therapeutic measures.

Atraumatic arterial lesions, particularly rupture, is frequently accompanied by a similar involvement of a local vein. There are, however, isolated traumatic occlusions of veins without any damage to the arterial blood supply (Fig. 11.15). Venous blockage due to overloading must be considered a result of an acute trauma (Fig. 11.16). Venous stenosis, furthermore, can be caused by scar tissue from a neighboring region (Fig. 11.17).

Lesions involving the ducts of glands, in particular the parotid gland, are most often the result of stabbing, and cutting injuries during car accidents and, rarely, of blunt trauma. On the whole there is dilatation or obstruction of the main branch or one of the larger branches of the salivary ducts or a sialocele as well as secondary irregularities of its course or lumen (Fig. 11.18).

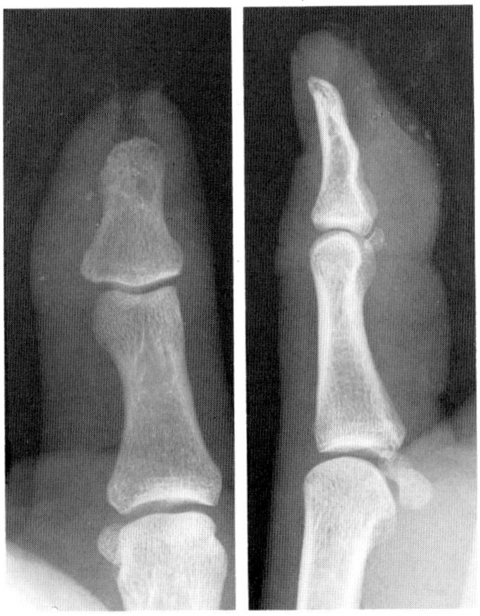

Fig. 11.1a b

Fig. 11.1a and b. Open soft-tissue injury of the tip of the thumb extending down to the bone. No visible involvement of bone. Superficial wound contamination by dirt and fine metal splinters.

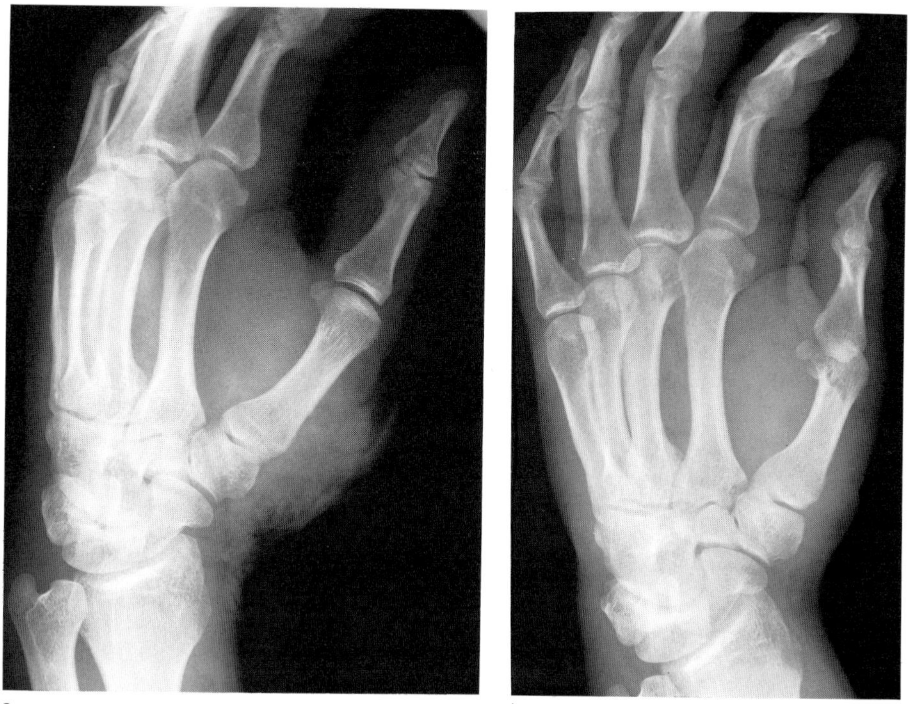

a b

Fig. 11.2a and b. A 36-year-old woodcutter with a severe soft-tissue injury by a motor saw. X-ray follow-up 3 months later does not show any reactive bony or joint alterations.

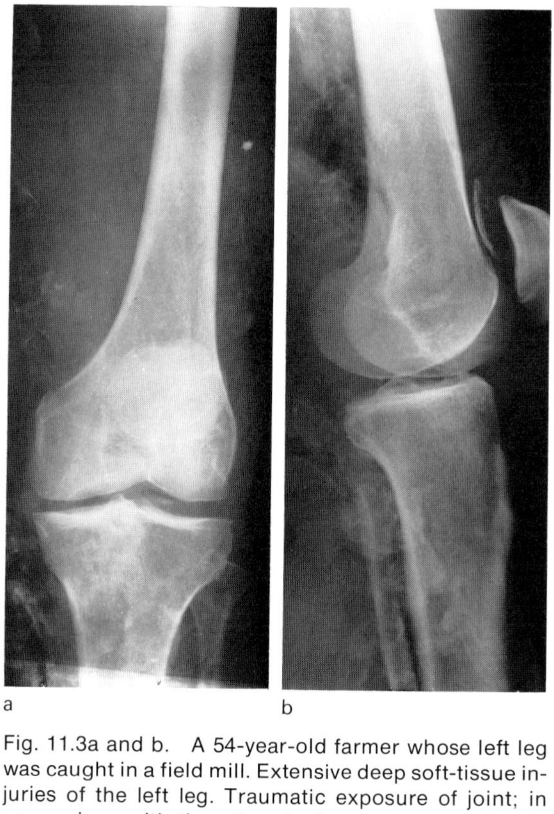

a b

Fig. 11.3a and b. A 54-year-old farmer whose left leg was caught in a field mill. Extensive deep soft-tissue injuries of the left leg. Traumatic exposure of joint; in comparison with the other findings, this is much less marked.

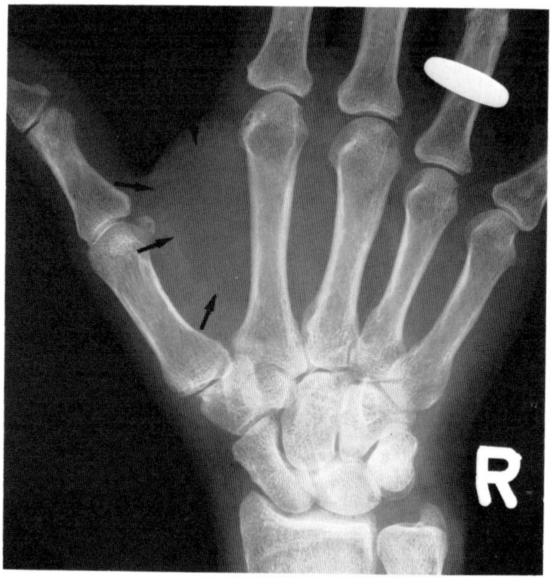

Fig. 11.4. A 60-year-old woman with a large traumatic epithelial cyst in the thenar.

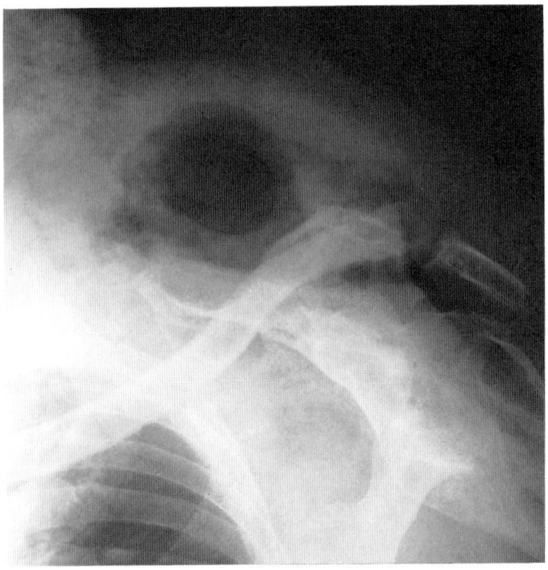

Fig. 11.5. A 60-year-old man with a gunshot injury 24 years earlier. Since then, there has been recurring local infection. Post-traumatic gas forming phlegmon (bacteriologically, *E. coli*) within the soft tissues of the right shoulder.

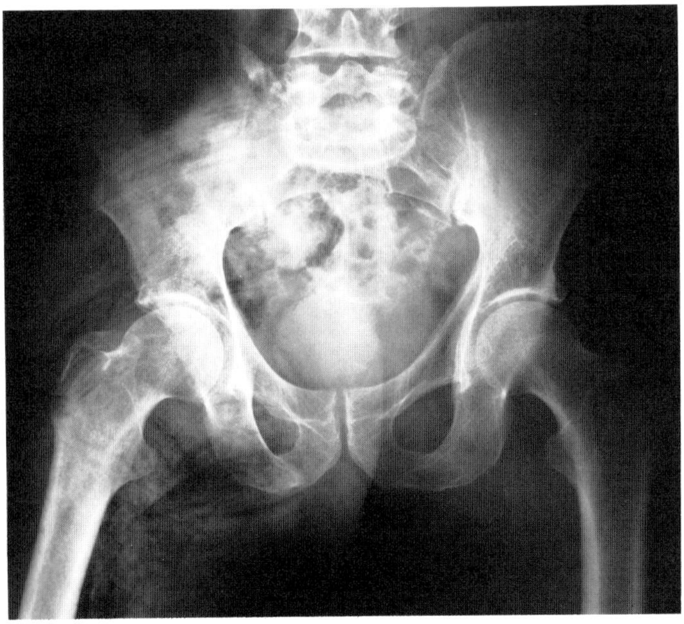

Fig. 11.6. A 61-year-old man 12 hours after an intramuscular injection of Irgapyrin. Extensive "feathery" gas formation within the musculature of the buttocks and thigh on the right due to clostridial infection.

Fig. 11.7. A 24-year-old woman with a traumatic interruption of the brachial artery as a result of a train accident. Simplified arteriography. Single cassette x-ray taken with portable machine.

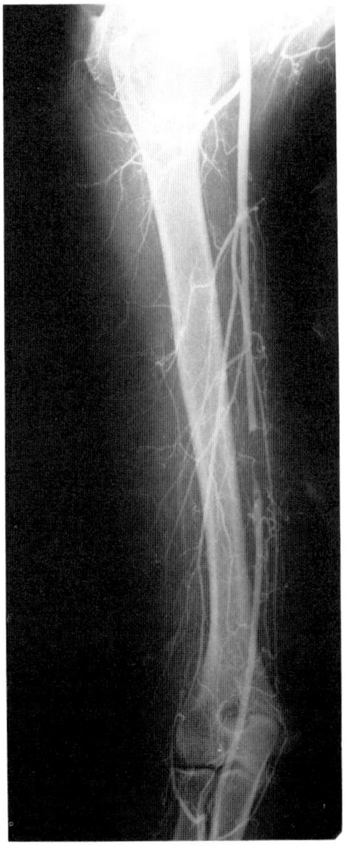

Fig. 11.7

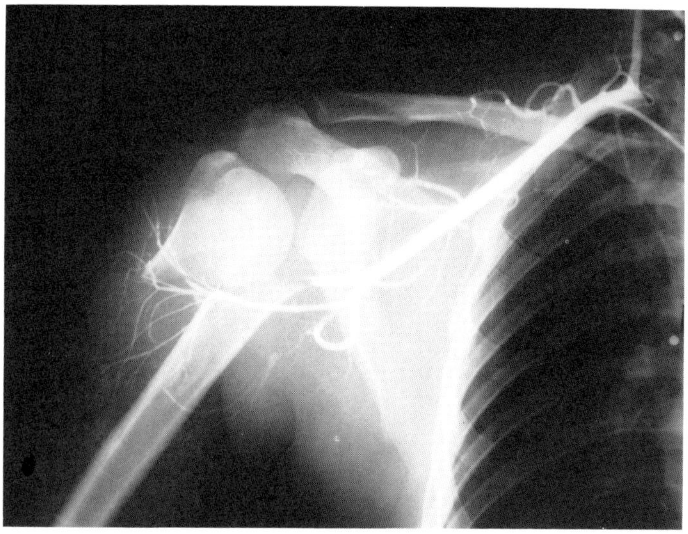

Fig. 11.8a

Fig. 11.8a and b. Occlusion of the brachial artery by compression.
a) After the accident.
b) Follow-up examination after surgery.

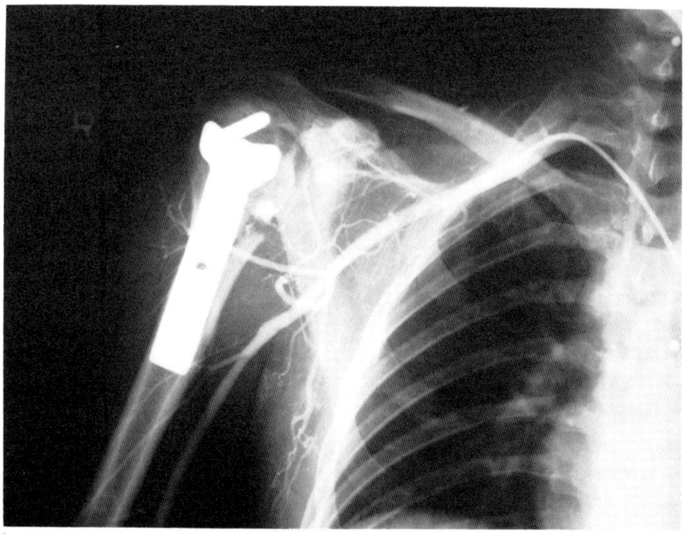

b

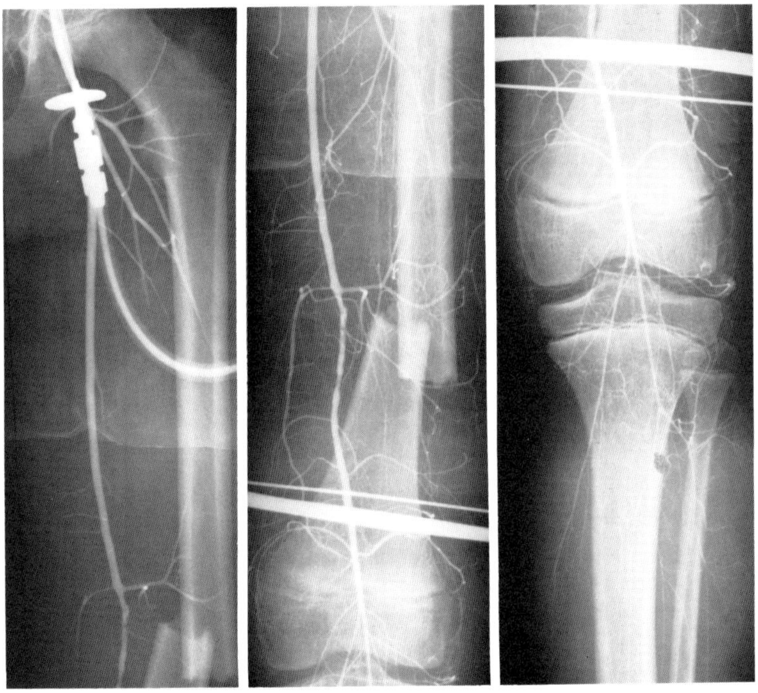
a b c

Fig. 11.9a–c. A 14-year-old boy after a skiing accident. Stenosis of the femoral artery extending over several centimeters in connection with a fracture of the femur. Marked functional narrowing of the popliteal artery and the vessels of the lower leg.

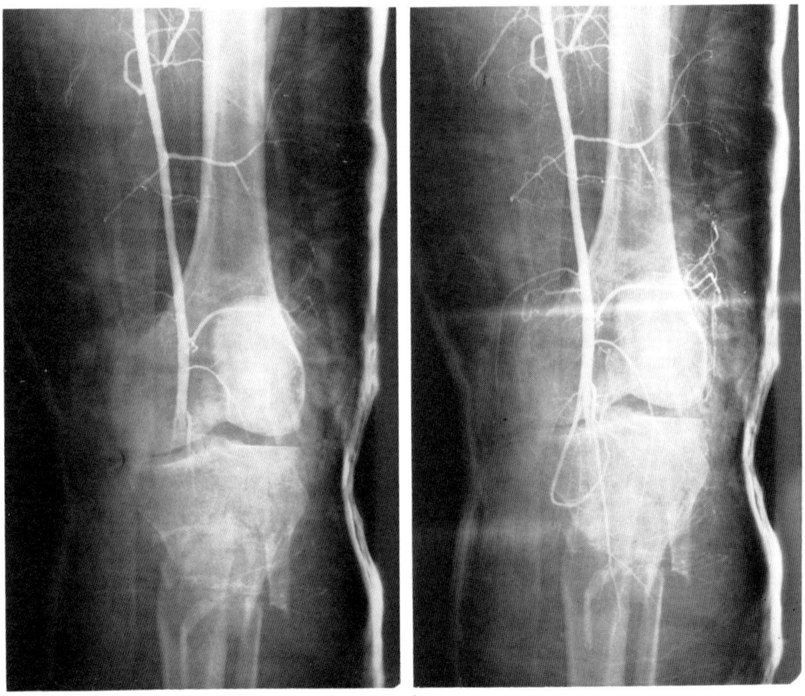
a b

Fig. 11.10a and b. A 40-year-old man after a motorcycle accident. Arteriography performed to check the disturbed circulation following fracture of the lower leg and its fixation in a plaster cast. Thrombotic occlusion of the popliteal artery. After surgical removal of a thrombus 3 cm. long, good circulation was reestablished.

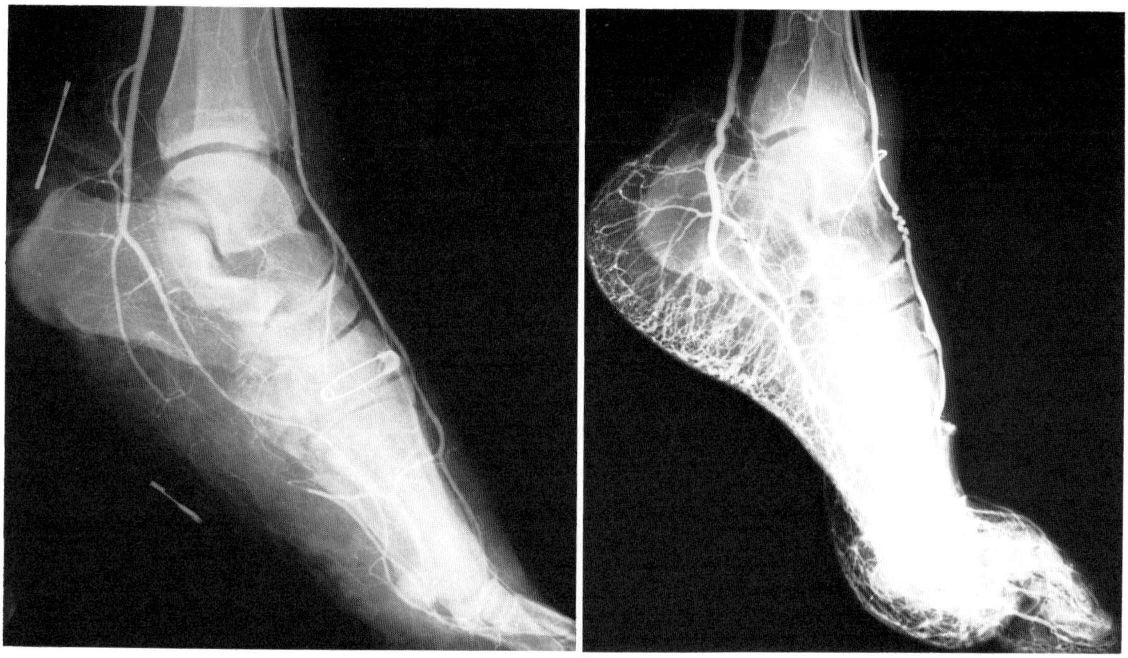

a b

Fig. 11.11a and b. A 22-year-old man with a degloving injury of the sole of the foot as a result of a traffic accident.

a) Traumatic disturbance of the arterial blood supply to the foot.

b) For comparison, normal blood supply to the soft tissues of the foot.

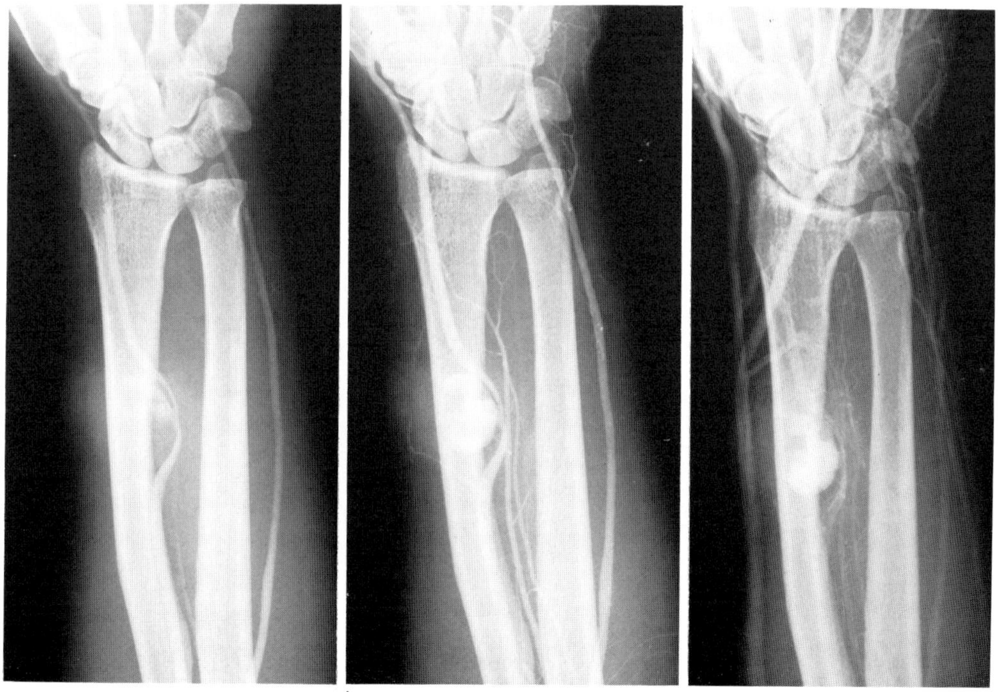

a b c

Fig. 11.12a–c. A 38-year-old man after an accident at work. Spurious aneurysm of the right radial artery. Arteriogram 5 weeks after stabbing injury.

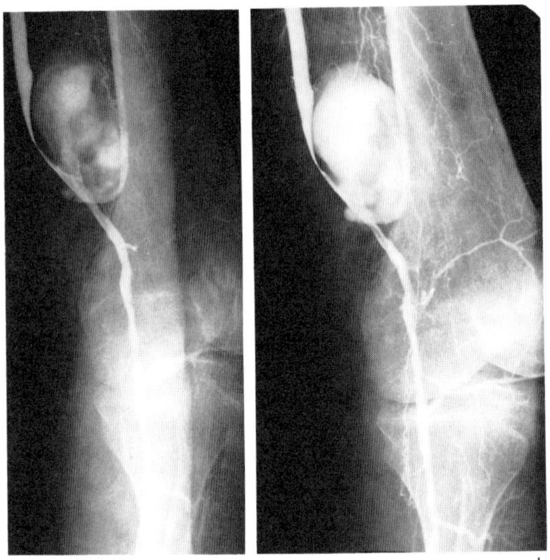

a b

Fig. 11.13a and b. A 60-year-old man with a spurious aneurysm of the left femoral artery.

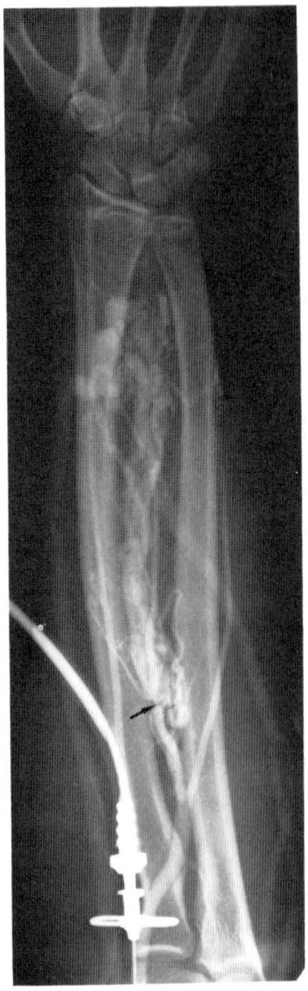

Fig. 11.14. A 15-year-old girl with an arteriovenous fistula on the forearm after an injury by a glass splinter. ▶

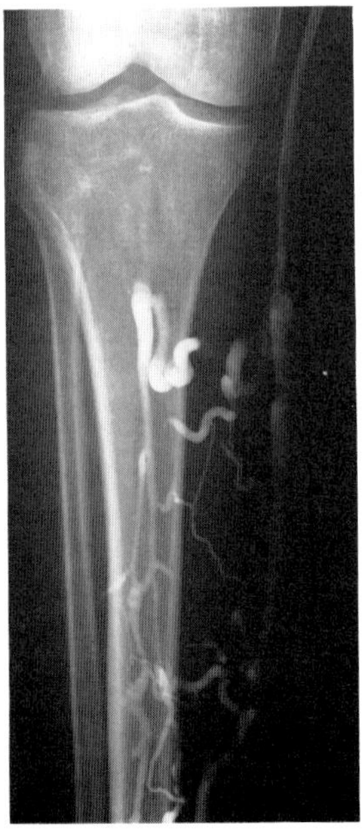

Fig. 11.15. A 40-year-old woman who fell from an agricultural vehicle and was run over the knee by one wheel. Occlusion of the popliteal vein.

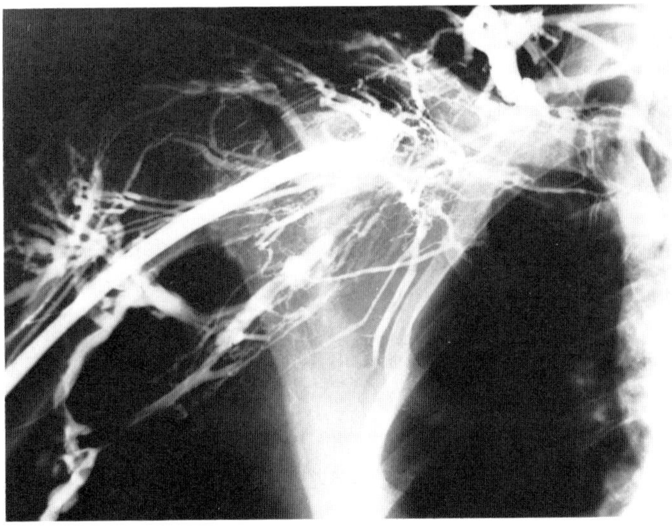

Fig. 11.16

▲

Fig. 11.16. A 48-year-old man who made the descent from the Parsenn Run in Davos eight times on skis. Developed sudden pain, soft-tissue swelling and visible widening of the veins in the area of the right shoulder. Acute traumatic blockage of the axillary and subclavian veins on the right by overexertion of the right shoulder.

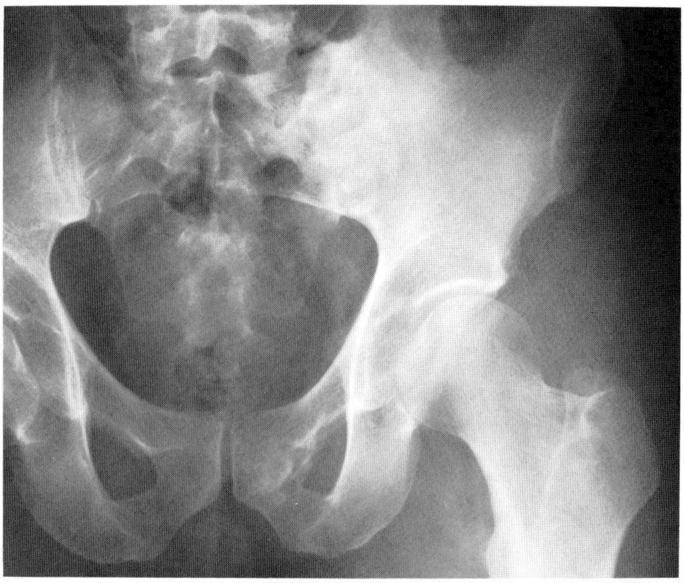

Fig. 11.17a

Fig. 11.17a and b. A 46-year-old man with post-traumatic stenosis of the left iliac vein after a posterior fracture of the pelvic ring on the left.
a) Survey film of the pelvis. Alterations in form and sclerosis in the area of the left iliosacral joint after fracture.
b) Venogram: stenosis of the iliac vein at the level of the left iliosacral joint. At surgery, extensive scarring in front on the left side of the sacrum.

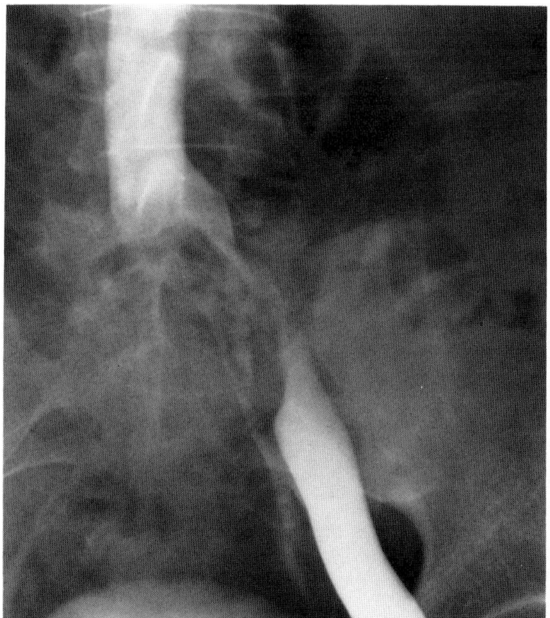

b

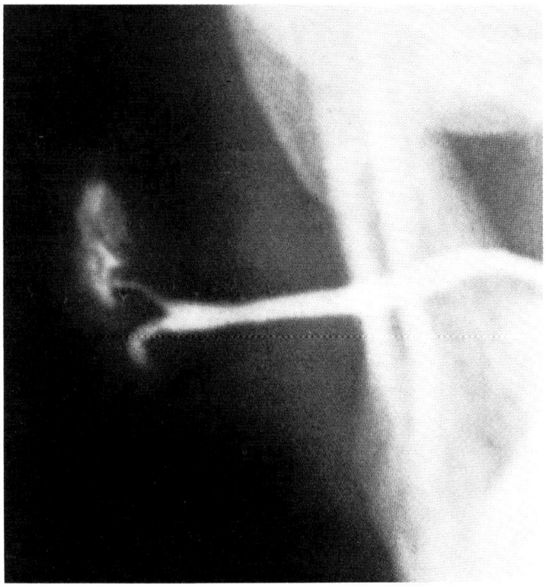

Fig. 11.18a

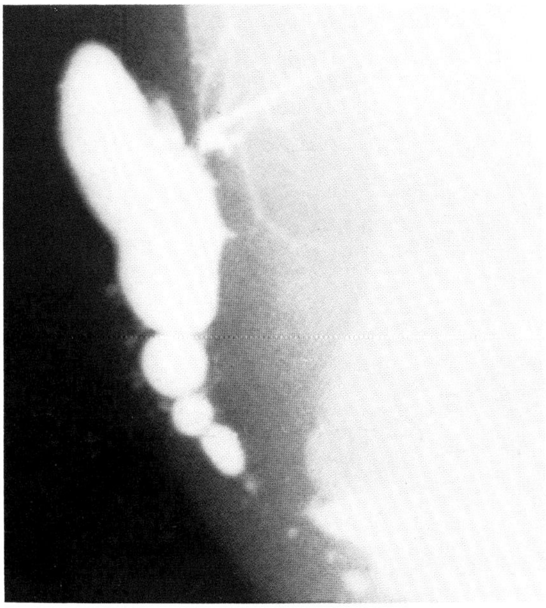

b

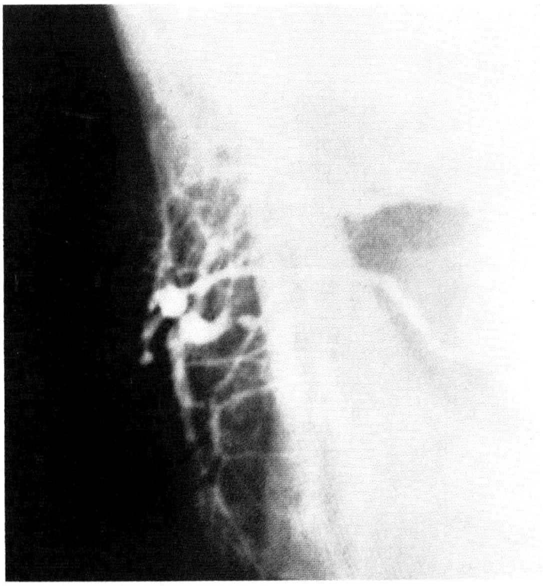

c

Fig. 11.18a–c. a) An 18-year-old man with occlusion of the inferior ramus of the parotid duct. Sialogram 9 days after a knife injury.
b) A 36-year-old man with a sialocele 7 days after a knife injury.
c) A 21-year-old man with secondary dilatation and deformity of ducts 4 weeks after a knife injury. (From N. Joffe: Am J. Roentgenol. *100:* 656, 1967.)

12 Special Traumatologic Problems During Infancy and Childhood

Because of their carefree and spontaneous behavior, children are particularly accident prone. Most accidents occur during play or sports; together with the accidents around the home, they amount to roughly 60 per cent. The proportion of traffic accidents has dramatically increased in recent years to more than 30 per cent. From one country and state to the next, there are differences in the percentage of accidents occurring in school (0.8 to 3 per cent) and in agricultural endeavour (1 to 9 per cent). Babies and infants obviously are involved to a great extent in accidents around the home, whereas older children sustain their injuries more often during sports and play and in traffic accidents. Thus, the annual distribution curve will show a seasonal peak in accidents during the summer months. In all age groups and all types of accident, boys are involved at a significantly higher rate. A close analysis of traffic accidents reveals that children as pedestrians are most frequently involved, and on bicycles, about half as much. Among the injured parts of the body, the skull is the most frequently hurt, followed by the extremities, abdomen, thorax, pelvis and spine. The high incidence of multiple injuries due to blunt trauma to the abdomen should be emphasized (over 20 per cent). The abdominal organs are affected in the following sequence: kidney, spleen, gastrointestinal canal, liver, bladder and urethra, and pancreas. Injuries to the liver have the highest mortality (Hecker and Daum, 1969). In blunt trauma to the thorax, associated injuries (skull and brain trauma; injuries to the abdomen and extremities) are seen even more frequently; fractured ribs, however are observed relatively rarely. The most common complication of trauma to the thorax in the child is contusion of the lung (Sorsdahl and Powell, 1965; Kilman and Charnock, 1969). Multiple injuries are usually seen as the result of traffic accidents and those occurring in an agricultural setting (Grünagel and Junkat, 1967). Intentional or unintentional abuse may be the cause of traumatic damage not suspected from the history. The importance and responsibility of the radiologist in suspecting and confirming the battered-child syndrome (Kempe and Silverman, 1962) or the abused-child syndrome (Baker and Berdon, 1966) have been repeatedly stressed in the last few years.

Iatrogenic injuries in childhood occur most often as perforations (particularly of the rectum) by catheters, enemas and thermometers (Hofmann and Petrausch, 1968; Parker et al., 1965). Mention should be made of the frequent occurrence, during infancy, of ingestion and, rarely inhalation of foreign bodies. X-ray diagnosis and the investigative approach are not significantly different from those in the adult.

Traumatic injuries to the internal organs at birth, with the exception of central nervous system hemorrhage, occur quite rarely. Radiologically, symptoms of a ruptured spleen, a ruptured diaphragm or a perforation may be seen. Injuries to the skeletal system will be discussed later (see page 237 and 249).

The diagnosis, especially in infants, may be severely hindered owing to the lack of history and cooperation during the examination. For this latter reason, it may even be difficult to conduct relatively simple x-ray investigations. For almost every different age group, there are different exposure data and requirements for radiation protection. This should result in a much more differentiated radiologic investigative technique. Whereas in an adult x-rays prior to and after reposition of a fracture are sufficient, in children this is not the case since there may be additional alterations because of the growth potential. Since growth occurs in an irregular fashion, there is no definitive time element that can be firmly established for controls in order to recognize traumatic disturbance in growth. Thus Blount (1957) has recommended that x-ray follow-up examinations should be obtained after three and six months, including the uninvolved extremity and with the x-ray tube being maintained at a constant distance of 2 meters. It is frequently necessary to obtain, at the initial examination, an x-ray of the uninvolved side for comparison. Injuries to the thorax and abdominal organs are somewhat similar in the adult, but this is not so in the skeleton of the child. Thus one may encounter serious problems because of the many different stages of skeletal development; even the specialist is again and again surprised by the multitude of possibilities for error and misinterpretation when faced with the many ossification centers, cartilaginous zones and epiphyses (fracture lines). Only sound knowledge of the normal skeleton of the child during the many different stages of development and maturation will prevent serious errors (Figs. 12.1 and 12.2). No one should ever be too proud to consult the appropriate books when in doubt.

Fractures of the skull during childhood have increased in frequency in proportion to the increase in the number of licensed vehicles. Falls from a balcony, window and diapering table are well known types of accidents. There are also skull injuries at birth, especially if there is delivery by forceps.

X-ray investigation should usually await all measures to treat shock, hemorrhage and open wounds. The injuries and fracture types in the child are different from those in the adult and can usually be properly delineated only if one is very familiar with the x-ray anatomy, its specific peculiarities and variations in the normal findings. One can distinguish: the widening of sutures (Fig. 12.3) and the linear fracture (Fig. 12.4); among impression-fractures, there is the Derby-hat lesion or rubber-ball impression (Blount, 1955), the ping-pong ball impression (Grob, from Willich, 1968) (representing a traumatic impression of the elastic skull without a fracture [Fig. 12.5]), also the true impression fracture sometimes mimicking a greenstick fracture or rounded or punched out fracture. For the demonstration of an impression fracture, the views on two planes (Fig. 12.6) usually obtained may be insufficient and additional views may be necessary. This also applies to the radiologic investigation of cephalohematoma or its sequelae (Figs. 12.7 and 12.8). In fractures of the facial bones in a child six years of age and older, it is important to pay special attention to the relationship of the fractures to the sinuses (p.a.view with the chin to the cassette), opacification by a lesion of the mucosa and hemorrhage can be indirect signs of a fracture. Fractures of the ethmoid (cerebrospinal fluid from the nose) can usually be recognized only on a.p. tomograms. In order to diagnose fractures of the petrous bone, one should use the special views according to Schüller and Stenvers. Fractures of the base of the skull are hardly ever visualized even on good special views (see details in Chapter 1).

A very special type of fracture is the "growing" fracture of the skull (Pia, 1954). This can occur only as a result of an injury to the bone and dura, with a connection between the external cerebrospinal fluid space (CFS) and the subcutis. CSF pressure and soft-tissue interposition prevent bony union and healing and especially where there is increased intracranial pressure, there will be widening of the fracture (Fig. 12.9). "Growing" fractures of the skull almost always require neurosurgical management. In the therapeutic approach to fractures of the skull in childhood, the determining factors are the patient's general condition and the type and degree of injury to the brain. Even in the presence of a depressed fracture, it is not of paramount importance to institute surgical intervention immediately; rather, one should restore the patient to the best possible general condition until neurosurgical management is possible. Symptoms of intracranial hemorrhage sometimes will lead to further radiologic investigations (compare Chapter 3).

Among injuries of the spine during childhood, fractures and dislocations of the cervical spine are rare and are usually the result of diving headfirst into shallow water and hitting the ground (Fig. 12.10). More frequently seen are subluxations due to whiplash injury (Fig. 12.11) in traffic accidents. Fracture of the dens, usually also the result of traffic accidents, is more often overlooked in the pediatric age group, as compared to adults. If such a fracture is suspected, several views should be obtained and tomography is indicated in order to properly visualize the atlas and epistropheus. In an eight-year-old child, one must expect to see compression fractures of the thoracic spine due to a fall from a height or a direct collision in a traffic accident or in sports (Fig. 12.12). Lumbar vertebral fractures are unusual during childhood (Fig. 12.13). Compression of a child's vertebral body is usually minor and, in view of the incomplete ossification of the total vertebral body, is frequently difficult to recognize. Kyphotic alterations and early-forming spondylosis may be the result of an overlooked or neglected vertebral fracture. In differential diagnosis one must consider malformations such as the Klippel-Feil syndrome as well as, in infancy, vertebra plana and in the older child, Scheuermann's disease.

Fractures of the ribs occur rarely in childhood. If they are part of a contusion of the thorax, it must be remembered that, in the majority of cases, pulmonary contusion will be the most significant pathology. Greenstick or incomplete fractures may result from a direct hit or a blow (compare with the battered-child syndrome).

With the increase in traffic accidents, there has also been a parallel increase in pelvic fractures, which were previously seen almost exclusively as a result of falls from great heights (Figs. 12.14 and 12.15). They are not as important unless there is concomitant injury of the bladder, urethra and other internal pelvic organs. Furthermore, there is always the possibility of later problems as a result of bony lesions and persistent deformity of the pelvis. A clear differentiation is necessary between fracture of the ischium and the lesions of the symphysis (Figs. 12.16 and 12.17) as well as ischiopubic osteochondrosis (Fig. 12.18) with its predilection for appearing in children 4 to 8 years of age. The age group from 12 to 19 years old, particularly boys, has a high incidence of traumatic avulsion of the apophysis because of the strong muscular attachments (Fig. 12.19).

Fractures of the clavicle are commonly seen in the child. They result from birth trauma, a fall during play or a blow. X-ray diagnosis is inconclusive when there is minimal or absent dislocation (Figs. 12.20 and 12.21). If, despite marked local soft-tissue swelling and possibly pseudoparalysis of the involved arm, there is no visible fracture on an x-ray, it is recommended that the x-ray examination be repeated one week later because, within this period, callus will appear if there is a fracture. On a tangential view or upshoot film, it is often possible to confirm the fracture at the initial investigation (Fig. 12.22). The rare fracture of the scapula may be the result of a car accident, a fall directly on the back or a hard blow to the back with a solid object. Usually this is accompanied by other severe injuries.

In the presence of Erb's palsy, an x-ray investigation is always needed to exclude the possibility of a dislocation, epiphyseolysis or the unusual birth-traumatic fracture and dislocation with 180 degrees' rotation of the head. Frequently during a delivery with some difficulty in extraction, but sometimes even during a seemingly uncomplicated strenuous delivery, injuries to the metaphyses are visible radiologically several weeks later, because of a massive subperiosteal organizing hematoma (Geiger and Schmid, 1967) (Fig. 12.23). When there is the differential diagnosis of birth-traumatic lesions of the shoulder, one should not overlook the unlikely possibility of osteochondritis as an expression of congenital lues (Fig. 12.24). Fractures of the upper shaft of the humerus, frequently involving the epiphysis, are seen with a higher incidence in older children and adolescents (Fig. 12.25). Avulsion fractures should not be confused with synchondroses (Fig. 12.26). Fractures through the shaft of the humerus will not present any diagnostic problems to the radiologist; they occur also as greenstick fractures (Fig. 12.27).

Injuries to the elbow area occur very often. Because of the many different centers of ossification, there is a wide field here for error in diagnosis. Dislocation without fracture is seen more frequently in pediatric patients (Fig. 12.28). The external aspect of a supracondylar fracture occurring in a child between 5 and 8 years of age can appear to be clinically just like a dislocation. The distal fragment usually shows angulation dorsally with displacement; the fracture line may be only faintly visible on the a.p. view (Fig. 12.29). Massive formation of callus is often visible early and may make it nearly impossible to correct the position of the fragments adequately (Fig. 12.30). Follow-up examination during fixation by a plaster cast will be hindered considerably by the cast, the forced flexion position and the metallic gear for the extension (Fig. 12.31). A.p. views may be attempted on several projections once at an almost right angle with the central ray directed first toward the upper arm and then toward the lower arm. In all x-rays from the elbow downward, there is some danger of gonadal exposure to the direct rays. It is therefore mandatory to properly cone down to the minimal field size needed and to adequately protect the gonads with lead shields. Fractures of the lateral condyle may be difficult to recognize (Fig. 12.32). Local loss of density in the form of a sickle dorsal to the distal humeral metaphysis is often an indirect sign of a fracture and always an expression of a severe injury (Fig. 12.33). The dislocation or fracture of ossification centers usually occurs together with displacement of a larger or shell-like fragment of the metaphysis (Figs. 12.34 and 12.35). Fractures of the medial condyle are rare; however, one should always consider the possibility of dislocation of the ossification center of the medial epicondyle. Its dislocation into the joint is frequently overlooked; even when dislocated this structure may appear just like a usual ossification center (Fig. 12.36). The loss of this ossification center does not have any major significance; however, its persistence within the joint leads to severe deformity and functional disturbance (Fig. 12.37) Other rarely seen lesions are fractures of the head or neck of the radius (Fig. 12.38) and a fracture of the olecranon (Fig. 12.39). The latter should not be confused with a normal apophysis, the so-called cubital patella (sesamoid within the tendon of the triceps muscle), or a divided ossification center for the olecranon. In the adult the tendency today of surgically removing a dislocated head of the radius cannot be applied in children because of the consequence of possible growth disturbance (Fig. 12.40). An entirely negative x-ray result will be, in any study of the so-called Chassaignac's subluxation (dislocation of the radial head from the annular ligament), frequently seen in infants resulting from a sudden strong pull at the forearm or hand, with overextension of the elbow.

In patients under six years of age, the most commonly observed fracture is that of the forearm or above the carpal joint – a greenstick fracture of the radius or both bones of the forearm just above the joint (Fig. 12.41). The typical greenstick fracture of the radius in the somewhat older child may appear just as a small dorsal crack or minimal protrusion of bone beyond the normal contour (Fig. 12.42). If there is a complete fracture (Fig. 12.43), it is necessary to obtain roentgenographic control of the position several days and two weeks after reposition.

In traumatic epiphysiolysis (Fig. 12.44), the epiphyses may spontaneously return to their normal position and then will only be visible because of the appearance of small metaphyseal avulsions (Fig. 12.45). In view of a possible growth disturbance follow-up x-rays are indicated three and six months later. If x-rays, from the time of an accident are not available, it may be impossible to distinguish between sequelae of trauma, epiphysiolysis and/or Madelung's deformity.

A well-known injury to the forearm is the so-called "wringer" injury caused by a laundry wringer. The great speed and marked force of the machine cause a rotational injury of tissues, usually also resulting in a fracture (Fig. 12.46). Because of the danger of secondary damage to bone, follow-up x-rays are needed after several weeks to months.

The most common childhood fracture is that of a finger caught in a door, toy or household tool. Early deformities of fingers may be the result of neglect of such "insignificant fractures" (Fig. 12.47). Minimal epiphysiolysis should be recognized because of the fine marginal avulsions at the metaphysis (Fig. 12.48). Fractures of the ground phalanx and metacarpals often occur during sports in older children and adolescents (Figs. 12.49 and 12.50); injury to the head of the metacarpal bones and Bennett's fracture are also known as boxer's fractures. The frequently occurring dislocation of the ground joint of the thumb cannot be overlooked.

Fractures of the carpal bones are seen rarely; a fracture of the navicular bone is as difficult to recognize as in the adult (Fig. 12.51). A common error in interpretation is the identifying of multiple dense ossification centers within the pisiform bone as a traumatic lesion (Fig. 12.52).

Dislocation of the hip is seeen with extreme rarity during childhood. It occurs posteriorly and inferiorly in about 70 per cent of cases (Fig. 12.53). In 10 per cent, it results in a necrosis of the femoral head. Recidivating luxation of the hip after minimal trauma and spontaneous dislocation has been described in mongolism (Fig. 12.54). Traumatic epiphysiolysis (Fig. 12.55) and fracture of the femoral neck (Fig. 12.56) are always the result of severe trauma. There is always the danger, despite careful and expert treatment, of aseptic necrosis of the femoral head and, occasionally, a refracture.

Fractures of the femoral shaft are localized in the middle third in about 70 per cent of cases (Fig. 12.57); greenstick fractures are seen mostly in the distal third. In the area of the proximal femur, the observed disorder occurs mostly in older children; mainly avulsion fractures of the major and minor trochanter are seen. The common T- or Y-shaped fracture of the distal condyle of the femur of the adult is seen only rarely in children. Fractures of the distal epiphysis with involvement of the growth zone may result in a dramatic deformity of this growing zone (Fig. 12.58). After lesions of the epiphysis during adolescence, early closure of the growth zone, with subsequent shortening or angulation, will usually occur.

Fractures of the patella in children will be even more frequently confused with a patella partita than in adults. Small avulsions and fractures at the articular surface are often seen in the knee. Demonstration of small free fragments is important, because the actual size of the fragments, owing to an invisible cartilaginous part, may be much larger. Joint effusion and hemarthrosis are expressions of an internal injury to the knee joint. In order to exclude a fracture, additional x-rays and follow-up examination after 10 to 14 days may be necessary.

Greenstick fractures of the lower leg or spiral fractures of the tibia are often overlooked (Fig. 12.59). This refers particularly to the so-called "waddling fracture" of the distal tibia observed in the age group of 9 months to three years. Instead of a typical fracture of the ankle as seen in the adult, skiing or playing soccer will usually result, in such children, in a fracture above the ankle joint or in epiphysiolysis and dislocation, with avulsion of a large metaphyseal wedge (Fig. 12.60). In the tarsal bones, fractures of the talus are seen more often than those of the calcaneus (Figs. 12.61 and 12.62). Again, at x-ray follow-up, one should look for aseptic necrosis as a consequence of trauma.

Avulsion fractures can easily be overlooked (Fig. 12.63). A spontaneous aseptic necrosis of the navicular bone (Köhler I) is sometimes called a fracture (Fig. 12.64). On x-rays, one should always very carefully study the soft tissues (gasgangrene infection? foreign-body involvement?) Caused by local infectious processes the soft-tissues or local infection of the fracture-fragments there may be significant additional growth. Metal devices used for internal fixation often are soon completely surrounded by bone; local infection may result in rapid marked resorption in their immediate area. Sequestration occurs in children less frequently than in adults.

Of special significance is the x-ray investigation in the diagnosis of the battered-child syndrome. Despite the fact that the original description of the typical local changes was given by Caffey (1946) more than a quarter of a century ago, it must be emphasized that these signs are still not widely enough known. Since the majority of the children affected are less than 3 years old, it would be very difficult to obtain an adequate history if, radiologically, there are several fractures without any known causal accident. This is particularly true in the presence of metaphyseal lesions – periosteal reactions close to the metaphysis as a result of periosteal bleeding; the possibility of a battered-child syndrome must be entertained (Fig. 12.65). The differential diagnosis should include metaphyseal alterations such as in scurvy and congenital lues; both of these, however, are generalized processes. The metaphyseal "zone of fragmentation" in scurvy can be easily differentiated from the so-called "corner sign" which is diagnostic of the battered-child syndrome. In the differential diagnosis, the Cornelia de Lange's syndrome (infantile muscular hypertrophy with multiple fractures), which is clinically typical, must be considered. It may be necessary in an individual case to obtain x-rays of different regions of the body. Fractures of the ribs, clavicle and vertebral body, as well as epimetaphyseal lesions of the proximal femur in its distal area, are frequently seen, and additional findings that may help in establishing a diagnosis of battered-child syndrome are poor nutrition, signs of general neglect, frightened attitudes, dazed sensorium (question of subdural hematoma) and multiple hematomas located especially in the face, around the head and on the left side of the body. There is usually significant discrepancy between the clinical and radiologic findings and the historical information supplied by the parents, siblings or guardians. It is usually necessary to admit such infants to a hospital. Once the diagnosis is ascertained, the physician has the unpleasant duty of starting the chain of events that will prevent such an infant's being exposed to further abuse (incidence of further injury, 80 to 90 per cent) by informing the appropriate agencies for the care and protection of infant victims of the battered-child syndrome.

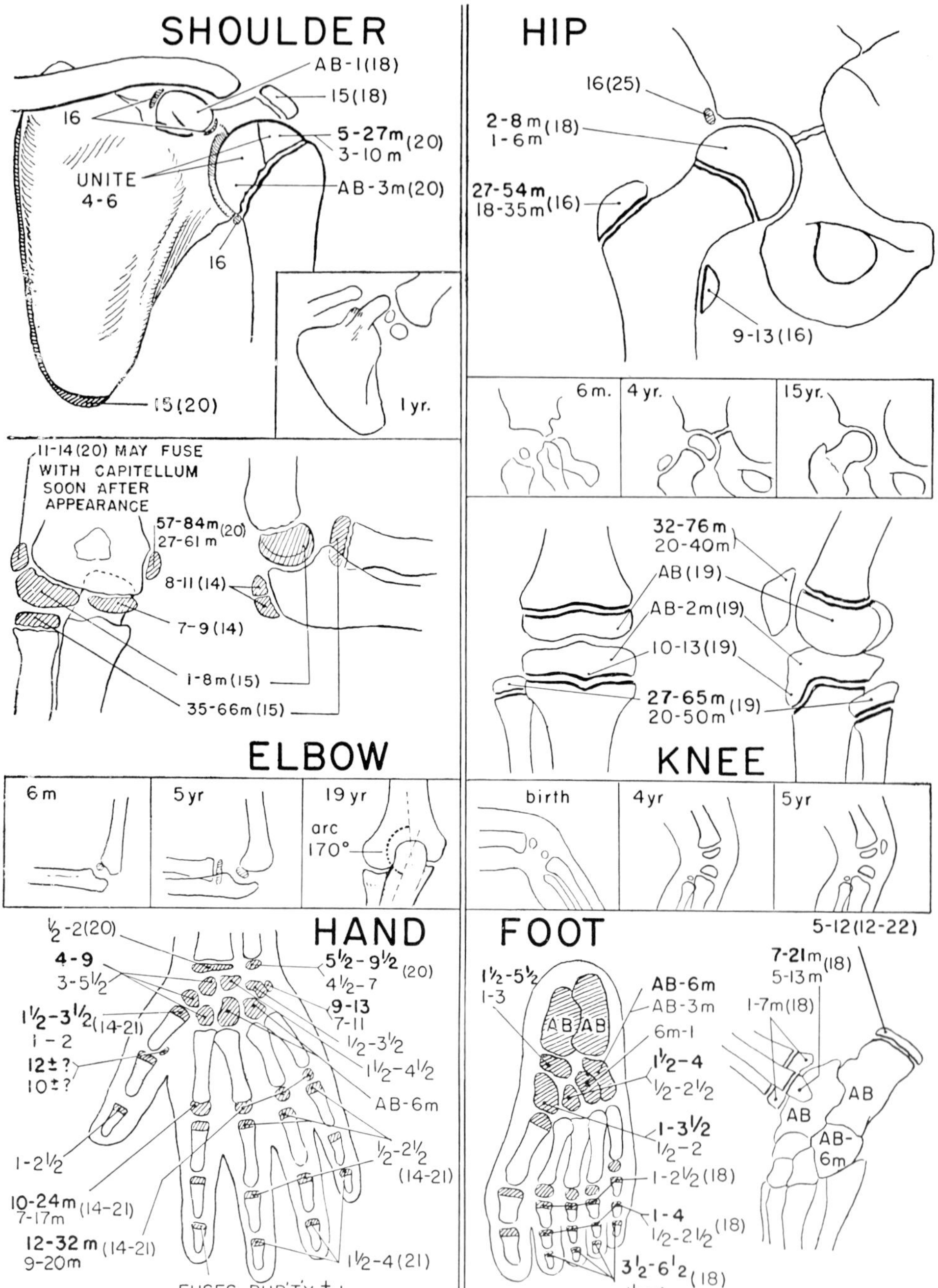

SHOULDER
AB-1(18)
15(18)
16
5-27m (20)
3-10 m
UNITE
4-6
AB-3m(20)
16
1 yr.
15(20)
HIP
16(25)
2-8 m (18)
1-6 m
27-54 m
18-35 m (16)
9-13(16)
6 m.
4 yr.
15 yr.
11-14(20) MAY FUSE WITH CAPITELLUM SOON AFTER APPEARANCE
57-84 m (20)
27-61 m
8-11 (14)
7-9 (14)
1-8 m (15)
35-66 m (15)
ELBOW
32-76 m
20-40 m
AB(19)
AB-2m(19)
10-13(19)
27-65 m (19)
20-50 m
KNEE
6 m
5 yr
19 yr
arc 170°
birth
4 yr
5 yr
HAND
½-2(20)
4-9
3-5½
1½-3½ (14-21)
1-2
12±?
10±?
1-2½
10-24 m (14-21)
7-17 m
12-32 m (14-21)
9-20 m
5½-9½ (20)
4½-7
9-13
7-11
½-3½
1½-4½
AB-6m
½-2½ (14-21)
1½-4(21)
FUSES PUB'TY ±1
FOOT
5-12(12-22)
1½-5½
1-3
AB AB
AB-6m
AB-3m
6m-1
1½-4
½-2½
1-3½
½-2
1-2½(18)
1-4
½-2½ (18)
3½-6½ (18)
1½-4
7-21 m (18)
5-13 m
1-7m(18)
AB
AB
AB-6m

Fig. 12.1

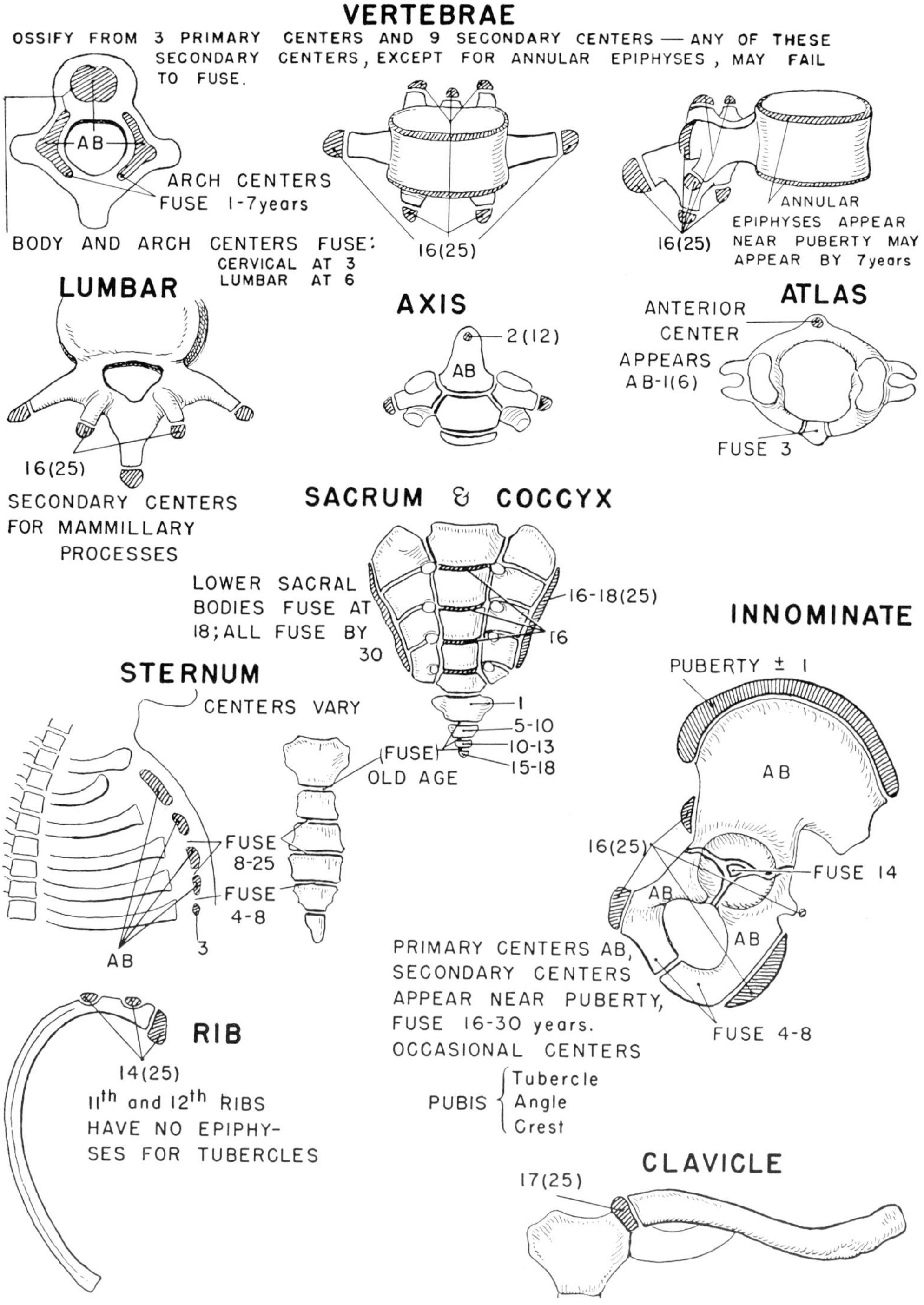

Fig. 12.2

Figs. 12.1 and 12.2. Timetable for the appearance of ossification centers. Numbers accompanied by a small "m" = months; otherwise, years. If there are two numbers given for a single ossification center, the upper one refers to boys and the lower one in lighter print refers to girls. AB = at birth. Approximate age at the closure of the epiphysis is given in parentheses. (From W. P. Blount: Fractures in Children. Williams & Wilkins, Baltimore, 1955.)

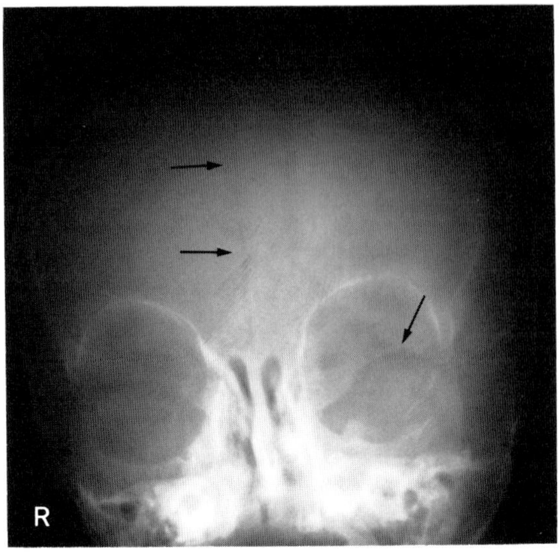

Fig. 12.3. A 4-month-old girl with widening of the lambdoid suture on the left *(arrow)*. Persistent frontal suture as a variant *(2 arrows)*.

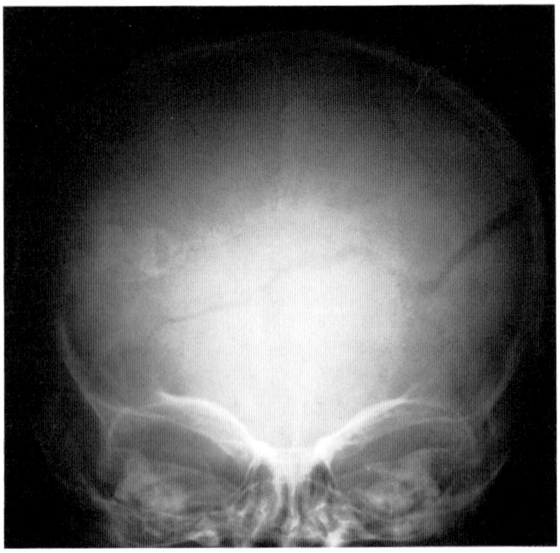

Fig. 12.4a

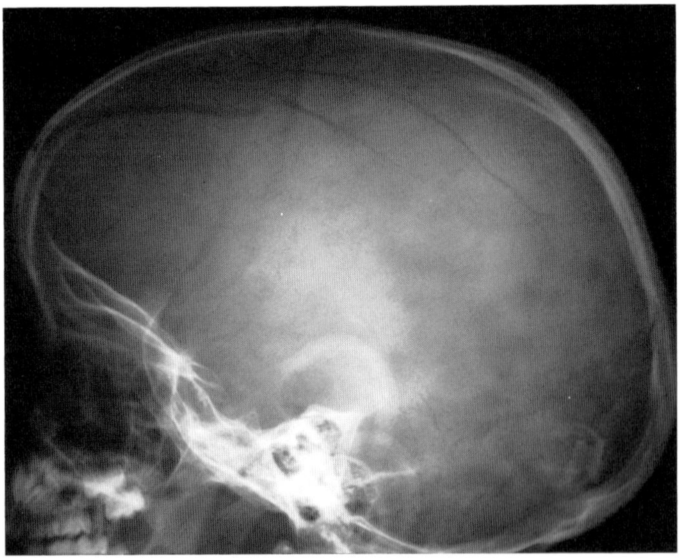

Fig. 12.4b

Fig. 12.4a and b. A 2-year-4-month-old child. Cause of the accident cannot be determined. No significant clinical symptoms. Investigated because of a suspected concussion. Linear fractures of the skull in the frontal region and in the parietal area on the left.

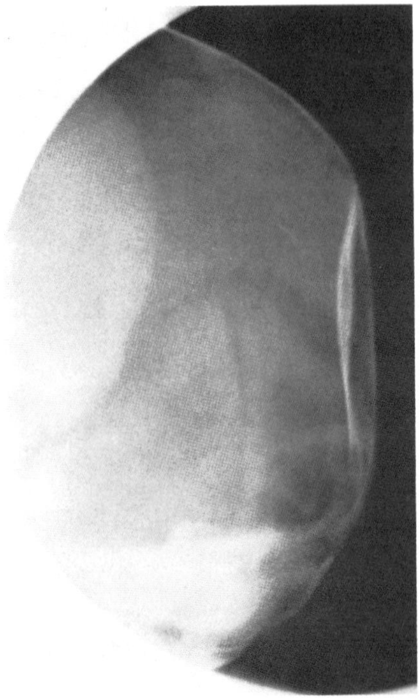

Fig. 12.5. Ping-pong ball fracture on the left 5 days after forceps delivery. (From E. Willich: Fortschr. Röntgenstr. *109:* 653, 1968.)

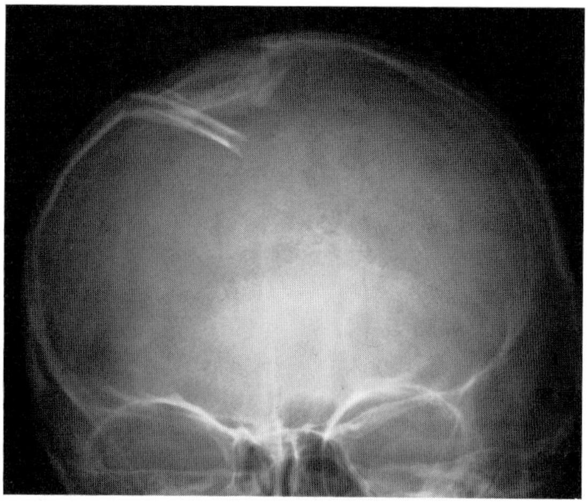

Fig. 12.6a

Fig. 12.6a and b. A 10-year-old boy who was hit on the head by a falling tile from a roof during a hurricane. Impression fracture of the right parietal bone.

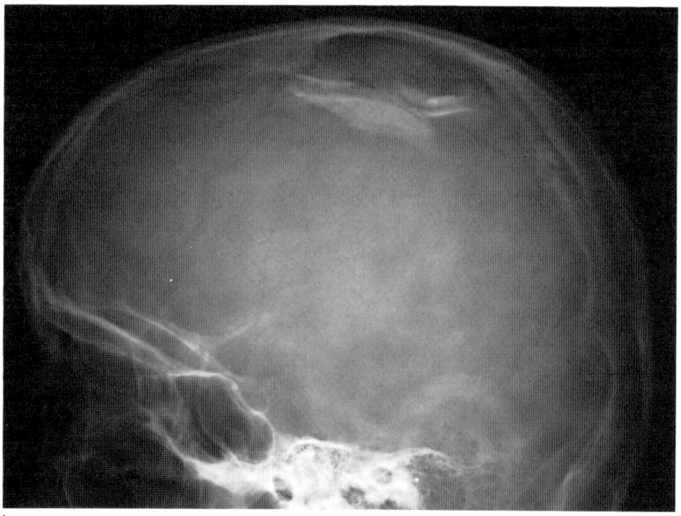

b

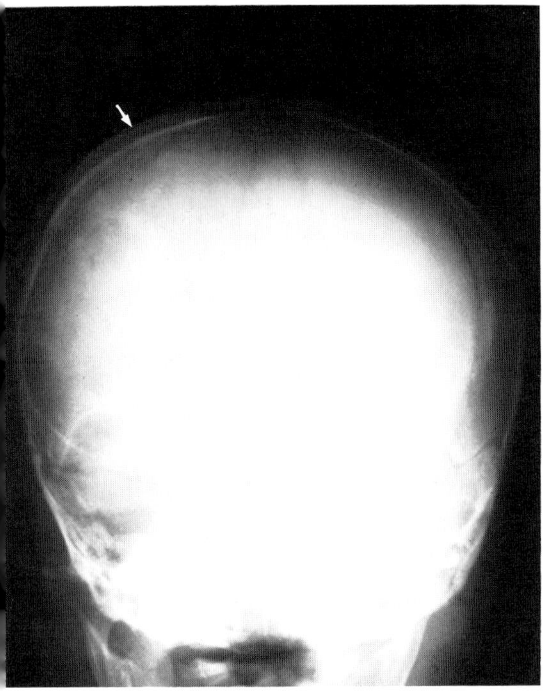

a

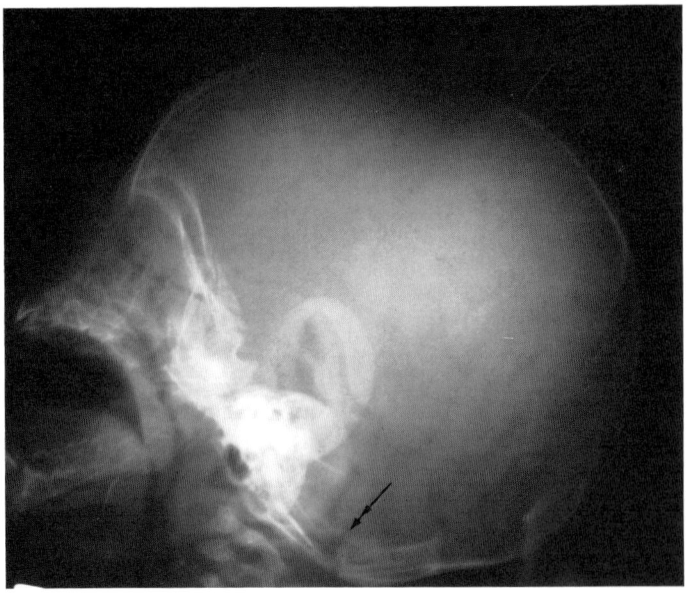

b

Fig. 12.7a and b. A 2-month-old baby after normal delivery; cephalhematoma *(arrow)*; note the interruption of the innominate synchondrosis *(double arrow)*. This is not a fracture.

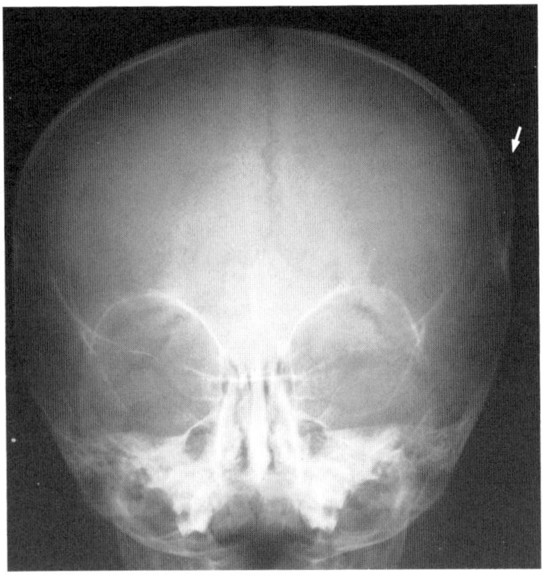

▲

Fig. 12.8. A 15-month-old girl with a smooth protrusion of the ossified cephalhematoma in the left parietal area.

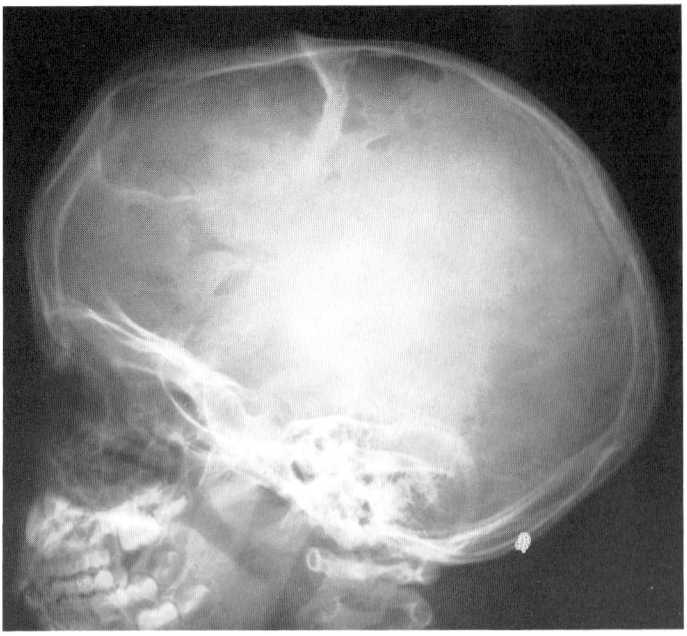

Fig. 12.9. A 4-year-8-month-old boy who was delivered by forceps. Growing fracture of the skull in front of the parietal region. Operative management.

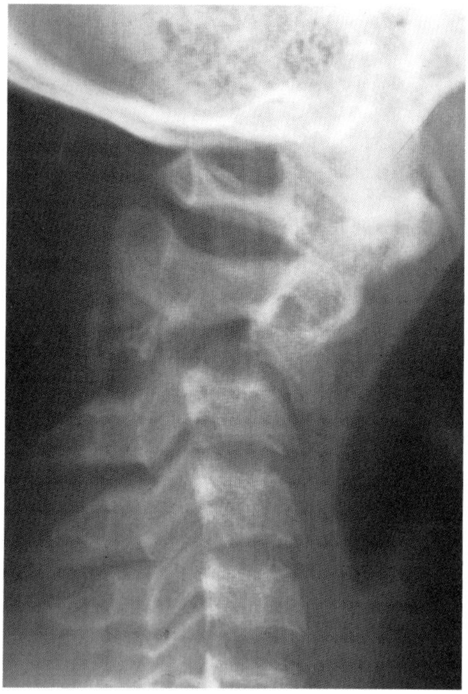

Fig. 12.10

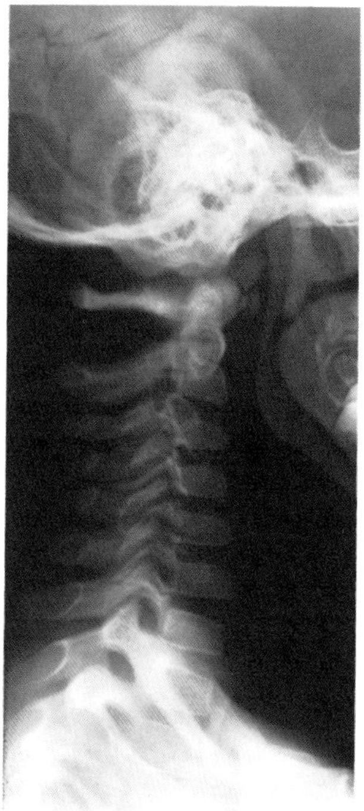

Fig. 12.11

Fig. 12.10. A 15-year-old boy after diving into a shallow pool and hitting the ground. Dislocation of the cervical spine at the level of C2/3, with a fracture of the articular processes.

Fig. 12.11. A 4-year-old boy who fell from a train going at about 80 km/hour. Kinking and slight displacement of the cervical spine at C2/3 by the crash mechanism.

Fig. 12.12. A 13-year-old boy who fell about 10 to 15 m while mountaineering. Compression fracture of the 5th to the 9th thoracic vertebrae. Loss of height and wedging anteriorly of all the affected vertebrae. Prominent opacification overlapping the anterosuperior edge of the vertebral bodies. Massive paravertebral hematoma (on a. p. view).

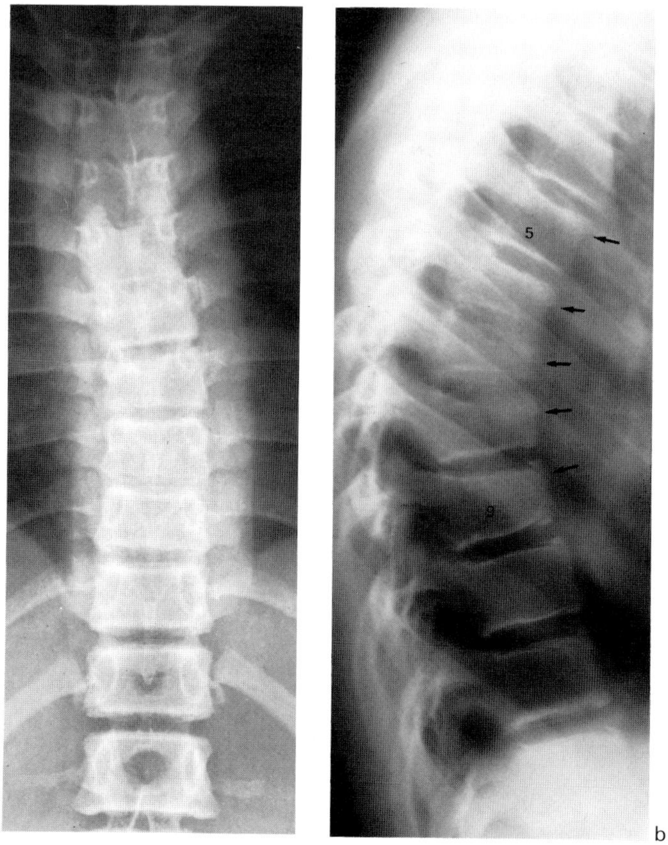

Fig. 12.12a b

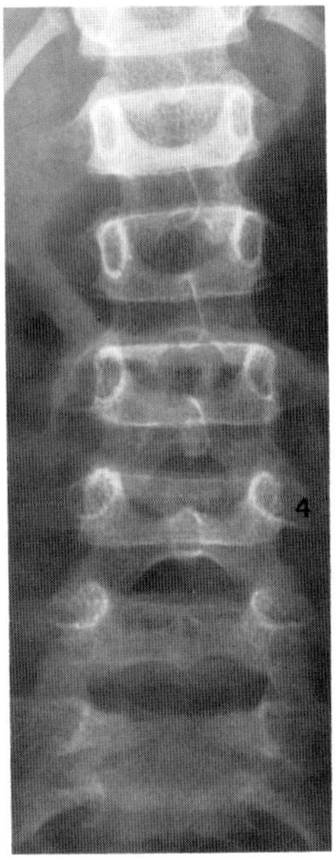

a

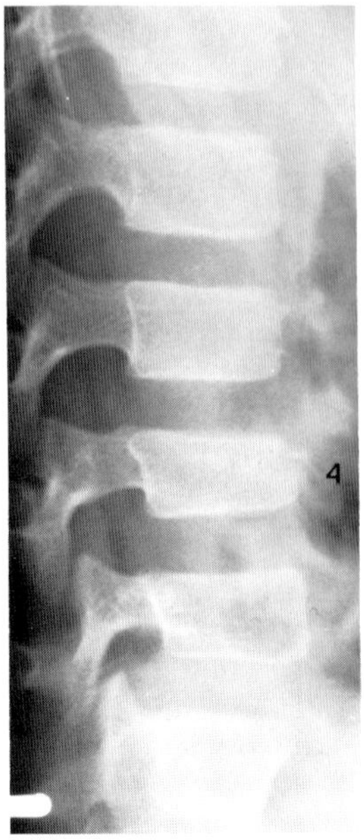

b

Fig. 12.13a and b. A 5-year-old girl who fell through a window on the 4th floor. Compression fracture of the 4th lumbar vertebra, with minimal deformity.

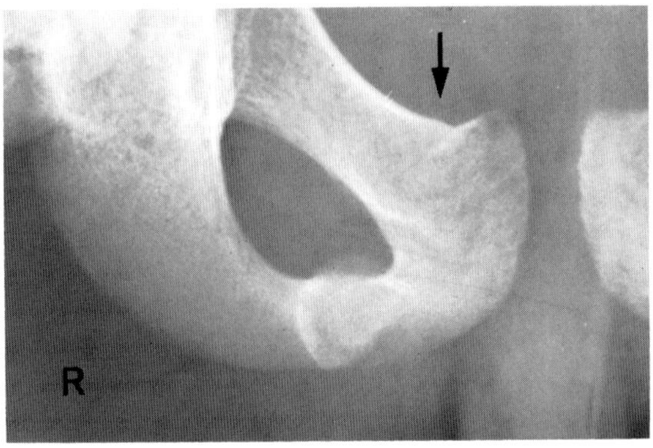

Fig. 12.14

Fig. 12.14. An 8-year-old boy who was hit by a car. Fracture of the right os pubis.

Fig. 12.15. An 11-year-old girl who fell about 4 m. from a haystack. Fracture of the os pubis on the right, and injury to the symphysis.

▼

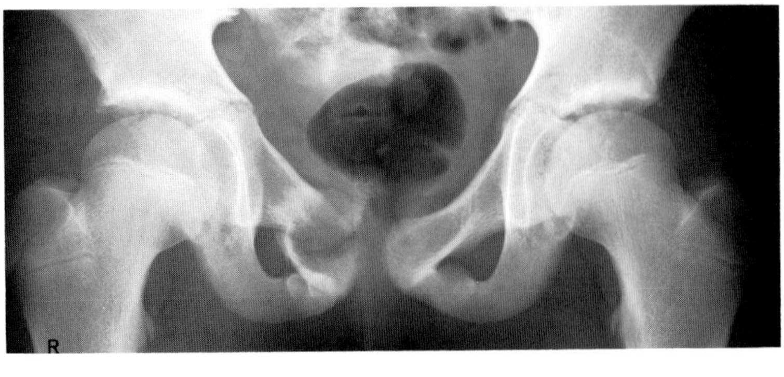

Fig. 12.15

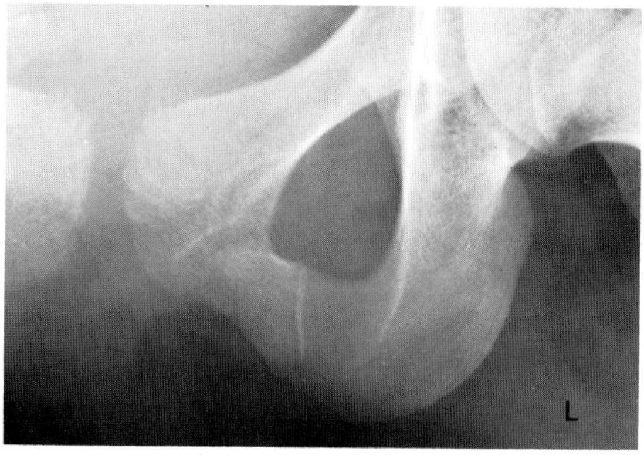

Fig. 12.16. A 14-year-old girl who fell through a window on the second floor. Fracture of the left ischium without significant dislocation.

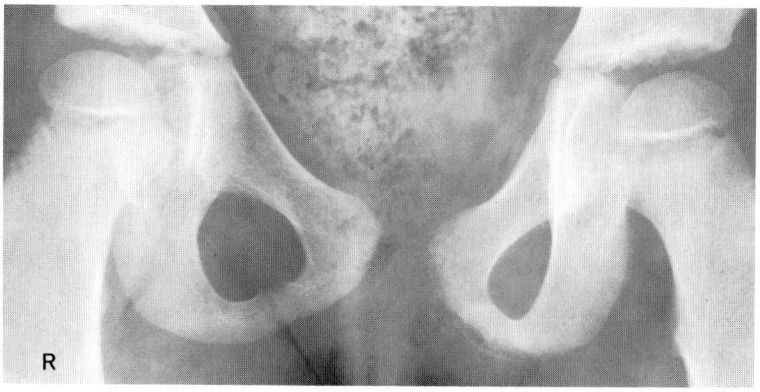

Fig. 12.17. A 5-year-old girl who was hit by a car. Three-week-old lesion of the symphysis, with periosteal reaction of the pubic and ischial bones (subperiosteal hematoma).

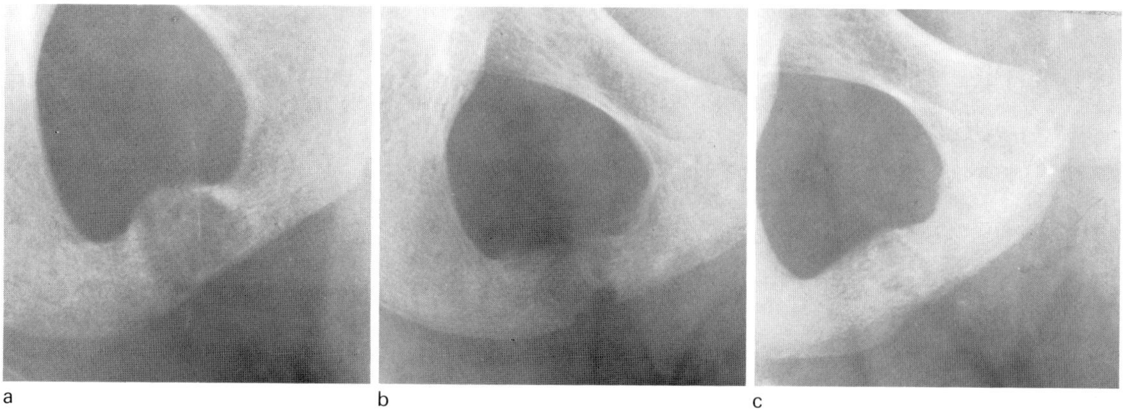

Fig. 12.18a–c. A 5½-year-old girl with ischiopubic osteochondritis; no trauma.
a) Early phase of the process.
b) Acute stage. Confusion with traumatic alterations is very possible.
c) Beginning of the healing process.

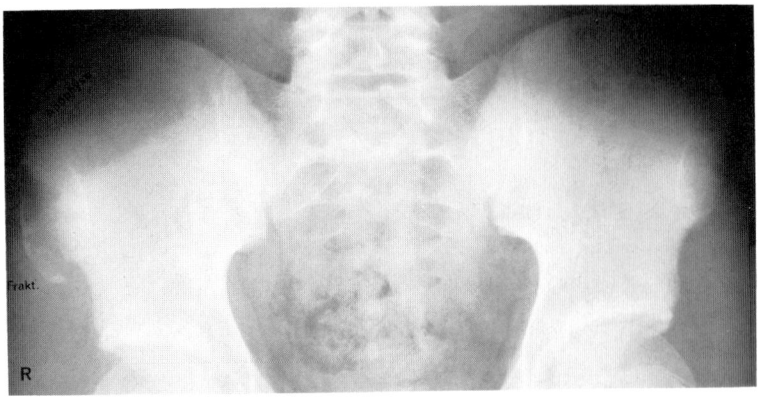

Fig. 12.19. An 18-year-old boy who, while running after a streetcar, suddenly developed pain in the right groin. Fracture of the right anterosuperior iliac spine.

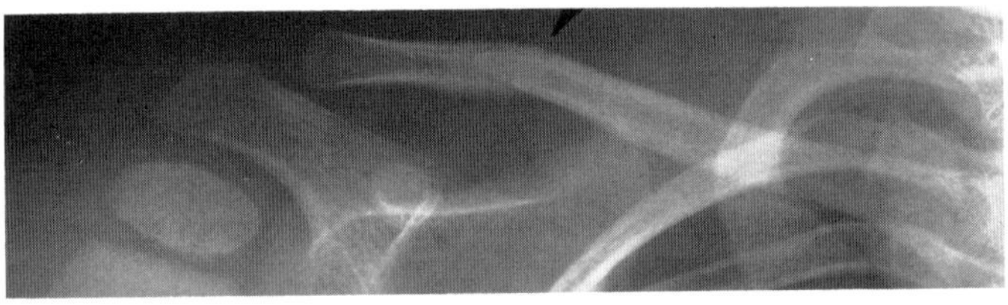

Fig. 12.20. A 1-year-7-month-old boy with no known trauma. Greenstick fracture of the right clavicle with minimal dislocation.

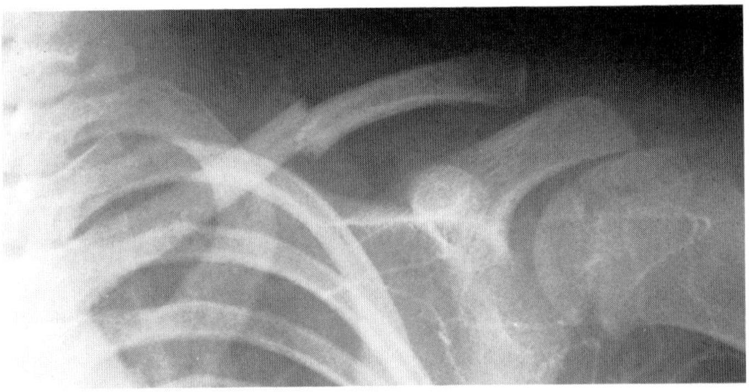

Fig. 12.21. A 3½-year-old girl who fell from a swing. Fractured clavicle with marked dislocation.

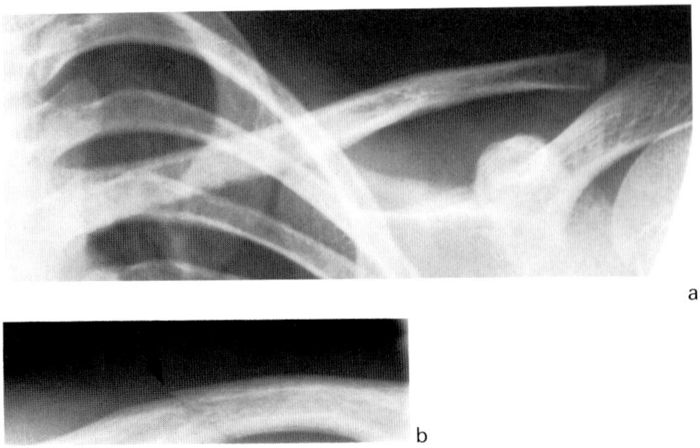

a

b

Fig. 12.22a and b. Fracture of the clavicle without significant dislocation.
a) No clear-cut findings on a.p. view.
b) Up-shoot film reveals fracture.

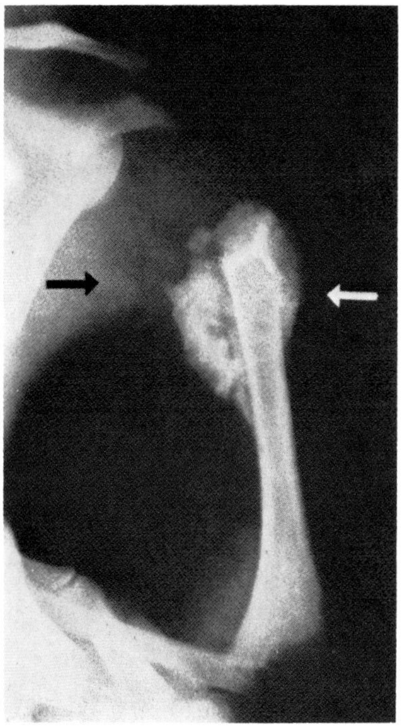

Fig. 12.23. Birth trauma to the metaphysis and massive periosteal ossification of a subperiosteal hematoma 4 weeks after delivery by manual extraction. (From H. Geiger and F. Schmid: Fortschr. Med. *85:* 321, 1961.)

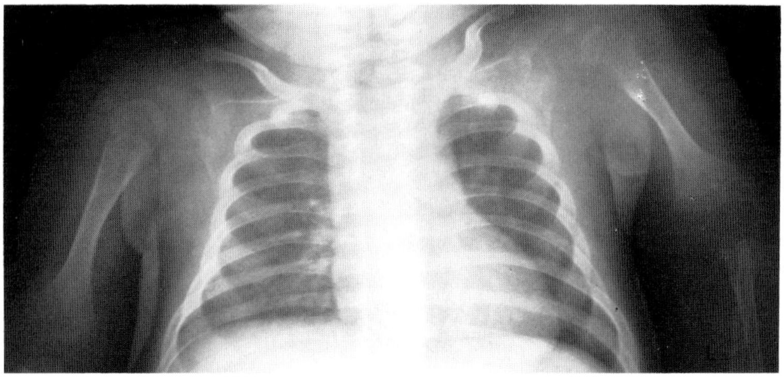

Fig. 12.24. A 3-month-old girl admitted for surgical management of a fracture of the humerus. This patient has osteochondritis as an expression of congenital lues.

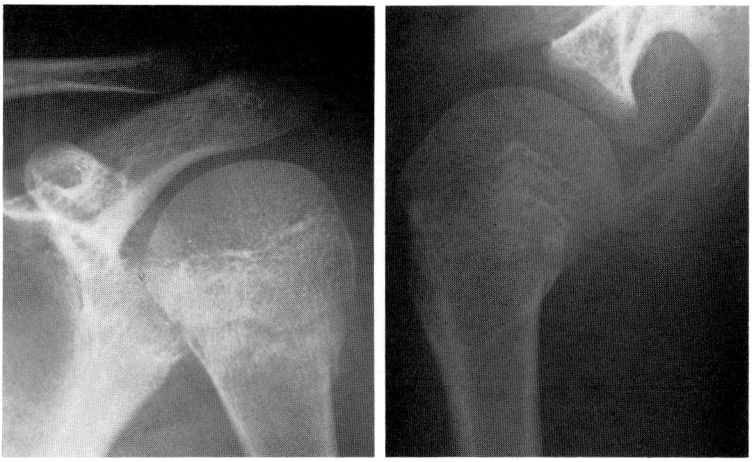

a b

Fig. 12.25a and b. An 11-year-old girl who fell from a horse. Fracture of the humerus involving the epiphysis.

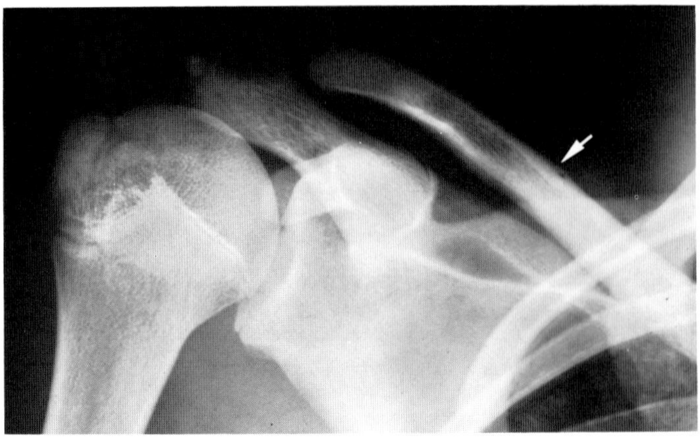

Fig. 12.26a

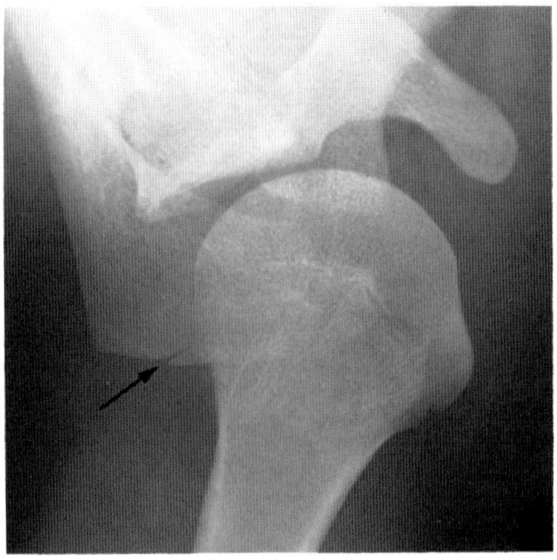

Fig. 12.26b

Fig. 12.26a and b. A 17-year-old boy after an accident with a motorscooter. A rare variant is a small bony channel for the supraclavicular nerve *(arrow)*. Avulsion fracture of a major tubercle and the acromion.

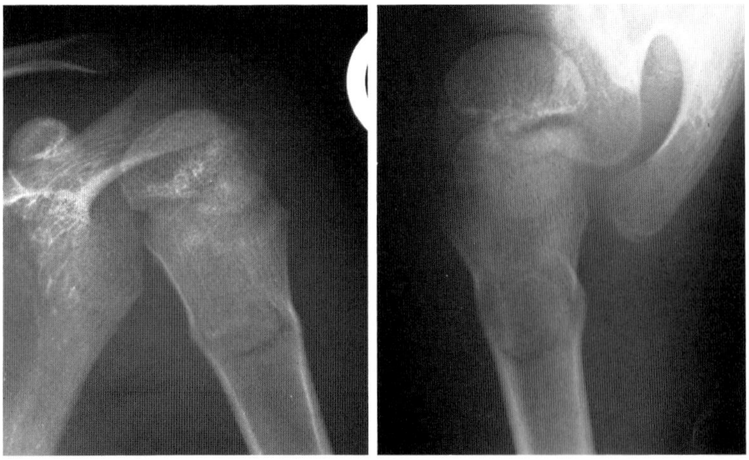

a b

Fig. 12.27a and b. A 5-year-old boy who fell from a wall. Greenstick fracture of the left humerus. In addition, transcondylar fracture.

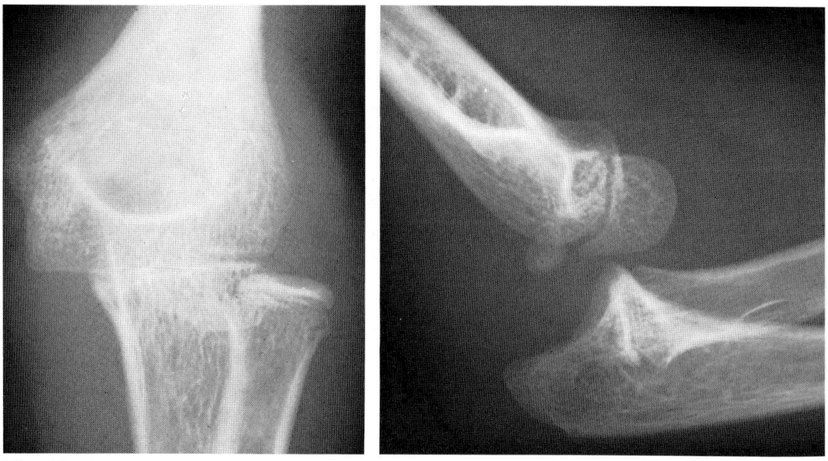

Fig. 12.28a b

Fig. 12.28a–d. A 12-year-old boy after a fall from a wall.
a and b) Dislocation of the elbow. Dislocation of the ossification center for the ulnar epicondylus.
c and d) X-ray follow-up after reposition. Note the completely corrected position of the ossification center for the ulnar epicondylus.

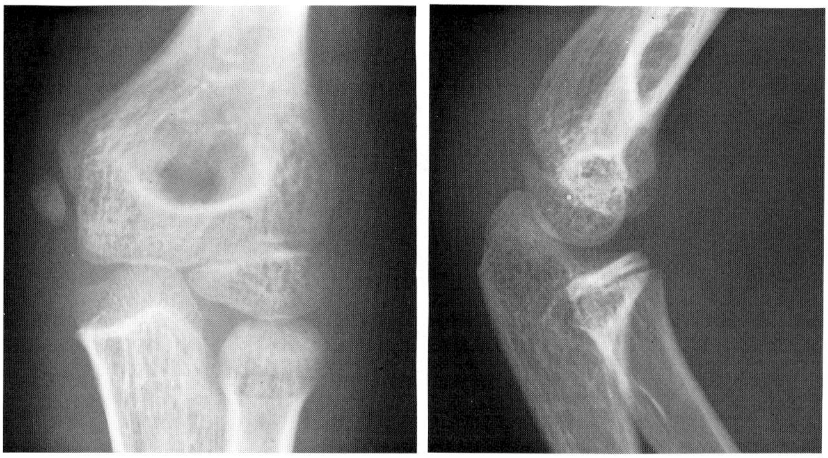

c d

Fig. 12.29a and b. A 7-year-old boy who fell while doing gymnastics. Supracondylar fracture of the humerus. Minimal dorsal angulation. Fracture line on a. p. view barely visible *(arrow)*. Infusion in the joint; no disability caused by displacement of the transparent recess dorsally.

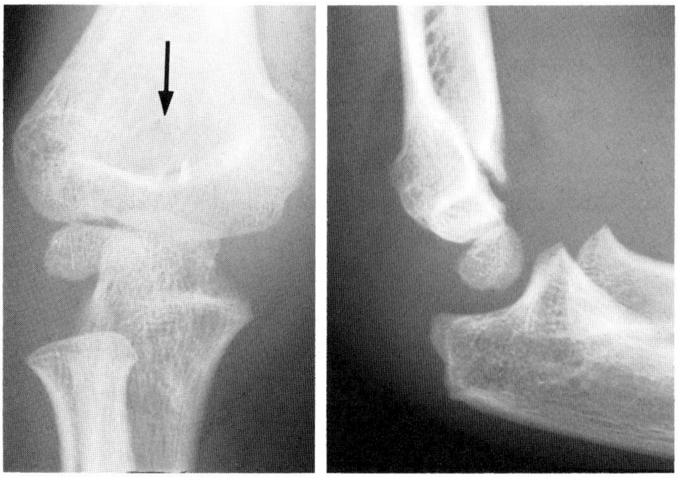

a b

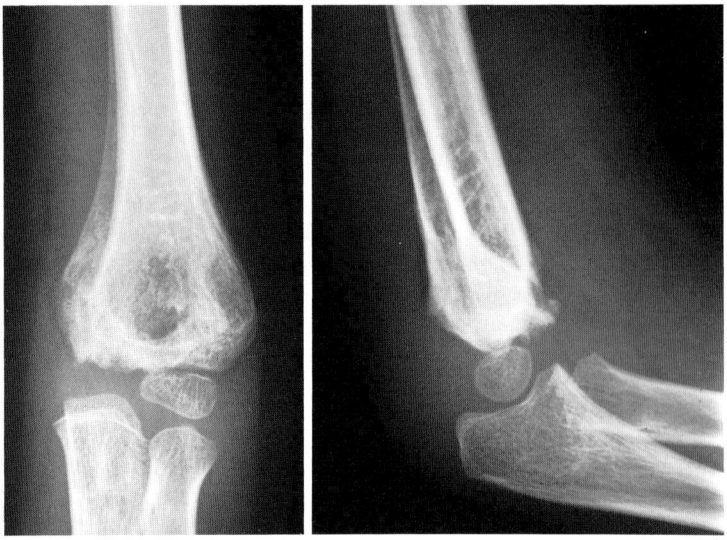

a b

Fig. 12.30a and b. A 6-year-old boy with massive formation of callus 6 weeks after a supracondylar fracture; dorsal angulation has not been corrected.

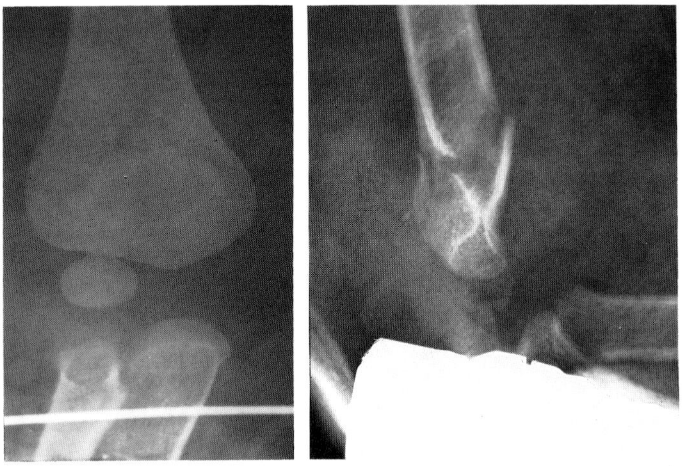

a b

Fig. 12.31a and b. X-ray follow-up through a plaster cast after a supracondylar fracture. The dorsal angulation has not been corrected. The joint is well visualized despite the overlap by a metallic device and can be properly evaluated.

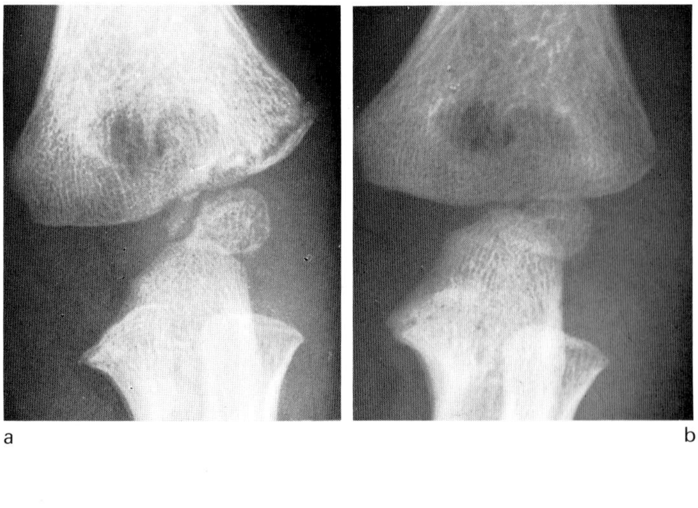

a b

Fig. 12.32a and b. A 5-year-old boy.
a) Fracture of lateral condyle.
b) X-ray follow-up 4 weeks later.

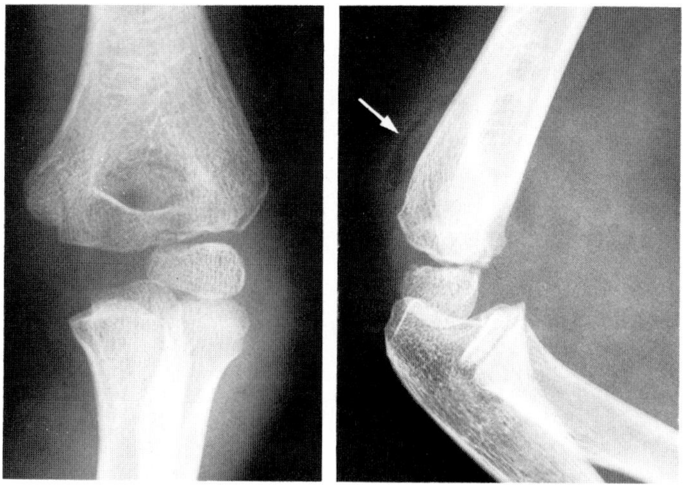

a b

Fig. 12.33a and b. A 7-year-old boy who fell on his left elbow. Sickle-shaped lucency dorsally *(arrow)*. Shell-like avulsion in the metaphysis on the radial side. Marked effusion of the joint.

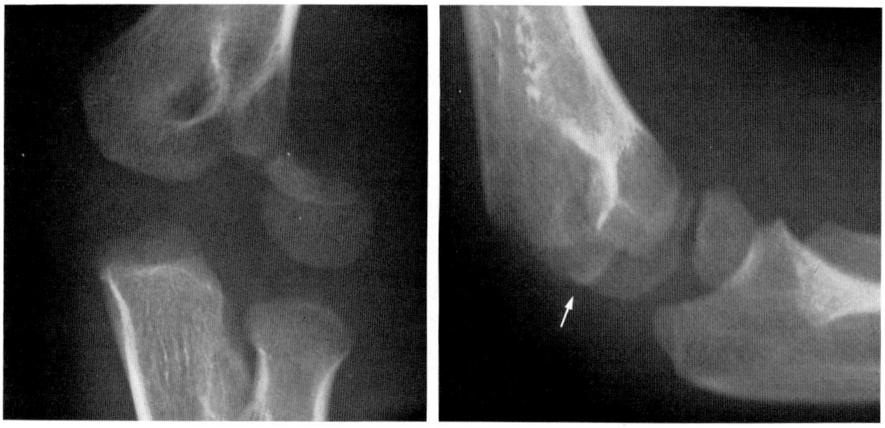

a b

Fig. 12.34a and b. Dislocation of the ossification center of the humeral capitulum, together with a large piece of the metaphysis itself. Subluxation. Note the still small ossification center of the medial epicondyle *(arrow)*.

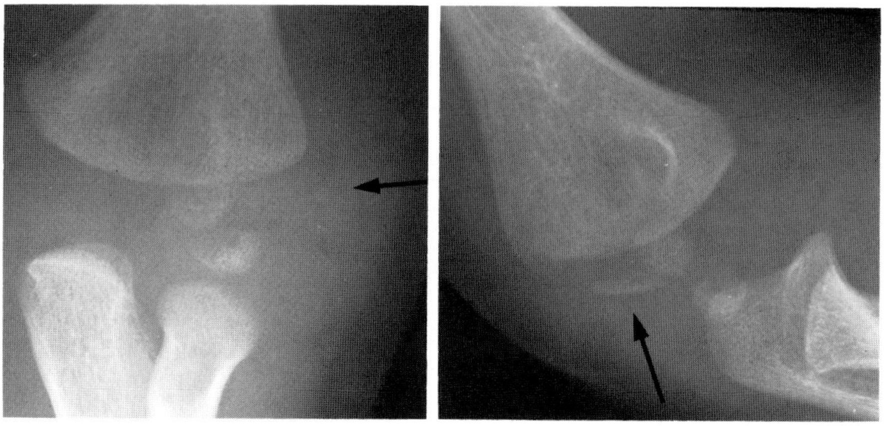

a b

Fig. 12.35a and b. A 3-year-old boy with a fracture of the ossification center of the humeral capitulum into two large parts *(arrow)*. Shell-like avulsion fracture of the lateral metaphysis *(arrow)*.

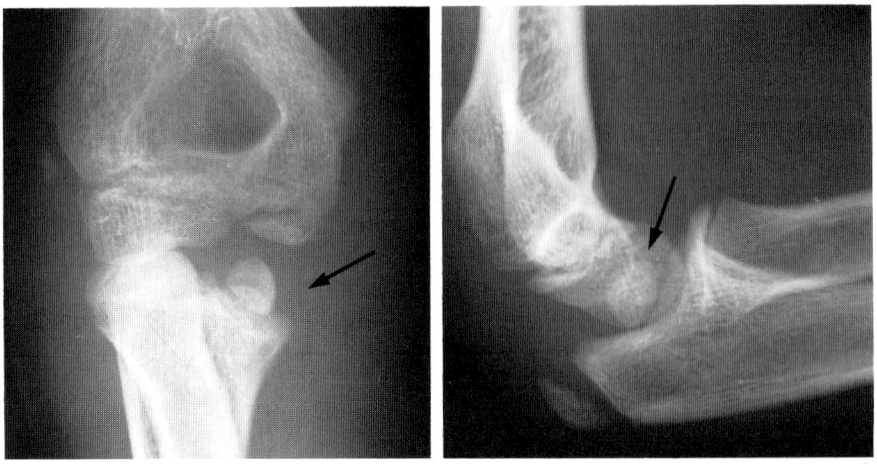

a b

Fig. 12.36a and b. A 13-year-old boy who fell on his right elbow. Dislocation of the ossification center of the medial epicondyle into the joint *(arrow)*.

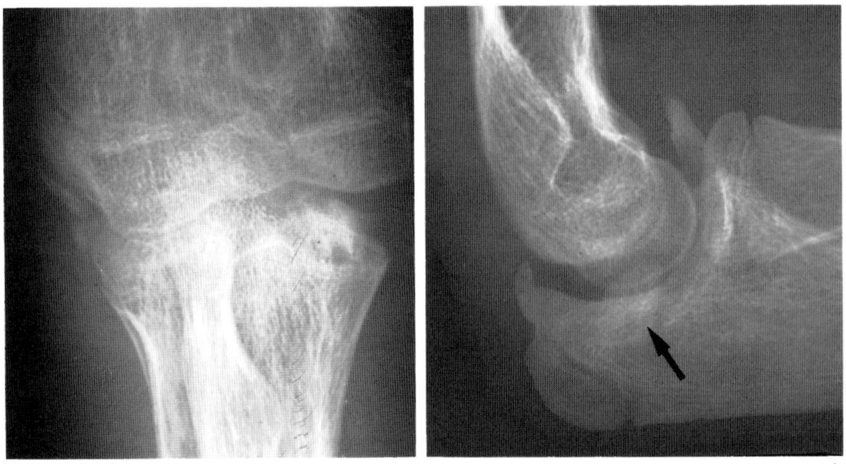

Fig. 12.37a b

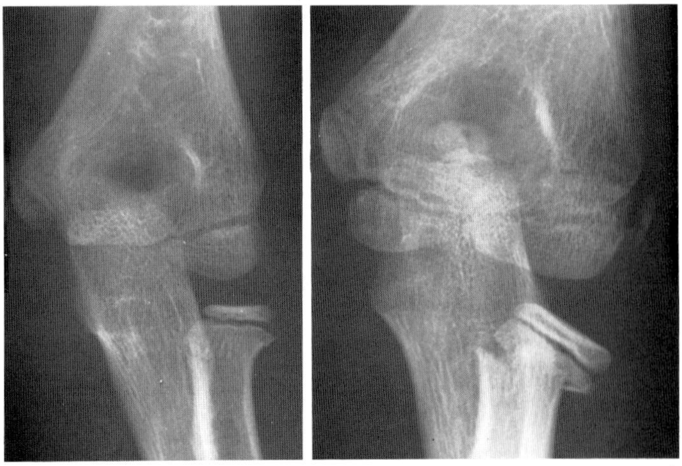

Fig. 12.38a b

▲ Fig. 12.37a and b. A 13-year-old boy who was referred to the orthopedic surgeon because of an unexplained limitation of extension. For 3 months, the ossification center of the medial epicondyle was caught in the medial part of the joint space. Avulsion of the tip of the coronoid process. Already significant deformity of the joint and atrophy of the bones.

Fig. 12.38a and b. a) A 7-year-old girl with a fracture of the neck of the radius and slight displacement.
b) A 12-year-old boy with a fracture of the neck of the radius and marked displacement.

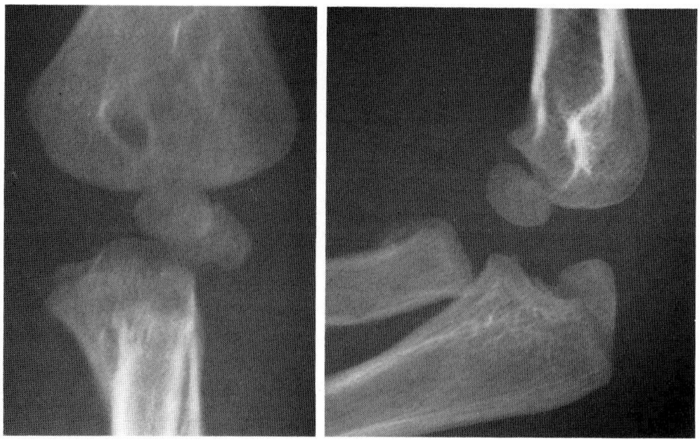

a b

Fig. 12.39a and b. A 4-year-old girl who fell from a haywagon. Fracture of the olecranon and displacement of the head of the radius, with an avulsion of the metaphysis (this is a frequent combination).

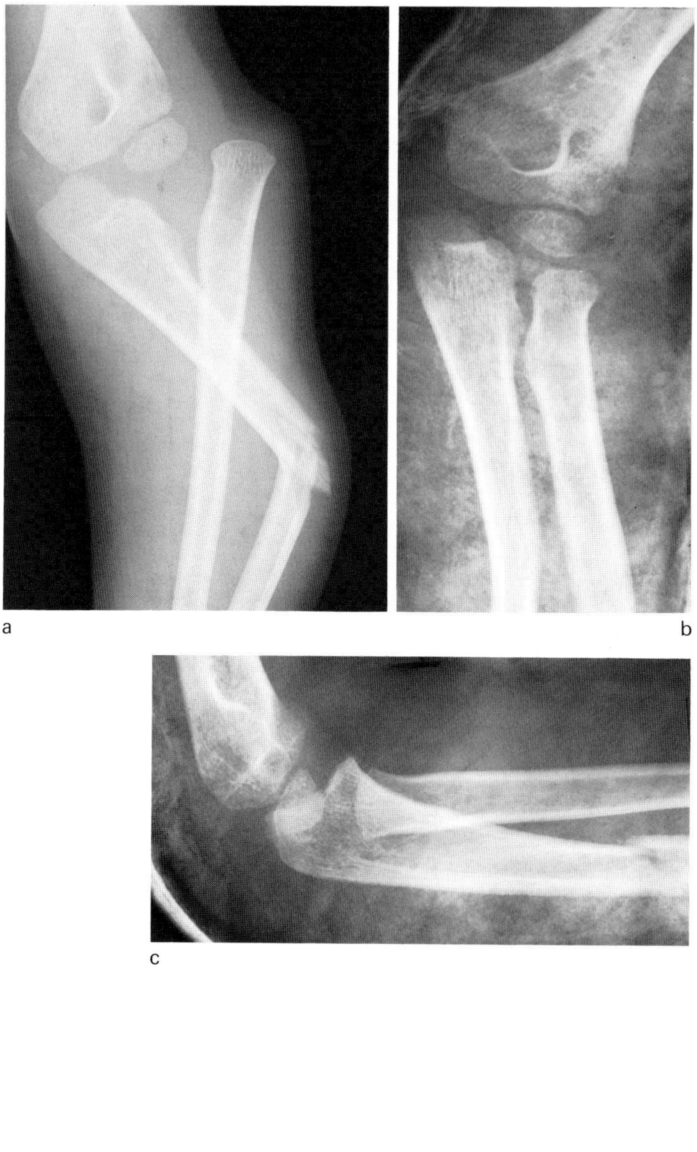

a b c

Fig. 12.40a–c. A 7-year-old boy who, during gymnastics, fell on his left arm. Monteggia fracture (fracture of the ulna with dislocation of the head of the radius). X-ray follow-up through a plaster cast shows a good joint.

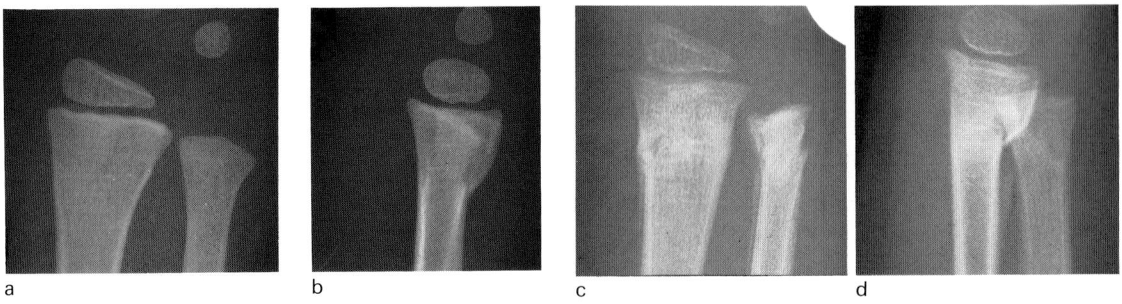

Fig. 12.41a–d. A 4-year-old girl who fell from a window and suffered a fracture of the skull.
a and b) Greenstick fracture of the forearm in a typical location. Minimal dorsal angulation.
c and d) Follow-up 3 weeks later shows the fracture of the ulna more reliably placed.

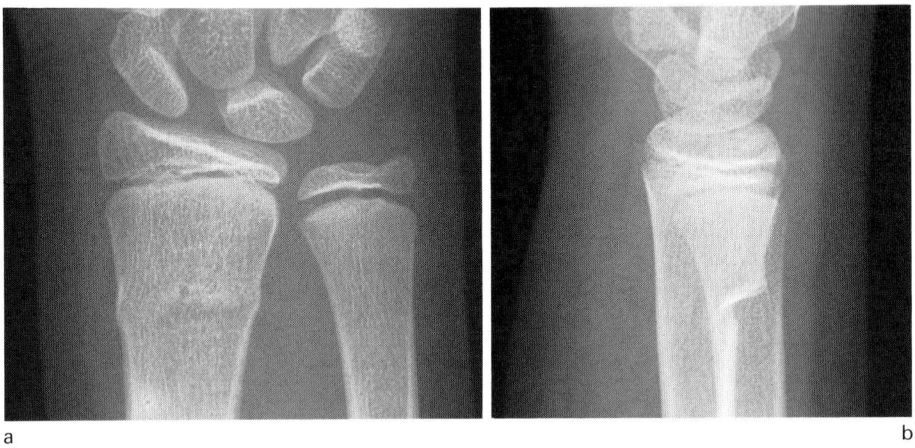

Fig. 12.42a and b. A 10-year-old girl after a sudden fall while sledding. Greenstick fracture of the radius, with typical dorsal buckling.

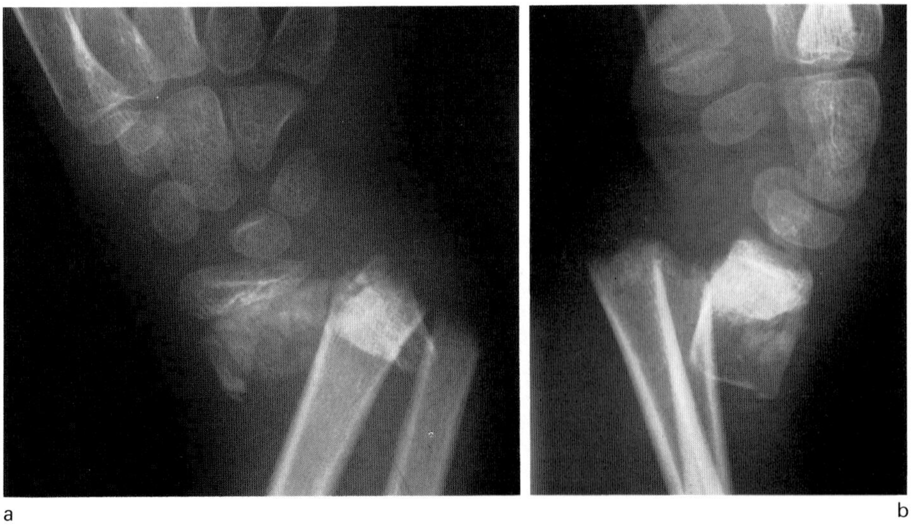

Fig. 12.43a and b. A 9-year-old boy who fell from the top of a triple-decker bed. Complete fracture of the forearm, with marked displacement.

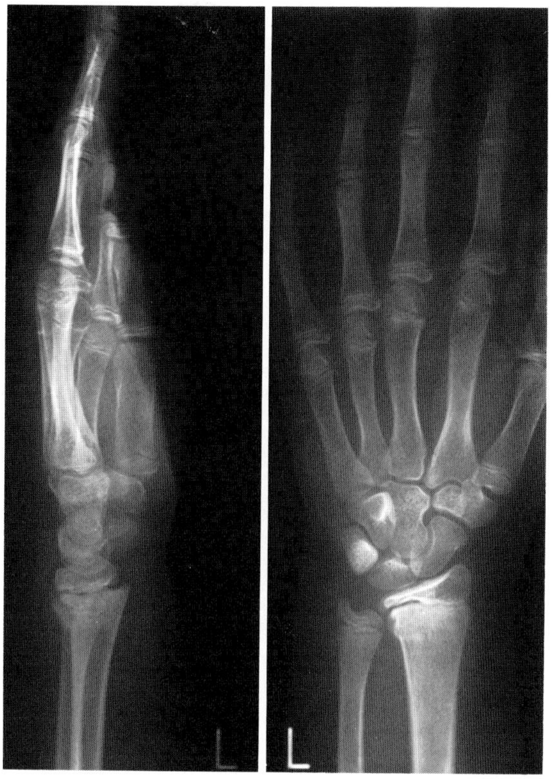

a b

Fig. 12.44a and b. 11-year-old boy with traumatic epiphysiolysis of the radius. Displacement of the epiphysis dorsal, together with a wedge of the metaphysis (most frequent localization).

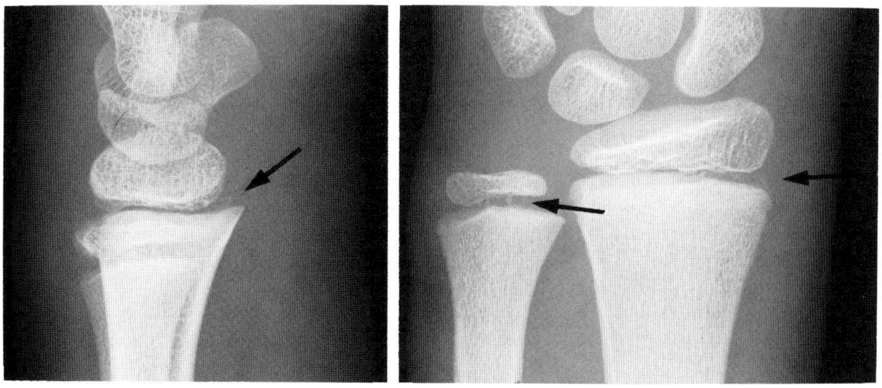

a b

Fig. 12.45a and b. A 12-year-old boy with small metaphyseal avulsions as a sign of traumatic epiphysiolysis.

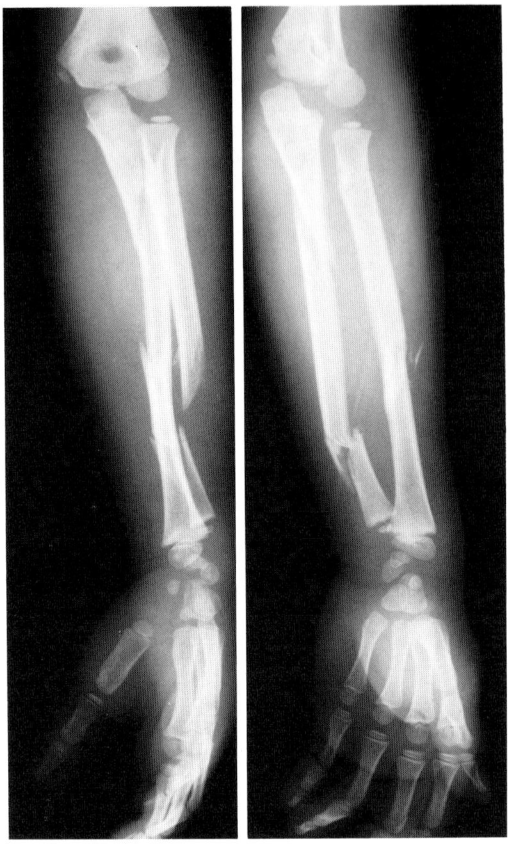

a b

Fig. 12.46a and b. A 7-year-old boy whose left arm was deliberately held in a laundry wringer. "Wringer injury" of the left forearm. Fracture of the radius; piece fracture of the ulna. Severe soft-tissue damage and disturbance of the circulation.

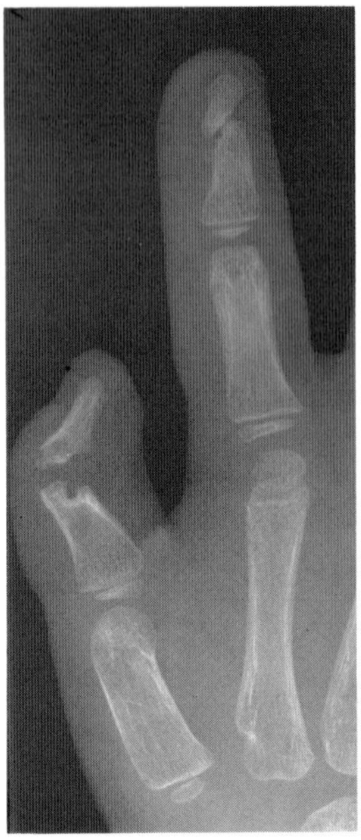

Fig. 12.47. A 5-year-old boy with early finger deformity as the result of a missed or overlooked fracture involving the growth center.

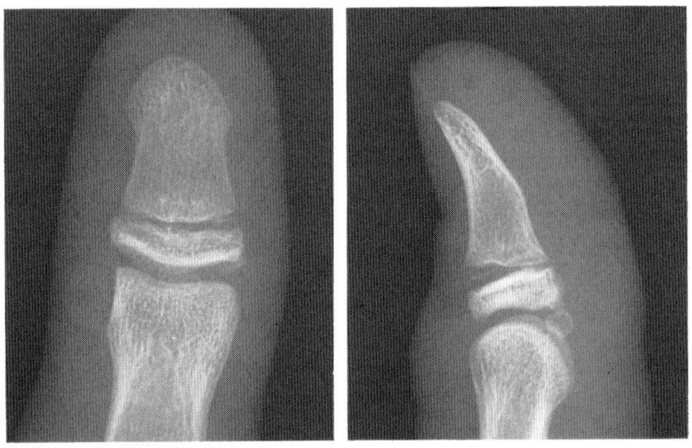

a b

Fig. 12.48a and b. A 17-year-old boy after an accident with a motorscooter. Epiphysiolysis with small marginal avulsions of the end phalanx of the thumb.

Fig. 12.50. A 16-year-old boy with a distal fracture of the second metacarpal bone sustained during boxing. ▶

Fig. 12.51. A 4-year-old boy who fell from about 150 cm, onto his left arm and hand (additional fracture of the olecranon). Fracture of the navicular bone without significant displacement. ▶

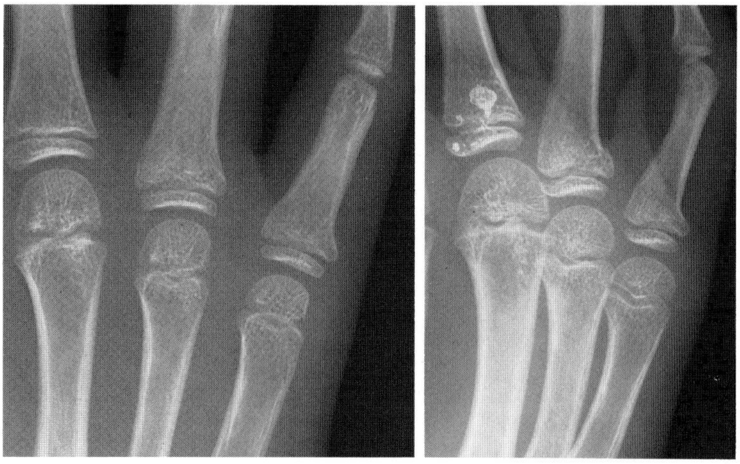

a b

Fig. 12.49a and b. A 10-year-old girl with a fracture of ground phalanges 4 and 5 at the base resulting from a fall while rollerskating.

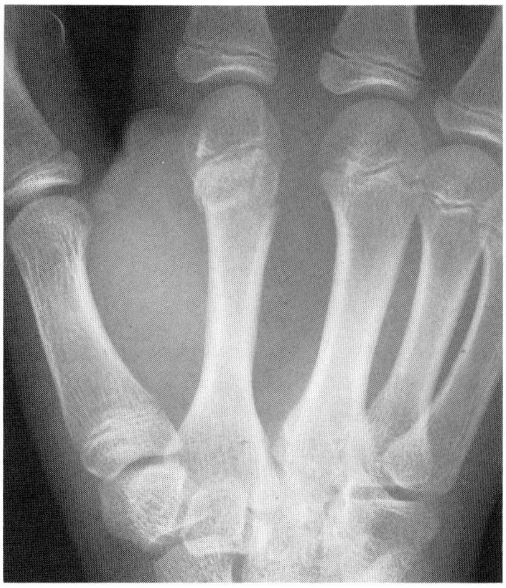

Fig. 12.50

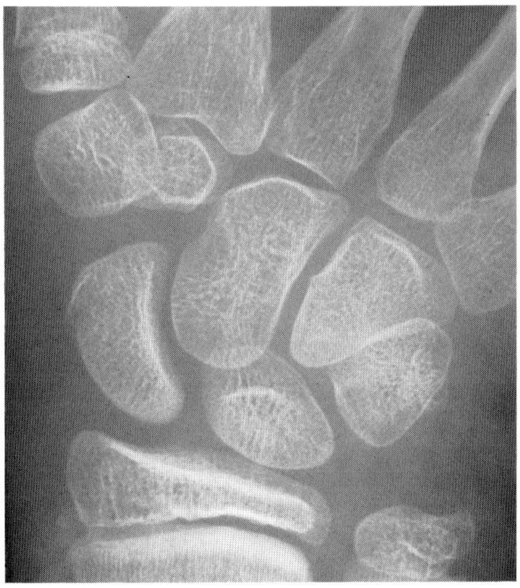

Fig. 12.51

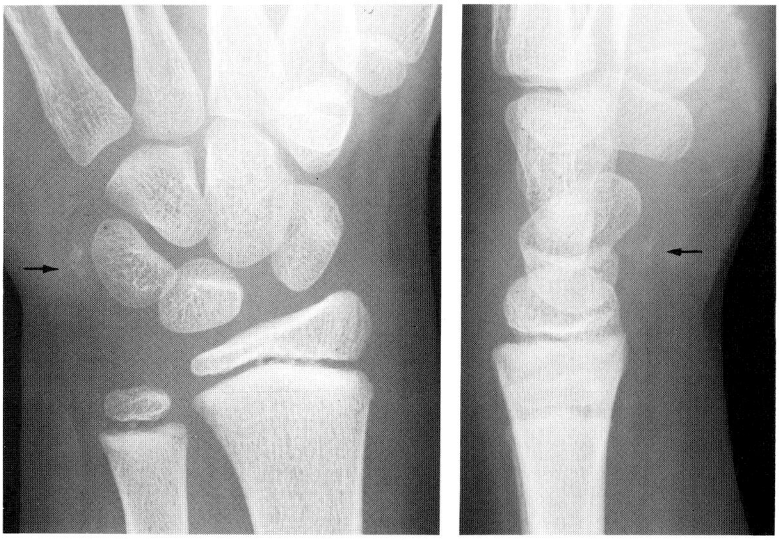

a b

Fig. 12.52a and b. A 9-year-old boy who was treated for a fracture of the head of the radius. Os pisiform has multiple beaklike ossification centers. This is not a traumatic lesion.

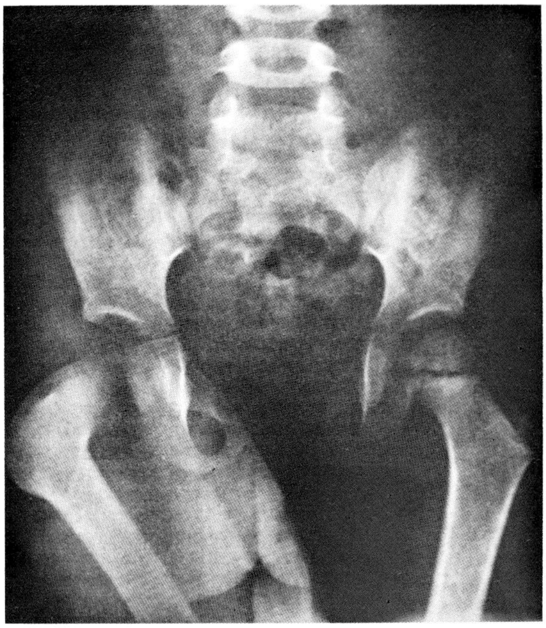

Fig. 12.53. A 7-year-old girl after a fall from a stairway. Posteroinferior dislocation of the hip. (From D. W. Wilson: J. Trauma *6:* 739, 1966.)

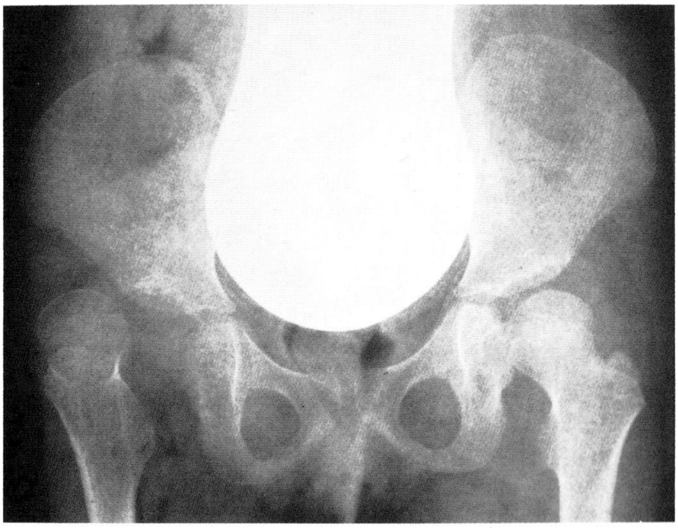

Fig. 12.54. A $5\frac{1}{2}$-year-old girl with no significant trauma. Dislocated hip on the right superiorly, with external rotation of the femur; mongoloid pelvis. (From H. Mau: Arch. Orthop. Unfall-Chir. *63:* 176, 1968.)

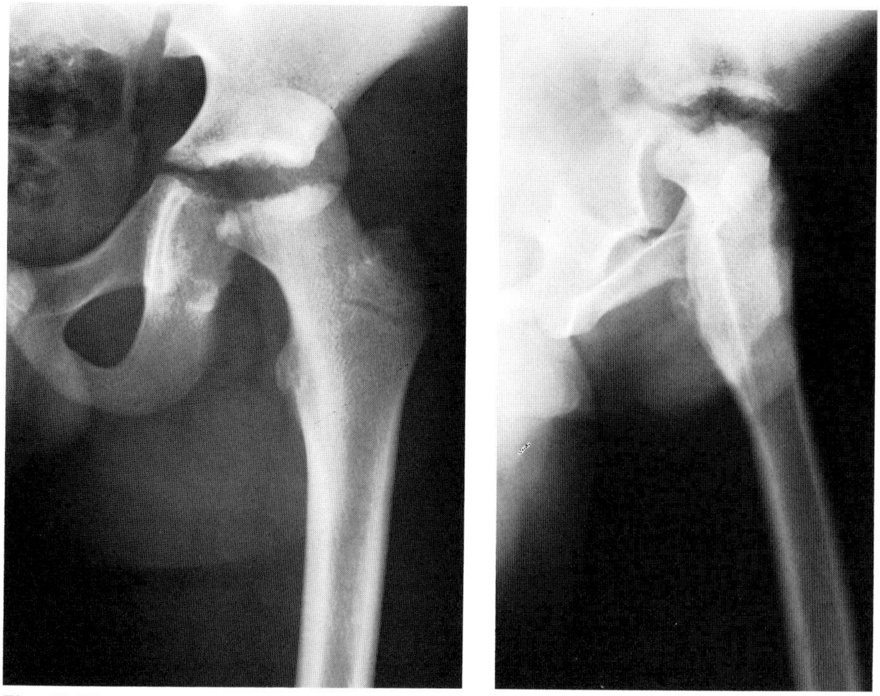

Fig. 12.55a b

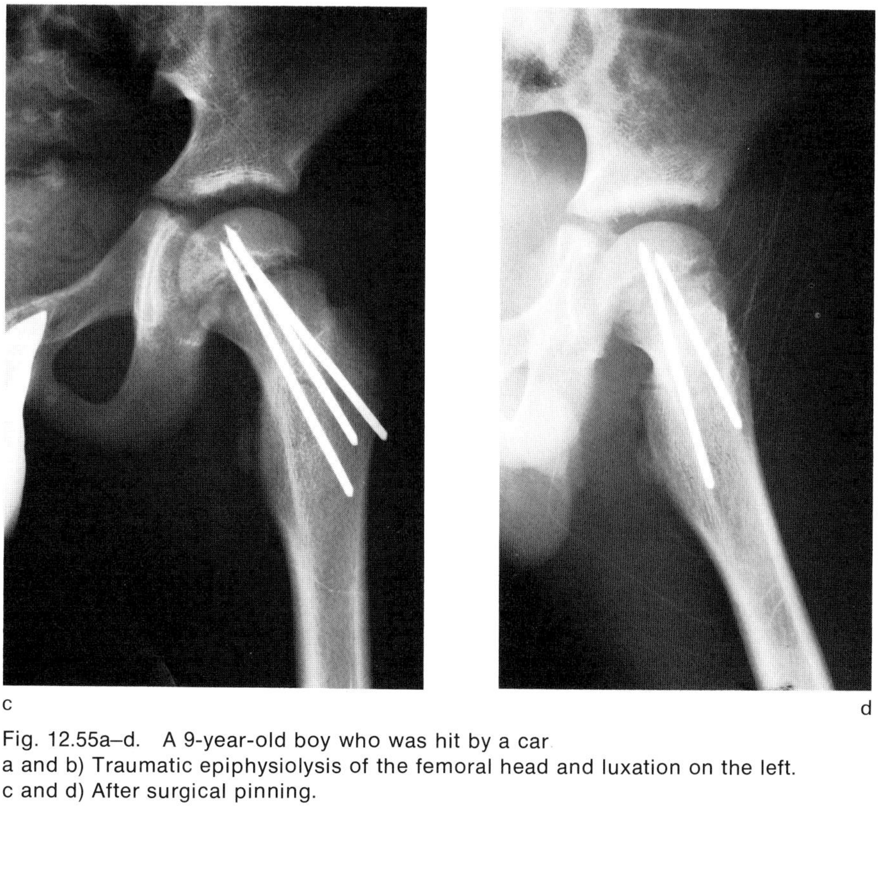

c d

Fig. 12.55a–d. A 9-year-old boy who was hit by a car.
a and b) Traumatic epiphysiolysis of the femoral head and luxation on the left.
c and d) After surgical pinning.

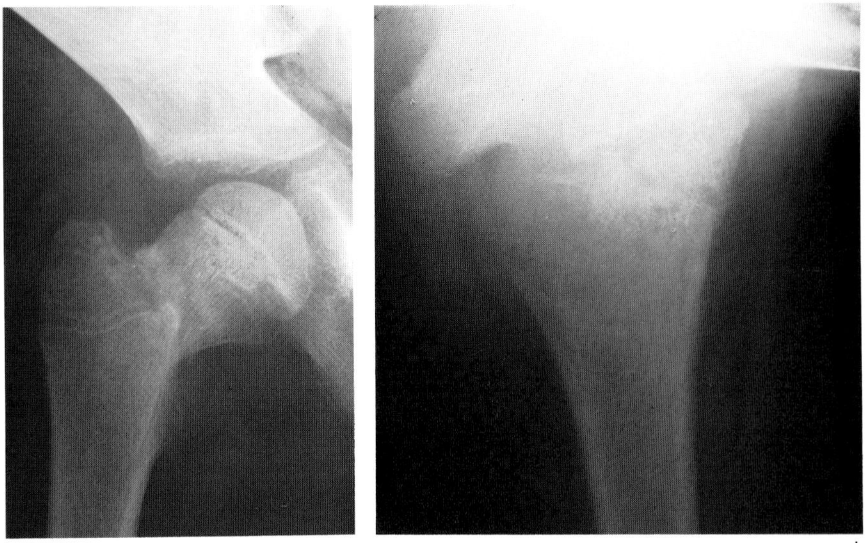

a b

Fig. 12.56a and b. A 6-year-old girl with a fracture of the right femoral neck sustained in a fall from some stairs. Dorsal angulation and wedging of the fracture fragments. Callus formation 6 weeks after the accident.

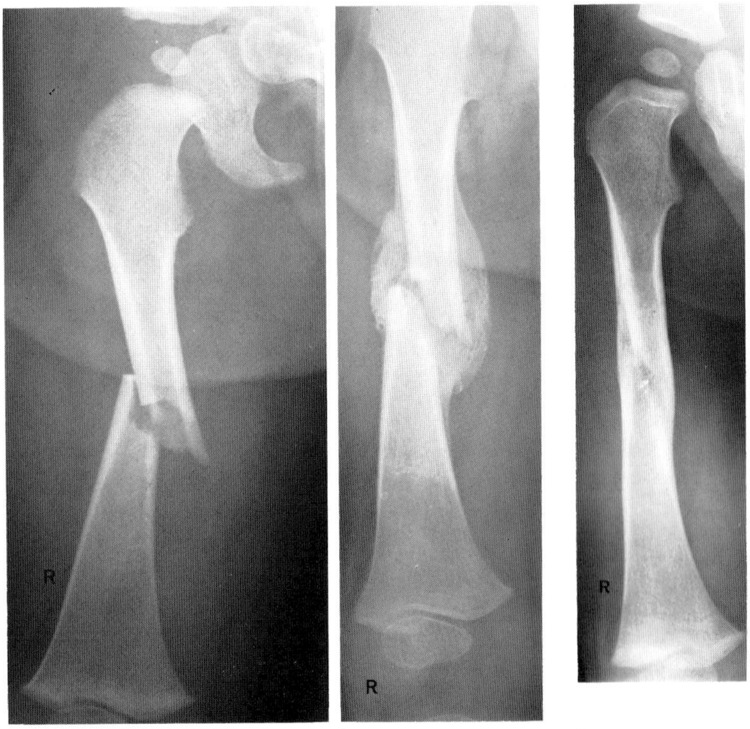

a b c

Fig. 12.57a–c. A 10½-month-old boy.
a) Fracture of the femur in the middle third.
b) After 1 month, bony consolidation with abundant formation of callus.
c) About 5 months after the trauma, only mild residual changes.

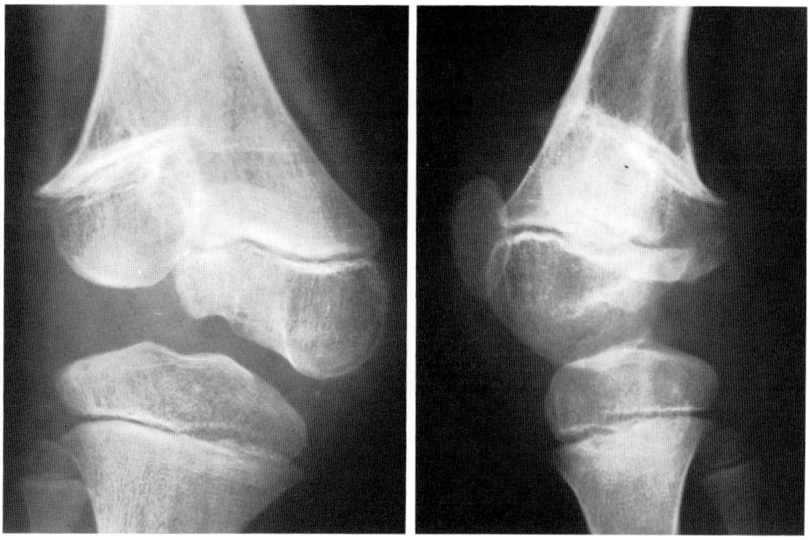

a b

Fig. 12.58a and b. A 6-year-old girl. Condition 1½ years after a fracture of the distal femoral epiphysis; partial involvement of the growth zone.

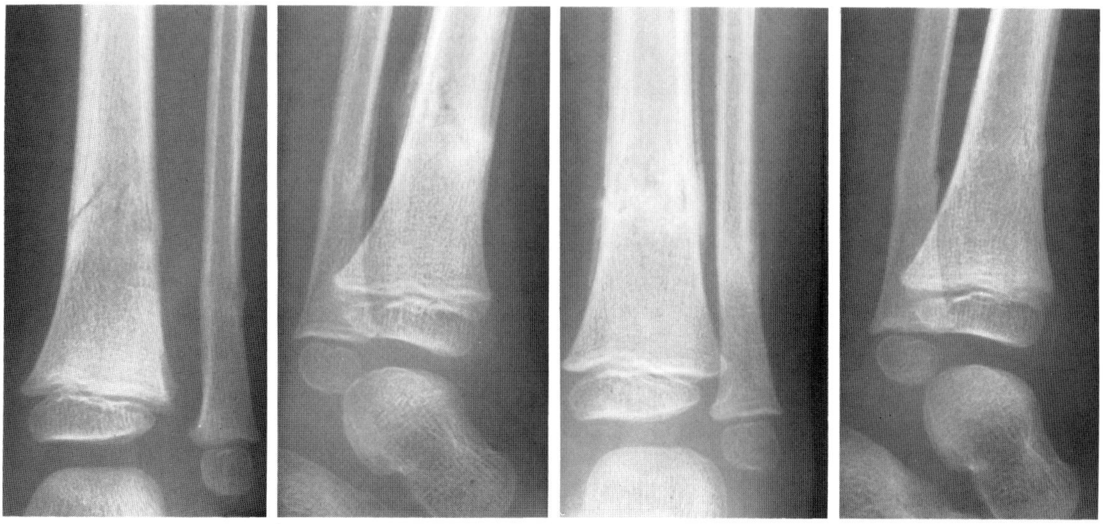

a b c d

Fig. 12.59a–d. A 3-year-old boy. a and b) Greenstick fracture of the left shank. c and d) X-ray follow-up 14 weeks later.

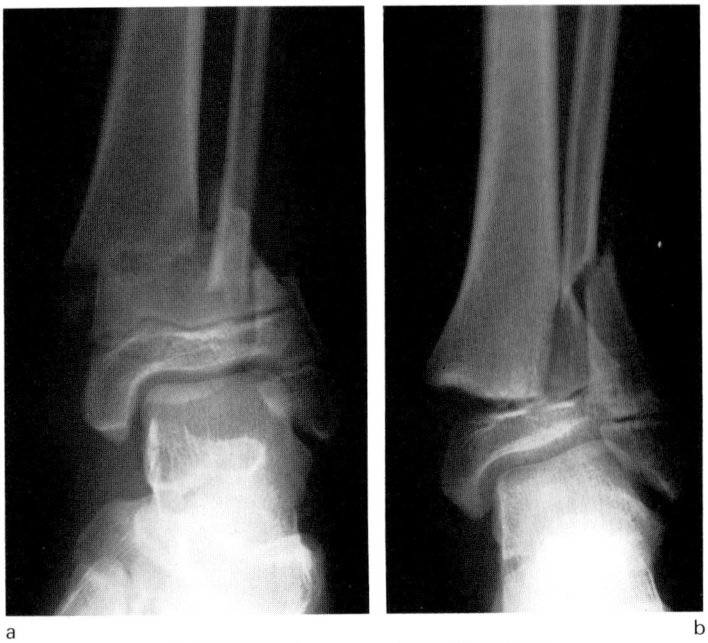

Fig. 12.60a and b. a) A 13$^{1}/_{2}$-year-old boy after a ski accident. Fracture of the tibia and fibula. b) A 7$^{1}/_{2}$-year-old boy after a ski accident. Traumatic epiphysiolysis, with a fracture of a large metaphyseal wedge from the tibia and a fracture of the fibula.

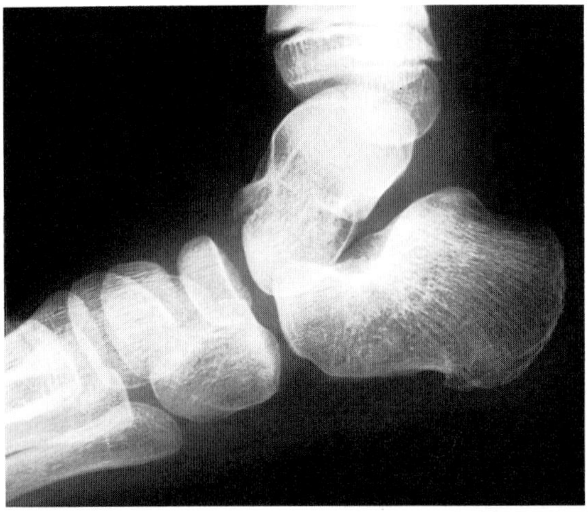

Fig. 12.61. A 5-year-old girl after a tractor ran over her right foot. Fracture of the talus.

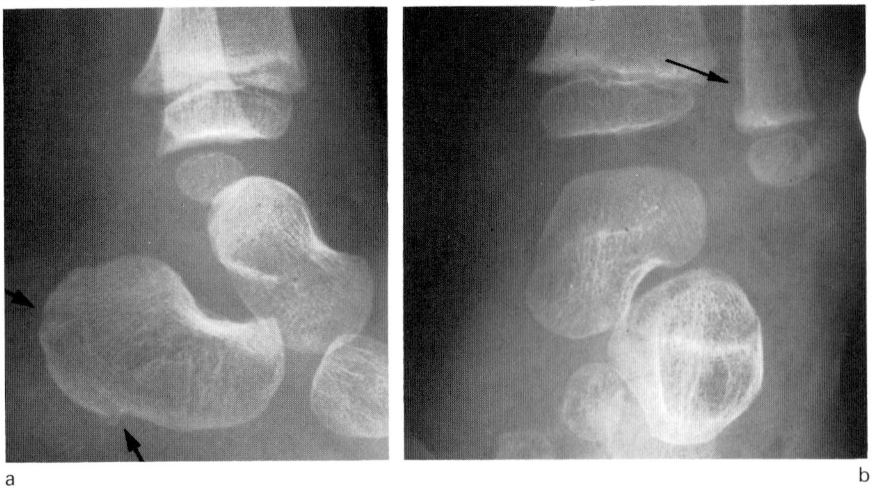

Fig. 12.62. A 2$^{1}/_{2}$-year-old boy with a fracture of the calcaneus and a fracture of the distal fibular metaphysis.

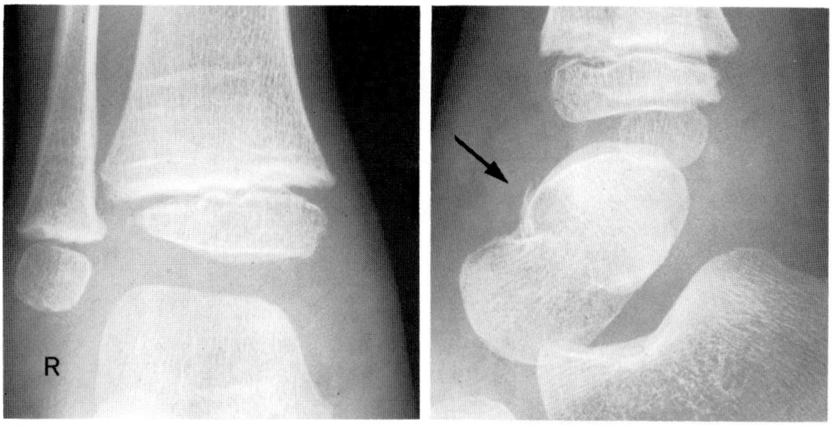

Fig. 12.63a b

Fig. 12.63a-d. A 4½-year-old boy after a tractor ran over his right foot. Avulsion fracture of the talus and the 3rd and 5th metatarsal bones.

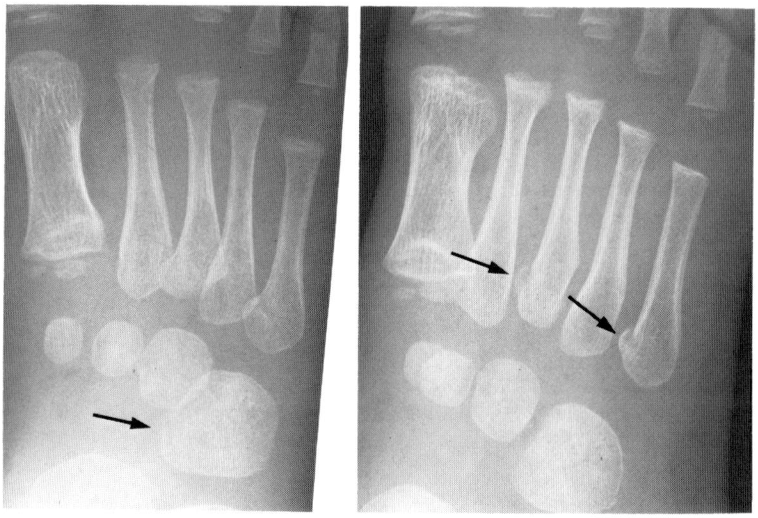

c d

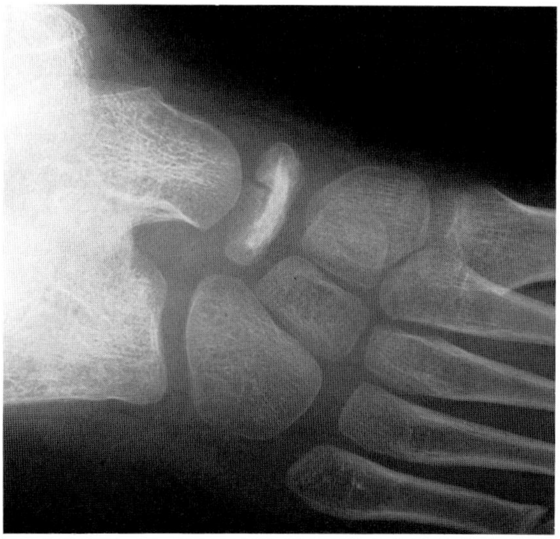

Fig. 12.64. A 7-year-old boy who was referred with a suspicion of a fracture. Deformity of the navicular bone (Köhler I).

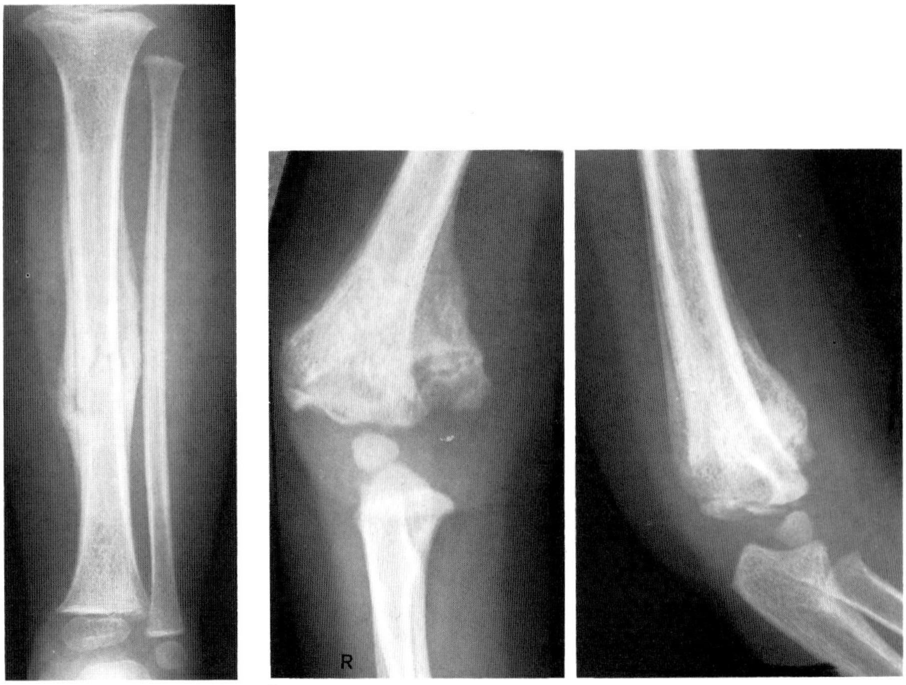

Fig. 12.65a b c

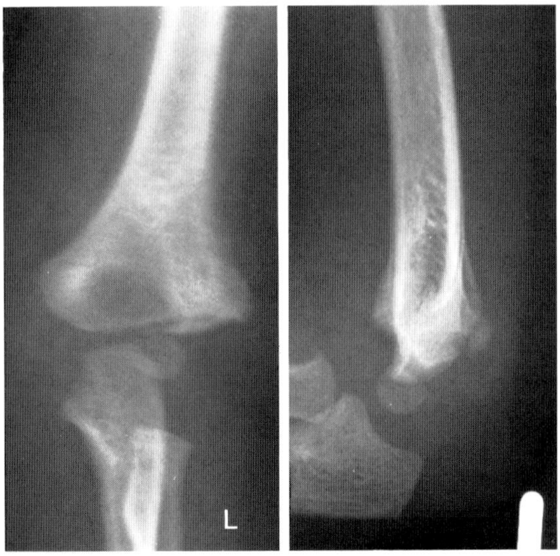

d e

Fig. 12.65a–e. A 1-year-10-month-old girl with the battered-child syndrome. Old fracture of the tibia on the left; deformity and massive periosteal reaction at the distal humeral region bilaterally, more so on the right.

13 Internal Fixation and Its Radiologic Evaluation

The evaluation of x-rays after internal fixation requires basic knowledge and understanding of the surgical techniques, the biology of bone healing and the most frequently utilized implants. In order not to limit oneself simply to a description but to arrive at a clear diagnosis, the following points and related comments must all be considered:

1. Implants
(Type of internal fixation and origin; biomechanical characteristics: tension band method, neutralization plate or compression plate, etc.)

2. Anatomy
(Position of fracture; eventually still noticeable degree of dislocation; bony defect and its significance on the stability of internal fixation.)

3. Quality of Skeleton
(Atrophy; osteoporosis; early post-traumatic or preexisting pathologic conditions.)

4. Stability
(Weight-bearing fixation or reduction fixation, primary instability?)

During the further course, one especially has to evaluate:

5. Healing of Bone
(Direct healing – without visible callus formation; or indirect healing – with callus formation.)

6. Bony Reaction
(Reactive callus, zone of lysis, atrophy, infection and others.)

Besides the conservative and functional treatment of fractures of bones, there has been a marked increase in the importance of surgical management of a fracture in the English-speaking world. The term used for these methods is internal fixation, whereas in French and German the term is osteosynthesis. This refers to all operative methods that produce varying degrees of effective mechanical stabilization of a fracture. Biologic healing and, therefore the real repair of the break in continuity will, however, not be effected as the result of surgery but only subsequently by a healing process.
In principle, there are two methods of internal fixation. These are stable internal fixation and reduction fixation.
Stable internal fixation can be brought about by intramedullary nailing, interfragmentary compression by insertion of screws or plates or the principle of a tension band plate. In special cases, there is the possibility of combining Steinmann pins and external tension to achieve the stability needed. The advantage of all these aproaches is that mechanically the fracture can be neutralized and the effected stability is great enough so that there is no need for additional fixation by bandages or casts. Furthermore, immediate active physiotherapy is possible. Older methods, particularly in the adult, may result in fracture disease (atrophy of muscles and of the skeleton, stiff joints, circulatory disturbances, etc.); this can be effectively avoided (Wieser and Allgöwer, 1962).
Intramedullary nailing, inaugurated by Küntscher (1940) and improved upon and further developed by Maatz (1943), Herzog (1953) and finally the Association for the Study of Internal

Fixation (ASIF), is an operative method with ideal characteristics fulfilling all the requirements postulated for a weight-bearing fracture fixation. The effective principle of this method is the insertion of an expandable intramedullary splintage (marrow nailing). Stability is not achieved by additional compression but by the homogeneous filling of the marrow space with the pin or nail at the actual level of the fracture. True adaptation would be significantly improved by reaming of the marrow cavity (Fig. 13.1).

One has to distinguish between remote and direct, open marrow nailing. The indirect, remote insertion of the nail is performed, without directly approaching the actual fracture, from a remote site. Reposition of the fracture and surgical intervention are usually done with the help of an image intensifier with television viewing. In the open method, the fracture is surgically approached and its exact position controlled. The nail, however, is inserted from a site away from the fracture.

Screw and plate fixation, as developed by the Swiss Association for the Study of Internal Fixation, is based on a different principle. The fracture will be placed under interfragmentary pressure either by a simple screw fixation or (according to the type and localization of the fracture) (Fig. 13.2) by an external plate applied to the bone with screws. Based on their function, one can distinguish between the following: neutralization plate, tension band plate, compression plate and buttress plate (Müller et al., 1969).

A neutralization plate is used (Fig. 13.3) when the fracture is first corrected by insertion of cortical lag screws with a subsequent bridging of the entire fracture area with a correspondingly sized plate. The latter is usually put under controlled tension so that there will be a resulting axial compression.

The principle of the tension band plate (Fig. 13.4) stems from the fact that any long bone, as a result of eccentric forces, does have a pressure and a tension side. The femur, for instance, has its tension side on its laterodorsal side, and the humerus, on its dorsal side. One must, however, be aware that in certain situations there may be exceptions to this. The humerus, for instance, has its tension side ventrally (its volar side) if there is a stiff elbow joint. All these peculiarities, as well as regional unfavorable soft-tissue conditions, are determining factors in the choice of and in the position of the implant.

The compression plate is usually inserted for transverse or short oblique fractures (Fig. 13.5). By temporarily inserting a tension device, the plate is put under tension so that there is pressure on the fracture. The characteristics of a neutralization plate have to be observed in its actual location on the bone.

The buttress plate is used in the area of spongy bone, for instance, to avoid the displacement of a fracture of the tibial plateau (Fig. 13.6). The application of the principle of a tension band plate can result not only from the use of a plate but also from the use of a simple or a figure-eight loop of wire (Fig. 13.7). The basic principle involved is that the wire loop is placed in such a manner that the existing tensile forces are neutralized and result in compression forces. It is to the credit of Pauwels (1940) to have added to the operative methods then available the principle of tension (Fig. 13.18). Particularly in the area of the olecranon, the patella as well as the inner and outer aspects of the ankle, this method has gained wide application (Fig. 13.8). It is of paramount importance that the wire inserted on the tensile side is, indeed, strong enough to resist the local mechanical forces. The internal fixation by tension is one method in the group of weight-bearing fixations. Its principle will be made effective by its function.

Irrespective of the method of internal fixation applied, it is important that, at least for the duration of the healing phase, there be full mechanical stability. The reason for this is the maintenance of circulation or the possibility of rapid revascularization; anatomic adaptation of fragments; proper position, size and quality of implants; the filling of bony defects with autologous and homologous spongy bone and, in rare instances, with bone cement (methacrylate, palacos and others); and finally prophylaxis of local infection (Fig. 13.9). For evaluation of the length of the plate, one must be familiar with the principle that, for instance, on the tibia each main fracture fragment should contain 5 cortical screws and, in the femoral area, 7 cortical screws. Broad plates are only inserted into the femur and the humerus (Fig. 13.10).

Internal fixation by adaptation is a method of treatment whereby the fragments are directly connected by Kirschner wires, screws, cerclage wires or similar devices after open reposition. This method does not result in a weight-bearing fixation. In all of these situations, it is necessary to apply an external type of fixation in the form of plaster splints or circular plaster casts. Its main application is for fractures of the growing skeleton; however, judicious criteria must govern its use (Kuner and Weyand, 1971). Disadvantages resulting from the immobilization needed must not be feared in the child, since fracture disease is practically unknown in this age group. In the application of internal fixation, one must pay careful attention to the peculiarities of the growing skeleton (Fig. 13.11). The physis should, if at all possible, not be crossed by Kirschner wires and, in a situation when this is absolutely required, it must be done at a right angle. Insertion of a screw across a growth plate is totally unacceptable. The implants must be removed soon – after 2 to 6 weeks. In adults, there may be reasons for the use of the adaptation type of internal fixation (extensive destruction, large defects and others). In such instances, it is also necessary to apply a plaster cast. To the radiologist, its presence is a good indication of this type of internal fixation.

Great importance must be attached to the x-ray in the evaluation of the course of healing. Certain criteria will determine whether there is undisturbed healing of a fracture treated by internal fixation and thus the timing of full resumption of normal activity, or possibly disturbed healing. Special knowledge of the biologic process of repair, biomechanical insight and knowledge of the implants are basic for full understanding. In this regard, it is equally important to be familiar with the different types of repair of bony discontinuity. On the basis of the x-ray symptoms, one has to clearly distinguish between direct and indirect healing of bone. This simply means that, under certain conditions, there will be healing of a fracture without any visible formation of callus, whereas in other conditions, there will be formation of callus. Terms frequently used are those of primary and secondary fracture healing.

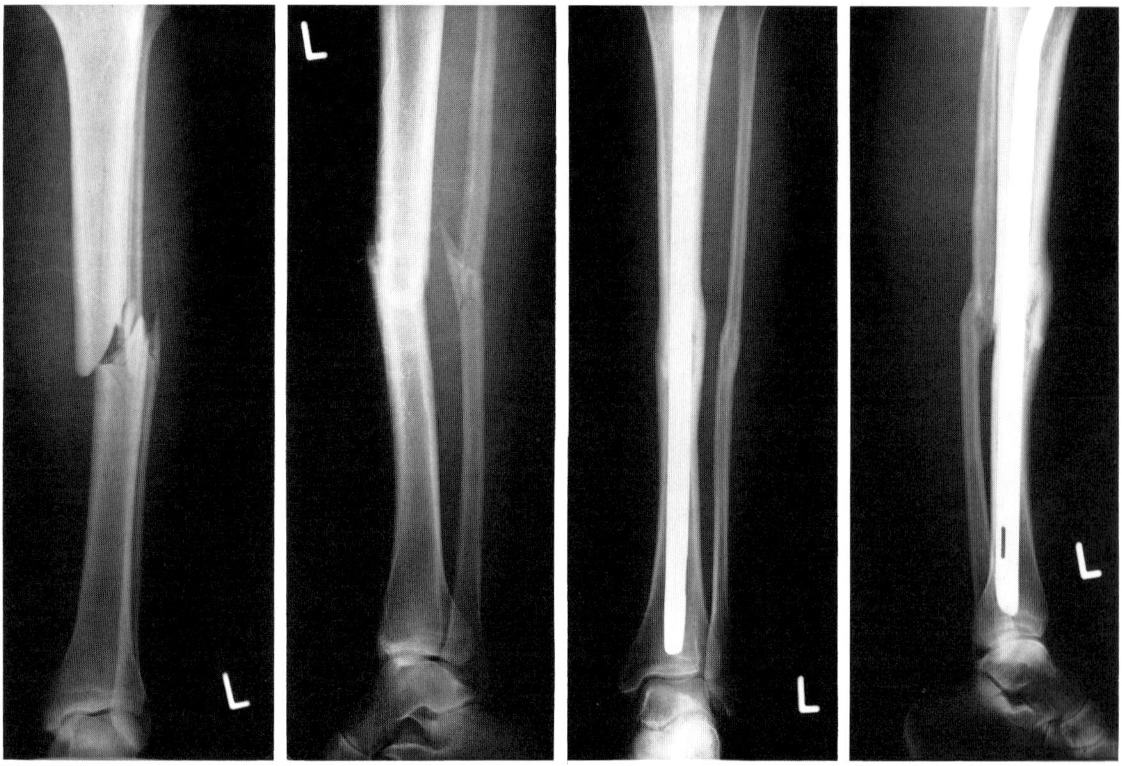

Fig. 13.1a b c d

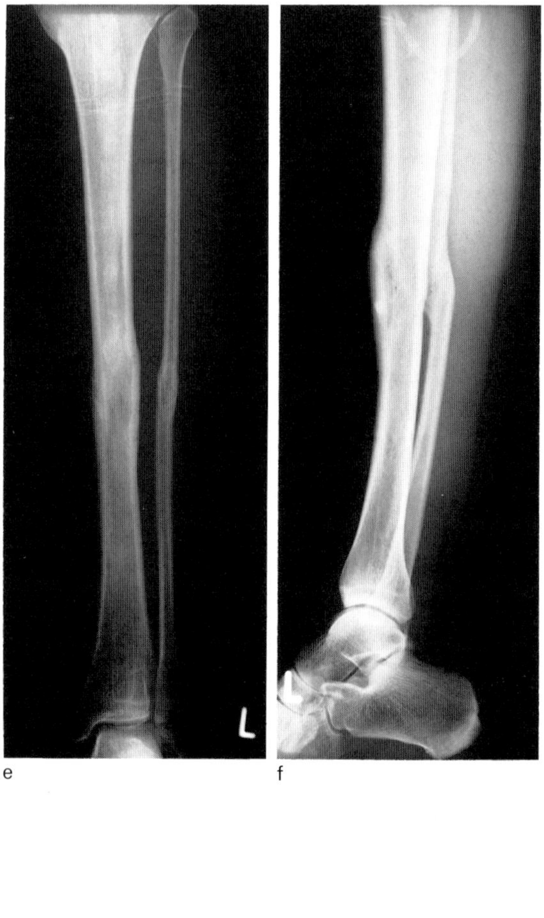

e f

Fig. 13.1a–f. a and b) Fracture of the lower leg in the middle of the tibia and fibula by direct trauma (bumper injury). Fracture with formation of a butterfly fragment in the dorsolateral region. The fibula shows a fracture at exactly the same level also with a third fragment.
c and d) Internal fixation by closed intramedullary nail (AFIP intramedullary nail). The x-ray shows the local condition 14 months after internal fixation. The fracture of the tibia is fully healed, with a moderate amount of callus. The fibula also shows excellent trabeculation through the fracture area, with marked callus formation. The anatomic condition, particularly the axis of both bones, appears excellent on both views.
e and f) Condition 2 years after the accident and internal fixation by closed intramedullary nail. The nail has been removed. The former fracture area is solidly healed, with a moderate amount of typical callus. (This shows the x-ray manifestations of the type of bone healing by secondary intention.)

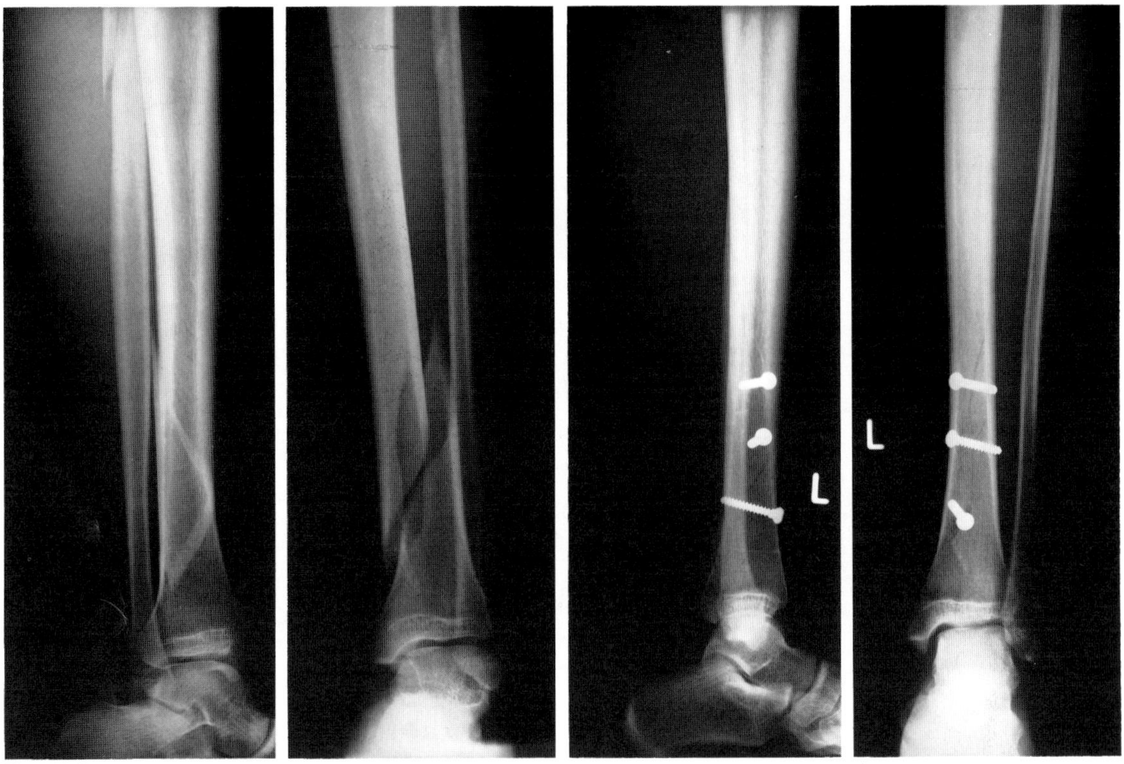

Fig. 13.2a b c d

Fig. 13.2a–d. Fracture of the left shank with spiral fractures involving the tibia in its middle to lower third and with a fracture surface larger than twice the width of the shaft. High spiral fracture of fibula; internal fixation using screws exclusively. Three cortical lag screws have been spacially arranged in such a fashion that they result in interfragmentary compression. Anatomically there is an ideal position with the fracture gap just visible. This fracture cannot yet be allowed to bear weight (4 weeks follow-up for control). The fracture of the fibula is left alone. Its position is good.

Fig. 13.3a and b. The large butterfly fragment was first connected by a cortical lag screw to the proximal and distal main fracture fragments (interfragmentary compression), with subsequent neutralization of the entire fracture area by insertion of a long plate. Bone healing by primary intention, note no radiologically visible formation of callus.

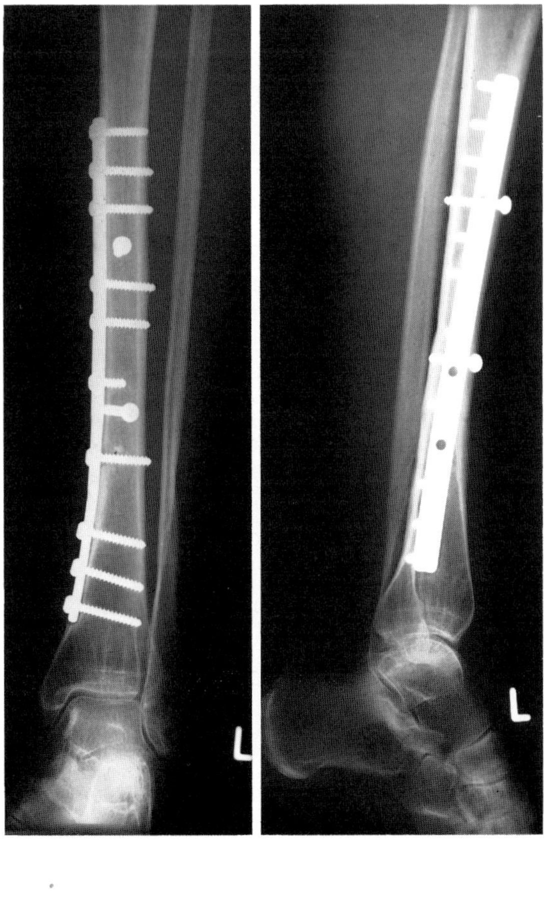

Fig. 13.3a b

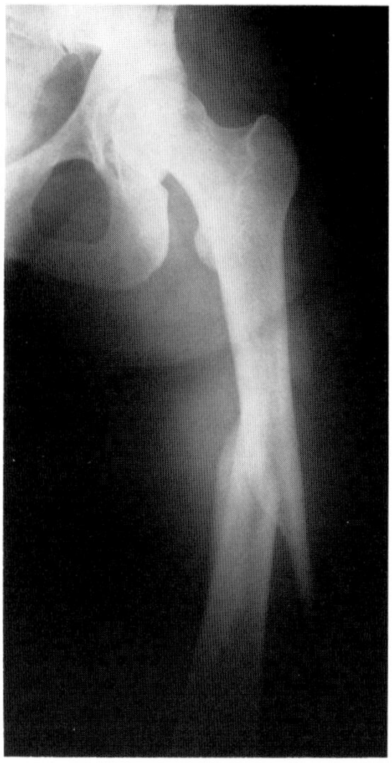

Fig. 13.4a

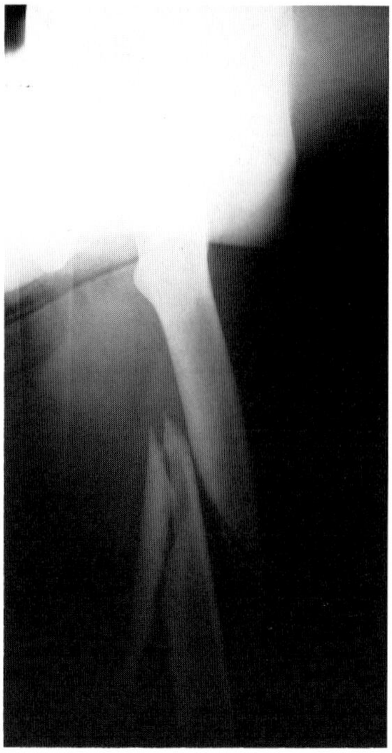

b

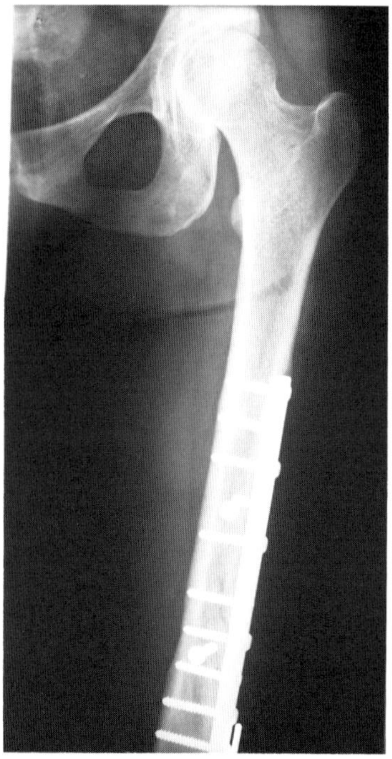

c

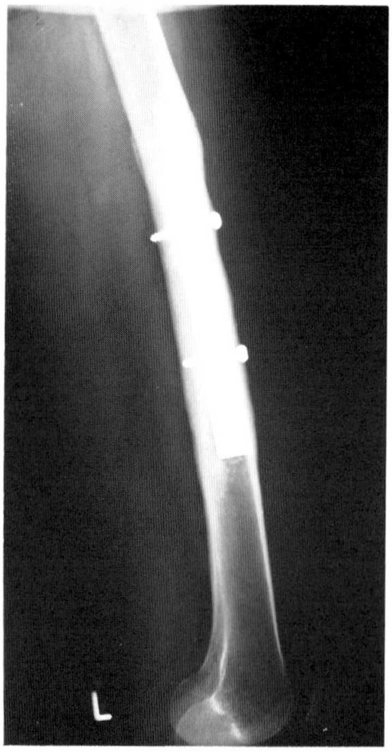

d

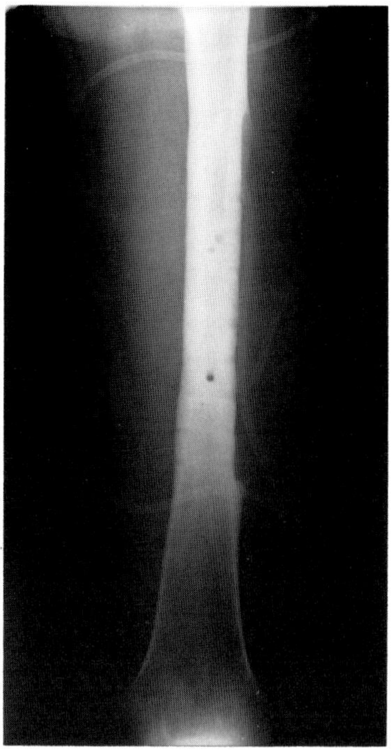

Fig. 13.4e

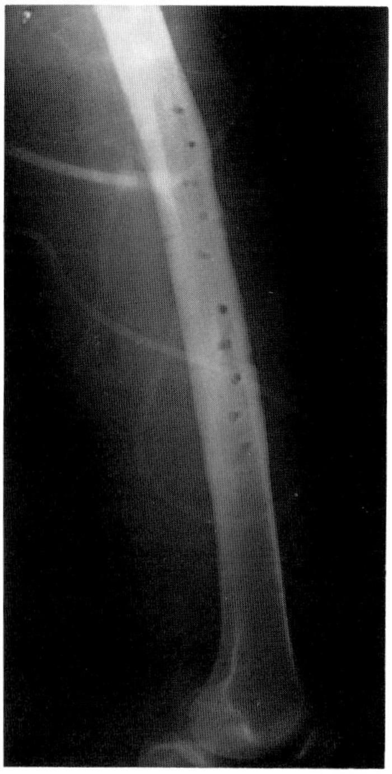

f

Fig. 13.4a–f. A 32-year-old woman with a ski fracture.
a and b) Fracture of the femoral shaft with a free butterfly fragment.
c and d) Internal fixation of the fracture of the femoral shaft applying interfragmentary compression by insertion of 2 cortical lag screws and a neutralization plate in the manner of a tension band plate placed in a dorsolateral position onto the femur. Compare Fig. 13.18, which shows the erector-set principle. Result: Bone healing by primary intention, without radiologically visible formation of callus.
e and f) Removal of metallic implants 26 months after internal fixation. Still recognizable are the different holes where the screws had been inserted in the midsection of the femoral shaft, as well as the old area where the plate was placed together with 2 Redon-drainage catheters.

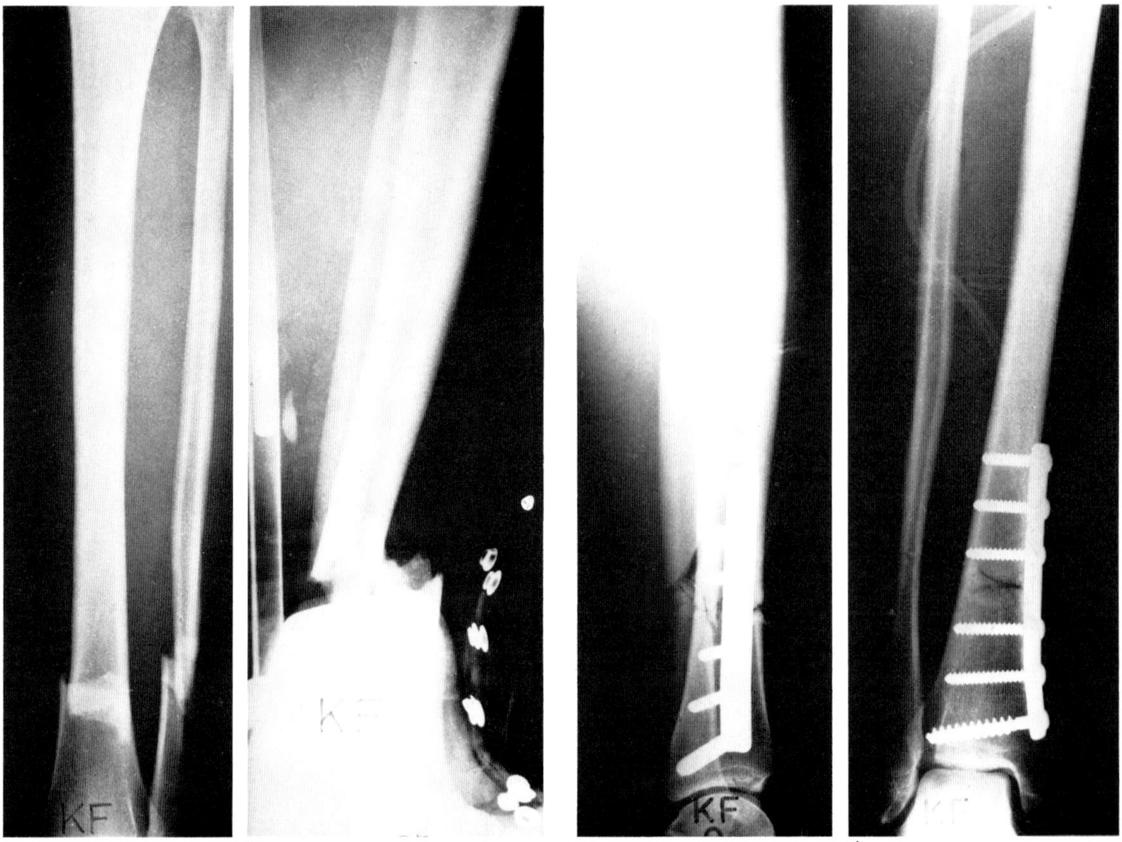

a b c d

Fig. 13.5a–j. A 20-year-old woman skier.
a and b) Boot-top fracture with injury to the Achilles tendon.

c and d) Internal fixation in the lower 3rd of the tibia by insertion of a 6-hole AFIP plate. The fracture line of the transverse fracture of the tibia is visible. The reposition of the surgically corrected fracture of the tibia as well as that of the fibula left to heal by itself seems to be excellent. On the a. p. view, there is an inserted Redon-drainage catheter (postoperative x-ray). Result: Weight-bearing internal fixation by plate of a fractured right tibia in its distal 3rd.

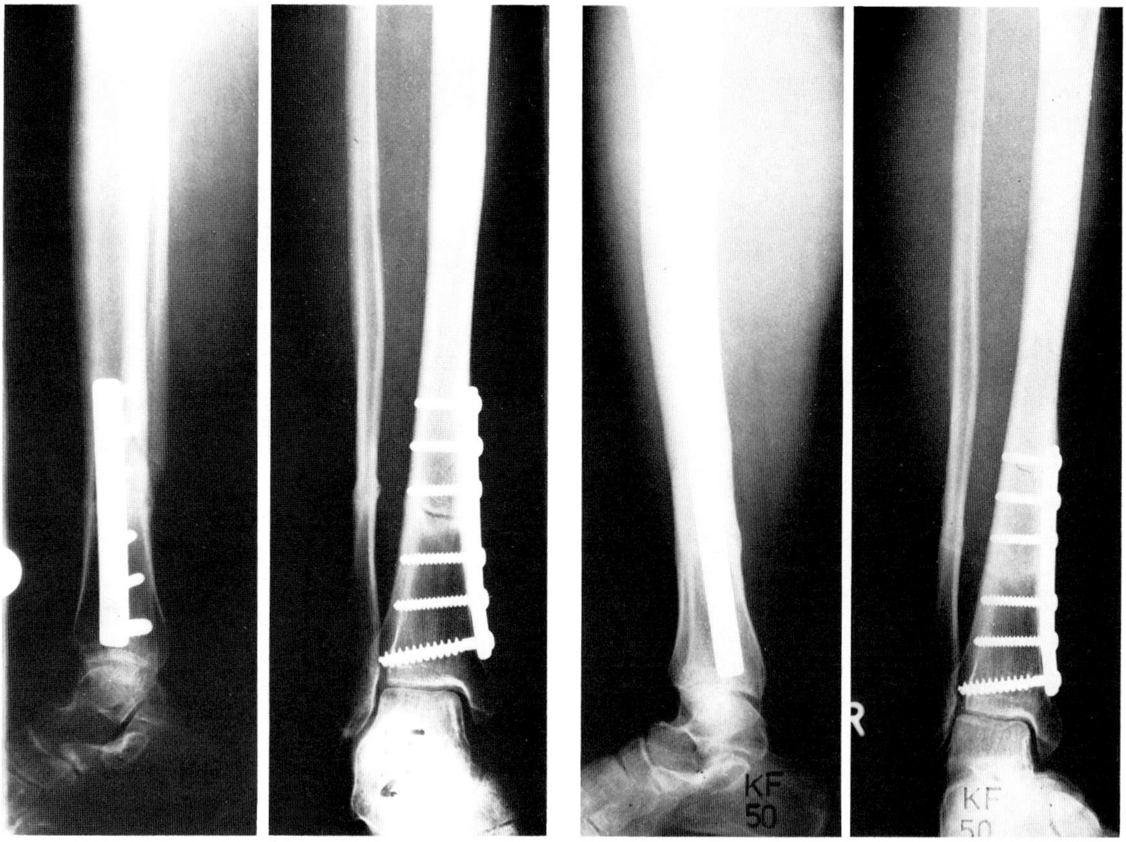

e f g h

e and f) 28 weeks after the accident, bone healing by primary intention (contact and gap healing). Medially and anteriorly, there is not as yet complete consolidation of the fracture. The internal fixation was considered ready for weight-bearing after 10 weeks.

g and h) After almost 1 year (50 weeks), the bony trabeculation across the fracture area is practically terminated as defined for bone healing by primary intention. There is no radiologically visible periosteal formation of callus. The material used for internal fixation is well tolerated in the bone. No recognizable areas of lysis around the screw threads.

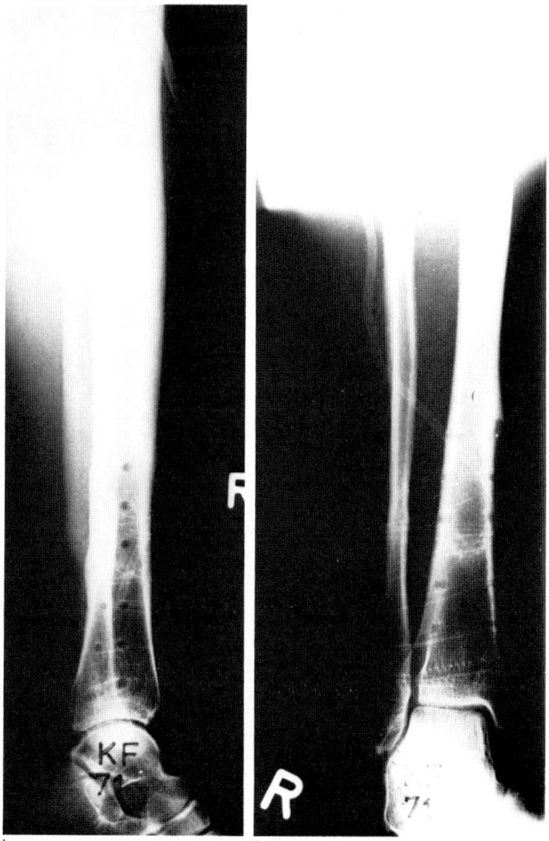

i j

i and j) Removal of the inserted metallic devices used for internal fixation 71 weeks after the original operation. An x-ray in the a.p. as well as the lateral view; bone healing by primary intention appears completely terminated without visible callus. The anatomic condition of the tibia as well as the fibula appears excellent. Some of the screw holes are still visible. From the presence of the Redon-drainage catheters, it can be concluded that this x-ray was obtained immediately after removal of the metallic implants.

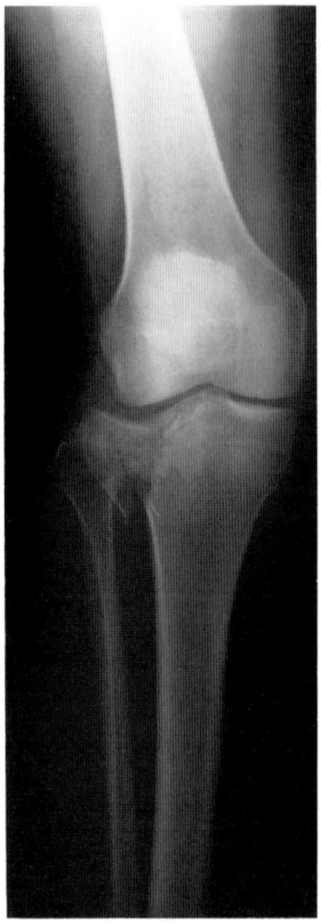

Fig. 13.6a

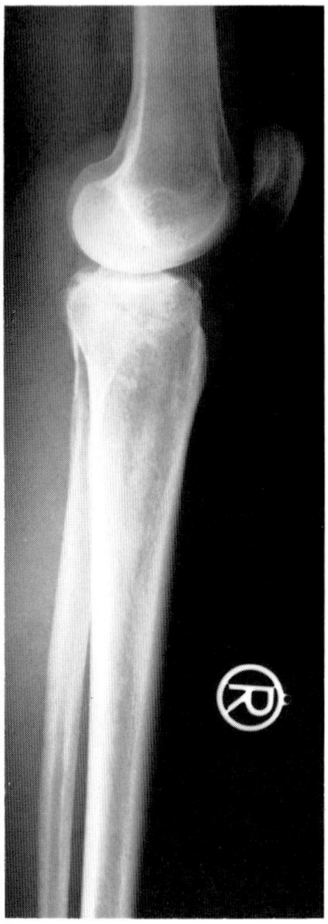

b

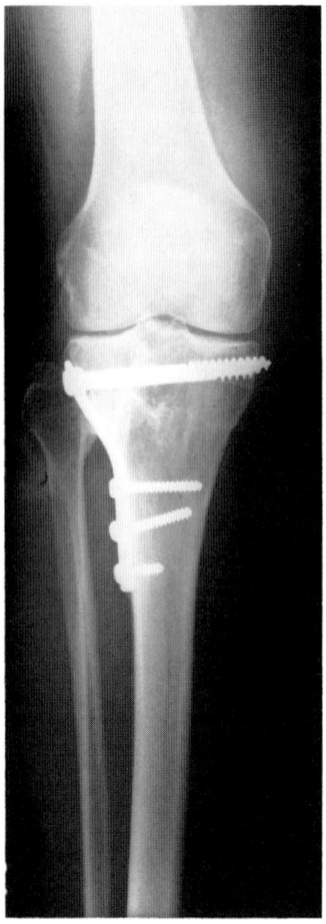

c

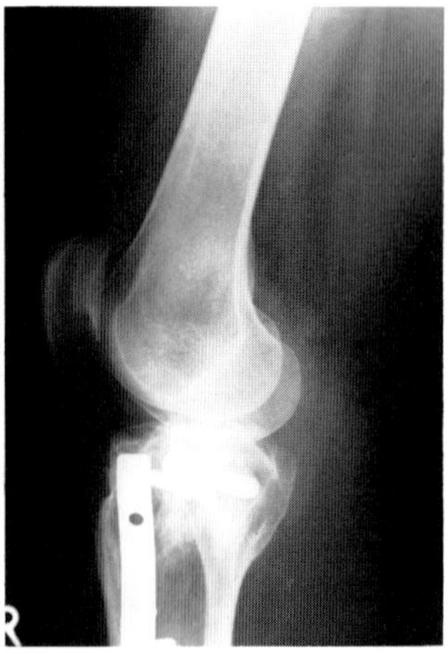

d

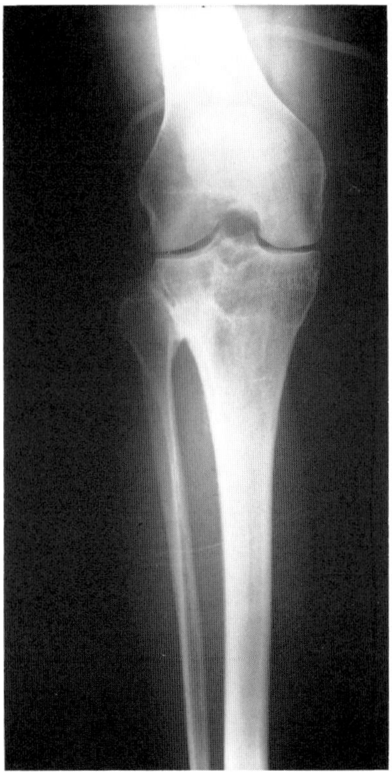

e

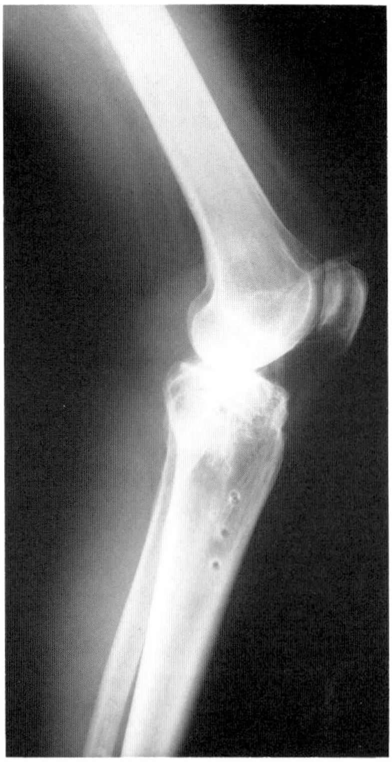

f

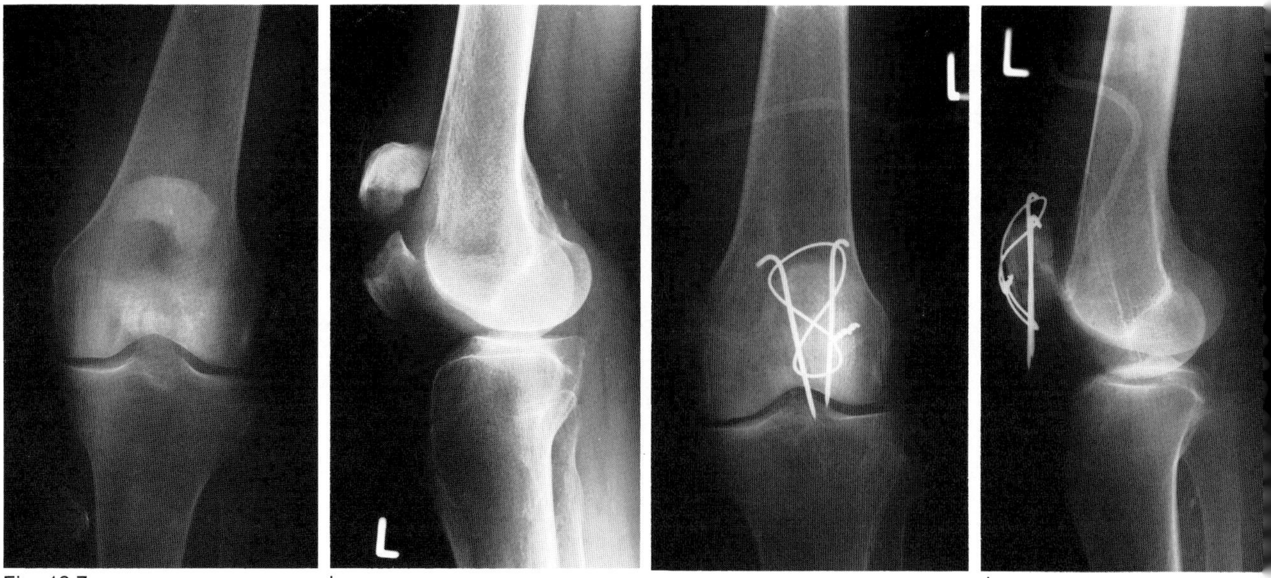

Fig. 13.7a b c d

◀ Fig. 13.6a–f. a and b) Compression fracture of the lateral condyle on the right with depression of the tibial plateau and marked dislocation laterally.
c and d) Internal fixation of the fracture of the tibial head. After elevation and repositioning of the lateral fracture fragment with a large area forming the joint, autologous spongiosa from the iliac crest is used to fill in the gap under the plateau. The good anatomic result is maintained by an exactly adapted plate (buttress plate). Additional spongiosa screws are applied dorsally.
e and f) Follow-up x-ray year after internal fixation, following removal of the metallic implants. The lateral compression fracture of the tibial plateau is solidly trabeculated throughout. Area of condensation in the region of the spongiosa transplant to plug a defect with loss of bone. Functionally normal joint.

▲
Fig. 13.7a–d. a and b) Transverse fracture of the patella on the left, with typical distraction of the proximal fragment.
c and d) Operative repair using a classic internal fixation of the tension type with the help of a ventrally inserted wire (smooth retropatellar articular surface). Thus the resulting forces of traction are neutralized particularly during active physiotherapy. Both cut wires will prevent a possible rotation of the fragments. The main feature of internal fixation of the patella by tension is that the tension wire must be located ventrally within the patella. It is not entirely necessary that it be inserted as a figure-8 loop wire. This type of internal fixation allows weight-bearing.

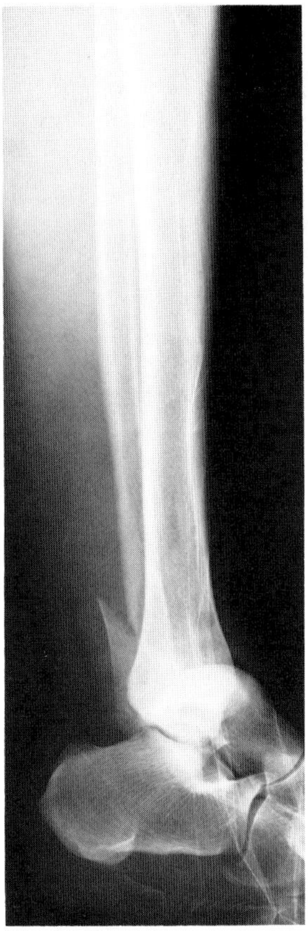

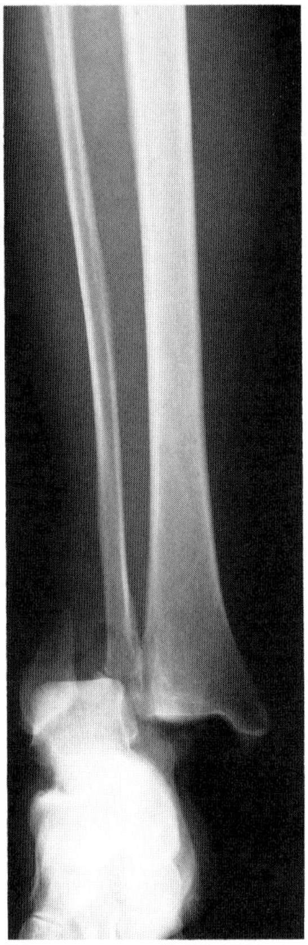

Fig. 13.8a b

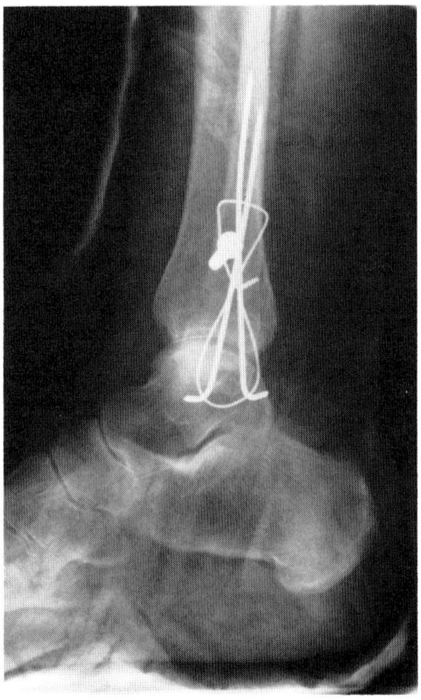

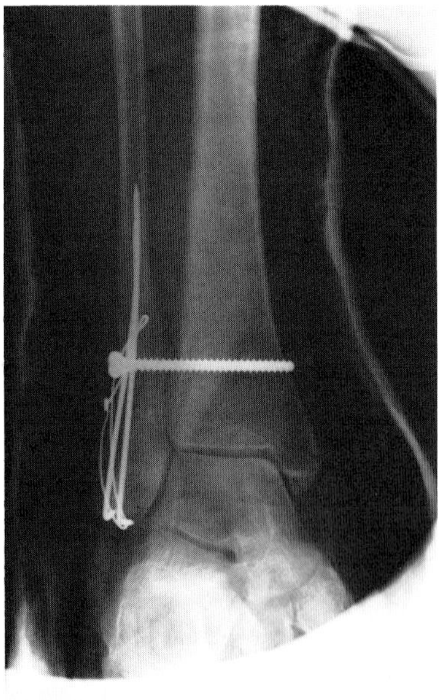

c d

Fig. 13.8a–h. a and b) Open fracture luxation of the ankle on the right with marked lateral position of the talus. Oblique fracture of the distal fibula at the level of the syndesmosis. Rupture of the internal ligament; air collection between both fragments of the fibula on the a. p. view.

c and d) X-rays after surgical management. There is good anatomic reconstruction of the ankle joint on both views. Stabilization of the lateral ankle using a typical tension fixation by inserting two cut wires and a figure-8 loop of wire. In addition, insertion of a suprasyndesmal set screw (to maintain the syndesmosis). U-splint to avoid the possibility of a drop foot.

e and f) Follow-up after 8 weeks. The anatomically good position of the ankle joint and the fibula is maintained without any change and consolidated in the absence of visible callus. The set screw has been removed in the meantime (this is usually done after 6 weeks, before weight-bearing). Tension fixation of the fibula remains unchanged. The metal implants have normally no reaction in the bone.

g and h) Final follow-up x-ray after complete removal of all metal parts 12 months after the accident and internal fixation. The fracture of the fibula has healed in good position. Normal joint.

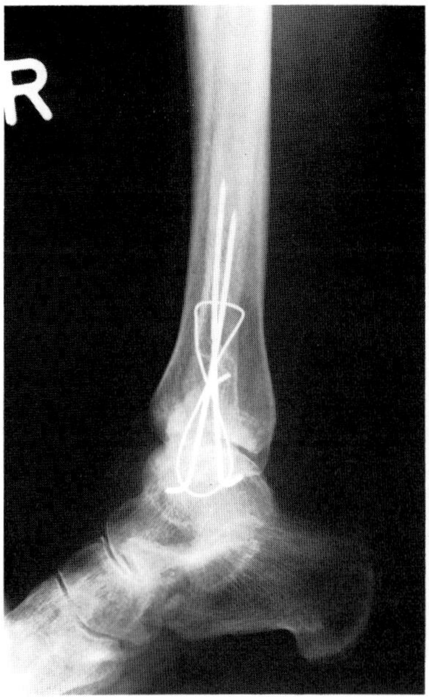

Fig. 13.8e

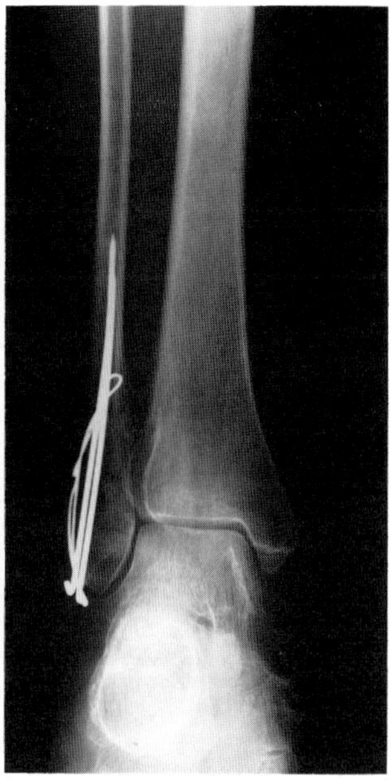

f

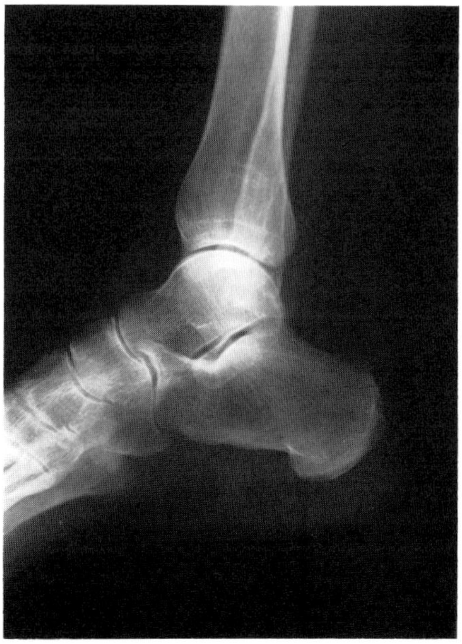

g

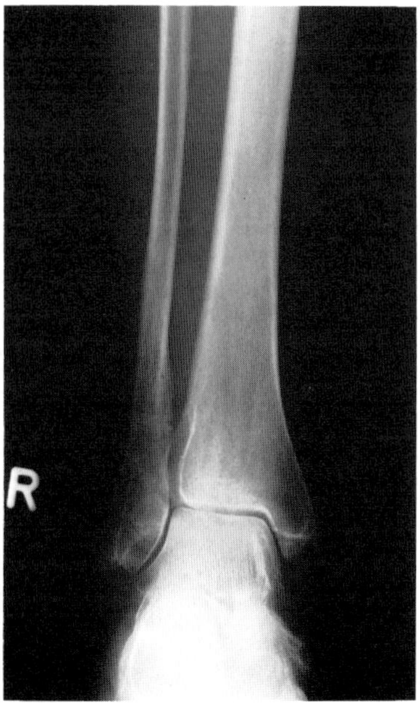

h

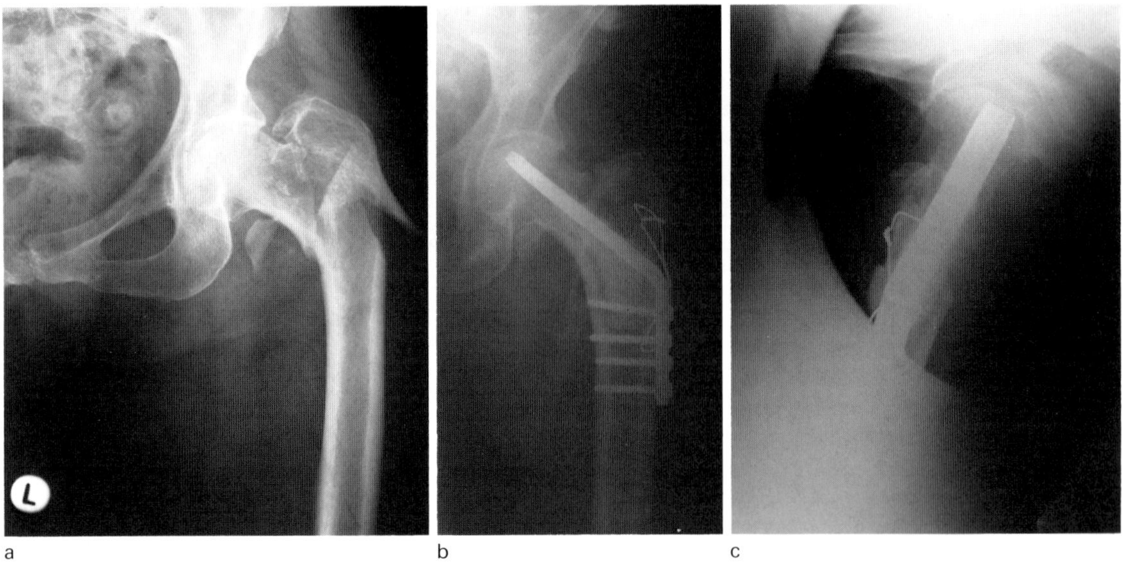

Fig. 13.9a-c. An 88-year-old patient.
a) Peritrochanteric comminuted fracture with avulsion of the minor trochanter and dislocation of the peripheral fracture fragments cranially.
b and c) Combined fixation using a 130-degree angle plate with a 4-hole shaft. The defect, caused by compression of the spongiosa medially and dorsally, has been filled with bone cement (methacrylate). A contrast agent has been added to the bone cement. The major trochanter has been fixed after insertion of a tension wire. With this combined fixation (bone cement and metallic implants), it is possible in many instances to bring about weight-bearing fixation. This is a particularly useful method in the handling of pathologic fractures.

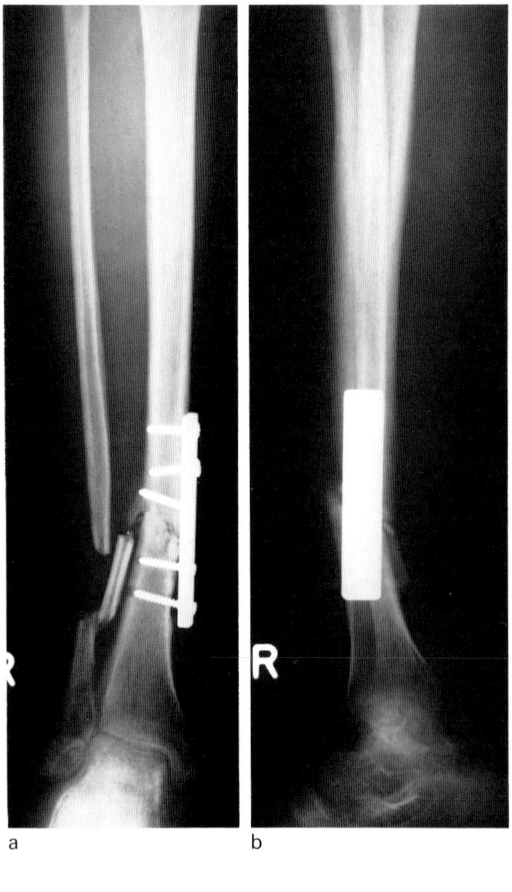

Fig. 13.10a and b. Nonhealing distal shank fracture on the right. Internal fixation with a short and broad plate. Abnormal position with valgus and antecurvation. Formation of an irritation callus on the lateral side of the tibia. Zone of lysis around the two lowermost screws indicates unstable internal fixation. Comment: One should not use wide internal fixation plates when dealing with fractures of the shank.

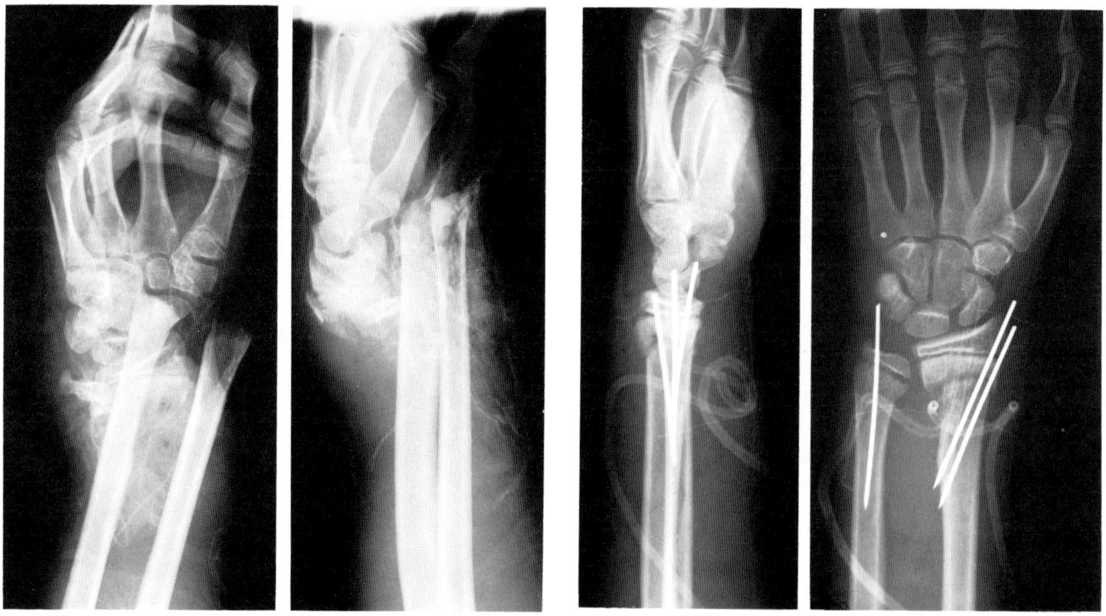

Fig. 13.11a b c d

Fig. 13.11a–d. A 12-year-old boy.
a and b) Open distal fracture of the radius and ulna.
c and d) Immediate internal fixation with revision of the wound, vessels, nerves and tendons. The method used here is a reduction fixation always requiring, in addition, a plaster cast.

Primary (Direct) Healing of Fractures

In all probability, this term was coined by Lane (1914) when he proposed to refer to bone healing by primary intention under those circumstances when by x-ray examination there is no visible formation of callus (Willenegger et al., 1971). Danis (1949) has confirmed this phenomenon during stable internal fixation of the forearm. He has concluded that the process of reparation must take place primarily within the cortical bone ("soudure autogène"). It must, however, be stressed that basically the terms healing by "primary intention" and "secondary intention" do not have any relationship with the healing processes of the skin and underlying structures; they are only borrowed. They simply indicate that a fracture can heal with, as well as without, a solid "bony scar."

The breakthrough in clarification of the histologic and morphologic events during primary bone healing results from the studies of Schenk and Willenegger (1963) in osteotomy of the radius of the dog. They could demonstrate that in a perfectly adapted fracture, with stable fixation after insertion of a compression plate, there is, within the fracture line immediately below the plate, fracture healing occurring within the osteons themselves, and that there is no local reaction such as filling in of a fissure (Figs. 13.12 and 13.13). Within the cortical region opposite the inserted plate, however, there is usually a slight gap with a certain distance between both fracture fragments. Correspondingly, there is also a marked difference in the histologic appearance of this region. On the one hand, one can see direct contact healing and, on the other, gap healing. The common basis for both of these possibilities of primary healing of bone is an absolute mechanical stability.

Contact healing (Fig. 13.14) is a process that occurs in a single phase. There is no resorption at the edges of the fragments at the fracture line, so perfect contact is maintained. By this type of adaptation, the possibility of blood vessels and tissue elements entering the fracture line is avoided. Because of the longitudinally regenerating osteons, there is an interlacing of the fracture fragments. The most significant event in this type of healing is the regenerating osteon with its typical structure (compare with Fig. 13.14c). At the tip of such a "cutter head", there is always an osteoclast. From its activity results a channel corresponding to the future diameter of the osteon (roughly 150 μ). The "cutter head" is followed by a rich blastema, with the decisive development of a blood vessel as well as the early phase of osteoblasts and the osteoid seams along the walls. They must be understood to result from the activity of osteoblasts.

Using tetracycline marking, Schenk (1972) was able to document that the speed for the daily longitudinal advance is roughly 0.1 mm.

Gap healing (Fig. 13.15) is a process that occurs in two phases. An initial phase is the plugging of the remaining gap with primary bone formation at absolute mechanical rest. From the periosteum and from the marrow cavity, sometimes also from Havers' channels, vessels grow into the gap. They are very delicate and are accompanied by perivascular cells differentiating along the fracture fragments into osteoblasts. It must be emphasized that the bone formed within the gap is not produced by the usual chain of events, namely, preformed cartilage with connective tissue, but that this is primary bony plugging of the gap. In a second phase, there is the longitudinal organization of the fracture by the osteons' growth in either direction from one fragment to the other. Thus results a very intimate interdigitation of both fracture fragments.

In a fracture treated by insertion of screws or internal fixation by plates, both of these types of primary bone healing will occur side by side. The final result and the stability of such primary bone healing are dependent on how many osteons can regenerate in a given amount of time. Schenk (1972) has determined, by tetracycline marking of the dog radius, that after 8 weeks over 60 per cent of the osteons will have regenerated as part of the healing process. This would correspond to a stability of roughly two-thirds of the initial value.

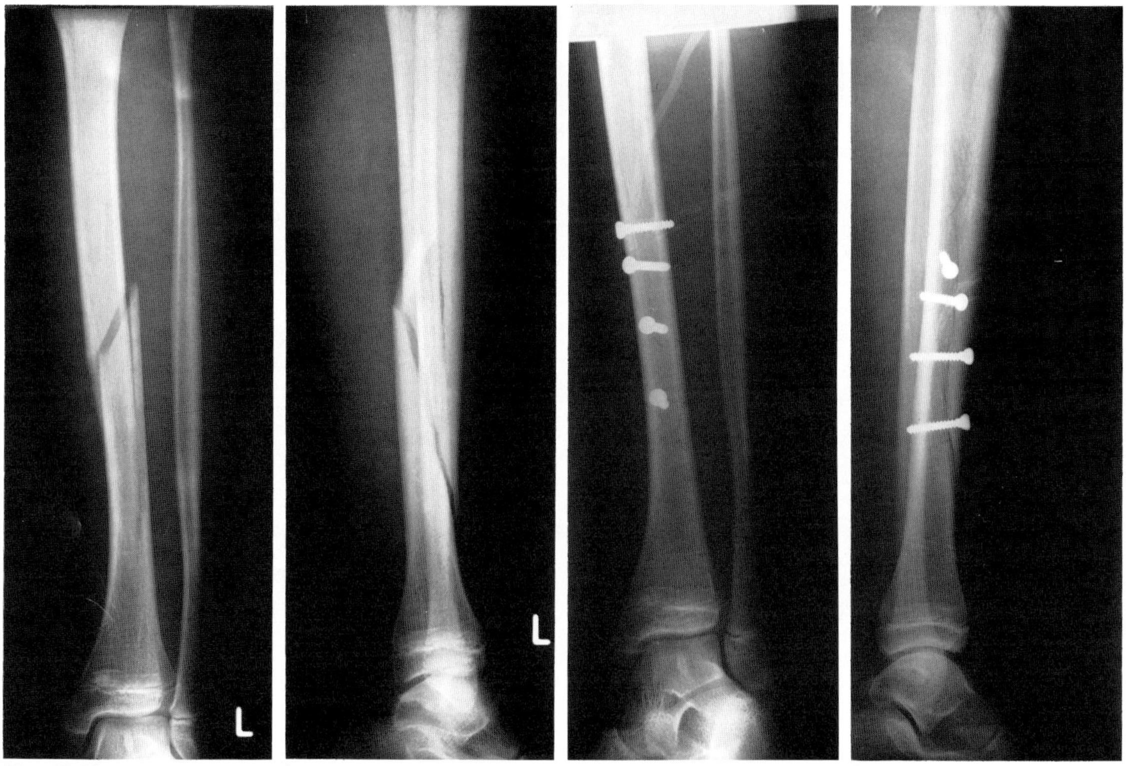

Fig. 13.12a b c d

Fig. 13.12a–h. A 15-year-old patient.
a and b) Isolated spiral fracture of the tibia.
c and d) Internal fixation by insertion of 4 cortical lag screws corresponding, in their spacially arranged insertion, to the fracture line. Result: anatomically exact reposition and weight-bearing fixation. In the upper area, there is a Redon drain. The a. p. view, but especially the lateral film taken on the day of surgical intervention, still reveals a thin fracture line.
e and f) Four months later, it is impossible to recognize the fracture line even on the lateral view. There is no visible callus. The structure of the entire former fracture is homogeneous. There has been weight-bearing of this extremity for ten weeks. Result: Primary fracture healing in a simple internal fixation using screws for an isolated spiral fracture of the left tibia.

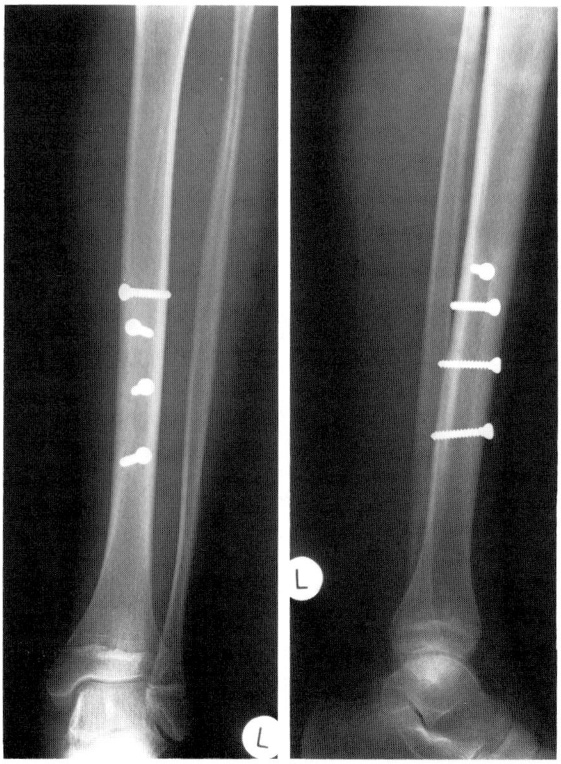

e f

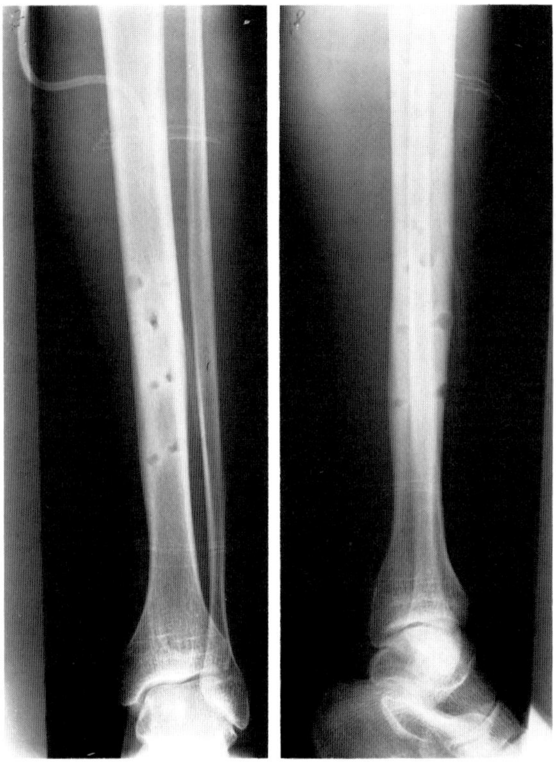

Fig. 13.12g h

g and h) Follow-up x-ray after removal of screws (left tibia) 15 months after the accident and internal fixation. The screw holes and channels are visible. Redon drainage since this is a case of mainly gap healing (compare with postoperative x-ray); this offers a good explanation for the minor degree of thickening of the cortical bone in the area of the former fracture.

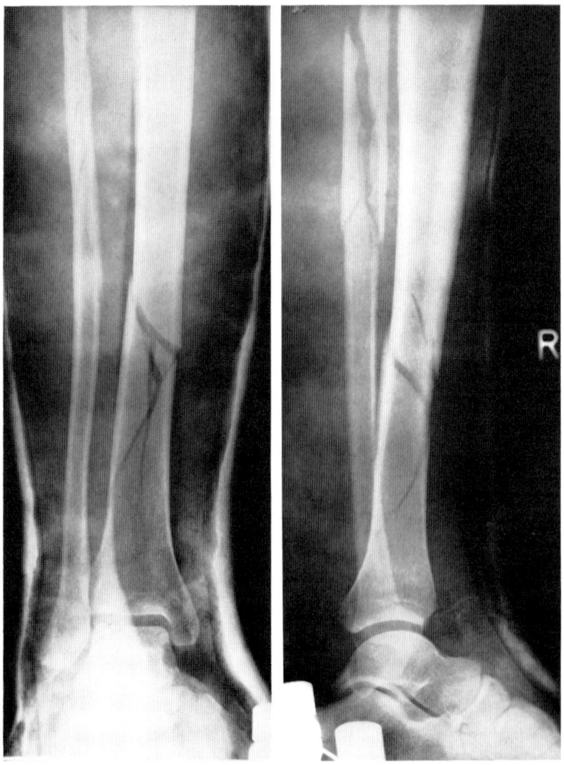

Fig. 13.13a b

Fig. 13.13a–j. a and b) Shank fracture on the right, with a large free butterfly fragment of the tibia in its transition from the middle to the lower 3rd. Fracture of the fibula is also of the spiral type, with a free 3rd fragment in its transition from the middle to the proximal 3rd. In a plaster cast there is reasonably good maintenance of axis on both views. There is an inserted extension wire through the calcaneus.
c and d) Internal fixation with 2 cortical lag screws, with interfragmentary compression and neutralization plate medially onto the tibia and a slight degree of axial tension. This is the additional hole created above the plate and is explained by the insertion of the tension apparatus. The fracture is anatomically adapted, with a minimal strip effect visible on an oblique view. This fracture extends all the way into the ankle joint close to the internal malleolus. The fracture of the fibula is left alone. Comment: It is not necessary to treat the fibula with such a fracture.
e and f) 8 weeks after internal fixation of the tibia, there is still a fracture line on the a. p. view. There is, however, no increase of this finding in this area. There is no demonstration of a lytic zone around the threads of the screws indicative of loosening or instability. All implants are in unchanged good position. No visible periosteal callus formation. Mild degree of atrophy of bone, especially ot the distal part of the fracture. Only partial weight-bearing of the extremity (about 20 kg) has been permitted.
g and h) 16 weeks after internal fixation of the tibia by interfragmentary compression and neutralization plate. In comparison with the aspect 8 weeks previously, there is significant disappearance of the fracture line (roughly in the middle of the film) Only in the area of the minimal step effect at the upper tip of the butterfly fragment is there a minimal periosteal callus. No zones of lysis. Reduction in the degree of skeletal atrophy. The extremity is now exposed to full weight-bearing.
i and j) 34 weeks after internal fixation of this fracture of the tibia, there is complete consolidation. Primary healing of bone after interfragmentary compression with 2 cortical lag screws and neutralization plate medially applied to the tibia. There is no recognizable fracture line or gap. Between the 2nd and 3rd screws, there is a minimal periosteal reaction as the result of a step effect. There is no reaction to the implanted metal parts within the bone. No changes in position. The fracture of the fibula has healed. Minimal atrophy of bony parts. Results: Primary bone healing of a fracture of the tibia on the right after internal fixation by interfragmentary compression and insertion of a neutralization plate. complete bony healing of the fibula in good position without foreshortening.

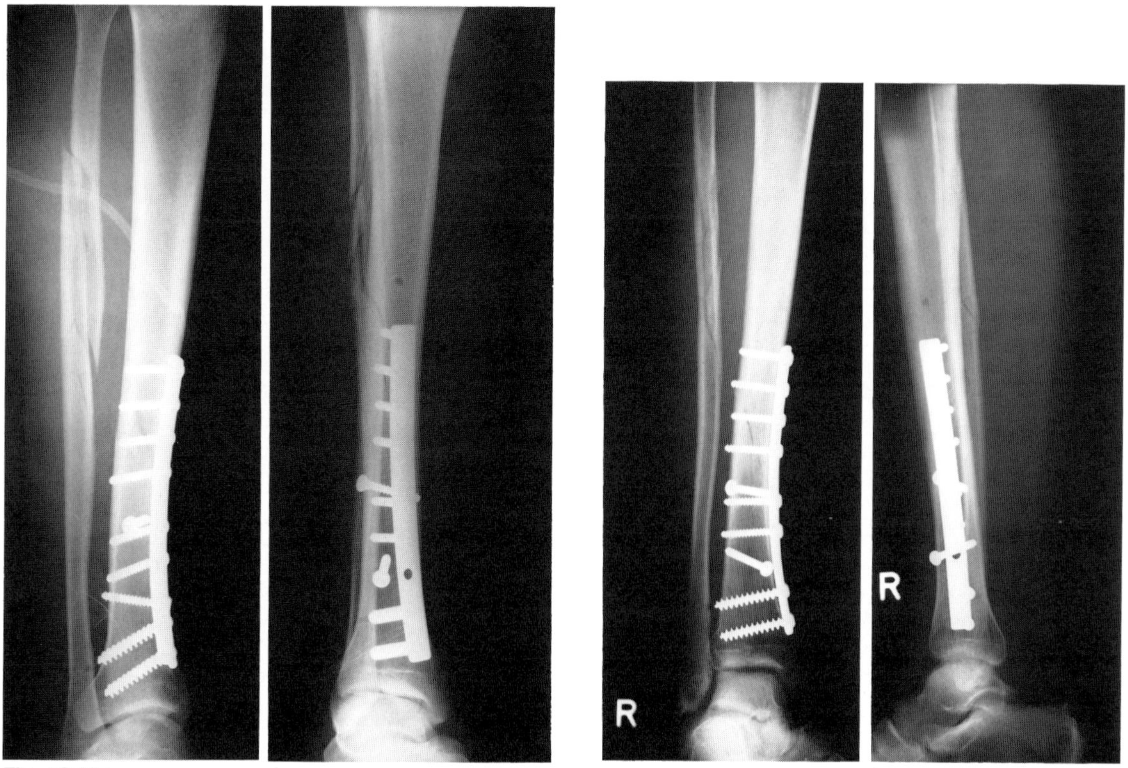

Fig. 13.13c d e f

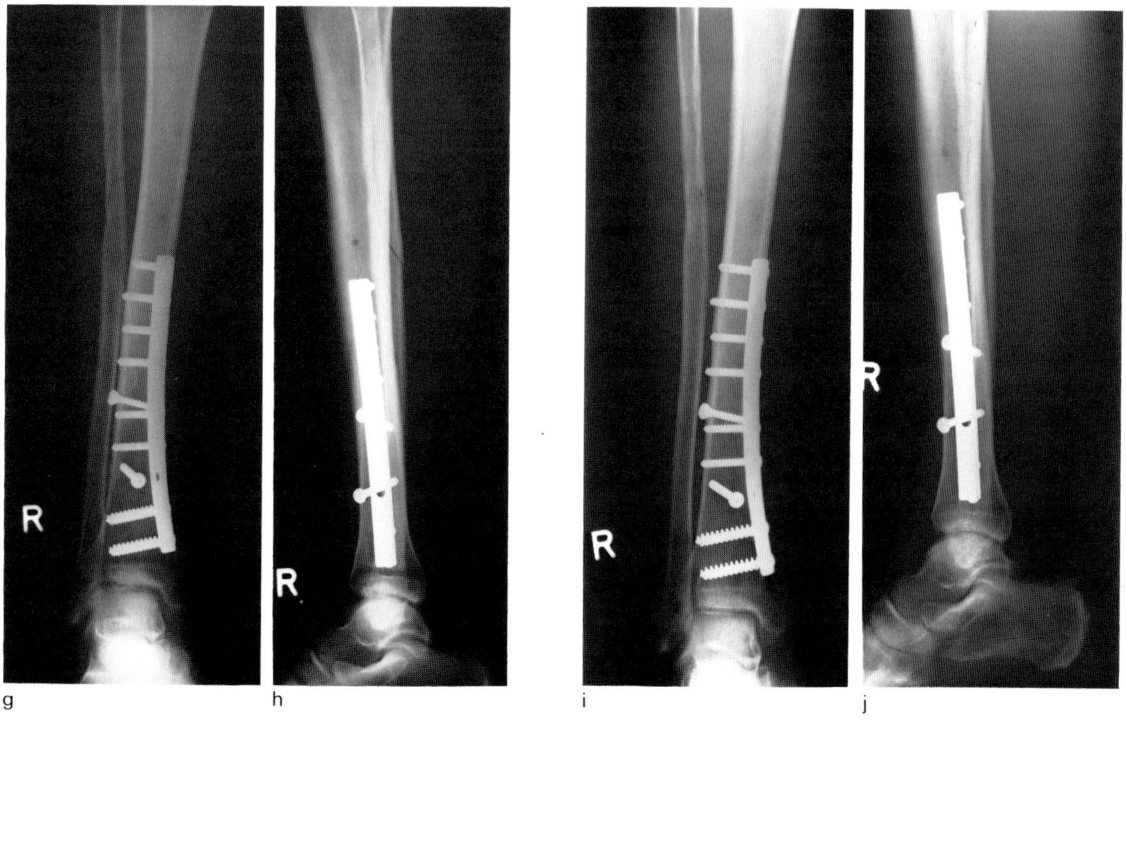

g h i j

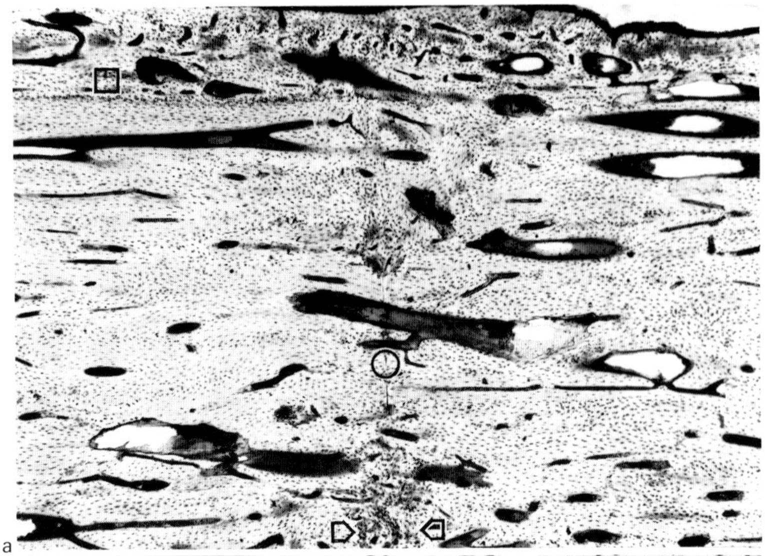
a

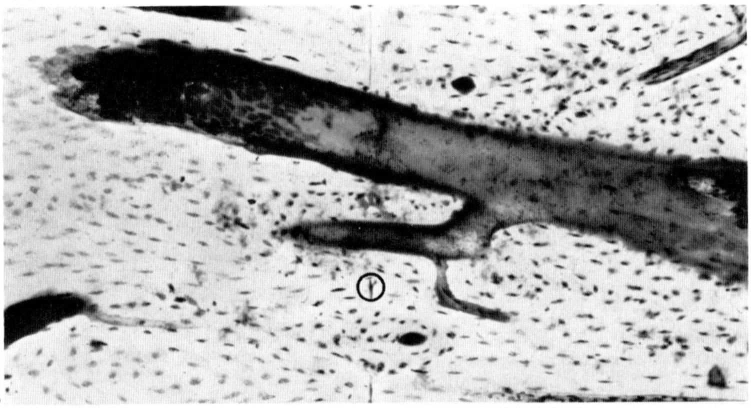
b

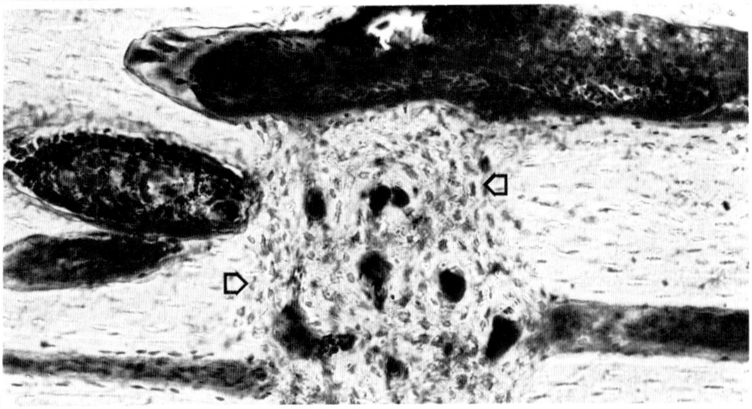
c

Fig. 13.14a–c. Primary healing of an osteotomy in a dog under stable conditions.
a) External view of the area of osteotomy 10 weeks after intervention. The circle marks the region with perfect adaptation, leading to direct intimate contact between both fracture ends. At the base of this figure, there remains a slightly gapping area filled b a primary plug of bone *(between arrows).* The *square* at the upper margin on the left designates the original surface of the diaphysis. Within this area, there has been a periosteal reaction.
b) Detailed view of the area marked by a *circle* (contact healing); the intimate line of connection between the two fragments has been crossed by a regenerating osteon branching immediately adjacent to the osteotomy.
c) Detailed view of gap healing 6 weeks after osteotomy of the radius of the dog; the *arrows* point to the original extent of the osteotomy gap which has healed, with primary bony regeneration. At its upper margin, this figure shows a regenerating osteon. Its formation has been initiated by a resorption channel cut by osteoblasts. Immediately thereafter, it is filled by newly formed bony lamellae (nondecalcified longitudinal section, fuchsin staining). (From H. Willenegger, S. M. Perren and R. Schenk: Chirurg *42:* 241, 1971.)

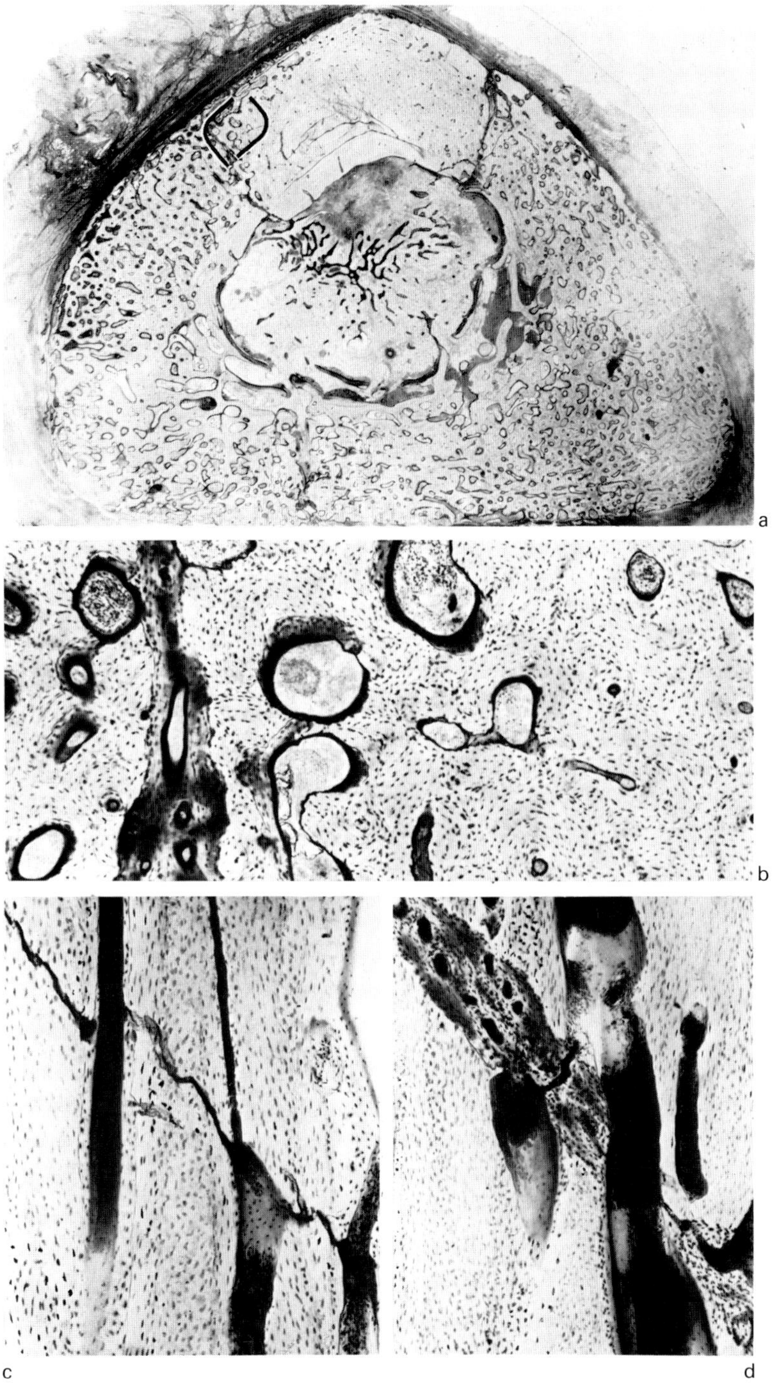

Fig. 13.15a–d. Primary fracture healing in man. The material for this investigation is from a 17-year-old girl after stable fixation of a fracture of the tibia. 12 weeks after her accident, this patient succumbed to a cerebral hemorrhage.
a) Survey view of a cross-section of the tibia; the anterior butterfly fragment is revitalized only at its fracture edges. In the other parts of the compact bone, there is dramatically increased regeneration involving more than two-thirds of all osteons.
b) The marked area in Figure a shows the image of gap healing under stronger magnification. The bony reparative process has proceeded to involve the devitalized butterfly fragment.
c) Contact healing with 3 regenerating osteons in a portion of the fracture that was perfectly congruent.
d) Longitudinal friction throughout a mildly gapping fracture area; healing in the manner of gap healing in two phases. The gap has already been filled by the primarily formed bony tissue and, in one place, it is already crossed by one single regenerating osteon (nondecalcified longitudinal section, fuchsin staining). (From H. Willenegger, S. M. Perren and R. Schenk: Chirurg *42:* 241, 1971.)

Secondary (Indirect) Healing of Bone

Fracture healing with radiologically visible formation of callus can also be called secondary healing of bone. This type of repair is found under conditions of conservative or functional management but also in several surgical methods of fracture treatment. Under the latter condition, it can be seen after inframedullary nailing and adaptation fixation. The formation of callus will begin in regions far from the fracture line and originate from parosteal tissues (Fig. 13.16). Among parosteal tissues, we should consider the periosteum, the tissues of the marrow cavity and the contents of the Haversian canals. There is callus formation in the periosteal area; in the marrow cavity between both fracture fragments, however, there is formation of connective tissue and fibrocartilage. The enormously increased inner restructuring of the compact bone corresponds to a revitalization so that healing is thus significantly influenced. New formation of bone follows the preformed fibrocartilaginous tissue. This can be compared, to a large degree, to the condition in the embryo because of its analogy to desmal ossification. Comparable to a matrix, there is development and local activity of osteoblasts resulting from an advance of blood vessels between the connective fibrous tissues. Thus osteoid can be formed which will eventually calcify (Schenk, 1972).

Pauwels (1940) had made an earlier attempt to interpret these phenomena as a biomechanical concept. A fracture with unstable fixation is consequently exposed to minimal movements, so that the blastema which has to develop from osteogenic tissue is constantly exposed to mechanical forces. The result is that formation of bone under these circumstances can only occur at a certain distance from this zone of unrest. The mechanical stress further results, on the side of traction in the formation of connective tissue and, on the side of pressure, of cartilage. Only slowly will there be a transformation of these intermediary tissues into bony material. Biomechanical factors and physical influences are not limited to healing of bone during conservative management but are equally important after surgical intervention. Perren et al. (1969), with the help of a specially developed measuring plate, demonstrated that in internal fixation with a compression plate, the initially induced interfragmentary compression remains effective over many months and does not revert to zero by a so-called pressure necrosis. A loss of pressure of about 10 per cent in the first week is explained on the basis of the viscoelastic properties of bone. Subsequent and slowly occurring reduction in pressure is largely the result of transformation of the osteon structure, which takes place by simultaneous and mostly axial resorption and regeneration of these units. Mechanical rest maintained at the exact location of the fracture is of decisive significance in this respect. This is the main factor favoring early vascularization (Rhinelander, 1965; Ganz and Cole, 1970). In experiments Rhinelander and later also Ganz et al. were able to show that the main narrow artery will resume its original size after complete cross-sectional osteotomy and subsequent stable internal fixation by plate, and that as early as 8 to 14 days afterward it fully bridges the site of the osteotomy.

Interfragmentary pressure resulting from lag screws or from a pressure plate does not by itself form a stimulus for the formation of new bone, it only increases stability (Mueller, 1971). However, the application of the pressure principle by the creation of axial compression using a tension plate device or a dynamic compression plate (DCP) (Allgöwer et al., 1969), on the creation of interfragmentary pressures using the principle of the lag screw, will not guarantee the required stability. Particularly in long bones, the adaptation achieved will decide the result, whether the internal fixation is stable or unstable for the duration of healing (Fig. 13.17). A typical example is fracture of the proximal femur with a medial defect (missing medial buttress). Here the laterally placed tension band plate adjacent to the shaft will be permanently subject to bending forces in the direction of varisation (Fig. 13.18). Finally, a fracture must result (Schuster, 1972). In the majority of cases, the reason for an implant fracture has to be found in poor or incomplete adaptation and in overlooking some critical biomechanical defect rather than in a defective implant.

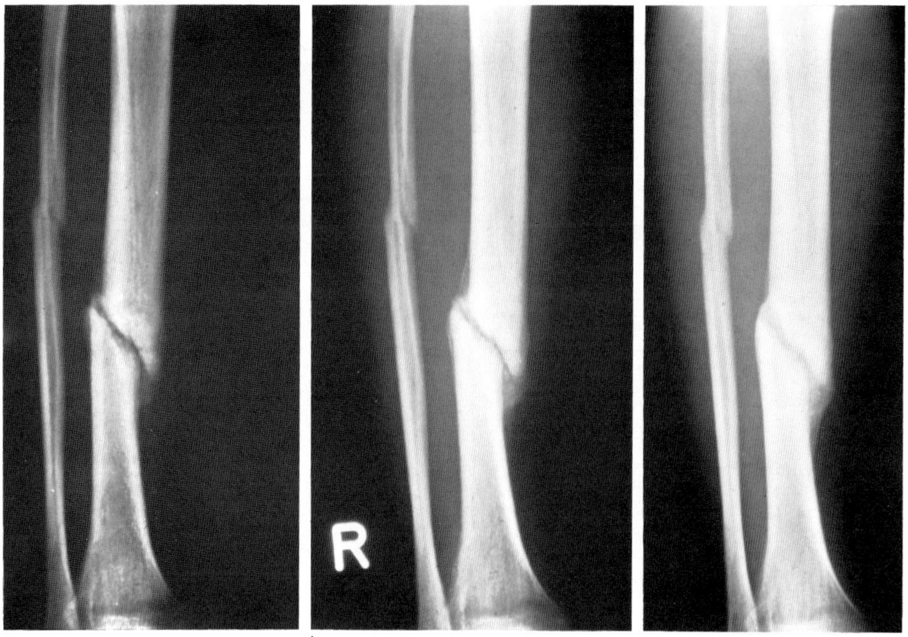

a b c

Fig. 13.16a–c. Healing of a fracture, with conservative management of a right shank fracture.
a) After 6 weeks, there is a fine callus with indistinct borders.
b) 4 weeks later, this is much denser and the fracture line appears vague; this is because healing occurs by periosteal as well as endosteal formation of callus and is visible on both planes.
c) An additional 4 weeks later, there is good consolidation of the fracture for weight-bearing. The structure of the periosteal callus can be clearly recognized; the area of the fracture has become denser. There is minimal varisation. Skeletal atrophy has already improved when compared with the previous examination.

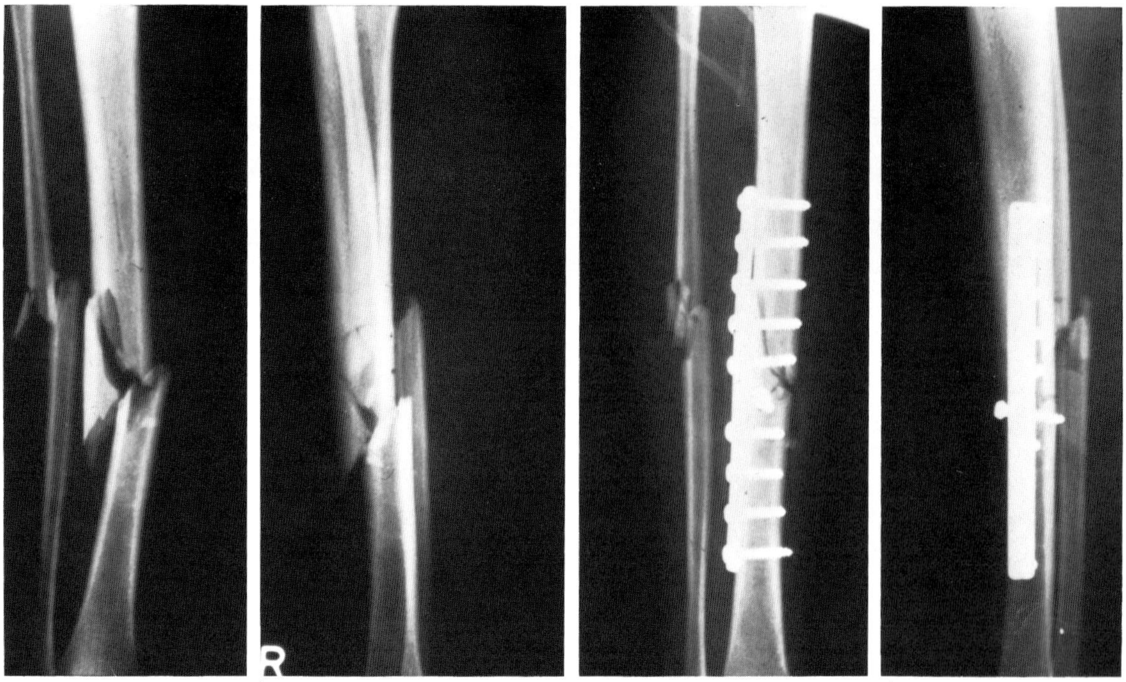

Fig. 13.17a b c d

Fig. 13.17a–j. a and b) Open fracture of the right shank in the middle, with a lateral butterfly fragment of the tibia. Fracture of the fibula at the same level.
c and d) Internal fixation by a lateral 9-hole plate. The butterfly fragment is connected by a solitary cortical lag screw to the distal main fracture fragment. Critical comment: No full anatomic adaptation and, therefore, a lack of bony support medially toward the plate. In addition to this, there is overexertion of the plate by bending forces so that a fatigue fracture of the implant must be feared and anticipated.

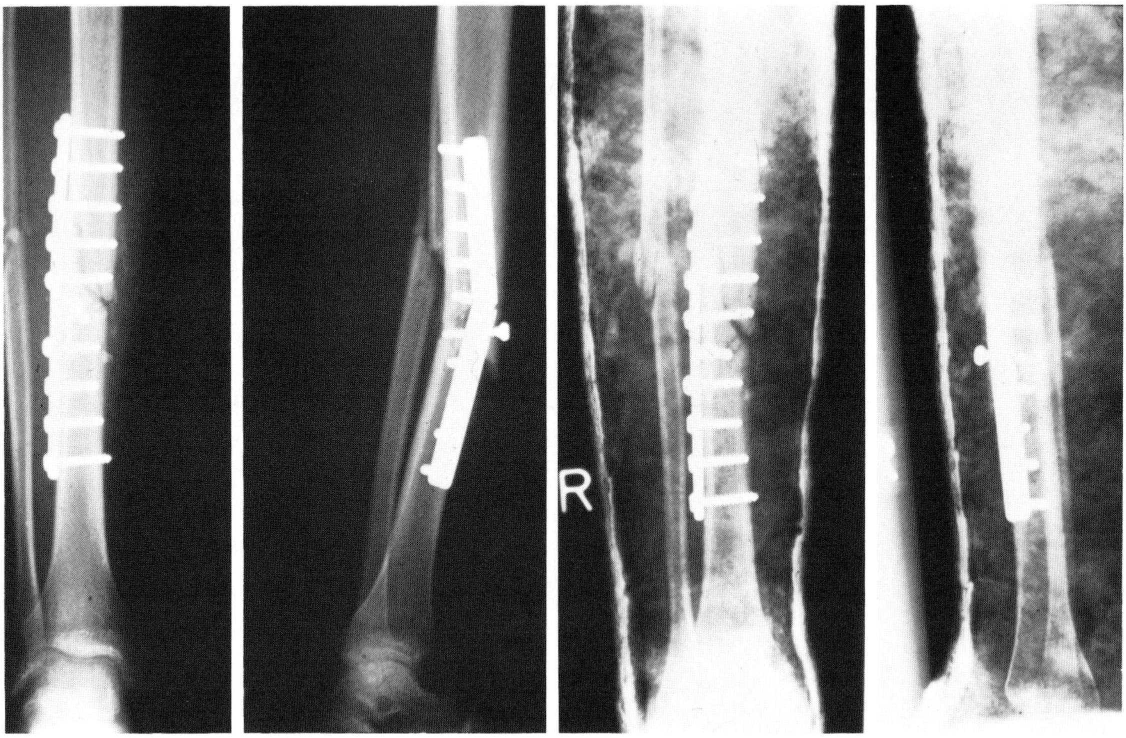

Fig. 13.17e f g h

e and f) As predicted, this fatigue fracture happened 7 weeks after internal fixation. The fracture occurred at the level of the 5th hole of the plate starting from above. The result is antecurvation of the tibia. The a. p. view reveals that medially at the level of the fracture, there is a poorly delineated, cloudy formation of callus which is the result of instability.

g and h) Reposition under anesthesia and plaster cast application. A new internal fixation was not attempted since the butterfly fragment was at that time largely excluded from nutrition.

i and j) 16 weeks after internal fixation and 9 weeks after fracture of the plate, with additional complete rest in a plaster cast, there has been consolidation of the fracture in an almost ideal position, with the visible formation of callus indicating secondary bony healing in the presence of an internal fixation by plate.

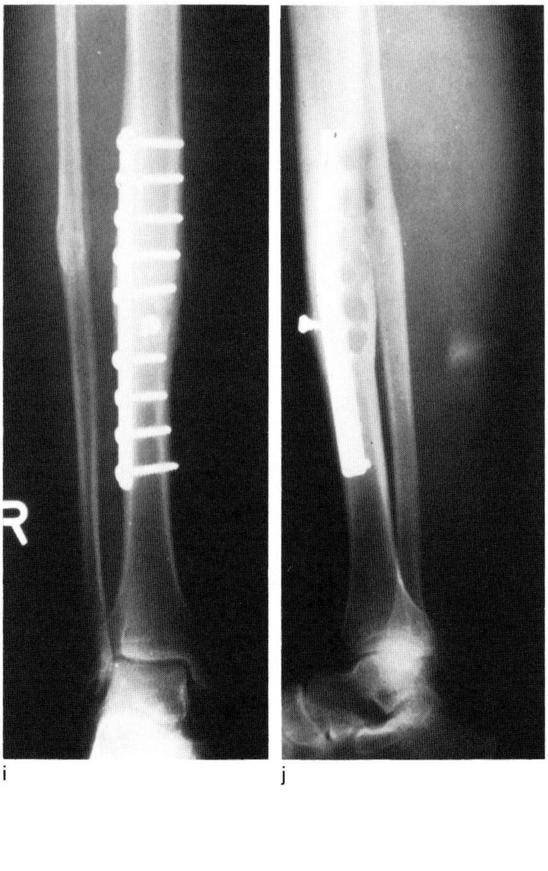

i j

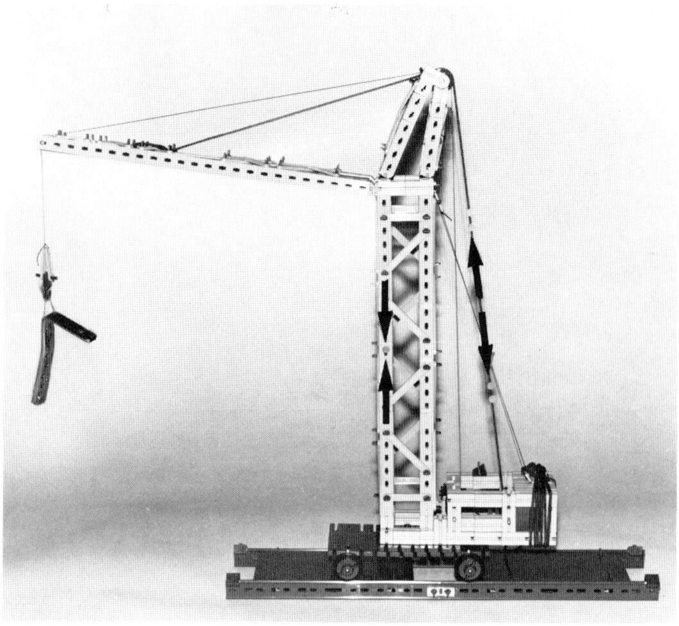

Fig. 13.18

Fig. 13.18. Photograph of an erector set carrying a condylar plate. Its construction allows one to recognize the mechanical principle of tension banding and, from this mechanical device, the principle can easily be transferred to the femur of man.

If there is centric weight-bearing by a column, this will simply lead to its being subjected to pressure, since the effective pressure lines will coincide with the axis of the column. The pressure tension will be equally divided over the cut section and is over all of the same magnitude.

If the weight is moved somewhat peripherally from the center of a column or exerts itself by an extended carrier beam, there will result maximal boundary tensions, and the pressure demands upon the column will no longer be simply direct pressure but there will also be the forces of bending. These unfavorable bending forces can be counteracted by counterbalancing or by the use of a tension band having the identical effect. The tension band will neutralize the bending forces to the column of the erector set so that its entire cross-section can again be subjected to pressure. The human femur is influenced by comparable mechanical conditions. Here the side subject to tension and bending is the laterodorsal aspect of the femur. This is the location of the iliotibial tract. During weight-bearing of the leg while standing, this tract is immediately put under tension and has the effect of a tension band. In fractures of the femur and when internal fixation by plate is contemplated, this plate will always have to be placed onto the laterodorsal surface so that it may be subject to tension (a tension band plate). If there were medial placement toward the inner surface of the femur, there would only be forces of bending affecting the plate, with fatigue fracture occurring very rapidly. This, incidentally, can also be the case if there is a properly placed and inserted lateral plate without adequate bony support as a result of bony defect. Internal fixation by tension banding is recommended not only for fractures of the femur but also for those involving the patella, olecranon and malleoli. In these locations, the best material for internal fixation is a wire (tension band wires).

Implant Material

Several specific requirements must be fully met by implant material used for internal fixation. It must possess optimal quality for mechanical stability, tissue tolerance, ability to be worked and must be economical. We must be honest about the fact that the ideal metal that meets all the stated criteria, combining the best tissue tolerance with the highest mechanical stability, has not yet been found. Today the frequently used implants are made from noble austenitic steel (type AISI 316) with chromium, nickel, molybdenum, manganese and silicium (Müller et al., 1963). Owing to its nonmagnetic characteristics, this metal has a high resistance to corrosion.
A survey of the presently most commonly used devices for internal fixation and endoprosthesis of the hip is given in Figs. 13.19 to 13.25.
The body will always respond to inserted foreign material with a local infection. This has been described also as a foreign body reaction. Under aseptic conditions, the metallic implant will soon be ensheathed in granulation tissue. Particularly on the side facing the soft tissues, there is somewhat dense fibrous capsule with the ability sometimes to calcify or even form bone.
If the implanted foreign body is chemically unstable, there will be an induction of increased infectious response in the area beneath the implant (Fig. 13.26), and this will persist with a mutually negative effect between the surrounding tissues and the metallic implant. This vicious cycle leads to a very complex result: corrosion metallosis (Allgöwer and Segmüller, 1965; v. Lüdinghausen et al., 1970). In such a case, the implant, instead of being surrounded by a usually avascular capsule of connective tissue, will be covered by granulation tissue. This will lead to resorption of adjacent bony tissue and will replace the latter eventually (Frank and Zitter, 1971). On the bone, it should be possible to demonstrate radiologically such resorptive phenomena resulting from the contact of bone with corroding metal. But the simultaneous use of different metals (for instance, austenitic steel screws in combination with V4A-plate) will, in the electrolyte-rich milieu of the normal organism, lead to the creation of a galvanic current. The result is massive corrosion. This in turn, together with the inevitable metallosis, will result in the loosening of the implant and thus lead to instability.
The term metallosis implies local damage and tissue alterations resulting from a metallic implant which exerts a foreign-body effect by pressure, displacement or destruction of tissue; and indirectly, by a chemical change of body fluids and by electrolyte activity with a direct galvanic interference with cellular vitality and impregnation of the surrounding tissues with ionized metal particles. Finally, part of this complex is a respective biologic reaction by the neighboring tissues around the implant (Contzen et al., 1967). Preferred locations for corrosion metallosis are areas with defective structure within implants, the point of immediate contact between screws and plates and particularly those parts of the implant located close to the fracture and, therefore, subject to very strong pressure forces. Metallic fatigue fracture is a complication, possibly the result of a biomechanically unfavorable constellation with an ensuing increased tendency toward corrosion. In the case of a trans- or supracondylar fracture of the femur and if on its medial side, there is a lack of bony support (compare Fig. 13.26), and this situation was corrected by internal fixation; the implant will be the sole mechanical support (Debrunner and Cech, 1969). The plate will be subject to a constantly alternating exposure by rapidly changing pressures on its cross-section (screw holes) for which it is not constructed. The monomolecular passivized layer formed by chromium oxide on the surface of chromium steels or chromium cobalt alloys will be destroyed by tension faults. Nickel corrosion will be the immediate result, with subsequent metallosis. On the other hand, instability will result in osteolysis, and tension faults of the metal are followed by bending and, ultimately, fatigue fractures (compare Fig. 13.17). Tension will also destroy the protective coating of the chromium oxide and thereby result in chemical corrosion and metallosis. This will be seen particularly in the areas where plates and screws or wires touch one another and where these are not intimately connected with adequate force (Scheuba, 1969; Schuster, 1972).
If there has been a fracture of an implant, there should be a detailed radiologic and, if possible, metallurgic analysis. The x-ray report should attempt to find answers or at least comments to the following: position of the implant in view of its biomechanical alteration; the dimensions of the plate; the degree and effectiveness of end-to-end adaptation of fracture fragments; determination of whether there are bony defects be-

cause of destruction of bone, absent fragments or spongiosa defects; and, finally, the determination if there is primary or secondary instability.

The term biomechanics implies the understanding of the characteristic alloplastic implants within the living organism under mechanical stress. For this reason, one should first decide whether the implant is placed in a manner that may well put it under stress. For an internal fixation plate, this would mean that the plate always has to be located on the tension side of the bone. In the femur, this is always its latero-dorsal aspect. A further and very important point is the radiologic evaluation of the degree of reposition of the fracture. One should always attempt to have full anatomic adaptation, which implies an exact end-to-end fitting of both fracture fragments. Only this will guarantee permanent stability. If bony defects are present in the region of the cortex opposite the plate, then severe bending forces will be exerted on the plate, eventually producing a fatigue fracture. This is the reason why autologous or homologous spongiosa or, in certain instances, bone cement (palacos, methacrylate) (Kuner et al., 1972). should be used to fill any defects (Fig. 13.32). Based on the mentioned facts, conclusions as to the existing stability are possible. An internal fixation shows primary instability if there is insufficient or incomplete adaptation of the fracture fragments, a significant bony defect has not been adequately filled and where the bony medial support is thus lacking or the implanted plate is too short. Secondary instability can be the result of bony resorption induced by activity (Willenegger et al., 1971) (Fig. 13.28) – either too early or too intensive weight-bearing on the injured extremity. The same can occur as a result of zones of lysis around screws, plates and intramedullary nails because of a localized circumscribed or generalized necrosis due to infection (osteomyelitis, osteitis). Primary tumors of bone but, more often, metastases in the area of internal fixation may lead to instability by a loss of substance, thus creating the milieu in which bending and sheer forces will alter the internal crystal structure of the metal and lead to tension corrosion.

In intramedullary nails, primary and secondary instability can also be the cause of metal fractures since, in such a situation, the cross-sectional loading of the nail is considerably larger than if there is a stable insertion of an intramedullary nail after cutting into the marrow cavity.

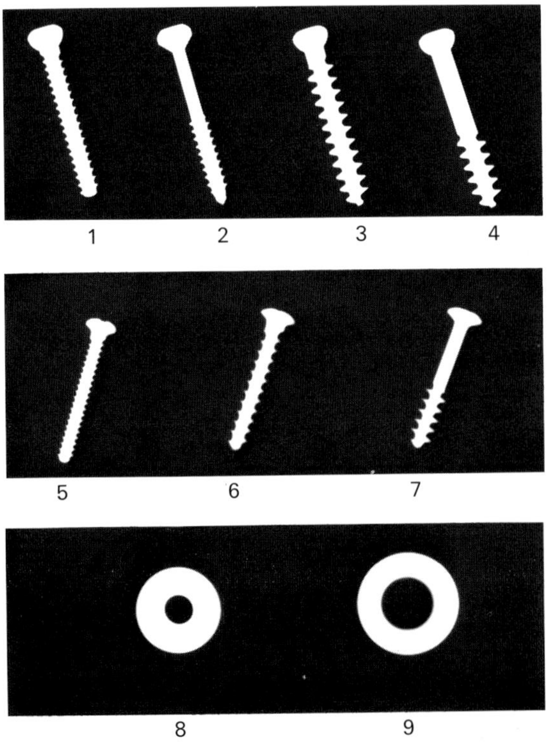

Fig. 13.19. Internal fixation screws of the ASIF on an x-ray:
1 Cortical screw
2 Malleolar screw
3 Spongiosa screw with long thread
4 Spongiosa screw with short thread (tension screw effect)
5 Smallest cortical screw
6 Small cortical screw
7 Small spongiosa screw (navicular screw)
8 Nut for cortical screw
9 Washer under head of screw
Comment: Screws 1 to 4 have a hexagonal recessed head; screws 5 to 7 have a cross-slit (Phillips head).

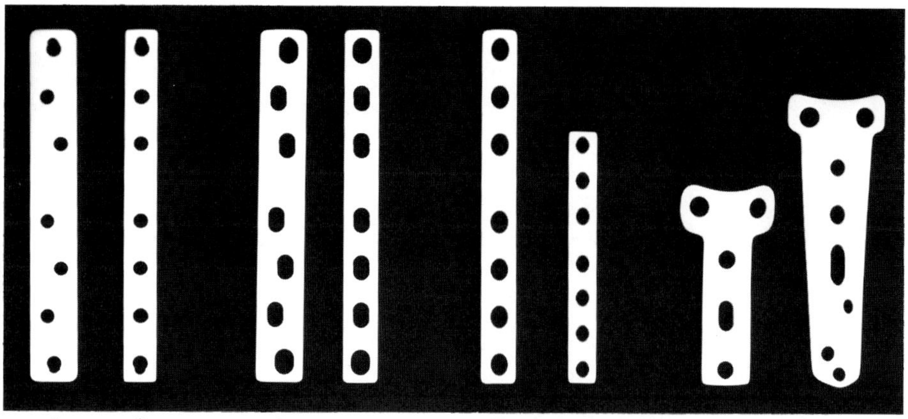

Fig. 13.20

1 2 3 4 5 6 7 8

Fig. 13.20. ASIF plates on x-ray:

1 Wide straight plate
2 Narrow straight plate
3 Wide self-tensing straight plate (DCP)
4 Narrow self-tensing straight plate (DCP)
5 Straight semitubular plate
6 Straight one-third tubular plate
7 T-plate
8 Spoon plate
9 Short straight plate (for internal fixation in the area of the hands and feet)
10 Small angled blade plate
11 Small T-plate
12 Small multiple fragment plate

Comment: All plates can be bent to adapt to an individual bony form.

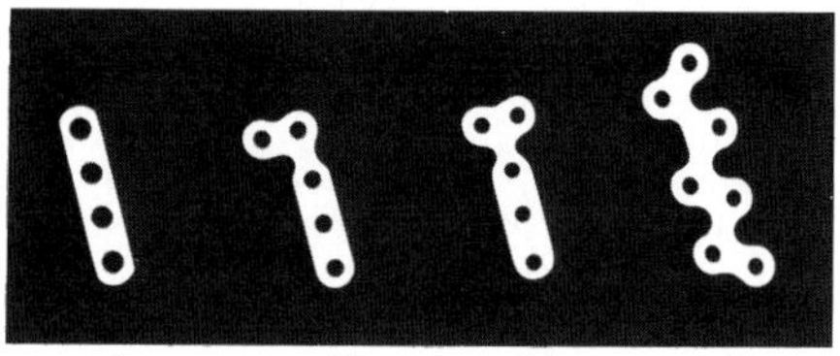

9 10 11 12

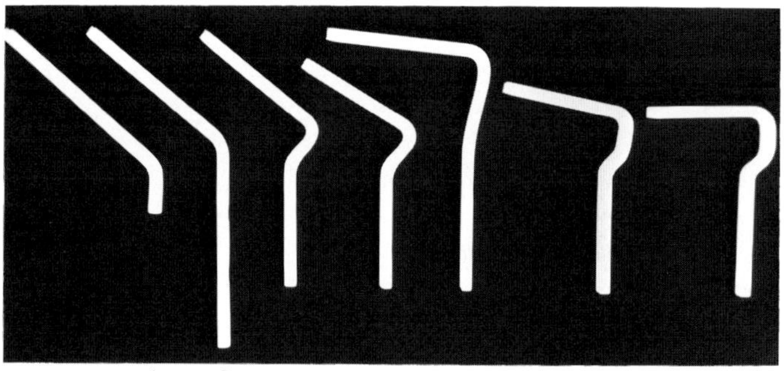

1 2 3 4 5 6 7

Fig. 13.21. Angle plates on x-ray:

1 ASIF nail (130-degree angle plate with one-hole shaft; femoral neck plate)
2 ASIF peritrochanteric plate (130-degree angle blade plate with multiple-hole shaft)
3 Hip plate (130 degrees)
4 Hip plate (120 degrees)
5 Condyle plate (95 degrees)
6 Double-angled plate (100 degrees)
7 Double-angled plate (right angle)

Comment: All ASIF angle plates have a U-profile of their blade.

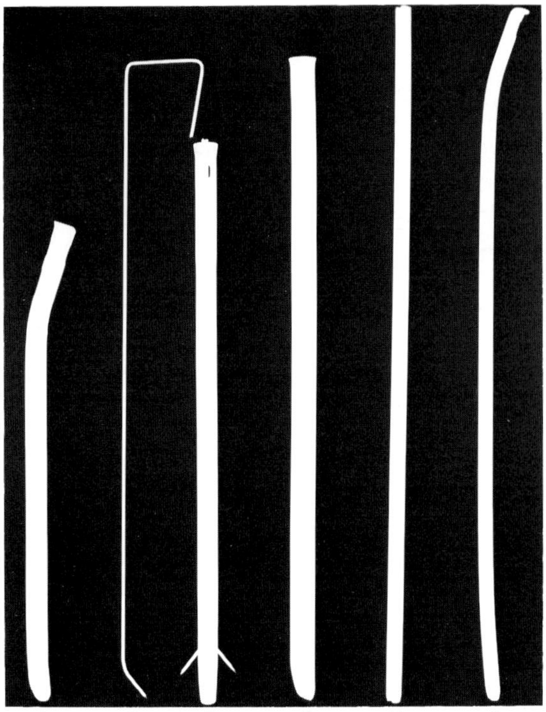

1 2 3 4 5 6

Fig. 13.22

Fig. 13.22. Bone marrow nails on x-ray:
1 ASIF tibial nail (lateral view)
2 Antirotation wires
3 ASIF-tibial nail (a.p) with antirotational wires introduced
4 ASIF femoral nail
5 Femoral nail according to Küntscher
6 Tibial nail according to Küntscher

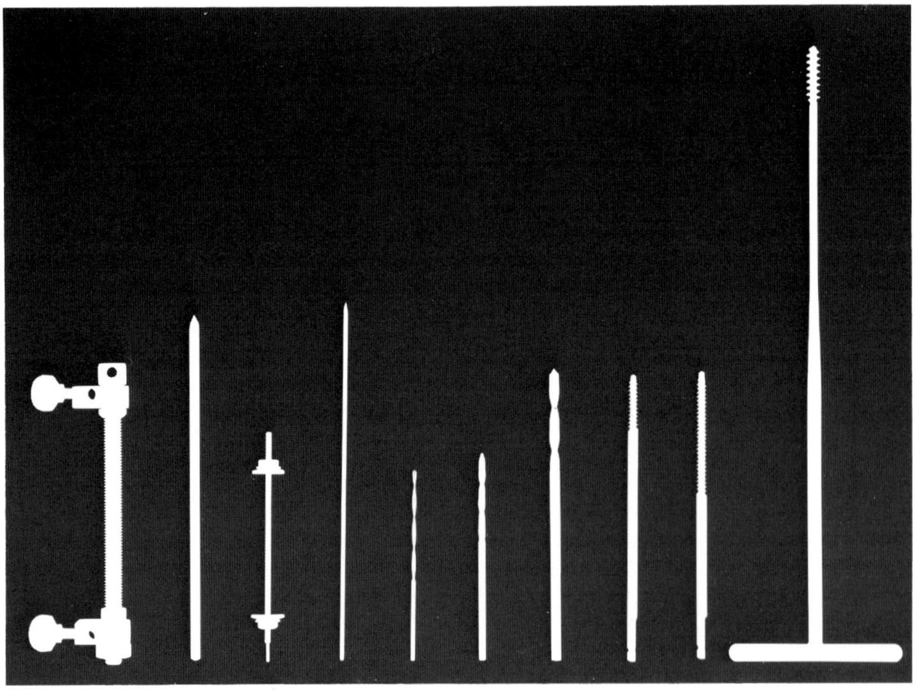

1 2 3 4 5 6 7 8 9 10

Fig. 13.23

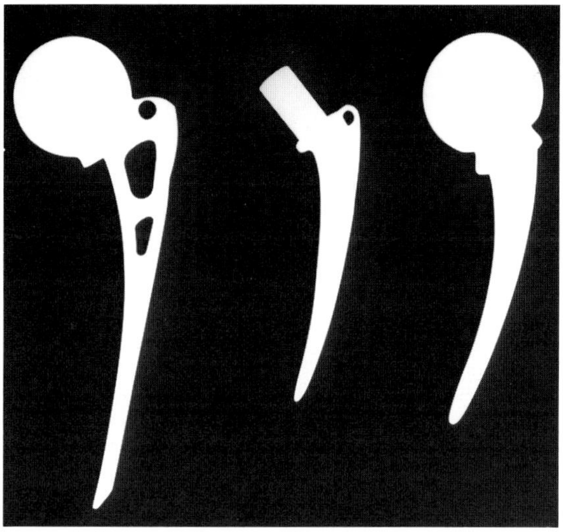
1 2 3

Fig. 13.24. Femoral head prosthesis:
1 Femoral head prosthesis according to Moore
2 Femoral head prosthesis system according to Weber/Huggler (the plastic head does not visualize on x-ray)
3 Femoral head prosthesis according to Thompson

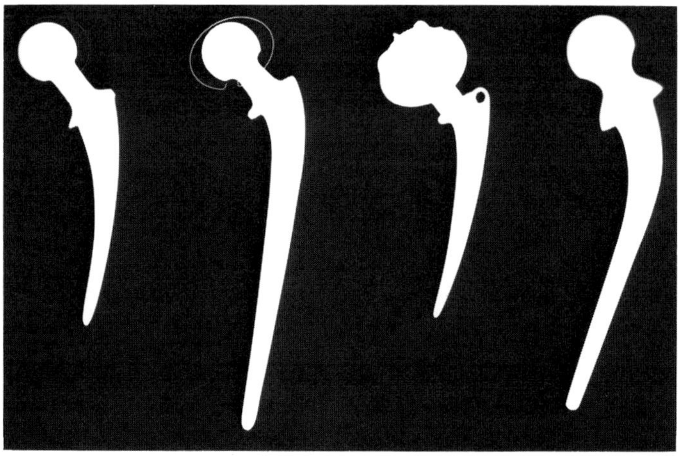
1 2 3 4

Fig. 13.25. X-ray appearance of various total hip replacements:
1 Total prosthesis, type Müller (acetabulum polyethylene)
2 Total prosthesis with a long shaft, type Müller (acetabulum polyethylene)
3 Total prosthesis system according to Weber/Huggler (rotation prosthesis)
4 Total prosthesis, model "St. Georg" (plastic acetabulum)
At present there are many more models in use.

◀ Fig. 13.23. Blunt instruments and implants on x-ray:
1 Outrigger compression device (Charnley type), usually used in combination with two or several Steinmann nails)
2 Steinmann nail (usually used in combination with outrigger compression device)
3 Andreesen screw or threaded bolt with two nuts and underlay disks
4 Kirschner wires (used for reduction fixation, particularly in children)
5 2 mm. ASIF cutter
6 3.2 mm. ASIF cutter
7 4.5 mm. ASIF cutter
8 Bone tap with short cutting portion (used for tapping when inserting cortical lag screws)
9 Bone tap with long cutting portion for cortical lag screws
10 Bone tap for spongiosa screws.
Comment: During internal fixation, there can be breakage of bone taps, cutters and other devices within the bone. These illustrations should help in their identification and localization.

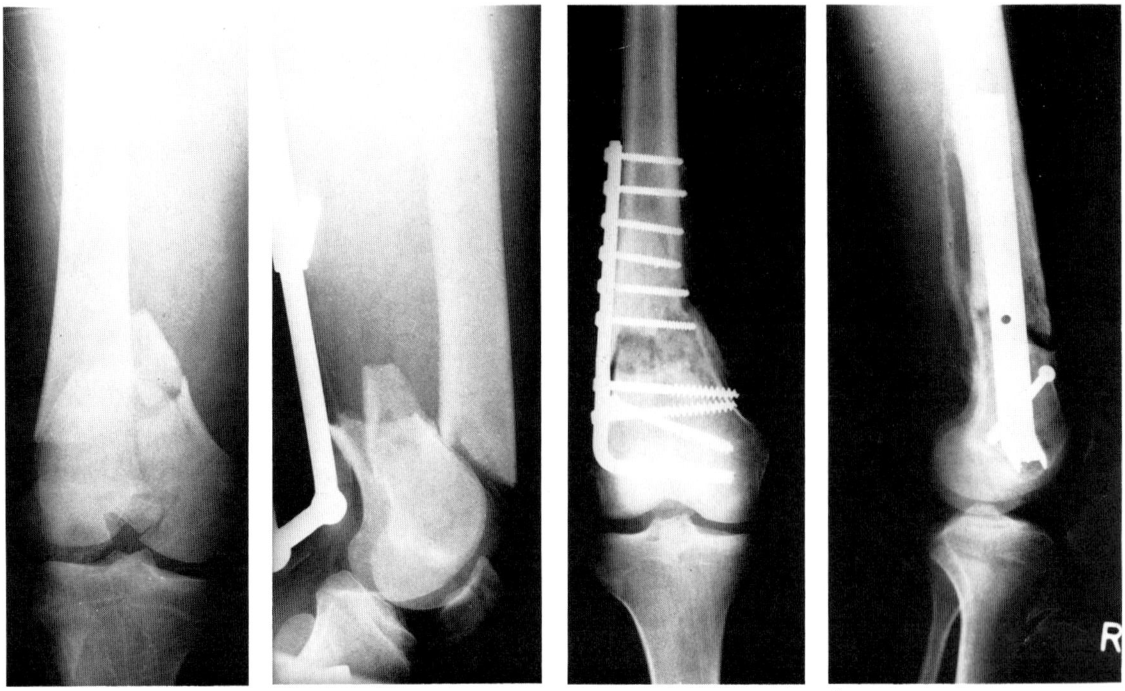

Fig. 13.26a b c d

Fig. 13.26a–l. a and b) Supra- and transcondylar fracture of the distal femur into the joint, with fracture of the patella.

c and d) Internal fixation by a 9-hole condylar plate and a lateral spongiosa screw. The 3rd hole of the plate has not been used. Adequate position of bony axis, with irritation callus dorsomedially and a bony defect on the other side. Condition 10 weeks after internal fixation.

e and f) As a result of the absence of bony medial support, there is a lack of bony healing (18 weeks after internal fixation) and, while there was only partial weight-bearing, there is now bending of the plate, with varix formation and avulsion of the uppermost screws, one of which is broken. Simultaneously, there are signs of osteitis. ▶

g and h) Internal fixation using a 12-hole condylar plate. Intraoperative x-ray shows the plate distally fixed by two screws and pulled with a bone-holding forceps proximally to the shaft, the cranially inserted compression device finally being used and compression being exerted on the pseudarthrosis. The fragments located within the tissue of the pseudarthrosis are not removed. ▶

i and j) An additional 12 weeks after the second internal fixation, there is consolidation with adequate bony structure. Dorsally there is a large callus. The position of the femur is good. The 3rd screw from above still remains from the first intervention. The infection is healed. ▶

k and l) After removal of the implants, there remains one broken screw. Complete bony trabeculation. ▶

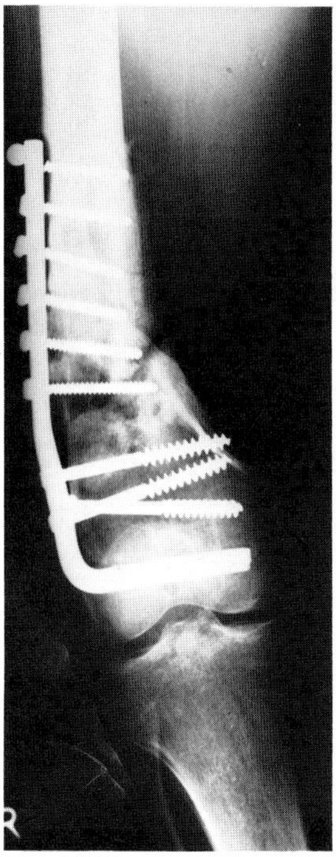

Fig. 13.26e

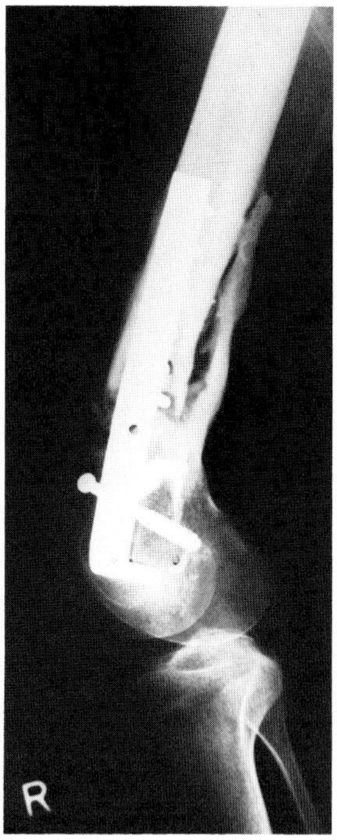

f

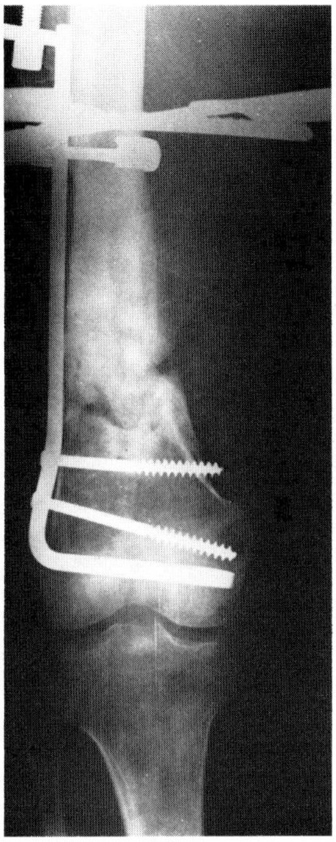

g

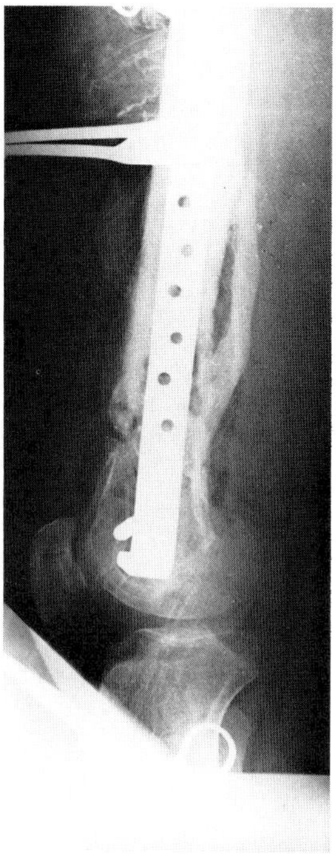

h

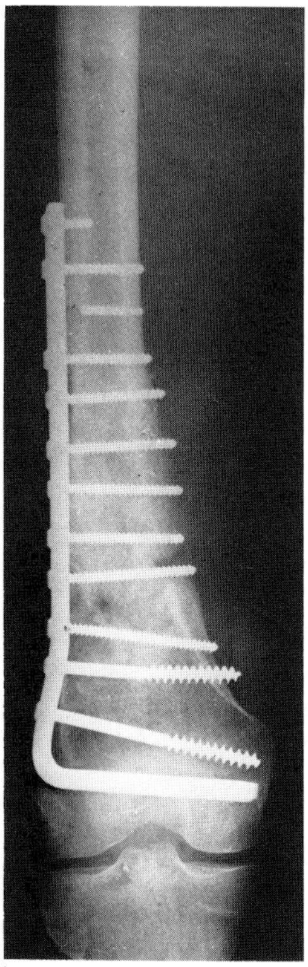

i

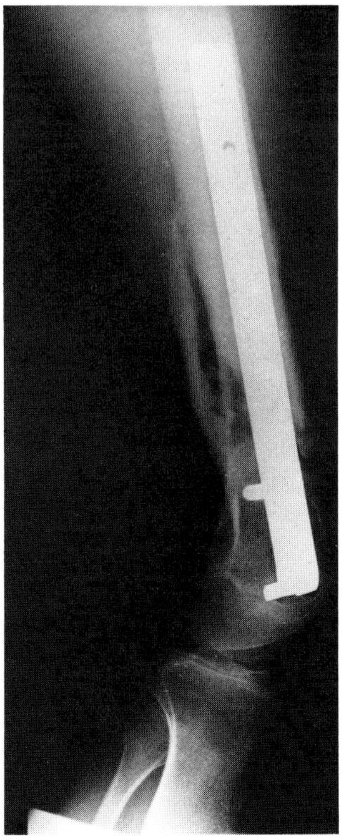

j

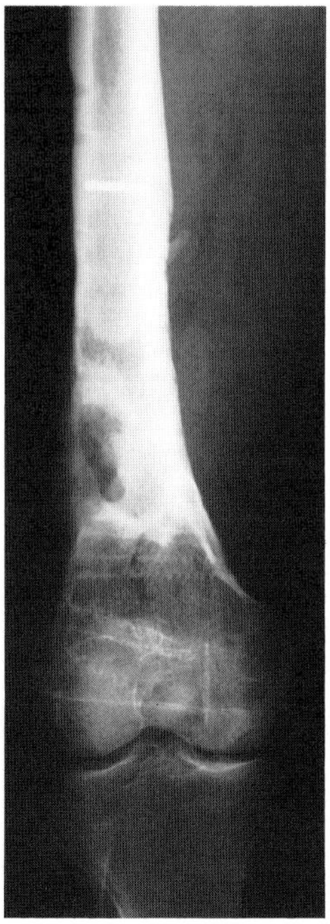

k

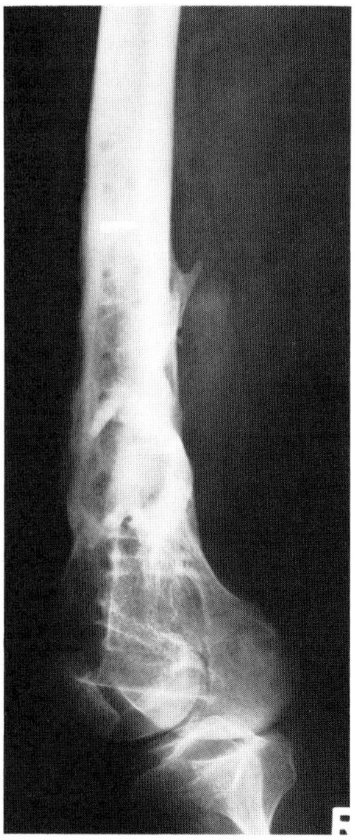

l

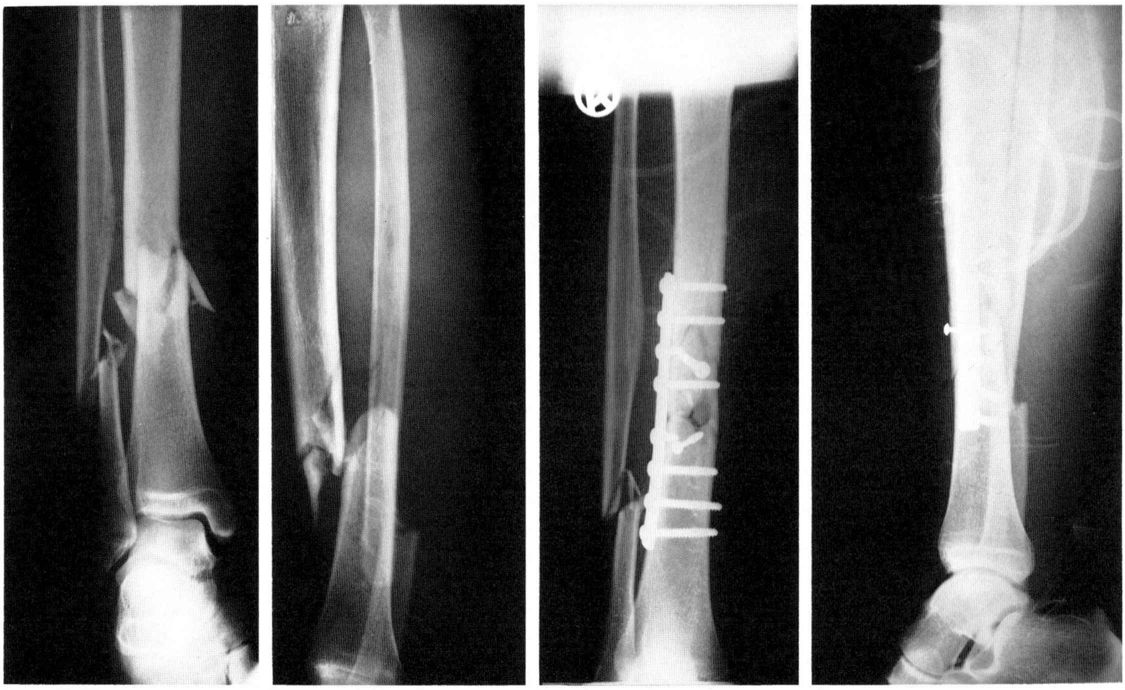

Fig. 13.27a b c d

Fig. 13.27a-h. a and b) Open shank fracture on the right; mainly oblique with multiple small fragments. Dislocation on the lateral view by the full width of the shaft. Within the soft tissues, there is an accumulation of air (perforation of the skin by bone is the first degree of an open fracture). The fibula is fractured about 8 cm. below the fracture of the tibia and also shows multiple small fractures of bones.
c and d) Immediate internal fixation by insertion of a narrow 8-hole plate into the tibia, with a cortical lag screw and a small spongiosa screw, further fracture fragments are fixed. There remains a mediodorsal defect. Autologous spongy bone was brought into this defect. The fracture of the fibula is left alone and does have a gap of half of the shaft on the lateral view, and one width of the shaft on the a. p. view. Medially and laterally to the shaft of the tibia, one recognizes Redon drainage (on postoperative x-rays). Results: Stable internal fixation by plate after an open comminuted fracture of the tibia with a mediodorsal defect. The anatomic axis is good in all directions. Comments: In open fractures, one has to be careful that the plate is covered by uninjured tissue. This is usually the case on the lateral surface of the tibia with its good musculature.
e and f) Six weeks after the accident and internal fixation, one still clearly recognizes the mediodorsal defect. On the lateral view, the transverse spongiosa is still not readily visible. Unchanged position of the implants, with no zones of lysis around the screws. The fracture is not ready for weight-bearing.
g and h) 11 months after the accident and internal fixation by a lateral neutralization plate for an open fracture of the first degree. Well-structured callus in the area of the formerly mediodorsally located defect filled with autologous spongiosa. In this case we are dealing with a visible formation of callus not as a sign of instability but produced by the transplanted spongiosa. All screws are located within the bone without reaction and without having changed their position. Only minimal atrophy of the skeleton; the fibula has healed with only minimal shortening, slight axis deviation and marked formation of callus. Comment: If spongiosa is introduced into a fracture, the visible formation of callus is not to be considered the sole expression of instability.

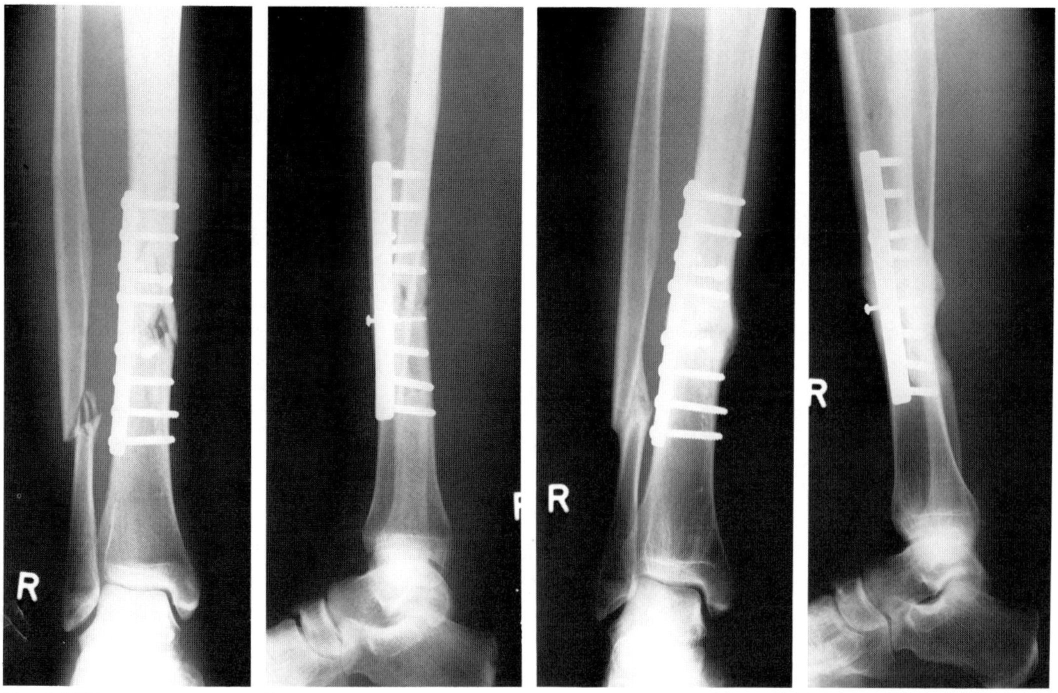

Fig. 13.27e f g h

Fig. 13.28. Zone of lysis in the tibia and fibula beside a suprasyndesmal set screw introduced 11 months earlier to secure the integrity of the syndesmosis in the treatment of an ankle fracture type C. Such screws in general should be removed 6 to 8 weeks after internal fixation. The lytic zone must be understood to result from mechanical irritation and not from infection.

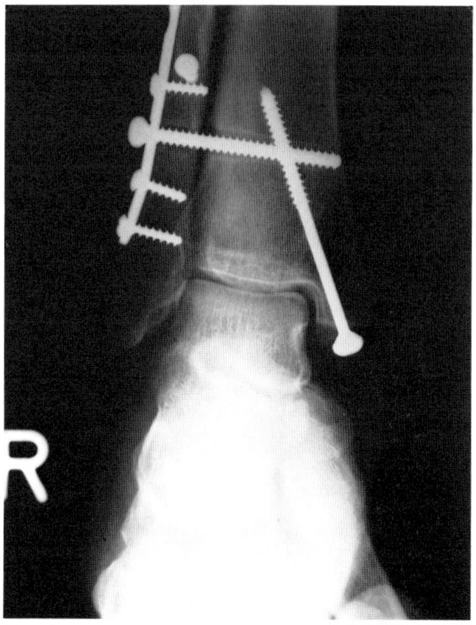

Fig. 13.28

The X-Ray Appearance of Primary and Secondary Bone Healing

Primary bone healing is characterized radiologically by the fact that during no phase of healing will there be visible formation of callus. This, therefore, is a direct angiogenic mode of bone healing consisting of two different types as described by Schenk and Willenegger (1963) – contact healing and gap healing (Figs. 13.14 and 13.15). The main active elements of the bone responsible for healing are regenerating osteons during absolute mechanical rest. The radiologic criteria for progressive healing are simply the gradual disappearance of the fracture line and the denser appearance of this zone. A direct type of bone healing is possible after internal fixation by screws and plates under interfragmentary pressure. The evaluation of this form of healing is difficult and requires great experience (Fig. 13.29).

All other radiologic signs during the healing phase of a fracture treated by internal fixation are indications of disturbed healing. An inserted internal fixation which does not allow weight-bearing will lead to the following three consequences:

1. The persistence and clearer recognition of the fracture line – fracture gap.
2. The visible formation of callus.
3. The appearance of zones of lysis around the screw threads.

The same triad is also seen if a weight-bearing fixation is exposed to full weight-bearing too early. Here we also must expect the danger of fatigue fracture of the metal (Fig. 13.17).

Primary as well as secondary instability will lead to the formation of additional callus. Because of its vague borders and the lack of structures within, it is also known as irritation callus (compare Fig. 13.30). The underlying cause can be eliminated by direct measures such as renewed avoidance of weight-bearing and use of additional plaster cast. This type of callus may rapidly change into one with more definite characteristics. It will then be readily recognizable within the surrounding tissues with a good bony structure. During this phase of consolidation, the fracture line will be filled in and trabeculation will be seen across it (Weller and Kuner, 1968).

The zones of lysis around the screw threads, plates or intramedullary nails complete the picture of unstable internal fixation (Wieser, 1964). This refers to a circumscribed defect in compact bone and spongiosa, respectively (bony resorption due to movement); the reasons for this are the abnormally intensive, intermittent, sheer and bending forces or, occasionally, a local bacterial infection (osteomyelitis, osteitis) with destruction of bone. In order to evaluate the radiologic symptoms listed, knowledge of the clinical condition is crucial because only by combining this information with the radiologic findings will it be possible to give a reliable interpretation. Any persistence of primary or secondary instability with signs of lack of bone healing indicates formation of a pseudarthrosis. Pseudarthrosis describes a fracture that has been present for 6 months without bony consolidation. If, after 3 to 5 months, there is no healing, we refer to this only as delayed bone healing or delayed fracture healing.

A pseudarthrosis can be subdivided into hypertrophic or atrophic types. A hypertrophic pseudarthrosis is characterized by marked expansion of the neighboring fragments. These appear to be sclerotic and represent an overactive bone formation with good vascularization. Because of its form, this type is sometimes called elephant-foot pseudarthrosis.

Chances of healing with complete rest are good because, by insertion of a tension band plate or a bone-marrow nail or other implant, the tendency toward rapid vascularization of the interposed cartilage or connective tissue will favor chondral or desmal ossification.

Atrophic pseudarthrosis is radiologically without any local reaction. The fragments at the fracture site are narrow and the calcium content is often significantly reduced. Circulation in this area is poor. Formation of the defect may be due to resorption or infection (defect or infectious pseudarthrosis).

Chances of healing are not nearly as good as in the hypertrophic type. The problems encountered and energies expended in closing the fracture are incomparably greater (stabilization, irrigation drainage, transplantation of spongiosa, etc.).

In this particular context the radiologist must be aware that implants for internal fixation (intramedullary nails, plates, etc.) should be left in place in the presence of infection of bone as long as they are capable of providing stability. This would ensure that there are no zones of lysis, no breaking or displacement of screws and, above all, no breaking of a plate or intramedullary nail.

Under conservative management, healing of the fracture occurs by desmal ossification. Since there is no absolute rest in the fracture, onset of ossification occurs at a certain distance from the zone of unrest. Radiologically, the progress of healing can be recognized when there is a deposit of apatite crystals. Calcification starts from an initial series of centers, which then will extend and meet one another, thus becoming increasingly dense. At this stage the callus can be seen on the x-ray as a vaguely delineated and irregularly dense tissue within the region of the fracture (Fig. 13.16). Within weeks and months, this zone is progressively better delineated and has a clearer structure so that there is a solid "bony scar" capable of weight bearing. The fracture line as such can no longer be recognized in this stage. There is even a bony structure in this region.

There are considerable differences between the radiologic criteria of a healing fracture of compact bone and those of spongiosa within a long bone. Whereas one can expect to see the "bony scar" in fracture healing of compact bone, there is a difference in the process in spongiosa in the form of an irregular condensation without a significant periosteal reaction. Only after complete trabeculation across the fracture is one justified in pronouncing this area as clinically healed. There are considerable difficulties in our approach to the evaluation of fractures in close proximity to joints as well as of fractures of vertebral bodies. Sometimes it is only possible to make a clear statement about the degree of healing after obtaining tomograms.

When using intramedullary nails, there are similar conditions as in conservative therapy (Fig. 13.31). After a corresponding time interval, there is formation of callus at the site of fracture, usually in the form of a spindle or a muff. This region is initially poorly delineated and shows a very soft structure that becomes progressively dense, finally having definite bony structure in its related function as a "bony scar." From a clinical viewpoint, intramedullary nails as a form of internal fixation, with cutting into the marrow cavity, do belong without question to the group of weight-bearing fixations. The usually seen, somewhat marked formation of callus is an indication that even by cutting into the marrow cavity in the area of the fracture, it is not possible to obtain absolute mechanical rest in this area. Callus formation resulting from minimal instability and bony material displaced at the time of the cutting of the fracture are not considered disadvantages, since the intramedullary nail, as an inner stabilizing element bearing the weight, is capable of mechanically neutralizing the fracture for the entire duration of healing.

Similarly, in both types of fracture healing – primary and secondary – as a sequela to trauma, there is a reversible diminution of bone density in the affected part of the skeleton. This is an expression of the very active processs of local repair intensified by metabolic events. This slight degree of traumatic bony atrophy usually can be recognized 3 to 4 weeks after trauma and, after 2 to 4 months, usually disappears. During therapy with weight-bearing fixation, it appears that this process is shorter and milder in character. Stable internal fixation, furthermore, will also prevent the complication of the Sudeck-Kienböck-type of atrophy or at least diminish the severity of its course (see Sudeck's atrophy, Chapter 14, page 321–322).

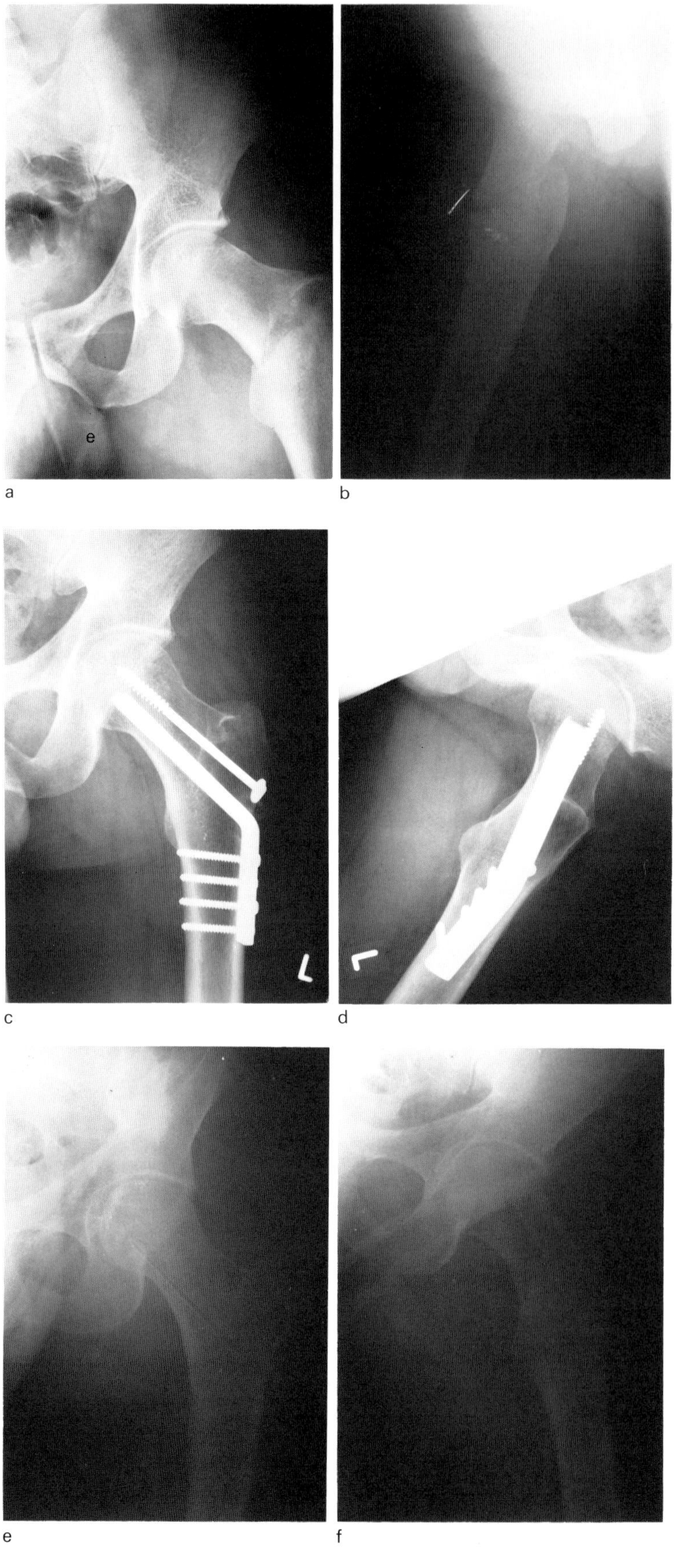

Fig. 13.29a–f. a and b) Lateral femoral neck fracture on the left, with diminution of femoral neck angle.
c and d) Internal fixation with ASIF 130-degree angle blade plate with a 4-hole shaft and an additional cranial spongiosa screw with underlay disk. This fracture 6 months later shows bony consolidation in good anatomic position without visible callus. Exact location of the implants; no zones of lysis; normal joints. Comments: The U-shaped cross-section of the blade in the femoral neck can be clearly recognized on both planes.
e and f) Two years after the accident and internal fixation, the implants are removed. The x-rays reveal the condition immediately afterwards, with the Redon drain still inserted. In the a. p. as well as the lateral view, it is easily seen where the blade was located in the femoral neck.

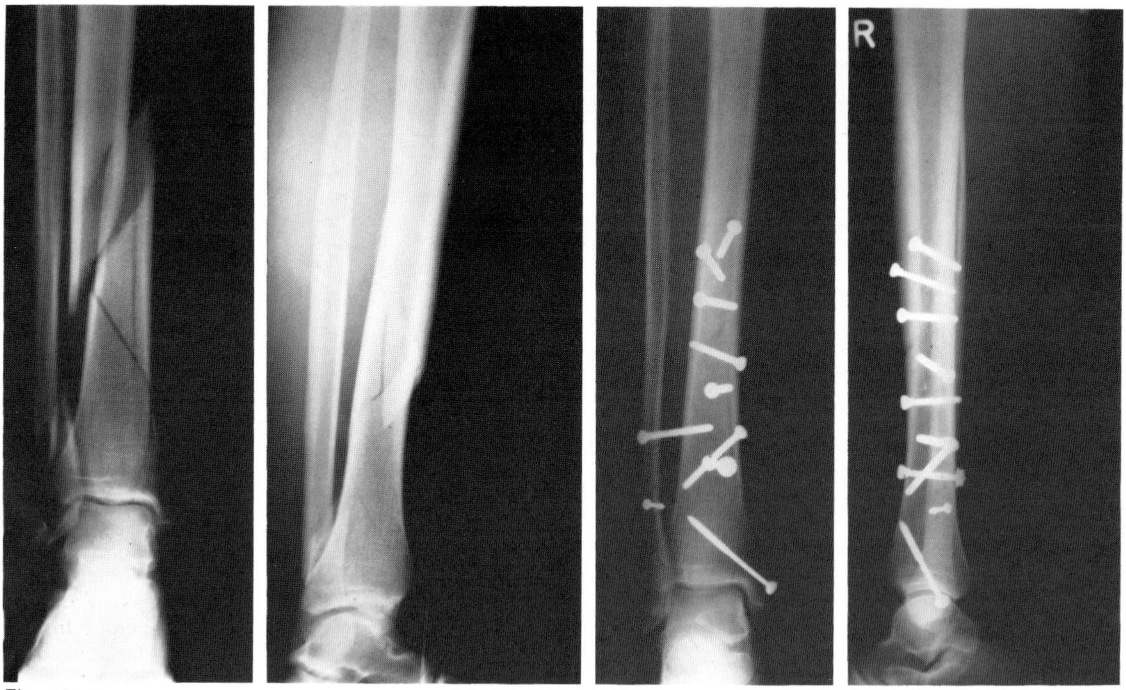

Fig. 13.30a b c d

Fig. 13.30a–h. a and b) Ski accident involving the right lower leg, with a long spiral fracture and a large butterfly fragment. The spiral fracture extends to the ankle joint (close to the inner malleolus). The fibula also shows signs of spiral fracture.

c and d) Internal fixation of the tibia and fibula by screw. Thus 8 cortical lag screws were inserted, along with one malleolar screw (the inner malleolus) and a small spongiosa screw in the fibula. The lowermost cortical lag screw in the tibia has a nut at its posterior end. Excellent anatomic reconstruction of the tibial and fibular fracture was achieved. Critique: Fractures with more than two fracture fragments do not lend themselves to a pure internal fixation by lag screws. It is not possible to obtain a weight-bearing fixation in this manner.

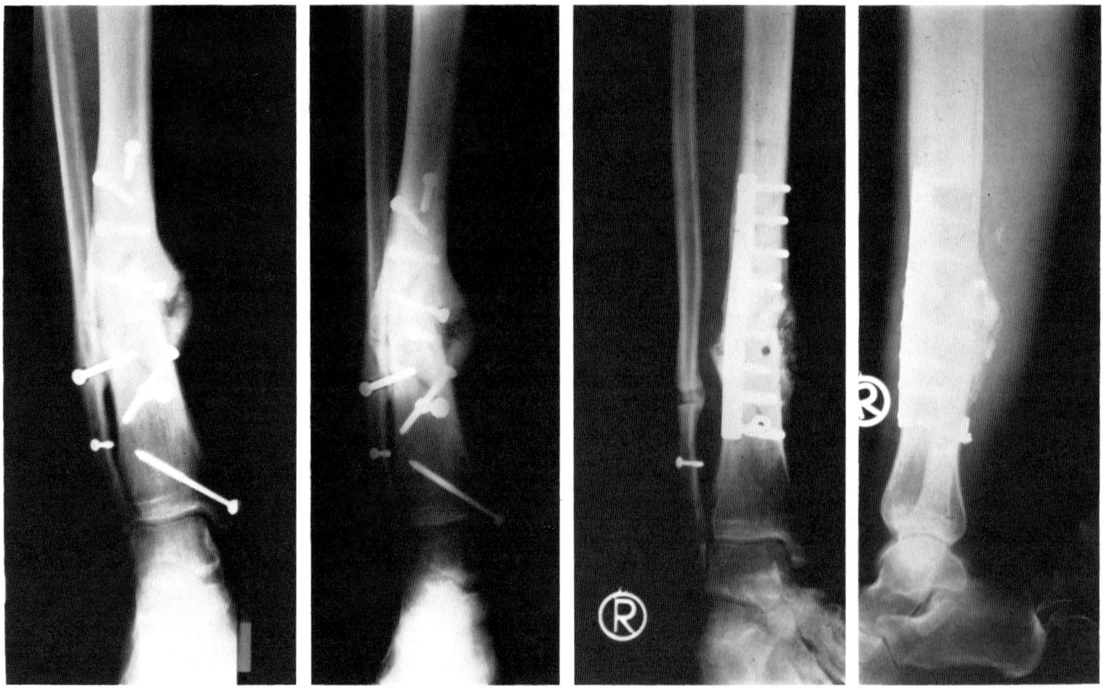

Fig. 13.30e f g h

Fig. 13.30
e and f) The existing instability due to a faulty indication for internal fixation by lag screws has resulted in the formation of an irritation callus and, finally, since neutralization of mechanical forces were absent pseudarthrosis developed in various positions.

g and h) Removal of metallic implants, with the exception of the small spongiosa screw in the fibula and the dorsal nut and stabilization of the pseudarthrosis by insertion of a narrow 8-hole plate at the convexity of the tibia, in this instance the lateral side, after setting the plate under tension this led to correction of the abnormal angulation and, as is visible on this x-ray 8 weeks after internal fixation by plate, ther is already a reasonable bony trabeculation across the former pseudarthrosis.

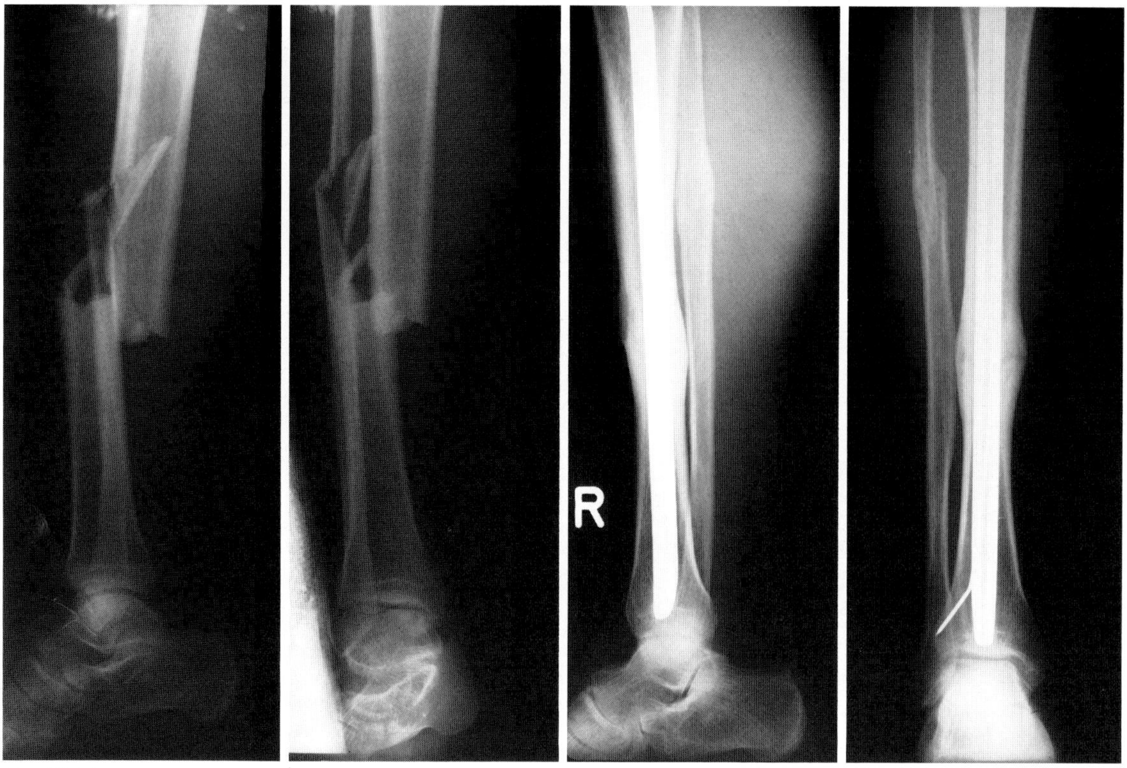

Fig. 13.31a b c d

Fig. 13.31a–f. a and b) Transverse fracture of both bones of the lower leg, with dislocation by a width of the midshaft.
c and d) Operative management by insertion, from a remote location, of an intramedullary nail with an additional antirotational wire.
c and d) The fracture is fully consolidated by a spindly well-structured callus. Anatomically the fragments are in excellent position. Implant within the bone without any local signs of irritation.
e and f) After removal of intramedullary nail and antirotational wire, excellent healing of fracture area.

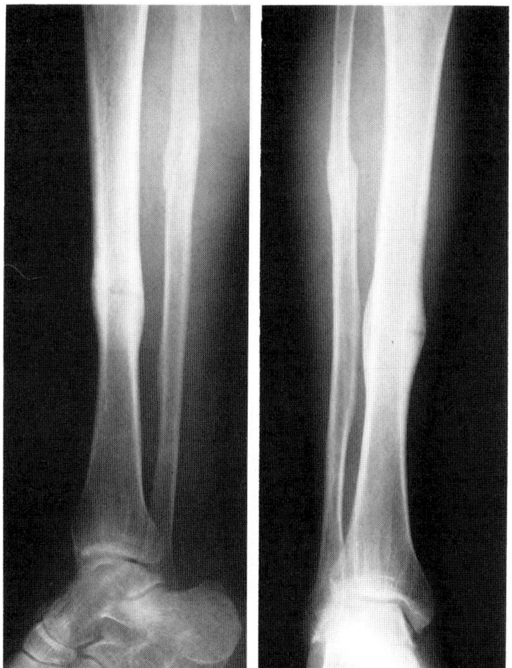

e f

Timing of X-Ray Investigations

In the therapy and management of fractures of bone, regardless of whether the therapy is conservative, functional or surgical, the x-ray will always assume central importance. Repeated x-rays on two planes will not only serve to evaluate the position of the fracture fragments but will also offer information on the progress of healing. The frequency and timing of x-ray examination are independent of the type of management and are directly determined by the type of fracture and its localization.

If a fracture is treated conservatively, there will be, after the original diagnostic investigation, the first follow-up examination directly after the conclusion of reposition and fixation. This radiologic investigation assumes special importance and must fully document the position of the fracture fragments on all planes necessary. This is also the case if the surgeon has had the benefit of an image intensifier to check his work in correcting the fracture. It is important in this regard to emphasize that, especially in the case of fractures of long bones, it is often impossible to form a reliable opinion on the exact position of the fragments with the image intensifier, and that, therefore, only x-rays showing the entire bone involved will suffice.

The second follow-up examination is usually done 10 to 14 days later. It is justified by the fact that, by this time, all local swelling will have disappeared and the plaster cast may now be too wide, with the inherent danger of secondary motion of the fracture. X-ray evaluation of rotation in fractures of long bones may pose a problem. A torsion of the tibia, for instance, if not extreme may be missed on the usual x-rays if the following sizes are used (15 x 40 cm or 20 x 40 cm), since these dimensions will only show one of the adjacent joints and never both simultaneously. Even on an excellent total survey film of the lower leg including both joints, measurement may not be fully reliable, since there are no firm points of reference (Spirig, 1966). It is for this reason that great importance must be attached to a clinical investigation.

Fracture x-rays are usually obtained in 4-week intervals. In addition to checking the position of the fracture, it is now increasingly important to evaluate the stages of healing. Primarily, one will have to watch the formation of the appositional callus bridging the fragments. In the course of its transformation into a progressively more defined structure, this will develop into a fixation callus, allowing the mechanical neutralization and increasing stability of the fracture area. If one can accurately see a fixation callus, it will no longer be necessary to have exterior immobilization. It is now possible to allow partial weight-bearing of the extremity.

In cases when there is a disturbance of fracture healing by instability or infection, x-rays must be obtained at more frequent intervals. The decision has to be made in every case on an individual basis.

When there is insertion of a weight-bearing fixation, an immediate postoperative x-ray control is indicated even if, during surgery, the procedure involved the use of an image intensifier or if during certain phases of the surgical intervention, x-rays were obtained. All further x-rays are needed for the supervision of healing. If this process is undisturbed, it is appropriate to obtain x-rays at 4-week intervals. Whereas one expects to see formation of callus within the fracture area starting about 4 weeks after insertion of an intramedullary nail, insertion of lag screws producing interfragmentary pressure or insertion of internal fixation by pressure plates demands painstaking observation for the possible formation of an irritation callus. Instability is the most frequent cause of such a development. If there is perfect stability, however, there will be a progressively dense appearance of the fracture line until there is a homogenous structure across it. In this regard, it is important that the radiologist be fully aware that there has been, for instance, transplantation of spongiosa (autologous or homologous) (Fig. 13.32); otherwise it could be misinterpreted. If healing has made such good progress that partial or later full weight-bearing can be allowed, an x-ray control 2 weeks later must be recommended in order to recognize early a possible secondary instability. If the entire healing phase has passed without complication, there should be a late follow-up after one year. If removal of the metallic implants is planned, a new x-ray examination is needed or there should be a film not older than 2 to 3 months. The final x-ray after removal of the implants for internal fixation terminates the management (Fig. 13.33).

During recent years, alloarthroplastic methods have assumed an increasingly important role. Despite the fact that these methods are not a part of internal fixation, they are frequently used in the management of fractures of joints, particularly the hip and knee. In particular, the use of a total replacement prosthesis for the hip (Fig. 13.34) after a medial fracture of the femoral neck is being advocated today. In earlier years, the simple replacement of the femoral head by a prosthesis if the patient was over 60 years old and required immediate mobilization was commonly performed. Nowadays, however, this is rarely done. The indications for such surgical procedures after trauma are mainly associated with complications after medial fracture of the femoral neck with necrosis of the femoral head or formation of pseudarthrosis or post-traumatic arthrosis.

For radiologic evaluation of such images, some criteria are important. They involve the appearance of the alloarthroplastic implants (for example, 1- to 3-part models), their anchorage within the bone (evaluation of the extent of the bone cement used; a line of methomethacrylate, palacos and others usually has the characteristic of an x-ray contrast) and finally the position of the bones (for instance, the position of the acetabulum in the pelvis or the varisation or valgus position of the head-shaft portion of the femur).

Operative management of fractures has made great strides by the use of novel methods, improvement of the material and technique used for internal fixation, and by dramatic lowering of the rate of infection as the result of careful aseptic management and the introduction of air turbulence-free operating rooms. Simultaneously, it has been possible to fully characterize the healing process under conditions of stable internal fixation and to recognize biologic types of healing as contact and gap healing, with their possible disturbance being recognizable on x-ray (Fig. 13.35). In hardly another organ of the human body is there such a simple and reliable evaluation of a surgical intervention available since it is now possible to detect mistakes in treating such lesions of bones. Only experience and critical judgment will permit one to fully recognize the essential points of reference and to attach new significance to the "x-ray cosmetic" of internal fixation. Besides this, there should be friendly cooperation and informed communication between the orthopedic surgeon and the radiologist. Only in this way will it be possible to manage difficult situations together, using optimal investigative methods.

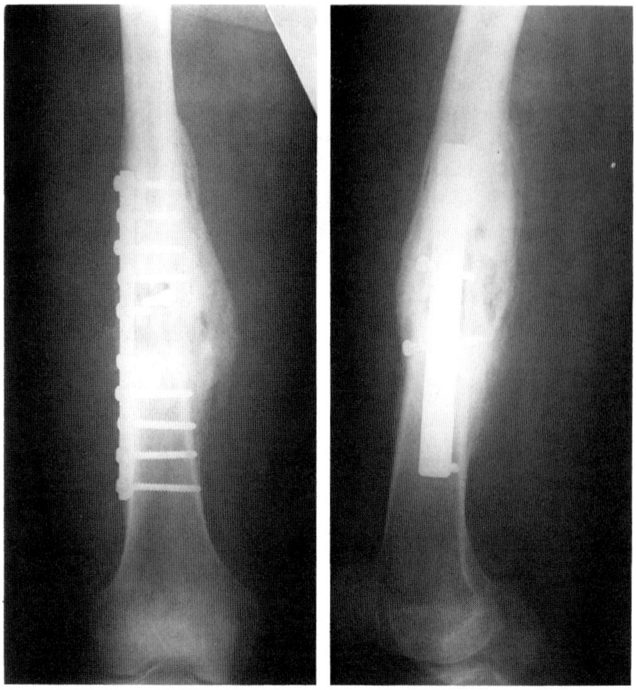

Fig. 13.32a b

Fig. 13.32a and b. Internal fixation of a comminuted fracture of the middle 3rd of the femur by insertion of a broad tension band plate (laterodorsal side of the femur), and fixation of a bony fragment by two specially arranged cortical lag screws. A large medial defect has been filled with autologous spongiosa transplant (operative report). Also, complete well-structured healing observed across the defect. Weight-bearing is possible. The inserted material for internal fixation is well tolerated by the local bone, without zones of lysis. Comment: This ist not an irritation callus, since there was a known transplantation of spongiosa.

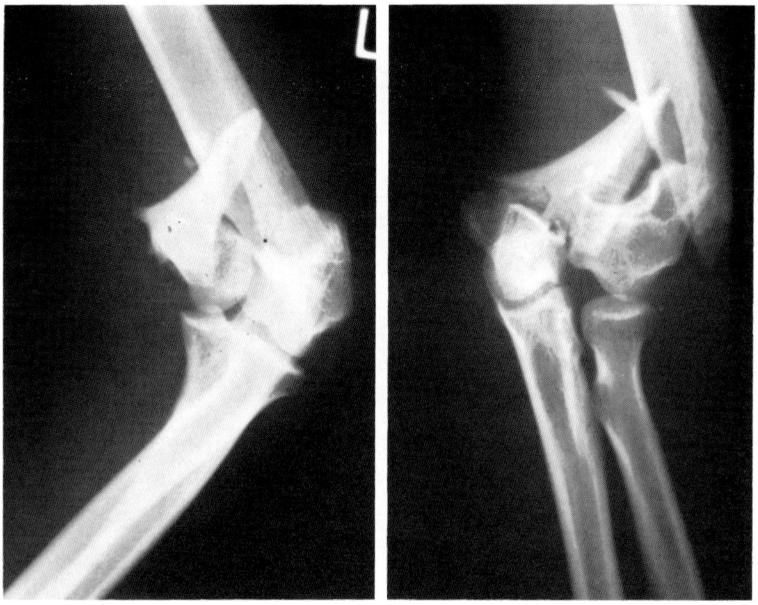

Fig. 13.33a b

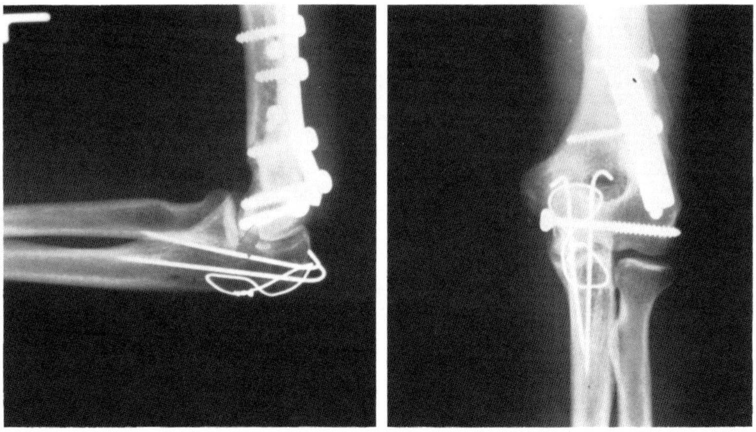

c d

Fig. 13.33a–d. A 17-year-old patient after a fall from a bicycle. Condition after poliomyelitis on the right.
a and b) Distal fracture of the humerus extending into the joint (Y-fracture).
c and d) Repair of all functions of the elbow joint using a weight-bearing internal fixation and applying the principles of the ASIF. To properly insert the internal fixation, the olecranon had to be subjected to osteotomy, with immediate stabilization by tension band insertion. The x-ray shows the condition immediately prior to removal of the metallic implants 18 months after surgery.

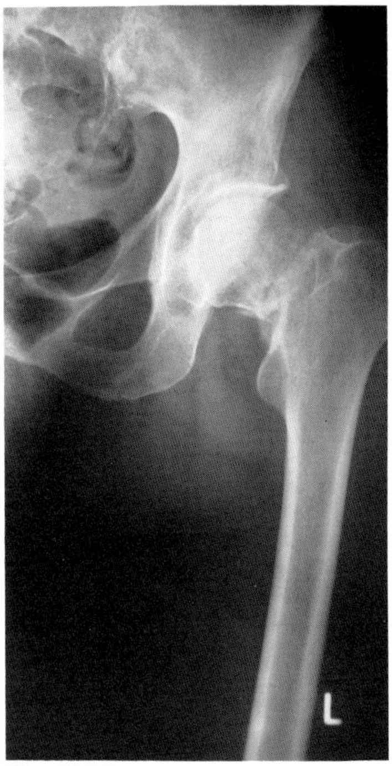

Fig. 13.34a

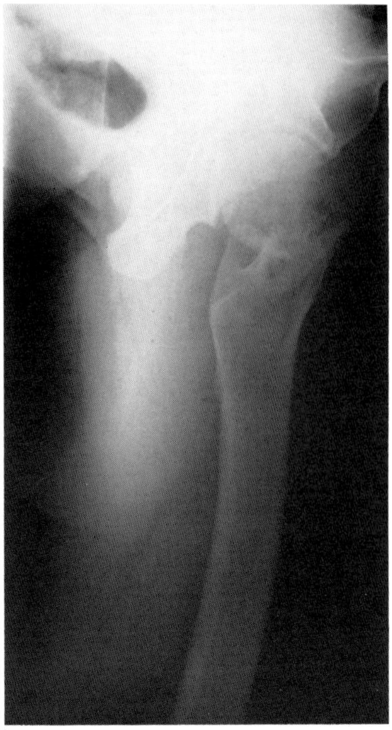

b

Fig. 13.34a–h. A 58-year-old woman after a fall in her own apartment.
a and b) Medial fracture of the left femoral neck, adduction type.
c and d) Operative management of the fracture, setting the femoral head in mild valgus position and fixation by a 130-degree angle blade platze with a 4-hole shaft and an additional spongiosa screw cranial to the blade of the plate. No local reaction to the implants. The head of the uppermost screw within the plate has broken off; the femoral head shows normal bony density and its form is round. Only minimal signs of coxarthrosis.

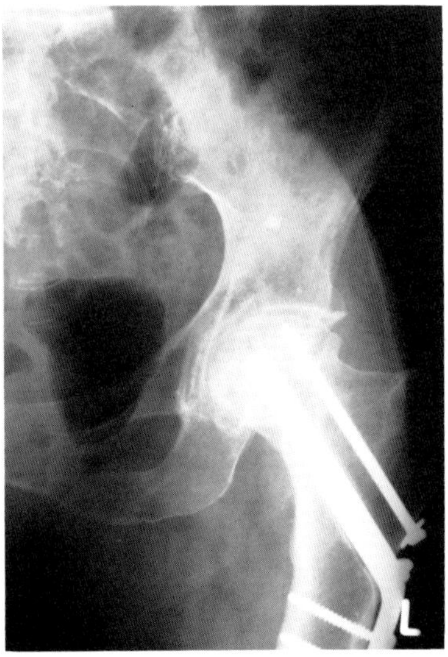

c

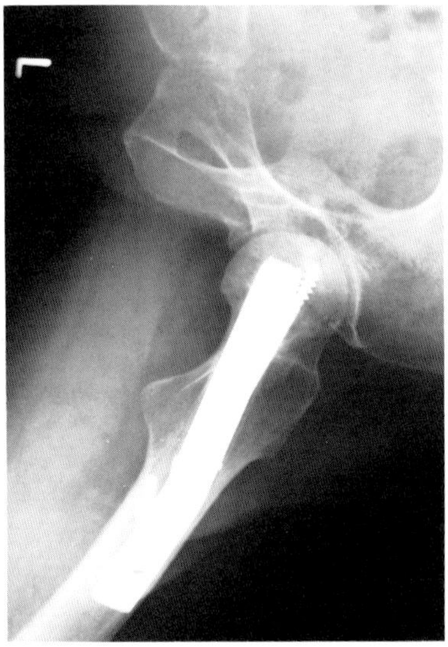

d

e and f) Almost 2 years after the accident and internal fixation, marked flattening of the femoral head, condensation and narrow bone space with simultaneous strong subjective complaints are observed.
g and h) Removal of the femoral head and total replacement of the hip, using the model of Müller. Exact location of the alloplastic parts of the joint and of the bone cement extending from within the femoral marrow space up to the tip of the shaft of the prosthesis.

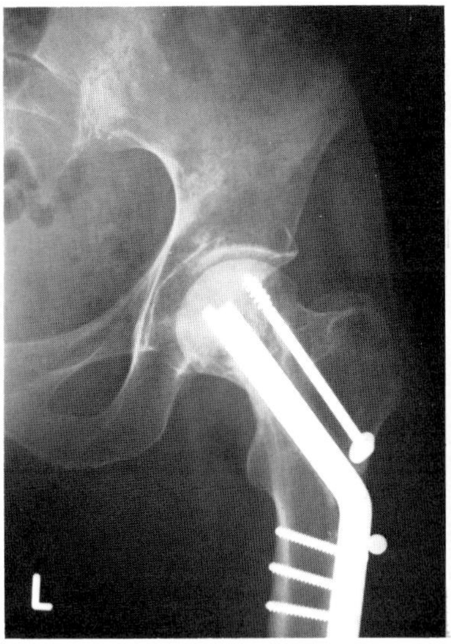

e

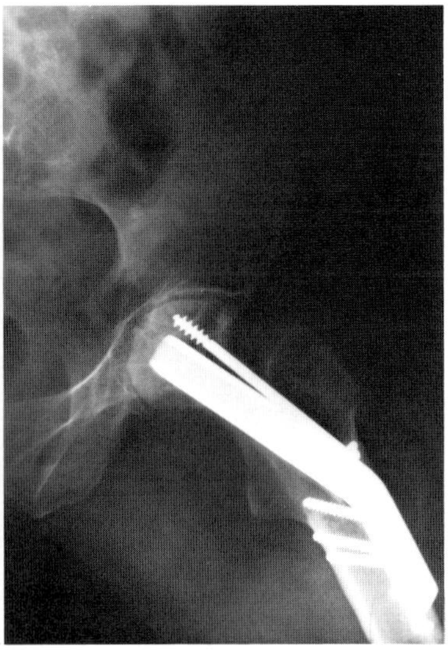

f

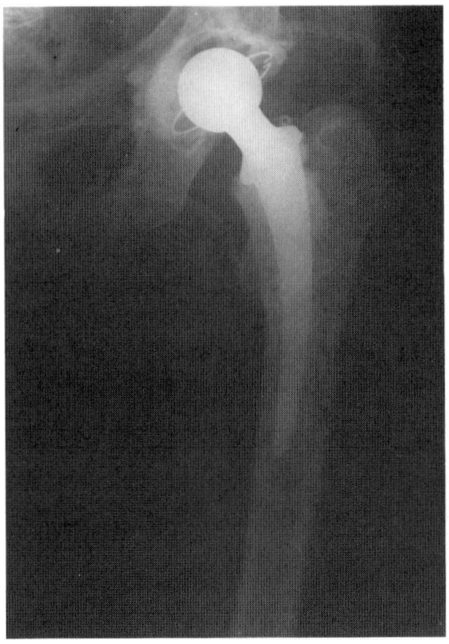

g

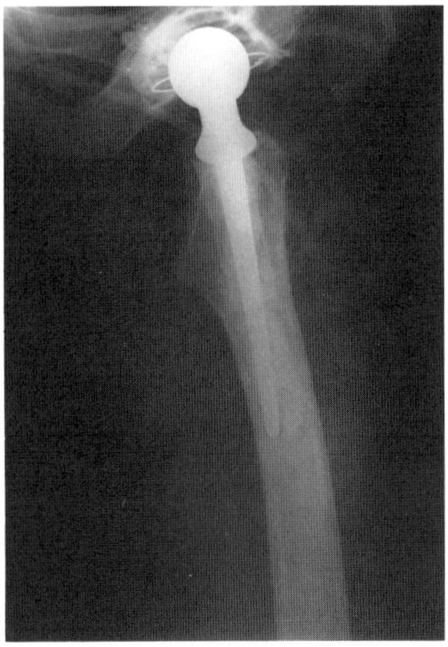

h

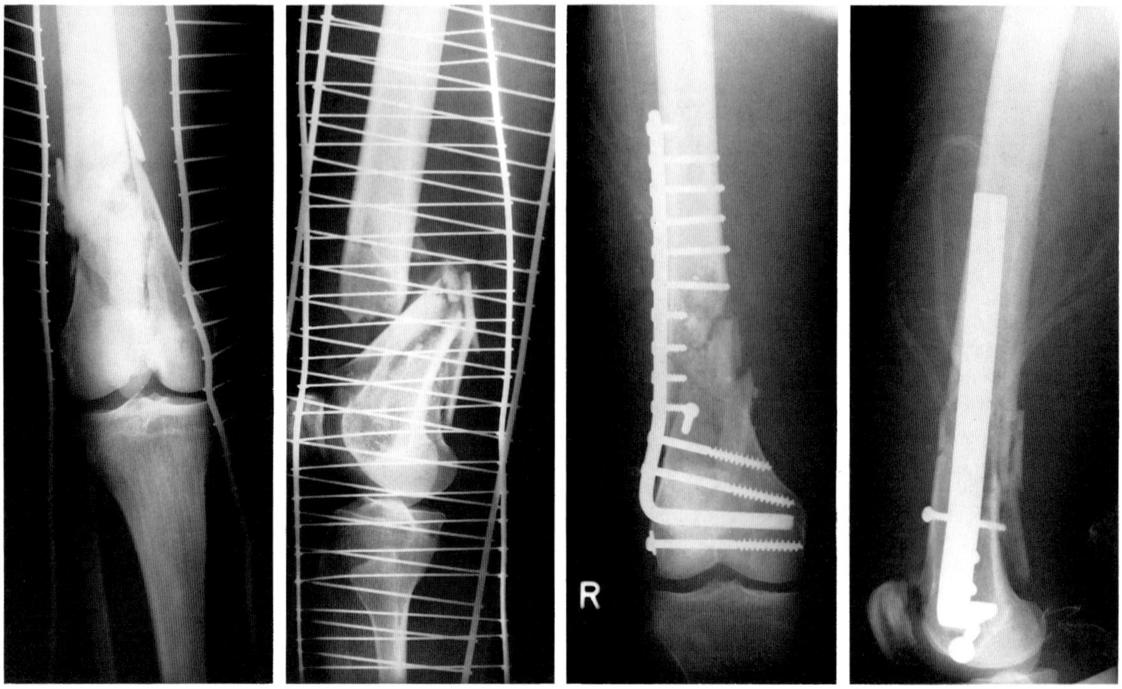

Fig. 13.35a b c d

Fig. 13.35a–l. a and b) Comminuted fracture of the distal right femur involving the joint. Typical dislocation of the distal fracture fragment dorsally. The bony fragments are individually well visualized on the lateral view.

c and d) Weight-bearing internal fixation after reconstruction of the femoral joint with insertion of distal, transversely placed spongiosa screws with washers, together with a 12-hole condylar plate. Because of the extensive mediodorsal area of fragmentation of the cortical bone and the filling of this area with homologous spongiosa transplant, it was not possible to have an exact reposition of these fragments. Only the large ventral butterfly fragment with its importance for the patella was attached by a cortical lag screw. In the upper area, one recognizes the Redon drains (on postoperative x-ray).

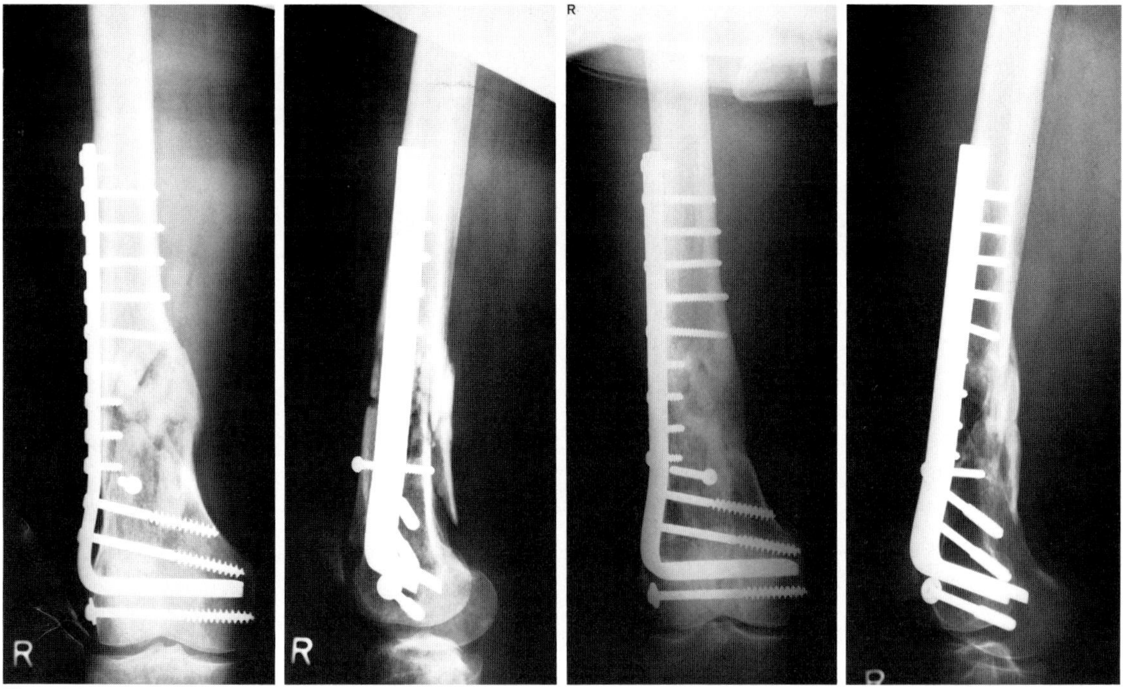

Fig. 13.35e f g h

e and f) 8 months after the accident and internal fixation, there is very active healing of the large bony defect. This process is not yet completed. The patient is bearing weight for the last three months.

g and h) 30 months after the accident and internal fixation, there seems to be radiologic healing of the fracture. Particularly on the a. p. view, complete bony trabeculation is observed across the former medially located defect. Also, on the lateral view there is now repair of the large, former butterfly fragment. The patient is asked to return for removal of the metallic implants. At this time, it appears that there is also a relatively large mediodorsal defect, so that there is a transplantation of autologous spongiosa, with replacement of the short screws in the area of the former comminuted fracture by long screws.

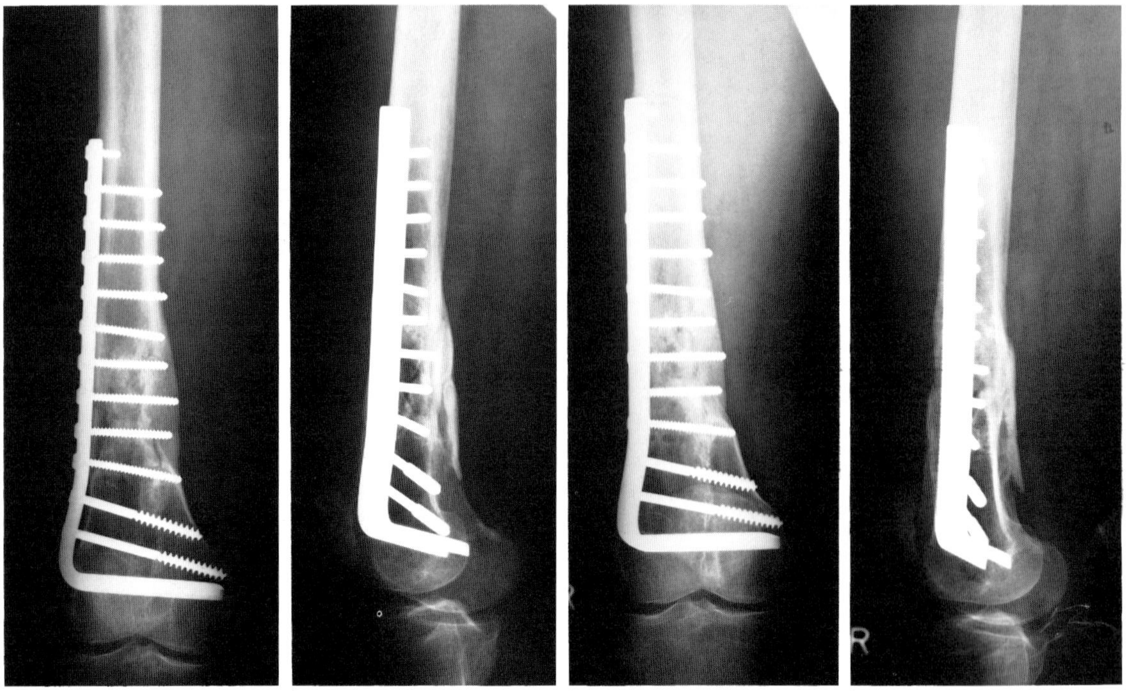

Fig. 13.35i j k l

i and j) Postoperative x-rays after renewed spongiosa transplantation and replacement of screws. The lateral view clearly reveals the local defect in the area of the 4th screw from below, now filled with autologous spongiosa transplanted from the iliac crest.

k and l) 5 months later, there is good bony stability in this area. The joint, as seen on x-ray and when clinically tested, is functional and back to normal. For the final removal of the metallic implants, it will be necessary to wait a further period of 7 months.

14 Sequelae of Trauma – Complications and Expert Reports

Normal Healing of Fractures

The purpose of repeated x-rays after fractures is not only to control the position of the fragments but, equally important, to determine the extent of healing of the fracture. Callus developing normally within several weeks will lead to an inner fixation of the fragments. As a result of this fixation, a complete bony reconstruction bridging the fractured area will occur during the following months. This so-called secondary type of bony healing of the fracture, with formation of a usually exuberant callus, is seen regularly during conservative management. For the eventual decision as to when the external fixation of a fracture can be terminated, it is important to consult the roentgenogram. Demonstration of well-formed periosteal bridging and, at the same time, the rounding and smoothing out of the originally indistinct, cloudy-appearing contours of the callus determine whether to let the patient start moving and bearing weight without a plaster cast. Until there is complete trabeculation across the fracture and the exuberant callus is reduced in size, eventually giving the bone a completely normal, functional appearance, this process will take about one year. The duration of this total healing process, before complete weight-bearing is fully reestablished, differs for the various types of fractures (Fig. 14.1). The normal duration of healing of an uncomplicated fracture, furthermore, depends in large measure upon the age of the patient; in children it is much shorter and quite a bit longer in middle-aged adults. The radiologic alterations after internal fixation of a fracture must be viewed and interpreted quite differently. During conservative

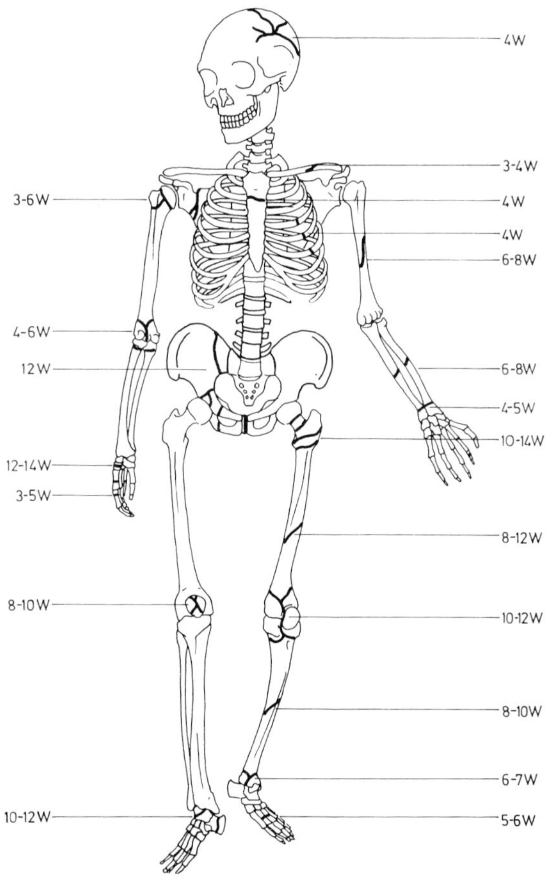

Fig. 14.1. Average duration of healing (W = weeks) of different types and locations of fractures. (From V. Schlosser: Traumatologie. Stuttgart, Thieme, 1968.)

management and in fractures with a tendency toward displacement of the fractured segments (typical fracture of the radius, shank fracture in extension, supracondylar fracture and forearm fracture), x-ray follow-up as a routine measure is needed more frequently than after fractures with a minimal tendency to dislocate and after a stable fixation.

As an expression of a metabolic reaction of the bone to trauma, there is, even during normal healing of a fracture, a reversible reduction in bony density associated with moderate structural rearrangement of the calcium-containing salts. This slight degree of posttraumatic bony atrophy is usually noticeable two to three weeks after the trauma and, within 2 to 4 months, it will completely disappear.

Complications

Whereas posttraumatic atrophy of bone is a regular parallel phenomenon, the so-called Sudeck-Kienböck's bony atrophy must be considered to be a real complication. According to Schinz (1952), this is a bony resorption and restructuring as a result of circulatory processes. Radiologically, Sudeck's atrophy must be differentiated from the usual posttraumatic atrophy of bone by its "patchy" appearance during the atrophic phase (Fig. 14.2) and its subsequent prolonged stage of diffuse atrophy (Fig. 14.3). When normal posttraumatic bony atrophy enters its healing stage, the density of the bone in Sudeck's syndrome will decrease and the stage of diffuse atrophy becomes more and more evident. The reparative changes and new formation of atrophic bony trabeculations, markedly more visible in the direction of weight-bearing, will be visible only after 6 to 12 months; this reparation will be terminated only after a long period of time. These structural alterations have also been termed hypertrophic bony atrophy and, since this is a persistent finding, also final atrophy (Fig.14.4). In long bones, the distal joints are usually involved early and to a greater degree than the proximal ones.

Sudeck's bony atrophy is seen not only after fractures but also after trauma to soft tissues, particularly injuries due to electrical current, together with aseptic necrosis (Barber, 1971); furthermore, it is observed after other types of burns, as well as during the course of infectious diseases or involvement of bone, joints or soft tissues. As a result of poor stability of a markedly atrophic bone, there is, especially during the stage of diffuse atrophy, the danger of a refracture or of a spontaneous fracture. A similar mechanism is seen at the base of Kümmel-Verneul's deformity of the spine (posttraumatic kyphosis) where, as the result of microfractures, there is a loss of height and wedging of vertebral bodies, with subsequent kyphosis.

As the result of mechanical and biologic factors, fractures can also result in the formation of pseudarthrosis. The tendency to form pseudarthrosis should be recognized at an early stage on the x-ray. Insufficient formation of callus, rounding and formation of callus at the ends of the fracture segments during conservative therapy are threatening signs (Fig. 14.5). After internal fixation, formation of a hypertrophic callus (as an expression of instability) and widening of the fractured area, with a zone of the fracture extending into the callus, are highly suspicious signs. The diagnosis of pseudarthrosis is usually simple (Figs. 14.6 to 14.8) but can be virtually impossible at the level of the navicular bone. With the use of tomography, visualization may be improved. One particular type is defect pseudarthrosis (Fig. 14.9).

An infection as a complication must be anticipated in open fractures and in injuries by projectiles but also after surgical treatment of a fracture. The difficulty of radiologic diagnosis is due to the fact that osteolytic zones within the tips of fractures and metallic implants cannot be differentiated, during an early stage, from simple resorptive atrophic alterations (Figs. 14.10 and 14.11). These are difficult to distinguish from an infectious periosteal reaction and an early formation of callus (Fig. 14.12). The later course, with a rapid increase in signs and symptoms until there is unquestionable formation of a defect, will confirm the diagnosis (Fig. 14.13). By using prophylactic antibiotics an infectious process can be masked for a long time (Fig. 14.14). Evaluation of an infectious activity in an old infectious alteration is often difficult and unreliable. The fresh appearance of a periosteal reaction, formation of a sequestrum, cloudy opacification and regional bony atrophy, as well as formation of fistulous tracts, are indications of an infectious activity (Figs. 14.15 and 14.16). Among infectious alterations, the infectious response to foreign bodies must be differentiated from the reaction to implanted metal parts (metallosis). This can also lead to the formation of fistulous tracts and, on x-ray, there may be occasional signs of corrosion after implantation of a metallic device (Fig. 14.17). Fractures of metal may be the result of too early weight-bearing or they may occur at a later time as so-called fatigue fractures of metallic implants. Bony fracture is always incompletely trabeculated at the time of such fractures (Figs. 14.18 and 14.19). Production flaws within the metal and injuries to the device, sometimes while the form is changed with the metal cold, cannot be recognized by medical roentgenograms.

Posttraumatic aseptic necrosis is most frequently seen in the femoral head. The sequence of the underlying disorders are: fracture of the medial femoral neck, luxation and dislocation of the hip and luxation-fracture and pertrochanteric fracture (Figs. 14.20 and 14.21). In the differential diagnosis, one must consider idiopathic aseptic necrosis of the femoral head, particularly in childhood, and the usually bilateral necrosis during hypothyreosis or following the intake of cortisone. The navicular bone of the hand, if fractured, will often develop an aseptic necrosis of the proximal fragment. In all cases, there is condensation or reappearance of the necrotic area as a reliable x-ray sign (Figs. 14.22 and 14.23). In osteochondrosis, this again can be considered the result of trauma or chronic trauma if there is a corresponding time interval and relationship, for instance, after prolonged work with an air-compression hammer.

During childhood, there may be traumatic damage to a growth zone, with resulting disturbance of growth, shortening and local deformity (Fig. 14.24).

Joints and the Spine

Arthrosis deformans may develop following fractures of the shaft that heal with an abnormal axis or fractures extending into a neighboring joint, and corresponds to the deformity after fracture or damage to the cartilage (Figs. 14.25 to 14.27). The onset of arthrosis deformans after trauma or the rapid increase of a preexisting arthrosis deformans can easily be determined by the x-rays taken after the accident, by the follow-up x-ray controls and by using the uninjured side as a control (Fig. 14.28). An older injury to a meniscus will be recognized by Rauber's or Jonasch's signs on a survey film, and if in doubt, arthrography will help clarify the finding (Fig. 14.29).

Dislocation involving the larger joints frequently results in posttraumatic flattening of the edges (Fig. 14.27). In the area of the shoulder, habitual luxation will cause a typical deformity (Fig. 14.30). A bony fixation of the joint is usually the result of an infection after an open fracture or a penetrating injury (Fig. 14.31).

Fractures of vertebral bodies usually will result in a deformity of the vertebral bodies and abnormal posture. Fracture of a single vertebra, with wedging toward its anterior or its lateral portion, will result in a kyphotic or scoliotic deformity. Fractures of several vertebral bodies lead to marked kyphosis, particularly if there is involvement of thoracic vertebrae . Usually, the more pronounced the deformity, the more severe is the posttraumatic spondylosis and the spondylarthrosis deformans. The differential diagnosis must consider Scheuermann's disease and a hemivertebra formation, particularly if there is no history of trauma. As the cause of Kümmel-Verneuil indirect posttraumatic kyphosis, one should assume abnormal osteoporosis and structural alterations by fusion of several vertebrae.

Periarticular calcification of soft tissues or ossifications is often seen following injuries to joints with or without dislocation or fracture, particularly after dislocation of the hip and shoulder Fig. 14.32). At the knee joint, the so-called Köhler-Stieda-Pellegrini syndrome, showing similar findings, is seen quite frequently (Fig. 14.33). Ossification within the muscle usually after a blunt injury is identified as posttraumatic myositis ossificans (Fig. 14.34). In the absence of current x-rays taken immediately after the accident, it may often be impossible to properly differentiate posttraumatic ossification from bony fragments of the fracture (Figs. 14.35 and 14.36). Posttraumatic humeroscapular periarthritis (Fig. 14.37) is feared because of its severe symptoms.

Traumatic epidermal cysts as a result of displacement of epidermis into the underlying tissues are occasionally observed in the soft tissues (Fig. 11.4) and, in much rarer instances, in bone, particularly the area of the terminal phalanges (compare Fig. 7.7).

To document late sequelae after injuries to vessels (stenoses, occlusions, aneurysms, arteriovenous fistulas) one should always use contrast injections of the respective vascular area. This may also determine whether there is a possible systemic disease (Fig. 14.38; compare Figs. 11.12 to 11.17).

In view of a possible confusion about the relationship between a trauma and a malignant disorder, the x-rays at the time of the accident will be very important; they will document the time, place and degree of local traumatic effects. For instance, the demonstration of subcutaneous or intramuscular hematoma will be of some importance in case of the later appearance of a sarcoma after a blunt trauma (Becker, 1966). The pejorative effect of trauma on a preexisting tumor – the acceleration of its local growth and the appearance of metastases – can be observed more accurately if there are traumatic alterations that can be proven radiologically. In the evaluation of a possible cause-and-effect relationship between trauma and tumor, the most important information is whether or not the tumor was present in a latent form. In early sarcomas (appearance within one year after trauma), particularly after blunt trauma, the assumption that the tumor was latently present at the time of the accident is reasonable (Stutz, 1954). The probability of a cause-and-effect relationship between the tumor and the trauma is acceptable if the latent period is more than two years, with an average of 12 to 13 years for soft-tissue sarcoma after penetrating injuries (Betzler, 1964).

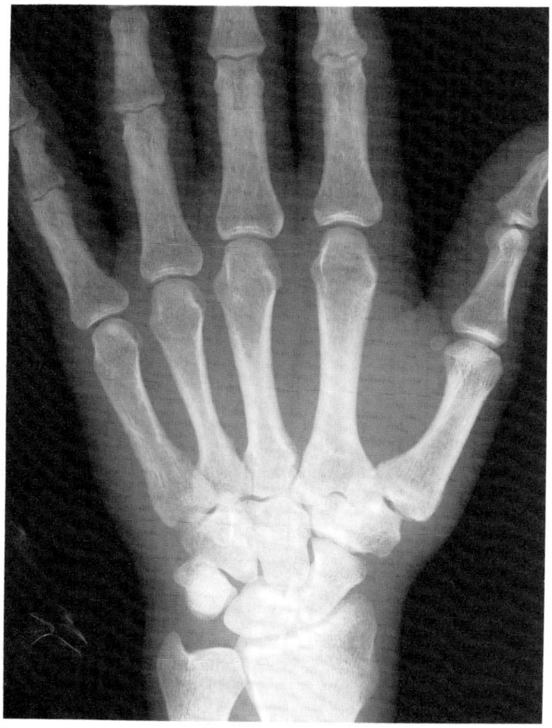

a

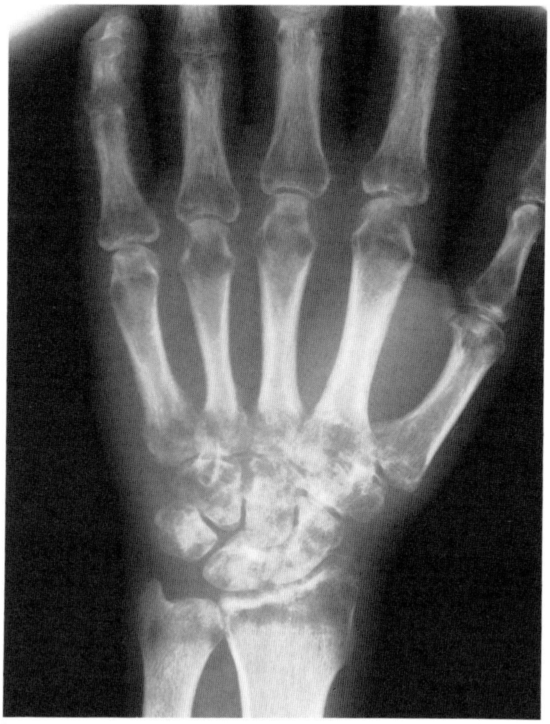

b

Fig. 14.2a and b. A 36-year-old woman with so-called "patchy" bony atrophy 2 1/2 months after a soft-tissue injury.

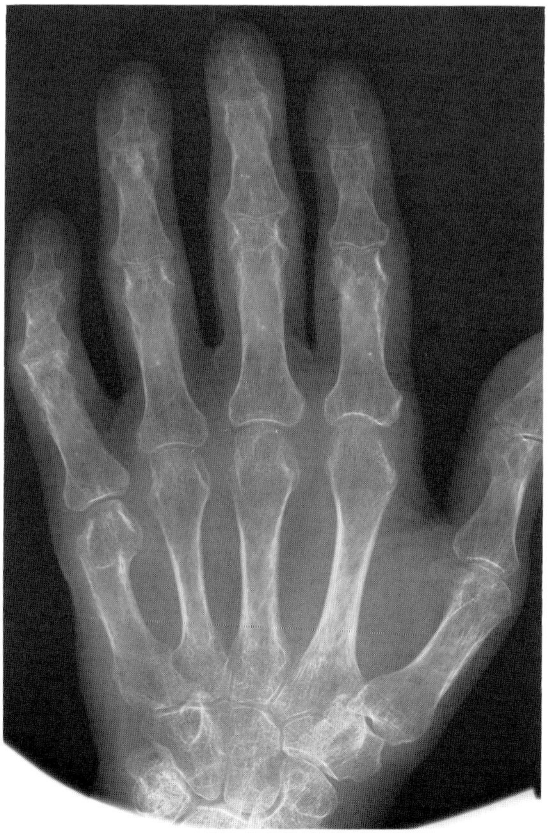

Fig. 14.3. A 68-year-old man with Sudeck's atrophy of the left hand. Transition from the diffuse to the hypertrophic stage 10 months after a fracture of the humeral neck.

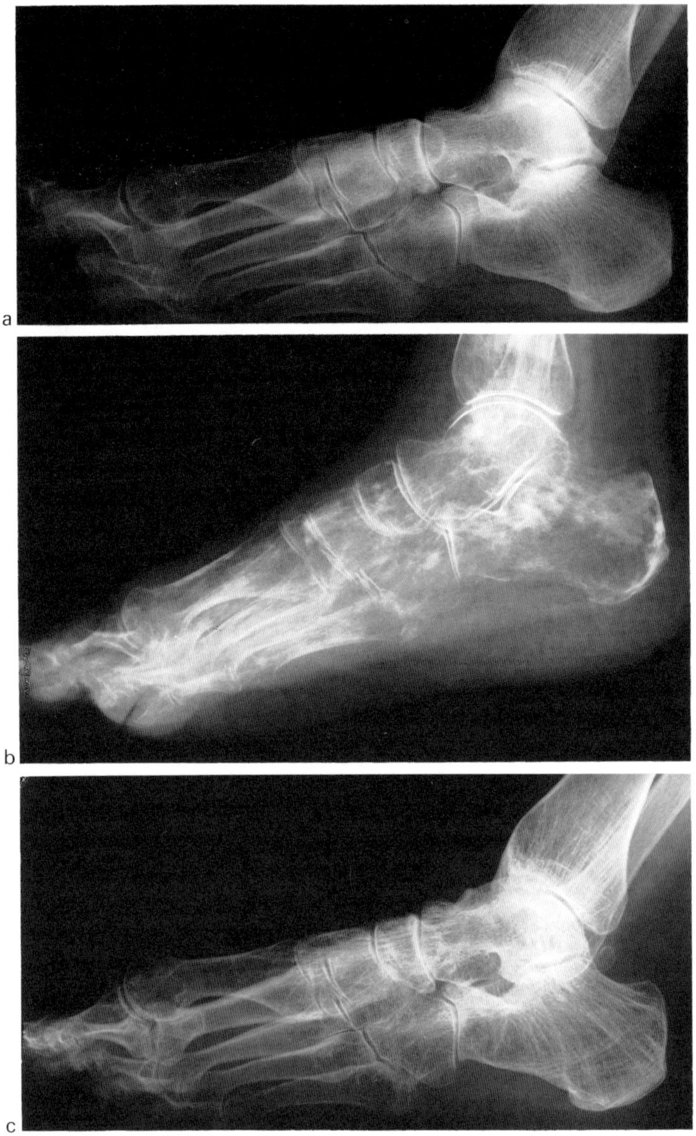

a
b
c

Fig. 14.4a–c. A 50-year-old woman with Sudeck's bony atrophy.
a) For comparison, x-ray of the uninvolved foot.
b) Transition from the patchy to the diffuse stage 14 months after the onset of atrophy.
c) Final stage of hypertrophic atrophy after 2 years.

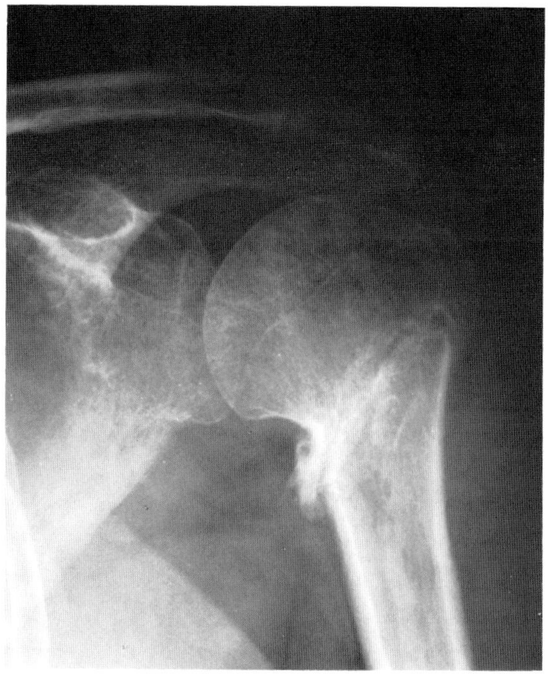

Fig. 14.5. A 43-year-old woman with early signs of a pseudarthrosis after a fracture of the humerus. Rounding and formation of cortical bone at the ends of the fractured fragments.

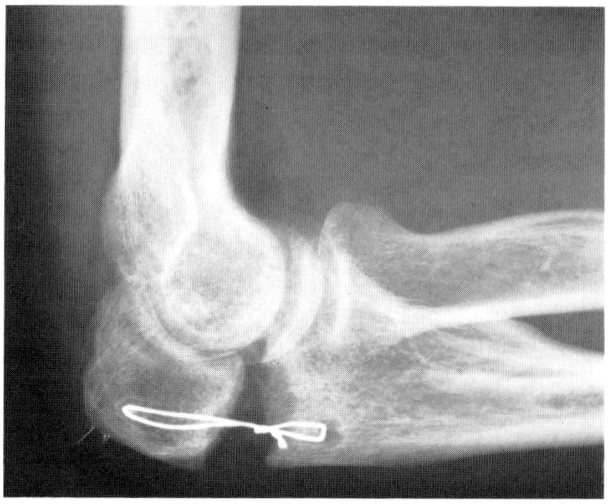

a

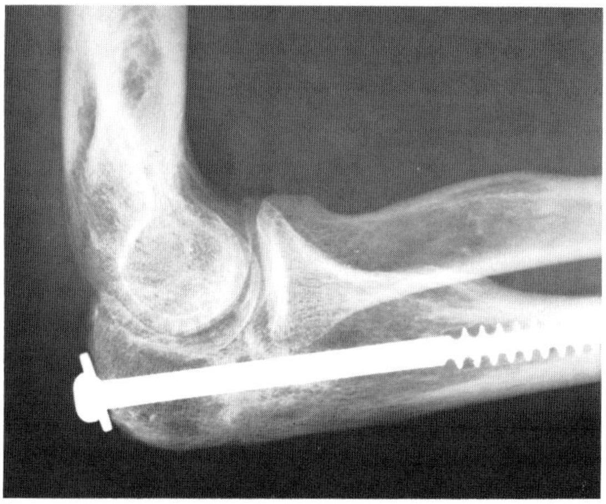

b

Fig. 14.6a and b. A 32-year-old man after an accident with a motorcycle.

a) Pseudarthrosis after a fracture of the olecranon and insertion of wire.

b) Bony consolidation after insertion of a screw.

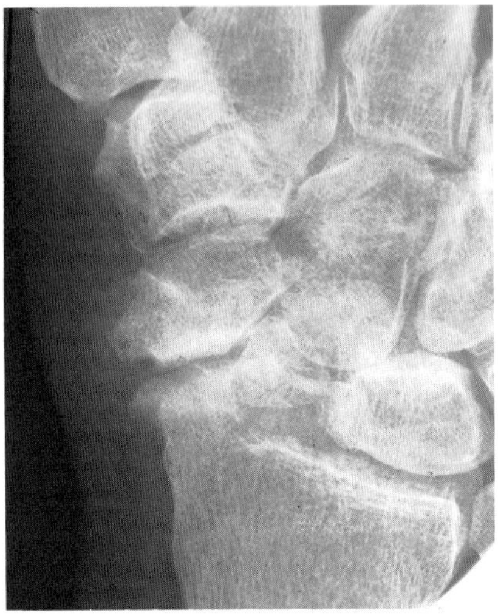

Fig. 14.7. Trauma 15 years earlier. Old pseudarthrosis of the navicular bone (frequently seen).

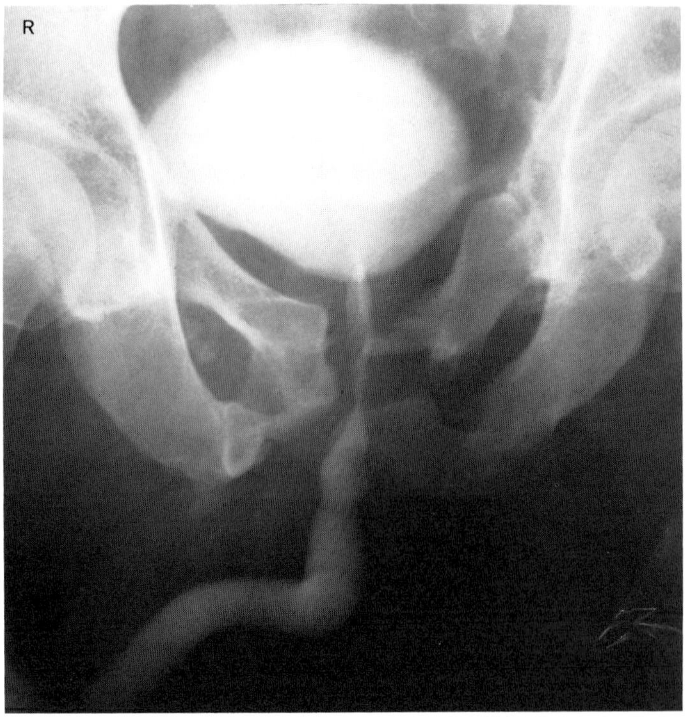

Fig. 14.8. A 35-year-old man with old pseudarthrosis of the pubic bone. Mild degree of urethral stenosis.

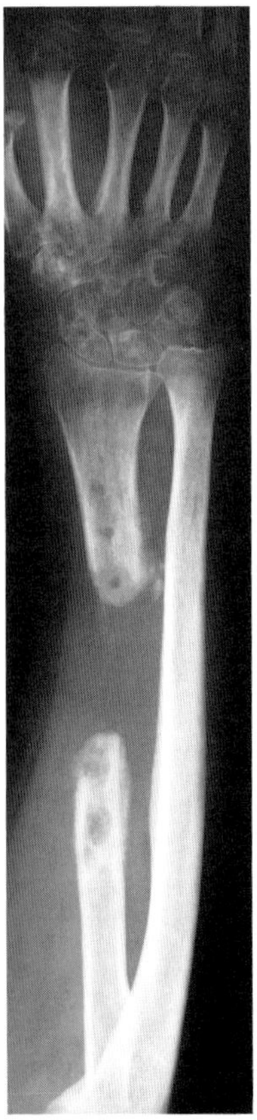

Fig. 14.9

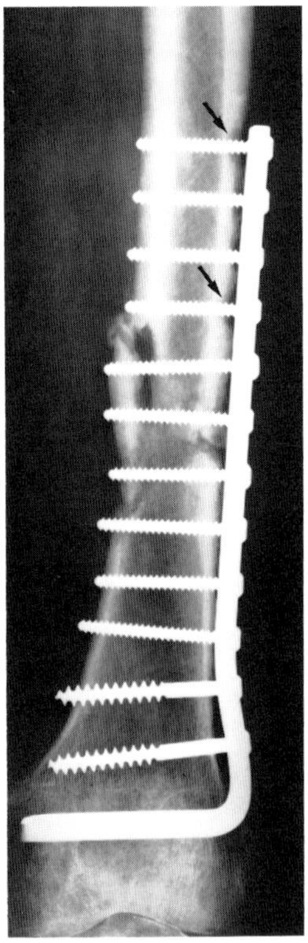

Fig. 14.10

Fig. 14.9. A 47-year-old man with defective pseudarthrosis of the radius after infected internal fixation under pressure caused by radial fracture. Sudeck's bony atrophy. Note bony atrophy of the styloid process.

Fig. 14.10. A 63-year-old man with osteolytic zones around the areas of the screws close to the plate in its upper area. Resorption at the fracture line of the fragment. Infectious process. Later, the metal parts had to be removed; formation of a pseudarthrosis.

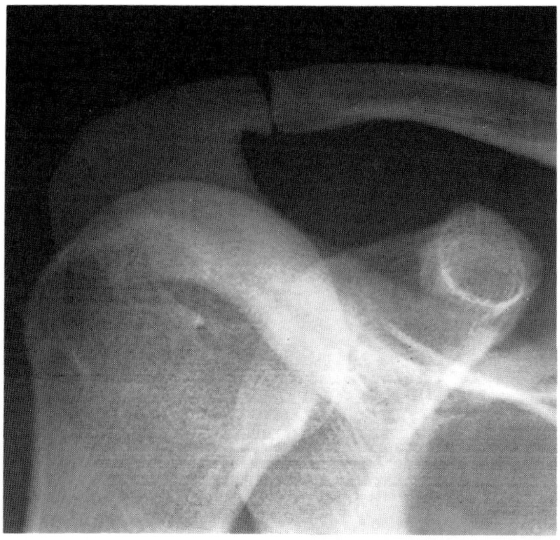

Fig. 14.11a

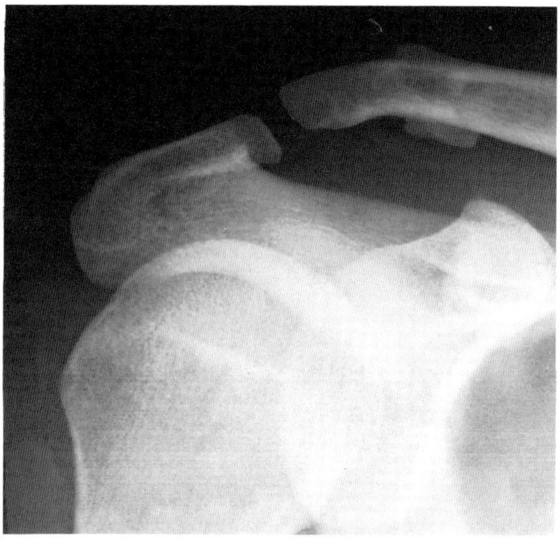

b

Fig. 14.11a–c. A 21-year-old man with posttraumatic resorption of the lateral end of the clavicle and posttraumatic ossification of soft tissues 5 months after contusion of the shoulder.
a) X-ray after an accident.
b) Resorptive defect; no local infection.
c) Final condition after 3 years.

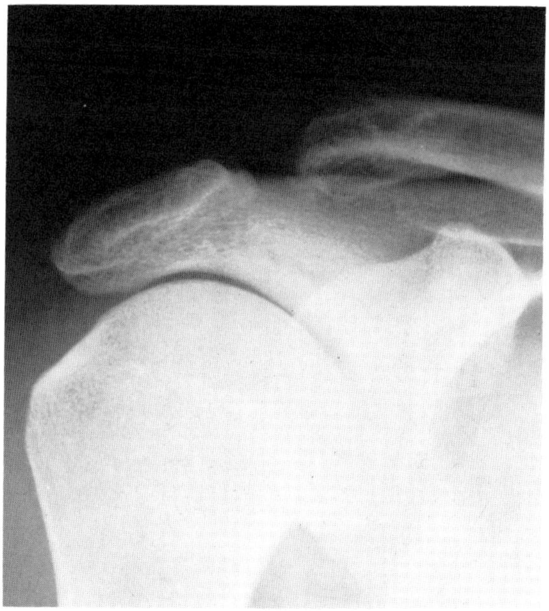

c

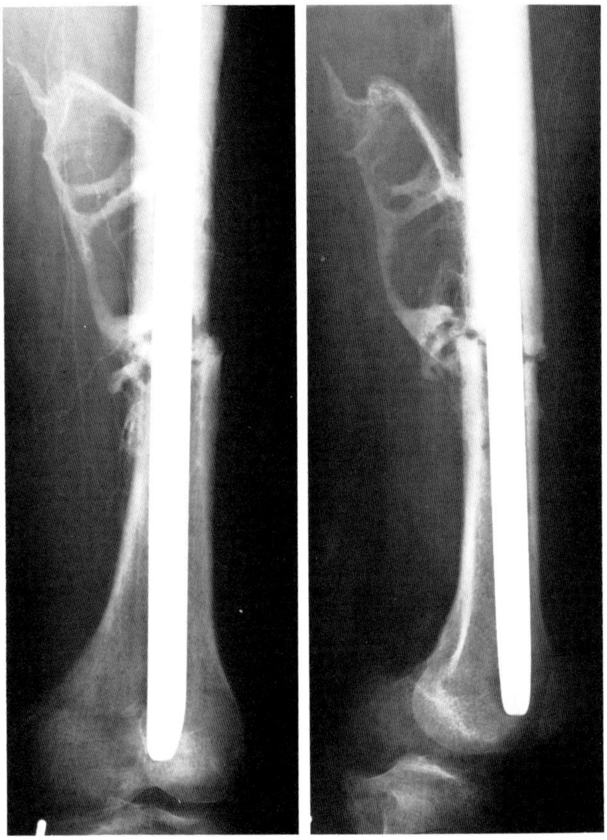

a b

Fig. 14.12a and b. A 40-year-old man with an open fracture of the femur. In addition to a bizarre callus formation, there is a mild periosteal reaction. Resorption at the ends of the fractured fragments. During the later course, there was local infection with formation of a fistulous tract.

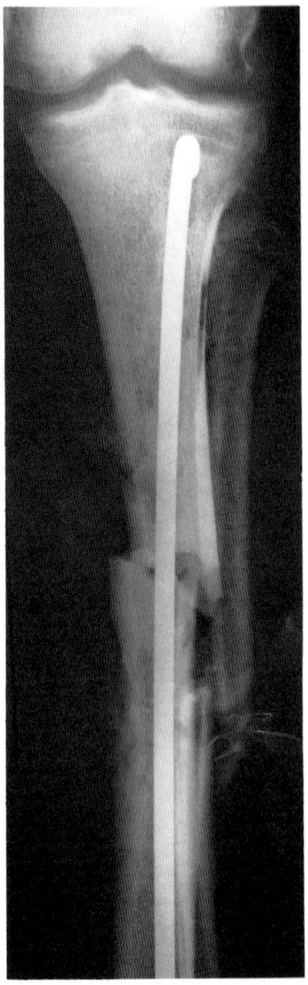

Fig. 14.13

Fig. 14.13. Active osteomyelitis of the tibia after a fracture of the shank and after insertion of a Rush nail into the tibia. Area of bony cortical defect; mild periosteal reaction. Early sequestration, particularly of the fracture fragment.

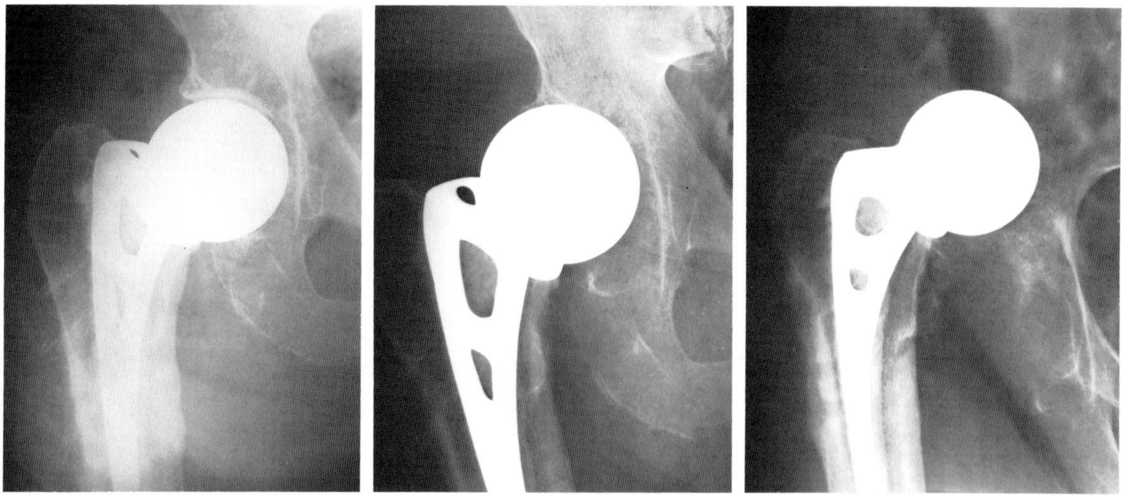

Fig. 14.14a b c

Fig. 14.14a–c. A 76-year-old woman with aseptic arthritis after insertion of a Moore prosthesis because of pseudarthrosis of the femoral neck.
a) Postoperative appearance.
b) 6 weeks later, defective contours of the joint. This was misinterpreted as being still compatible with a normal course.
c) Nine more weeks later, passive destruction of the acetabulum, with dislocation as a result of massive local destruction.

Fig. 14.15a–c. A 57-year-old man with reactivation of an old chronic osteomyelitis after a gunshot wound 24 years earlier.
a) Apparently quiescent phase.
b) Five months later, condition of a large sequestrum; infectious bony atrophy.
c) Defect-pseudarthrosis; further extension of the infectious process distally.
▼

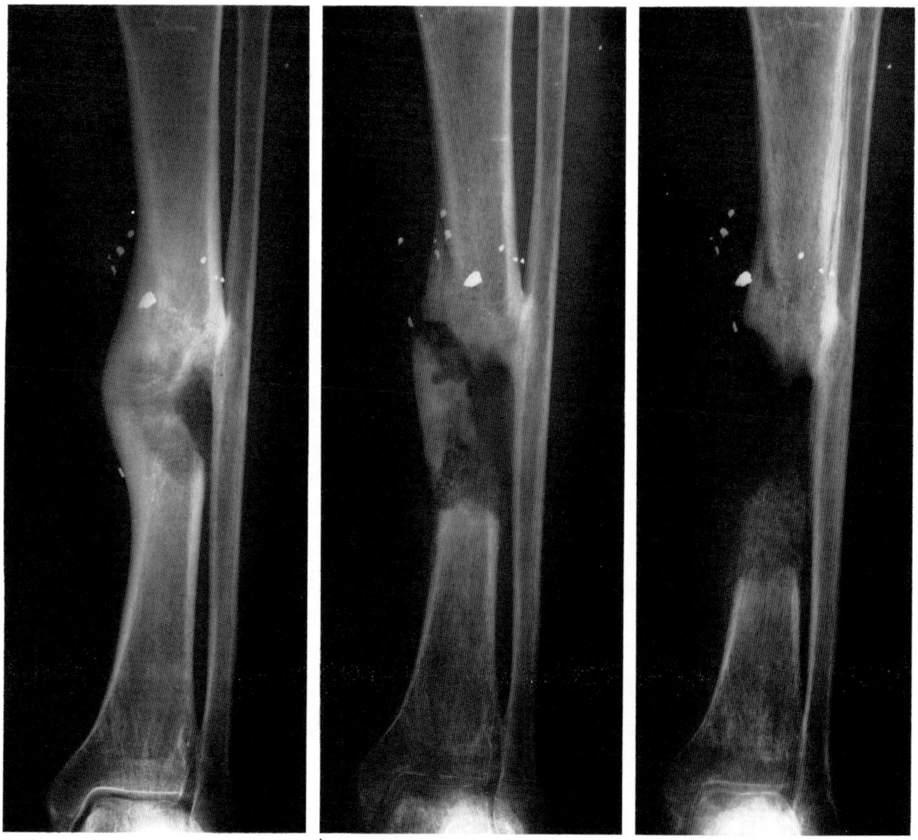

Fig. 14.15 a b c

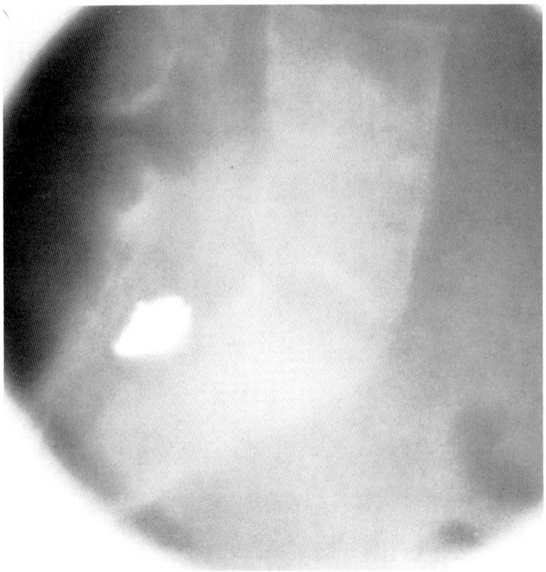

Fig. 14.16a

Fig. 14.16.a–c. A 39-year-old man who for years had a discharge of pus from fistulous tract openings in both inguinal areas and the left flank. Recent subileus; at surgery, a local postinfectious stenosis of the sigmoid and a large retroperitoneal abscess were found. Colostomy. Prior to a second surgical intervention for removal of a splinter, the patient died because of liver dystrophy. Late sequelae of chronic infection affecting the bones, joints, and soft tissues 17 years after grenade splinter injury.
a) Tomogram of the splinter located within the sacral canal. Corrosion of the dorsal aspect of the sacrum. Chronic infectious changes in the area of both sacroiliac joints and the immediate vicinity.
b and c) Fistulography; far-reaching fistulous connections with retroperitoneal extension. The splinter is located in the center of the fistulous tracts.

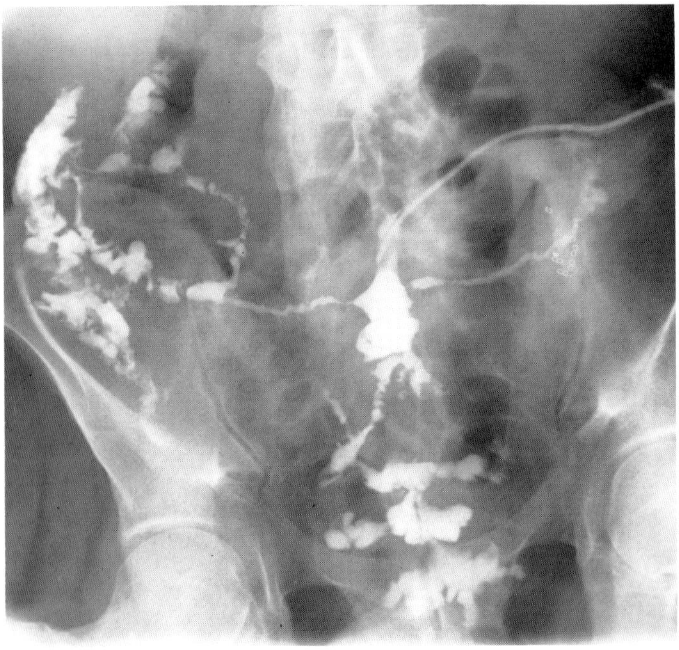

b

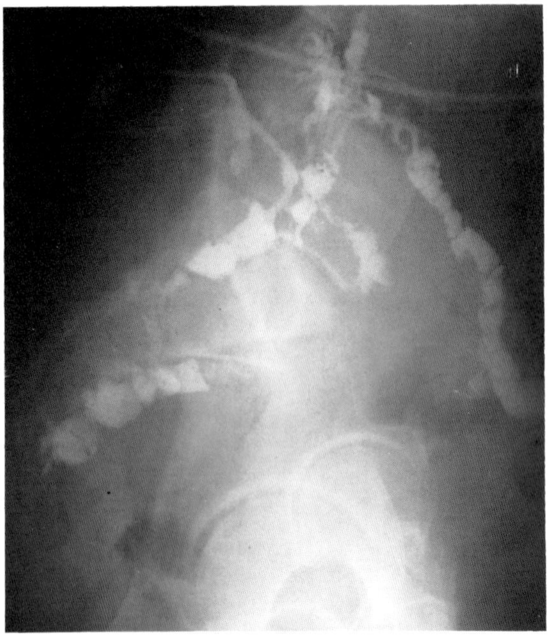

c

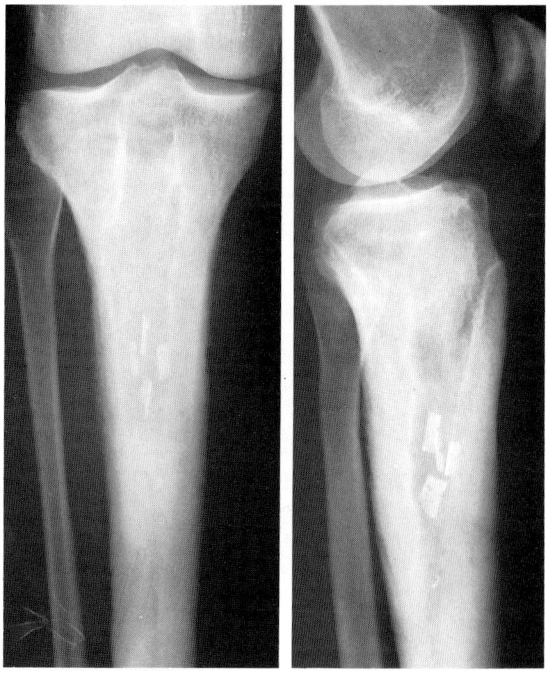

Fig. 14.17a b

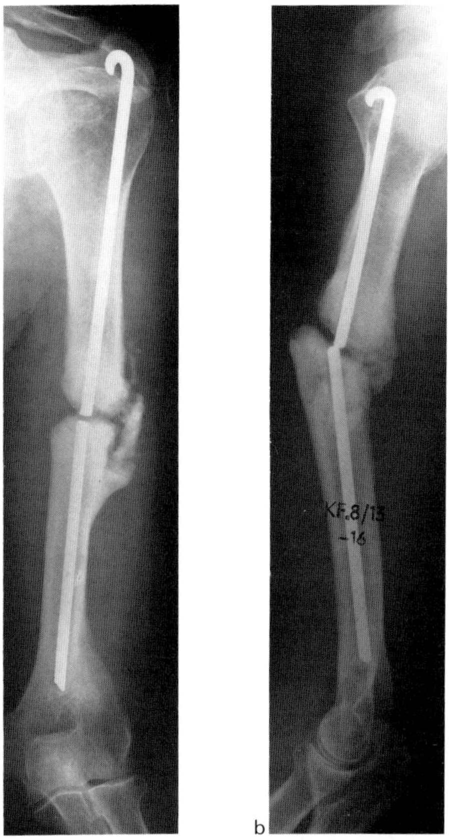

Fig. 14.18a b

Fig. 14.17a and b. A 30-year-old man who had a Küntscher nail removed 4 years previously after a fully consolidated tibial fracture. Owing to corrosion, metallic fragments remained in the marrow cavity after removal of the nail. Chronic infectious sclerosis response of the bone.

Fig. 14.18a and b. A 61-year-old man with Rush pin. It was attempted to stabilize the humeral midshaft fracture. Fracture of the pin; pseudarthrosis. After removal of the pin and insertion of an internal fixation by plate, bony consolidation.

Fig. 14.19. A 75-year-old woman who when boarding a plane, noticed a sudden cracking noise in the left hip. Fatigue fracture of metal one year after internal fixation. The fracture of the femoral neck does not show trabeculation across.

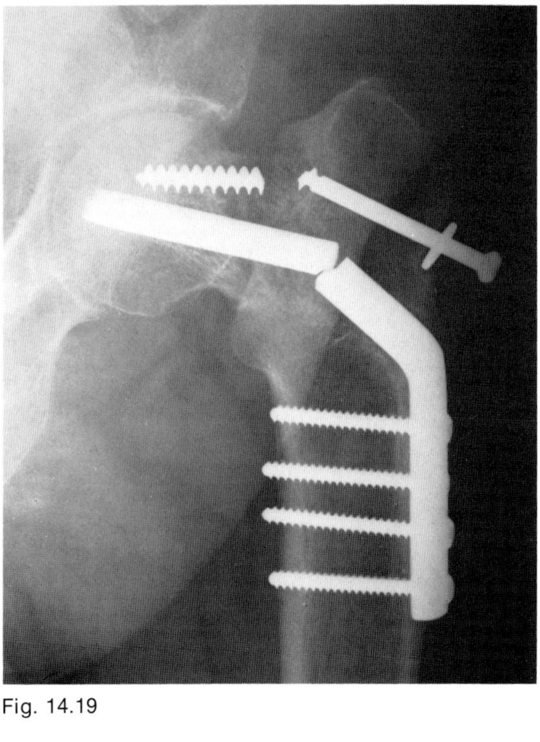

Fig. 14.19

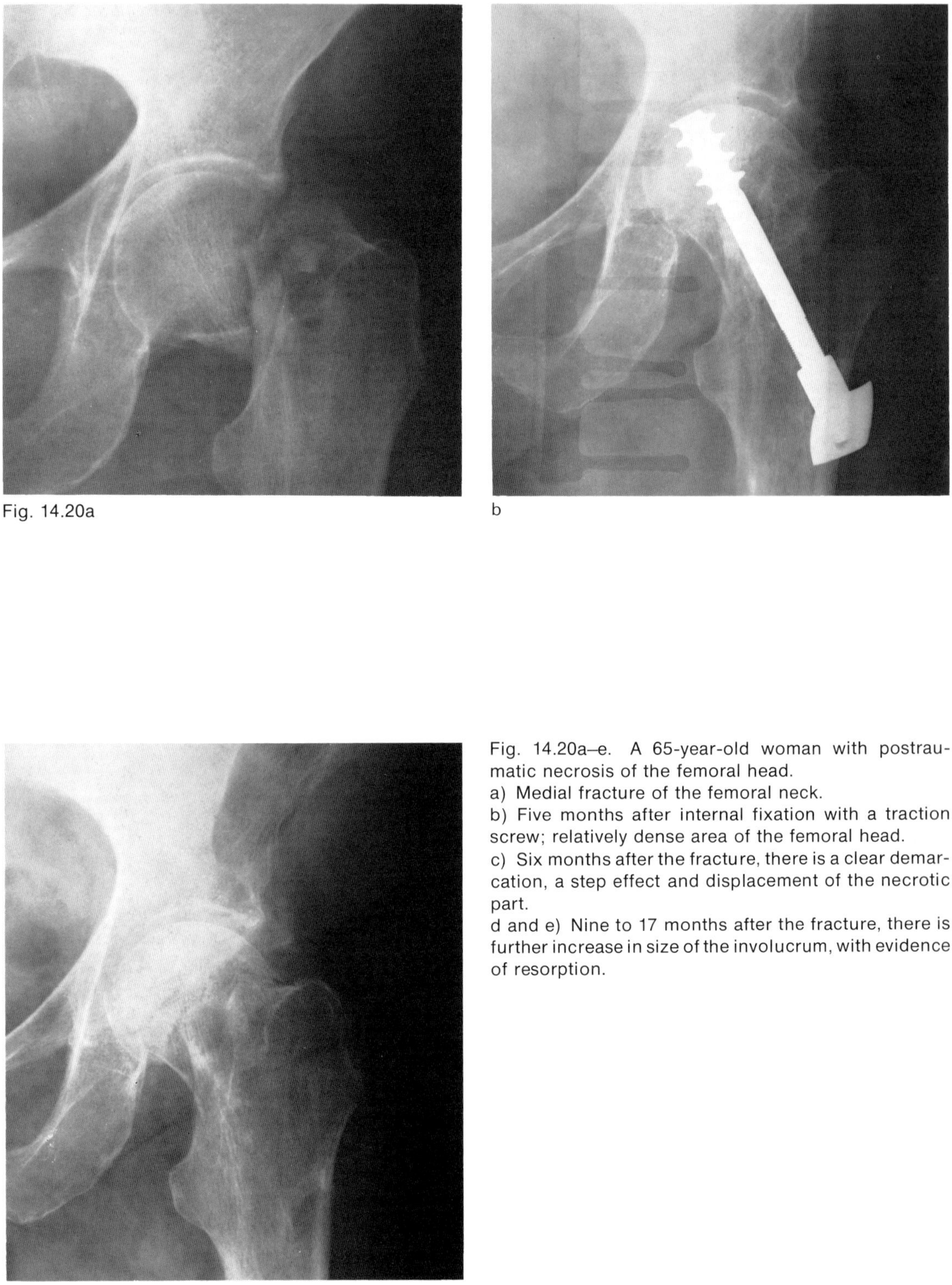

Fig. 14.20a

b

c

Fig. 14.20a–e. A 65-year-old woman with postraumatic necrosis of the femoral head.

a) Medial fracture of the femoral neck.

b) Five months after internal fixation with a traction screw; relatively dense area of the femoral head.

c) Six months after the fracture, there is a clear demarcation, a step effect and displacement of the necrotic part.

d and e) Nine to 17 months after the fracture, there is further increase in size of the involucrum, with evidence of resorption.

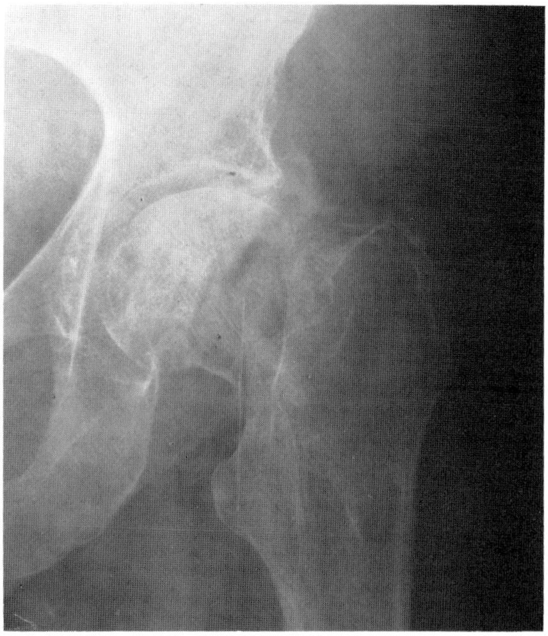

Fig. 14.20d

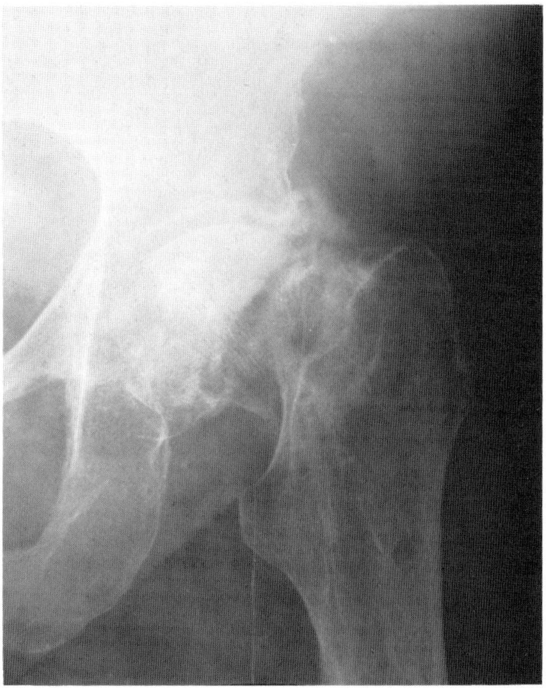

e

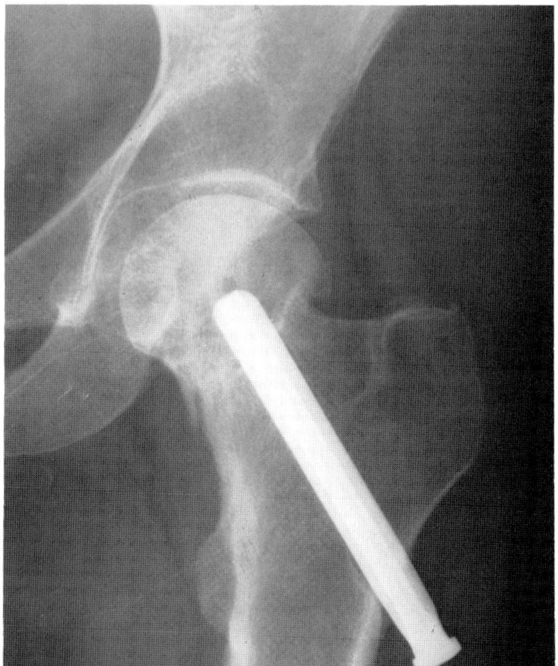

a

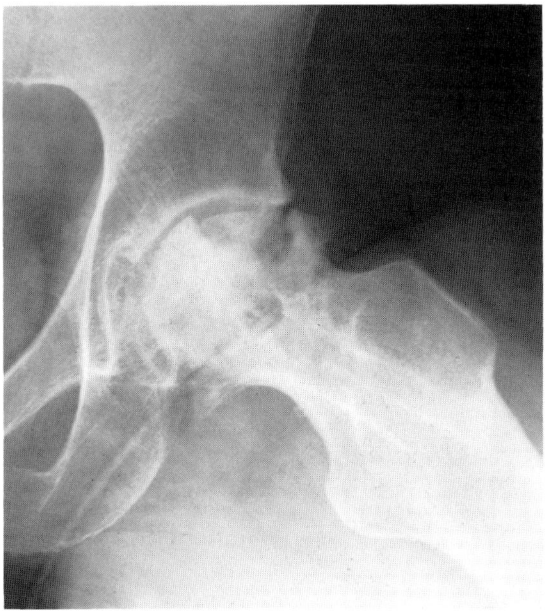

b

Fig. 14.21a and b. A 48-year-old woman with late necrosis of the left femoral head. Hip nail removed after one year when fracture looked radiologically healed. After almost 4 years, appearance of radiologic and clinical signs of necrosis of the femoral head. The onset of necrosis can be estimated at 3 years after the fracture.

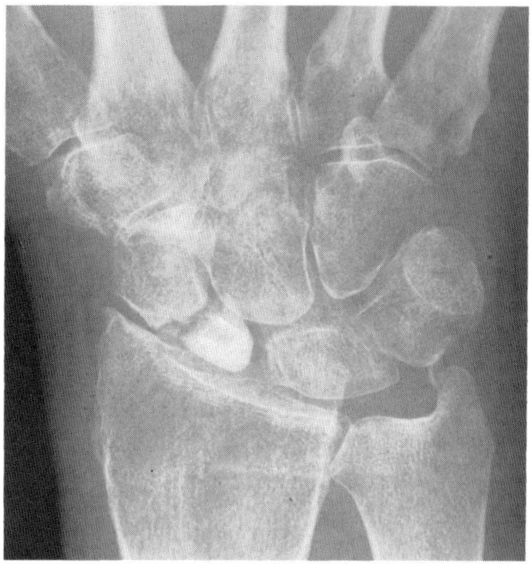

Fig. 14.22. A 43-year-old man with posttraumatic aseptic necrosis of the proximal segment of the fractured navicular bone 3 months after the fracture (fracture of the navicular bone, the radius and the ulnar styloid process).

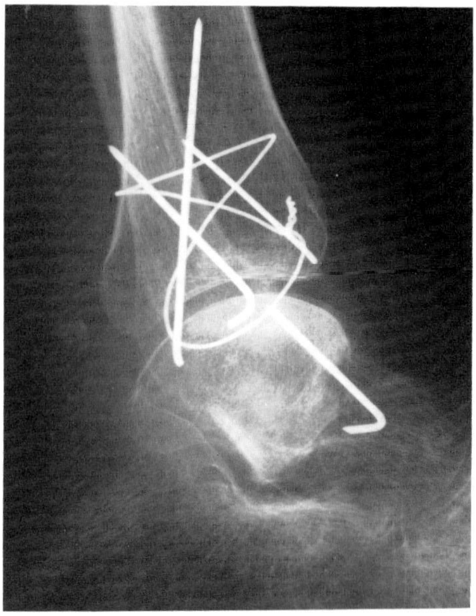

Fig. 14.23. A 20-year-old man after a fall from a scaffold 2 meters high. Early signs of necrosis of the talus 4 months after a fracture of the talus and luxation-fracture of the ankle joint. Relative density of the necrotic area.

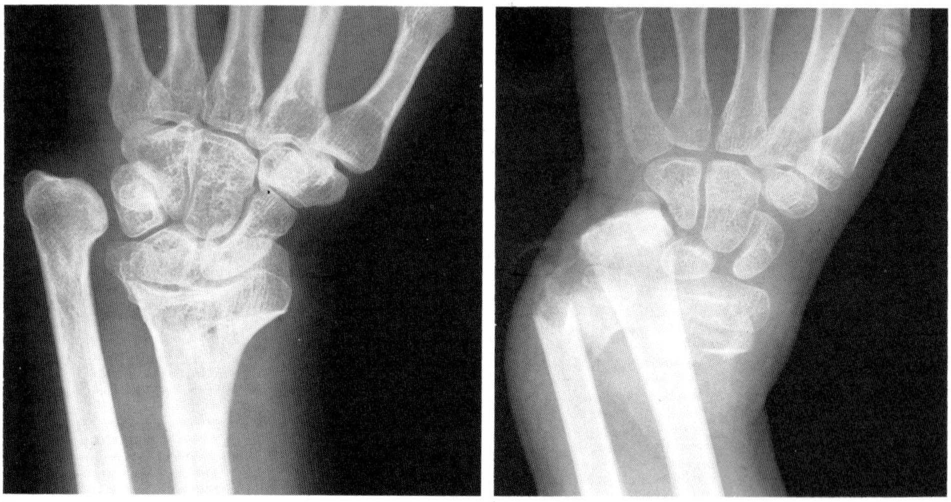

a b

Fig. 14.24a and b. A 28-year-old woman with severe deformity due to considerable shortening of the radius subsequent to an open fracture and epiphysiolysis at the age of 8 years.

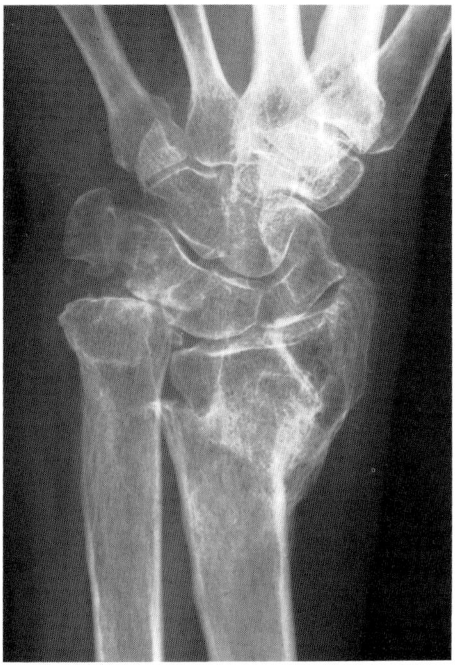

Fig. 14.25. A 65-year-old man with posttraumatic arthrosis deformans after a fracture of the radius with joint involvement.

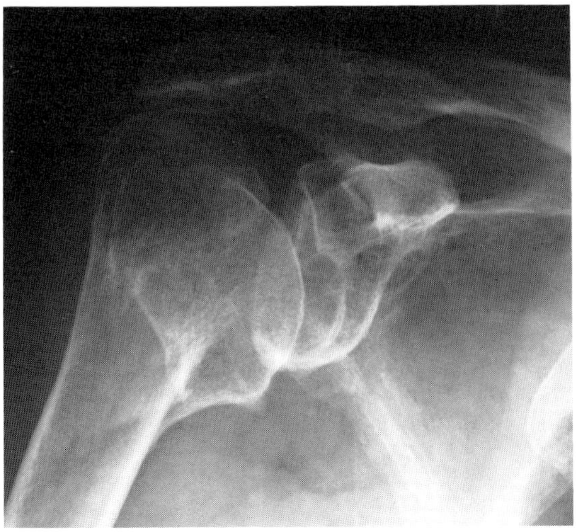

a

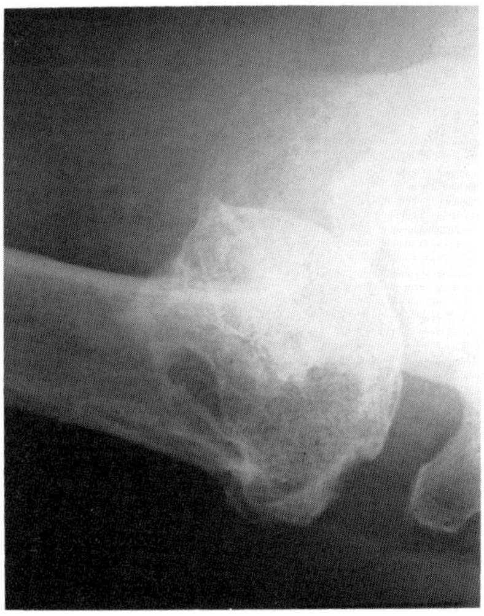

b

Fig. 14.26a and b. Posttraumatic arthrosis deformans of the right shoulder joint after a fracture of the neck of the humerus. The connection between the dislocation ot the humeral head and the deformity of the joint is obvious.

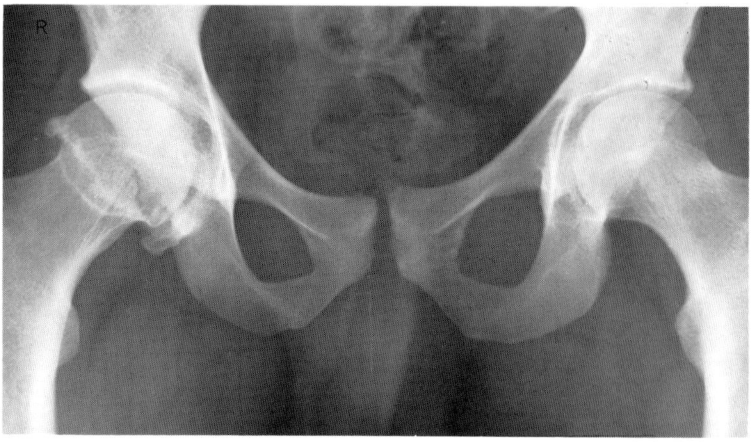

Fig. 14.27a

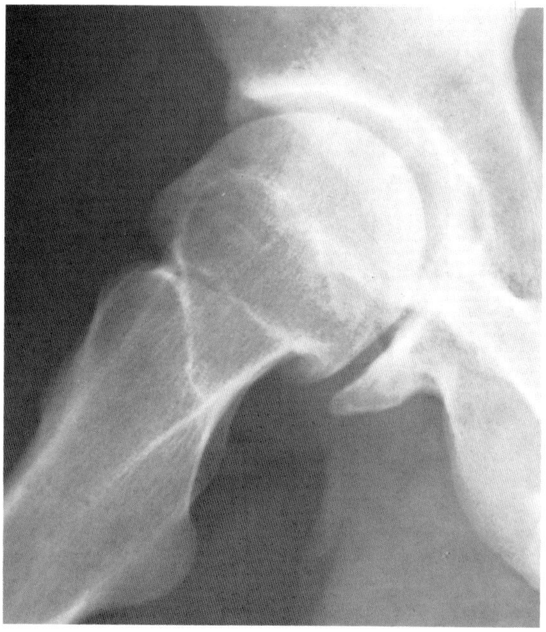

Fig. 14.27b

Fig. 14.27a and b. A 21-year-old man. Because of disturbed growth, there is a reduction in the size of the right ischiopubic segment. Severe arthrosis deformans of the right hip joint 5 years after luxation of the right hip during an accident at work.

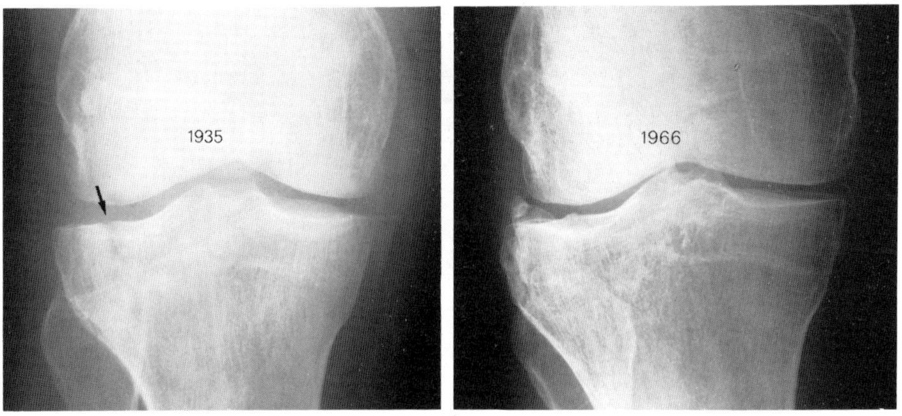

a b

Fig. 14.28a and b. Posttraumatic arthrosis deformans after a fracture of the tibial plateau, without significant displacement.

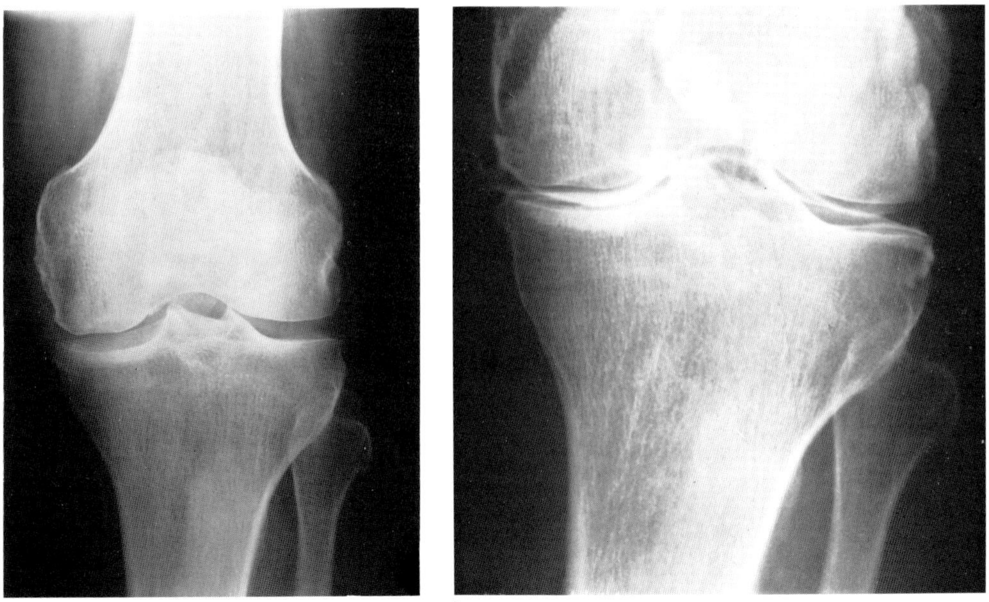

a b

Fig. 14.29a and b. Lesion of the meniscus as a result of distrotion of the knee joint.
a) On film, Rauber's sign (Console immediately below the articular surface) and marked Jonasch's sign (zone of rarefaction; thickening of the cortical bone at the medial tibial plateau).
b) Arthrogram: rupture of the medial meniscus.

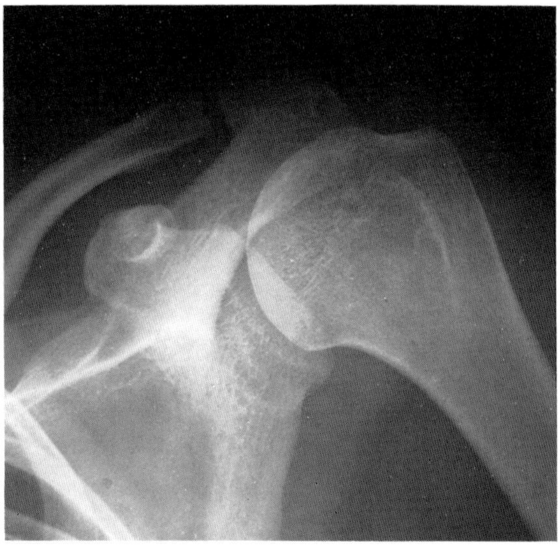
a

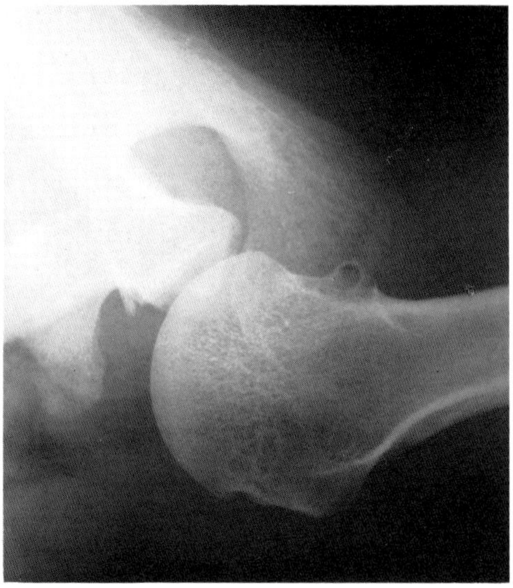
b

Fig 14.30a and b. A 23-year-old woman with an early appearance of arthrosis deformans in the shoulder joint; habitual luxation. Moderate degree of Hermodsson's sign.

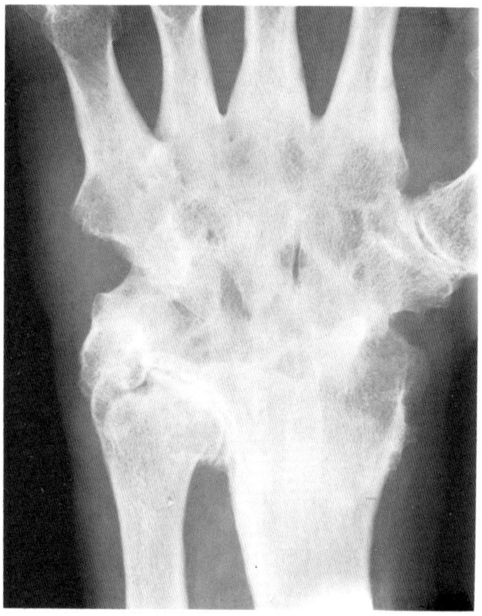

Fig. 14.31. A 85-year-old man with fixation (stiffening) of the carpus, including the radial carpal and metacarpal joints, after a gunshot wound during World War I. Recidivating fistulae.

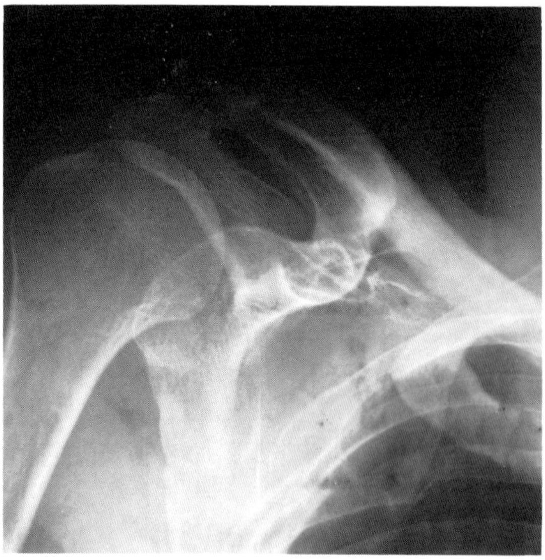

Fig. 14.32. A 44-year-old man with ossification in the coracoclavicular ligament after dislocation of the acromioclavicular joint. Old fracture of the 3rd and 4th ribs on the right.

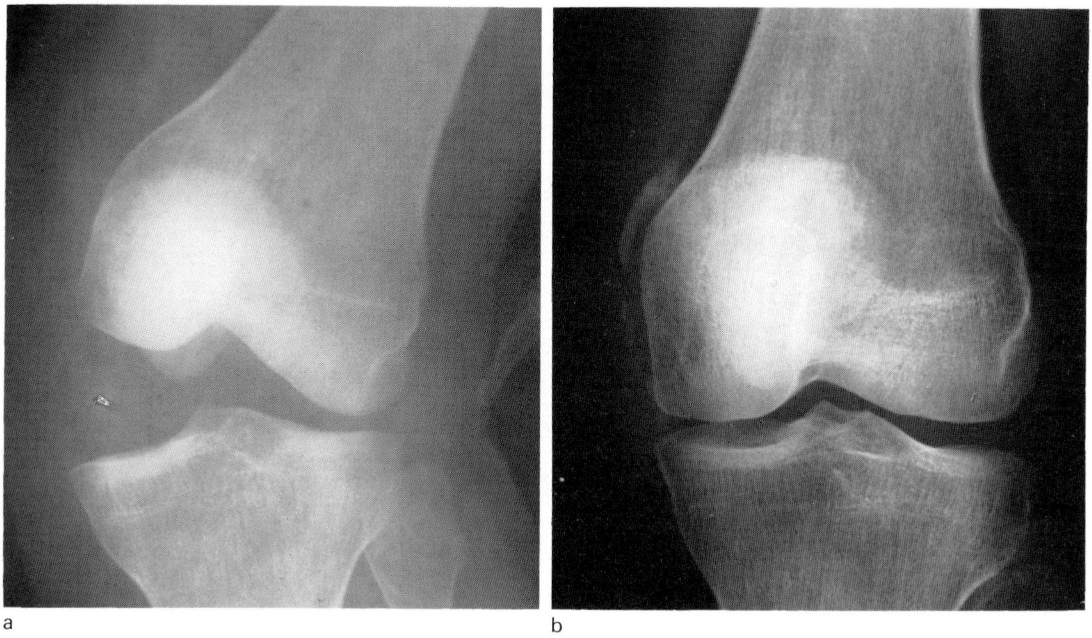

Fig. 14.33a and b. A 35-year-old woman, with Köhler-Stieda-Pellegrini's shadow and calcification in the medial lateral ligament. Rupture of the medial ligament while skiing.

a) After the accident: film while pulling at knee with wide opening of the medial joint space.
b) Two years after the accident.

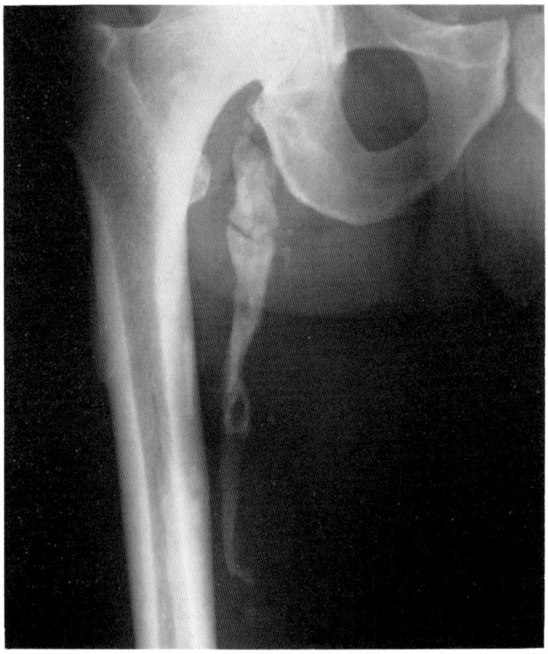

Fig. 14.34. Posttraumatic myositis ossificans of the adductor muscles.

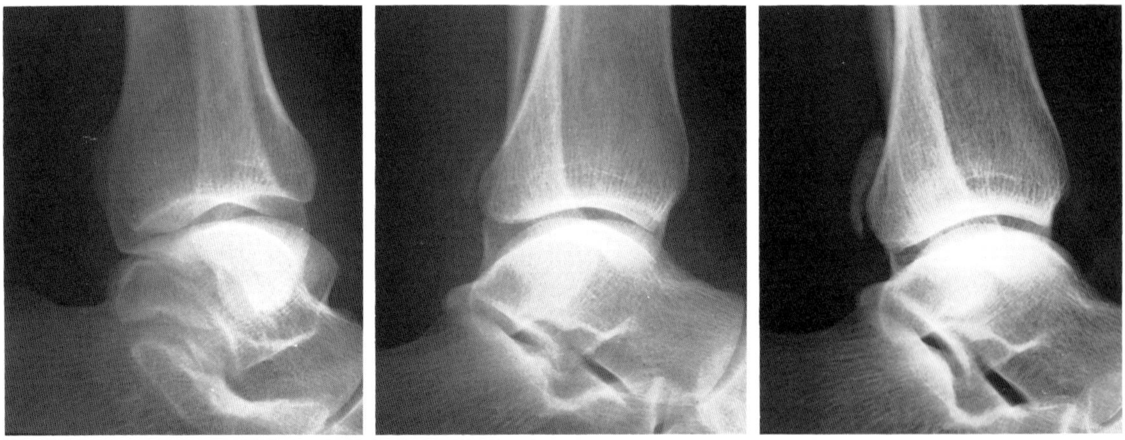

Fig. 14.35a–c. A 65-year-old man, development of a posttraumatic soft-tissue ossification over the distal and dorsal edges of the tibia.

a) Film after the accident.
b) One month later.
c) 6 months later.

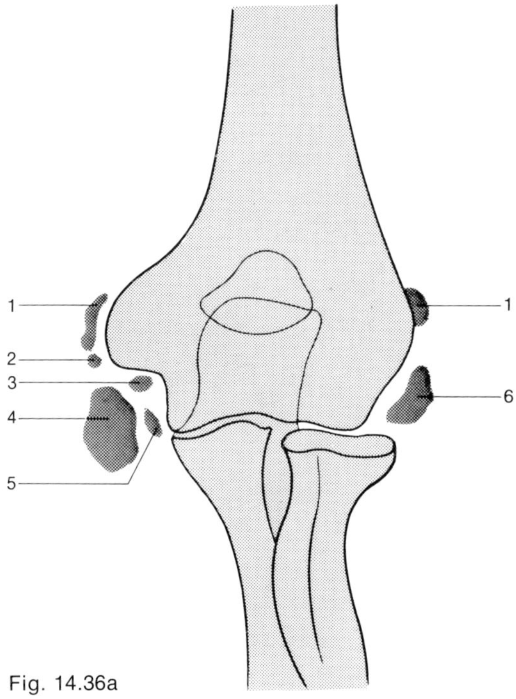

Fig. 14.36a

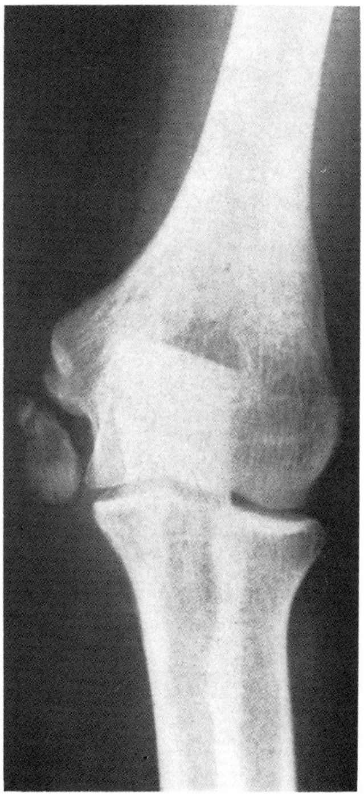

Fig. 14.36b

▲
Fig. 14.36a and b. Posttraumatic periarticular calcific and bony shadows in the area of the elbow.
a) 1 = soft-tissue calcification; 2 = persistent apophysis; 3 = calcific periarthritis; 4 = persistent posttraumatic apophysis; 5 = fragments; 6 = postraumatic calcific deposits in an hematoma.
b) Posttraumatic persistent apophysis. (From Z. Bánki: Fortschr. Röntgenstr. *101*:501, 1964.)

Fig. 14.37. A 22-year-old woman with a contusion of the shoulder 1 month ago. Posttraumatic humeroscapular periarthritis; also known by the term calcific peritendinitis with other joints.

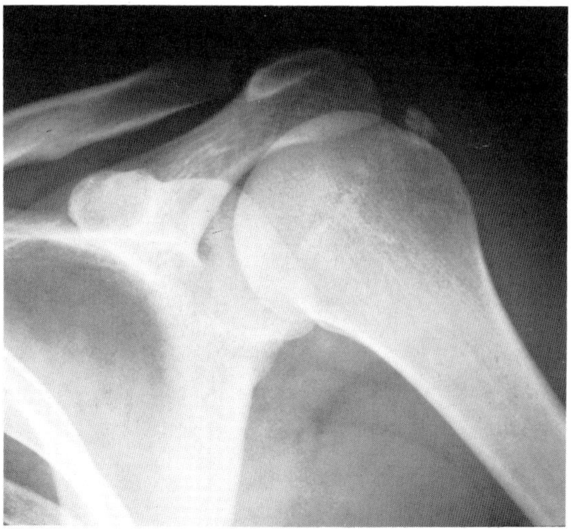

Fig. 14.37

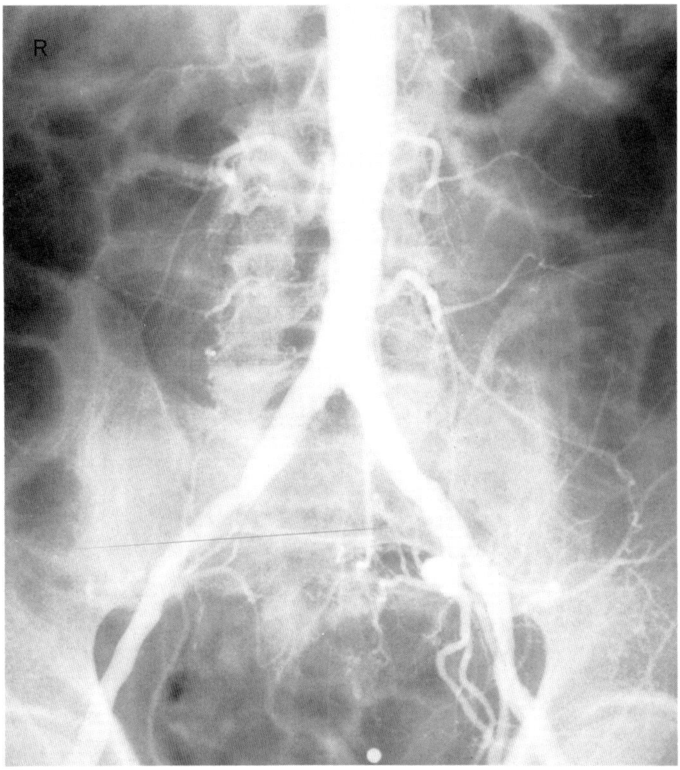

Fig. 14.38a

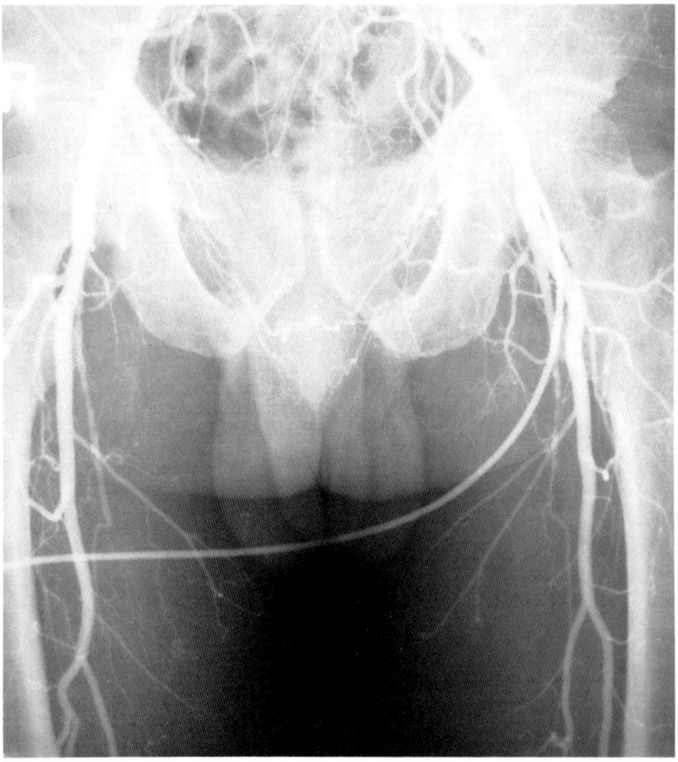

b

Fig. 14.38a–f. A 54-year-old man with interruption of the left posterior tibial artery and obliterating stenosis of the rest of the vessel after a gunshot wound and fracture of the fibula 27 years previously. In addition, there is a well-compensated arterial occlusive disease involving vessels within the femoral and pelvic areas.

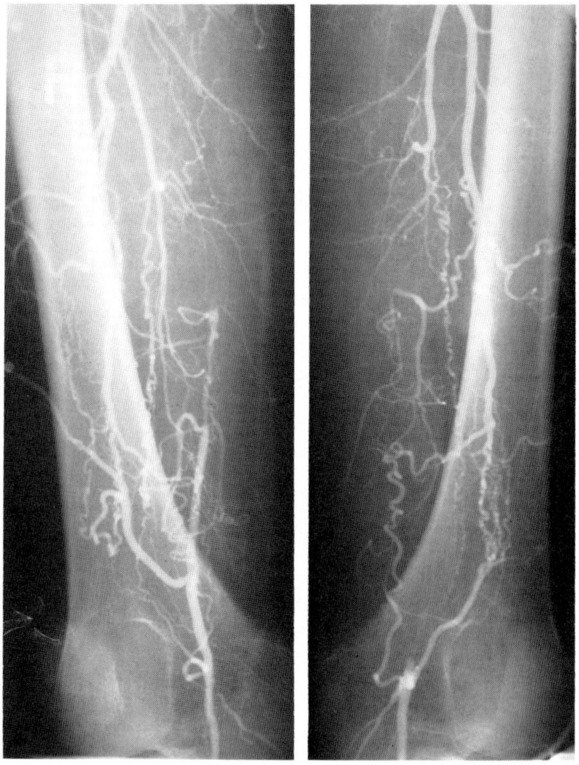

Fig. 14.38c

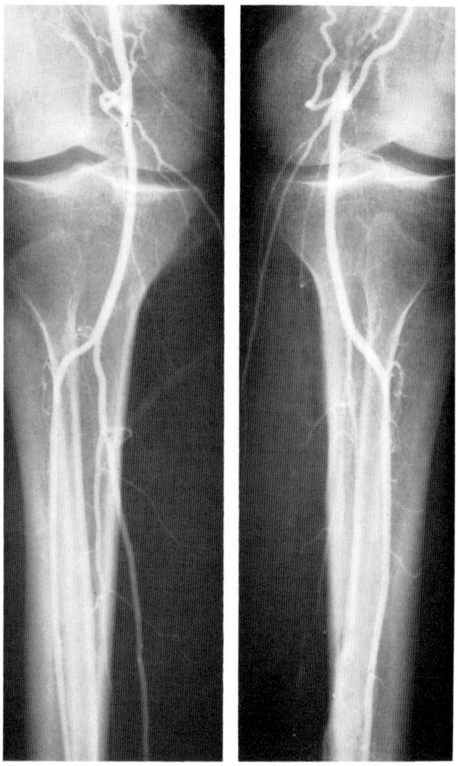

d

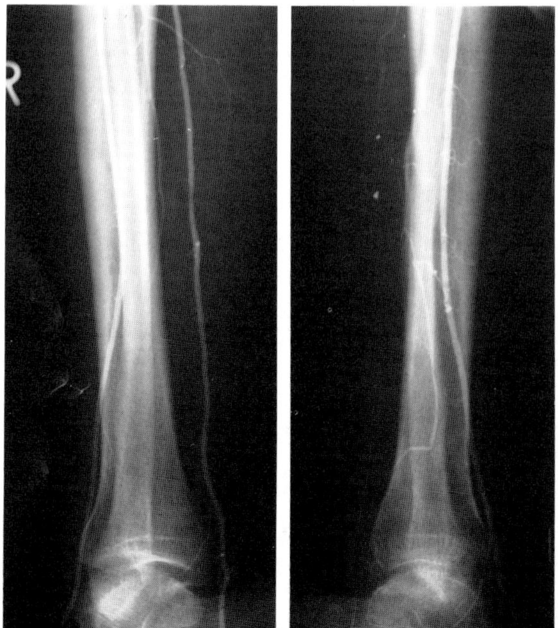

e

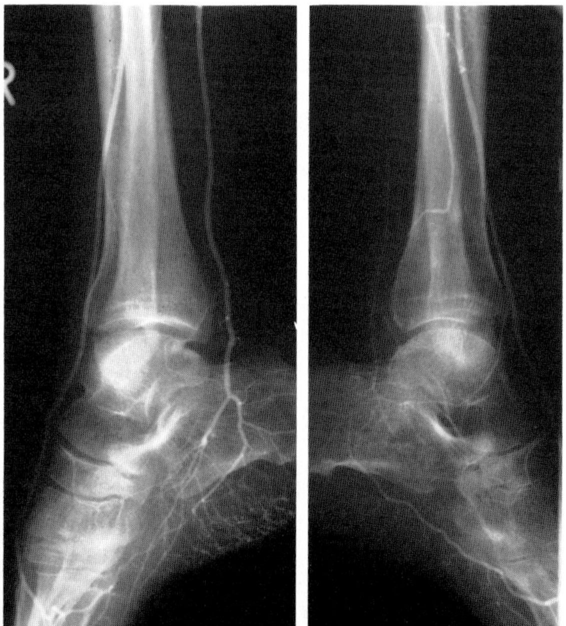

f

Internal Organs and Tissues

Trauma to the thorax, with involvement of the ribs and pleura, may result in more or less significant deformity of the bony thorax and differing degrees of scarring of the pleura (Fig. 14.39). Empyema, abscesses, chronic pneumonia and fibrous induration are radiologically recognizable as sequelae (Figs. 14.40 and 14.41). As a consequence of unrecognized rupture of a bronchus, after a temporary pneumothorax, a marked atelectasis may be found. Rupture of the diaphragm and diaphragmatic hernias are also often recognized quite late after the actual trauma (Fig. 14.42; compare Fig. 8.24); this is also the case in traumatic cysts of the lung. Esophagotracheal fistula as a complication after blunt trauma to the chest has been described (Heberer and Castrup, 1965).

Posttraumatic chylous effusion of the pleura is evidence of an injury to the thoracic duct. If there is a low lesion of the duct, the effusion will be on the right. However, the upper parts are affected on the left.

In an attempt to evaluate the consequence of trauma in the presence of cardiac damage, the ECG is significant. Radiologically, one can recognize deformity and enlargement of the cardiac silhouette, symptoms of increasing cardiac insufficiency or cardiac decompensation and dynamic effects of injuries to valves or the rare late complication of an aneurysm of the heart wall. It must always be considered that late traumatic injury to the heart is exceptional as compared to the incidence of degenerative disorders with similar symptoms. Unless there has been an immediate detailed radiologic investigation with a subsequent follow-up after trauma, it is unreliable to attempt to establish a case for traumatic damage after blunt trauma to the thorax (Rosenkranz, 1969).

X-rays are very important in the evaluation of pulmonary complications due to extrathoracic injury. Along with the further development of intensive care units, much needed radiologic information has become available in the last few years. X-ray diagnosis of pulmonary complications is based on consistently good and comparable portable x-rays taken at the patient's bedside. It is recommended that, in cases when time is of the essence, the most experienced x-ray technicians be charged with obtaining these films.

In tetanus, disturbed respiration is frequently the result of atelectasis or recidivating atelectasis (Fig. 14.43). Extensive infiltration of varying density and size is seen in massive fat embolization (compare Fig. 8.19). Focal or patchy and confluent extensive infiltration may be indicative of infectious disorders of the lung and may be predominantly circumscribed as in aspiration, or more diffuse as in sepsis (Fig. 14.44). However, it is impossible on radiograms to differentiate between infiltration due to bacterial sepsis and that due to Candida sepsis resulting from antibiotic immunosuppressive or cortisone therapy.

The effect of trauma-induced vasoactive agents (histamine, serotonin, catecholamine) on the pulmonary circulation may result in diffuse infiltration of the lungs, similar to that seen in overinfusion of fluids and electrolytes. In an actual case, this is quite frequently due to the coincidental effect of several factors; there may also be loss of blood and additional effects of medication. Research is still under way to learn more about the causes and effects of a disturbed microcirculation within the periphery of the vasculature of the lungs. It is generally accepted that the lung is an organ with a high degree of sensitivity to traumatic shock (Mills, 1968; Mittermayer et al., 1970; Vogel, 1972; Birzle et al., 1973).

Subsequent to blunt abdominal trauma, there is about a 10 per cent incidence of complications resulting from unrecognized causes or lesions impossible to detect at the initial investigation after the accident and affecting the inner structures of the body. An early complication is due to mucosal damage to the gut, to necrosis and to hemorrhage. The resulting scar with its stenosing effect can be demonstrated radiologically. Sooner or later, as a result of an incomplete rupture, there may be formation of an abscess, often of subphrenic localization (Fig. 14.45). A rare complication is that of abscess formation in the omental bursa after rupture of the pancreas (Bücheler et al., 1967) or the spleen (Fig. 14.46). The most common complication is an obstruction due to adhesions, the consequence of serosal lesions or peritonitis causing the extravasation of blood, bile, pancreatic juices or chyme into the abdominal cavity. During fluoroscopy and after intake of contrast material there will be insufficient or absent motility of individual bowel loops. Very extensive adhesions as well as stenoses resulting from scars may be the cause of ileus or subileus following damage of the mucosa or of the vasculature. Posttraumatic cysts appearing in parenchymatous abdominal organs are directly recognizable on roentgenograms if they contain calcifications in their walls; this is most frequently seen in cysts of the spleen. Pancreatic cysts can be recognized because of the displacement and posterior impression of the stomach (compare Fig. 9.20). In the diagnostic approach, the following contrast procedures are useful: gastrointestinal investigation (pancreatic and splenic cysts), intravenous urography (renal cysts), abdominal aortography, selective celiacography and renal angiography. Selective hepatic angiography will make it possible to demonstrate central subcapsular rupture as the cause of hematobilia (compare Fig. 9.10). Fistula formation in the abdomen most often results from a retroperitoneal injury to the duodenum. Here radiologic fistulography with a water-soluble contrast agent is indicated (Fig. 14.47). Obviously, fistulae are seen more frequently after penetrating injuries to the kidneys or similar involvement of one of the renal poles, with corresponding deformity of the collecting system (compare Fig. 9.23) and obstruction of the ureter due to retroperitoneal hematoma (compare Fig. 9.27). Intravenous urography, and possibly infusion urography, should always be the first mode of investigation to demonstrate low obstruction of the ureters. Occasionally retrograde urography may be necessary. Radiologic visualization of renal vasculature will, in addition to showing the renal arterial tree, also demonstrate the parenchyma (compare Fig. 9.26). As a consequence of traumatic renal damage, there may be hypertension and, in bilateral involvement, chronic renal insufficiency with hyperuricemia, and secondary gout. Stenosing lesions of the urethra are seen after injuries of the pelvis, particularly after fracture of the anterior pelvic ring (compare Fig. 14.8). Threatening late sequelae have been observed after the use of Thorotrast. Its storage in internal organs may lead, after 10 years, to cirrhosis of the liver with its well known sequelae and, after about 20 years, to the formation of malignant tumors (quite frequently hemangiosarcomas). Storage within the reticuloendothelial system has led to hemoblastosis. Instillation into the paranasal sinuses, its use in retrograde pyelography and perivascular injection have resulted in many cases of thorotrastomas and sarcomas or carcinomas (Fig. 14.48) (for literature, see Wenz, 1965; Wegener et al., 1971).

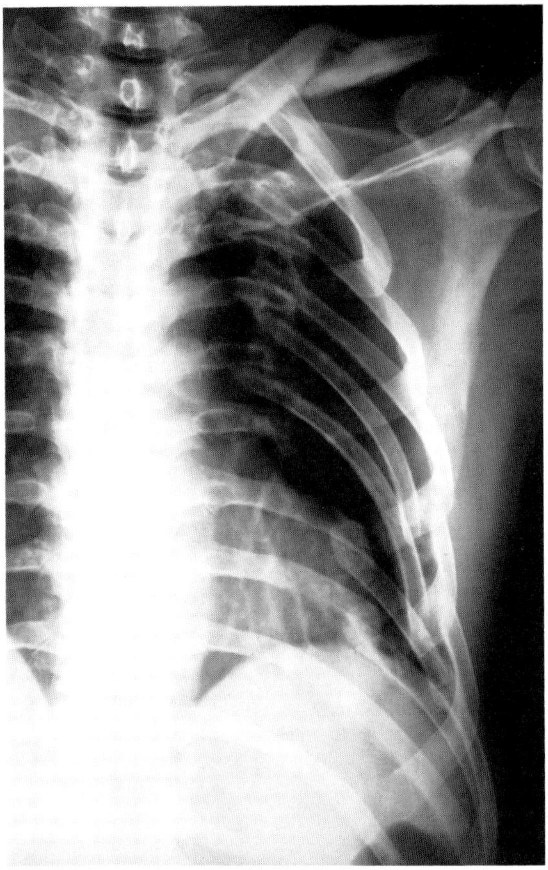

Fig. 14.39. A 46-year-old man with severe deformity of the left thoracic wall 4 months after a chest wall fracture. No visible residual findings of a large hematopneumothorax and of a surgically corrected torsion of the left lower lobe.

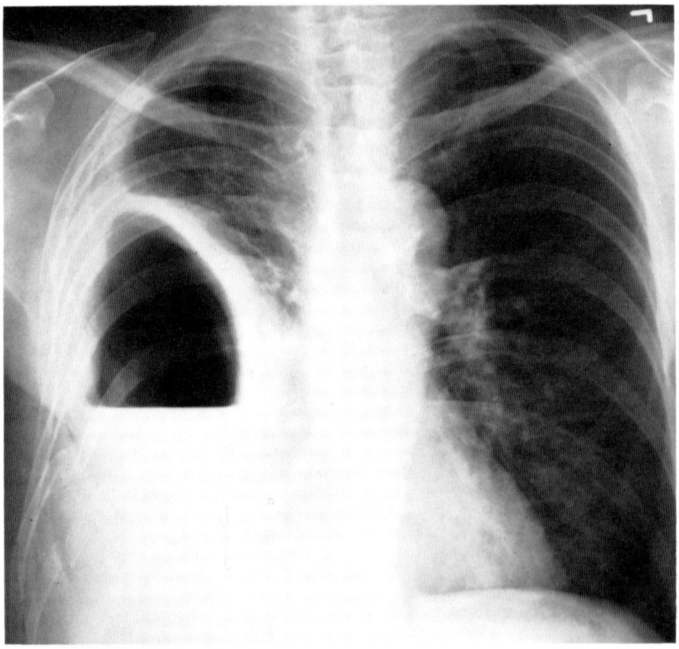

Fig. 14.40. A 59-year-old man with empyema of the right lower hemithorax as a late complication 2 years after a series of rib fractures.

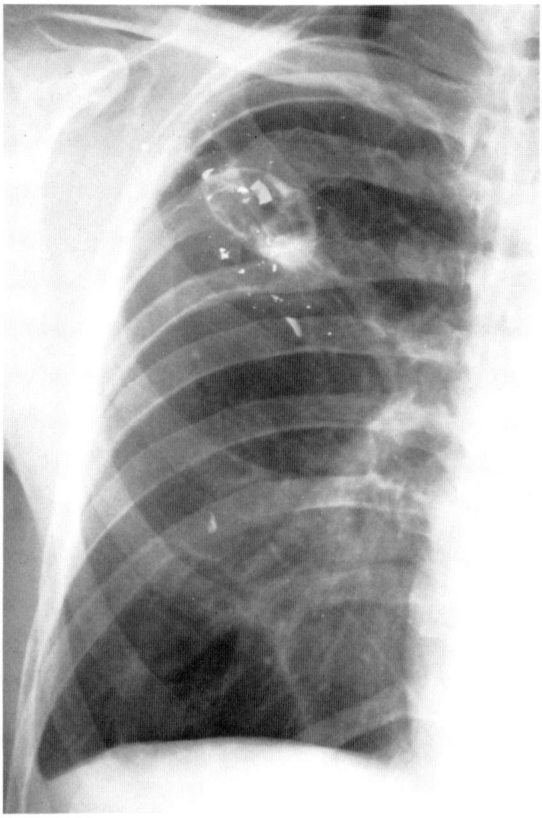

a

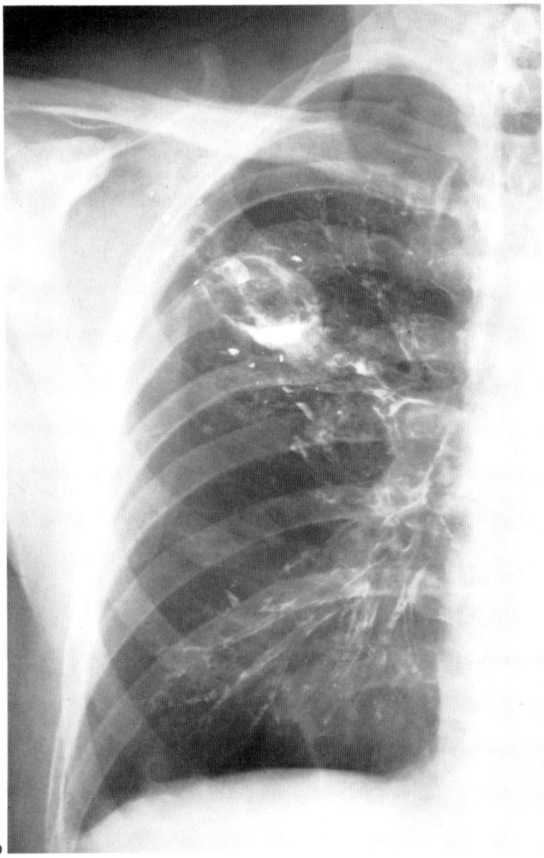

b

Fig. 14.41a and b. A 40-year-old man with a chronic lung abscess within the right upper lobe 20 years after grenade splinter injury.
a) Survey film.
b) Bronchogram; contrast agent enters the cavity.

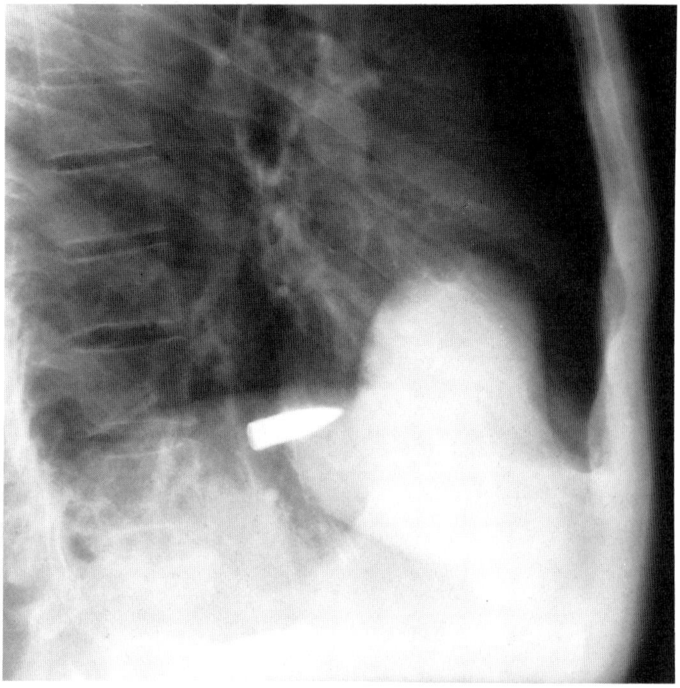

Fig. 14.42a

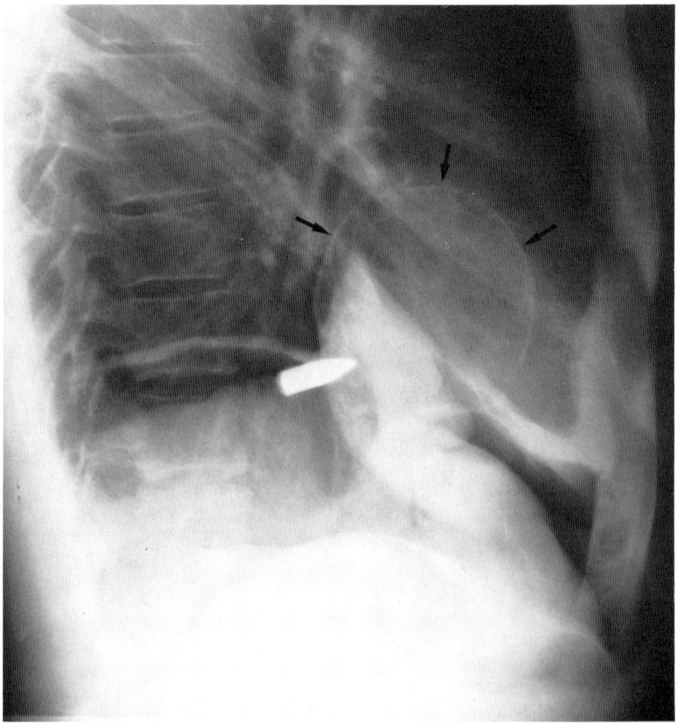

b

Fig. 14.42a and b. A 41-year-old man with a traumatic diaphragmatic hernia (true hernia), with mushroomlike prolapse of the liver 16 years after a gunshot wound. The rifle projectile is lodged within the posterior mediastinum.

a) Survey film, lateral.

b) Pneumoperitoneum. Demonstration of the peritoneal lining of the hernial sac.

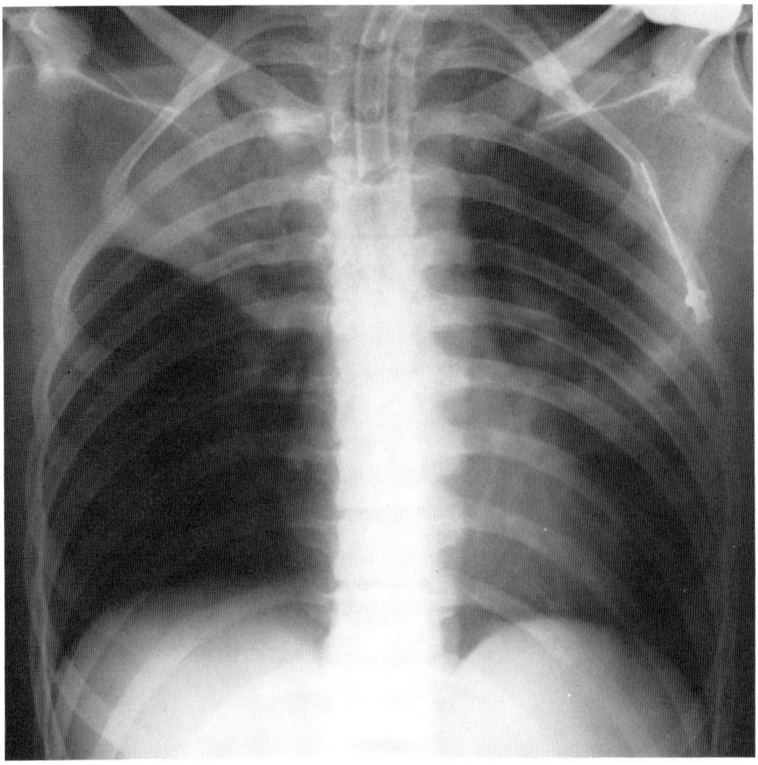

Fig. 14.43. A 16-year-old boy with recidivating atelectasis during tetanus. At this moment, atelectasis of the right upper lobe and partial atelectasis of the left middle zone.

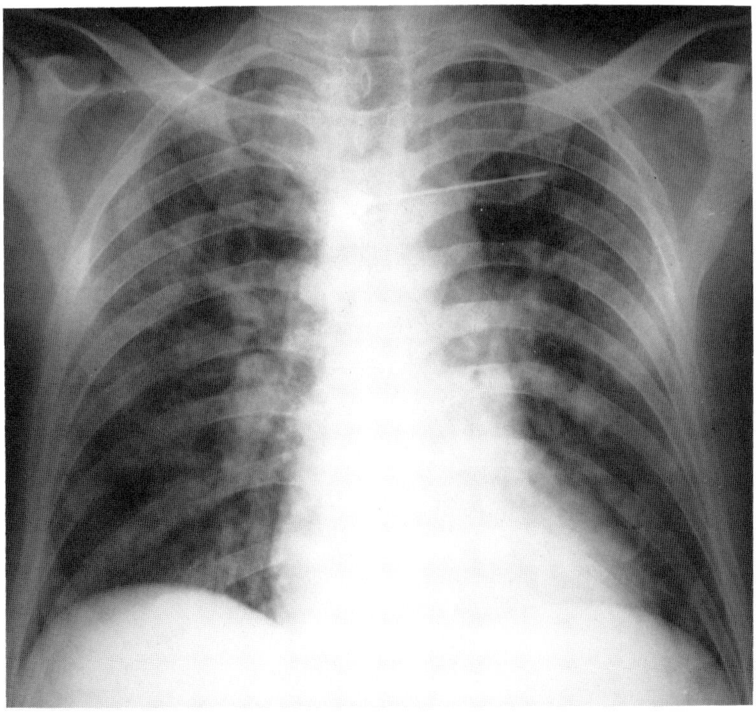

Fig. 14.44. A 40-year-old man with extensive infiltration throughout both lungs during Candida sepsis after burns and prolonged antibiotic therapy. After treatment with amphotericin, regression of infiltrations.

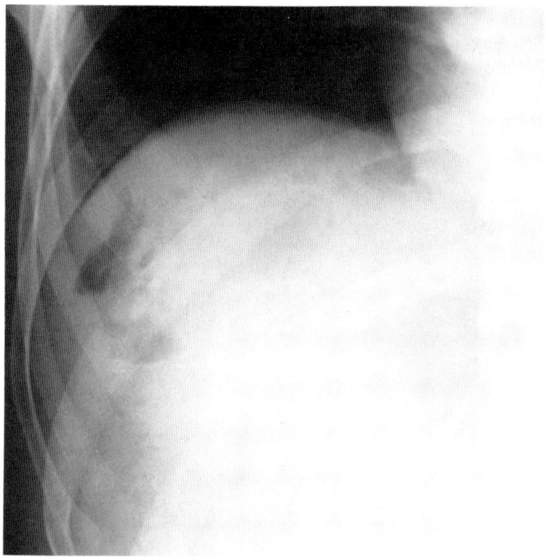

Fig. 14.45

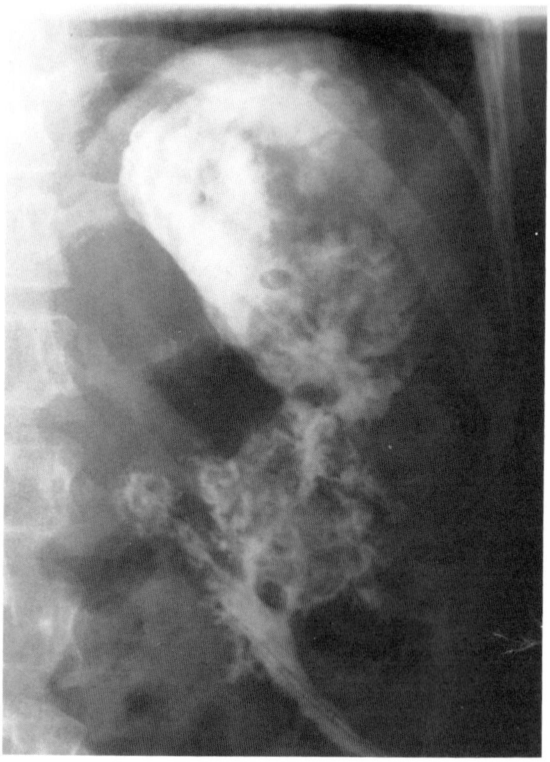

Fig. 14.46

Fig. 14.45. A 26-year-old man with a right subphrenic abscess several weeks after blunt abdominal trauma, with unrecognized rupture of the liver.

Fig. 14.46. A 23-year-old woman with severe multiple injuries due to a traffic accident (contusion of the thorax with a series of rib fractures; pneumothorax on the right; abdominal trauma with avulsion of the left kidney at the hilus; rupture of the spleen; and fracture of the left humerus, the left scapula and the left pubic bone). Formation of an abscess in the omental bursa associated with the ruptured spleen. Fistulography.

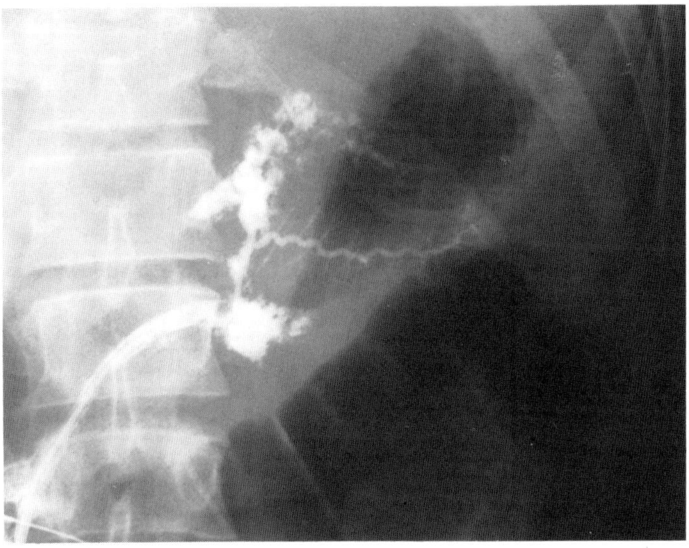

Fig. 14.47. A 21-year-old man. Condition after a ruptured pancreas and formation of a fistula. Fistulography with Urografin: demonstration of the pancreatic duct.

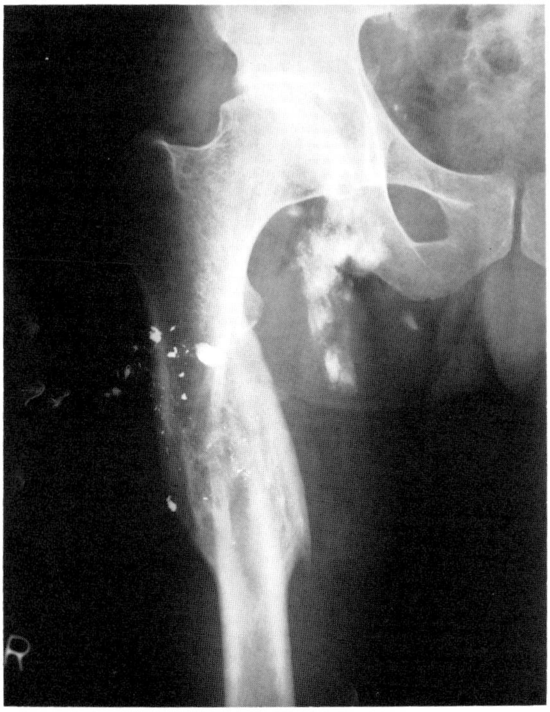

a

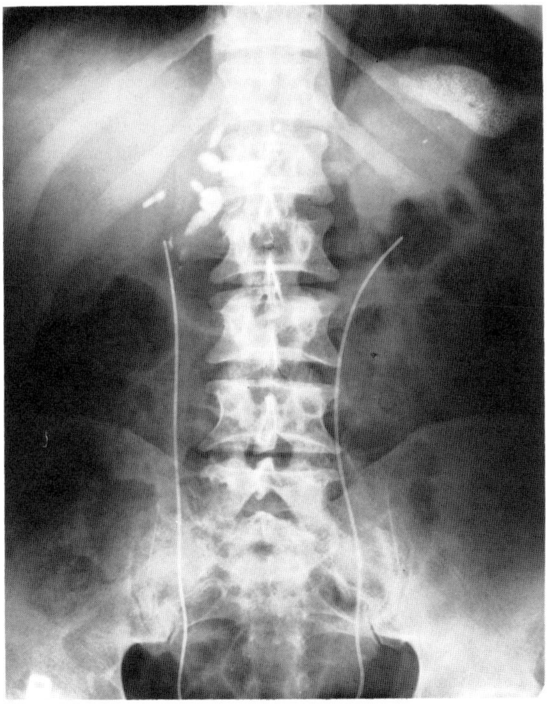

b

Fig. 14.48a and b. A 47-year-old man.
a) Thorotrastoma at the site of needle insertion 12 years ago for femoral arteriography.
b) Thorotrast is stored in the spleen and the lymph nodes of the hilus of the liver.

Approach and Principles in Compiling Expert Radiologic Reports

In virtually all cases of x-ray documentation of an accident, valuable information for objective evaluation will be obtained by a thorough x-ray investigation. It is always advisable to consult the early films taken immediately after the accident as well as the radiologic follow-up documents even though, admittedly, the many dozens of x-rays may make the job tedious.

The indication for specific x-ray investigations is determined by the type of injury and the particular questions confronting the examiner. The expert examiner, therefore, should fully familiarize himself with the existing documentation prior to requesting further x-ray studies. It is not essential to have a maximum number of films but to obtain the most pertinent ones as soon as possible. However, in order to demonstrate or exclude polyostotic or polyarticular alterations, several parts of the body will have to be x-rayed.

The optimal use of x-ray diagnosis by the expert examiner is only possible if the expert has sufficient experience and is well versed on the value and possibilities of radiodiagnostic measures.

In the course of an expert evaluation, the x-ray report may often form part of a surgical, orthopedic or urologic evaluation report. In many cases, it is a very important part and its content should, therefore, be factually sound and clearly formulated. In the first descriptive part, the recent traumatic alterations present at the time of the accident should be enumerated. Separate from this, reference should be made to old traumatic sequelae or other preexisting abnormal findings. If the cause-and-effect relationship is questionable, it is recommended that the date of the accident and of all the described x-ray films in the report be emphasized, especially if this refers to films obtained elsewhere. In simple cases, it is sufficient to then describe the condition at the time the new x-rays were obtained for the expert report; in difficult and problematic cases, however, it will be necessary to describe the course of the most important intermediate stages up to the present condition. In the summary of the evaluation, trauma sequelae evident from the x-ray investigations ought to be clearly emphasized. There is an advantage if, already on the basis of an x-ray report, it can be clearly concluded whether a cause-and-effect relationship with the incriminated trauma should be considered definite, possible or only conceivable.

Expert reporting based on x-rays will facilitate a strictly objective viewpoint for the expert examiner; still, there are ample opportunities for being tempted into a benevolent or negative wording of statements. One should always be fully aware that an expert report must be strictly impartial and that falsifications with intent are subject to prosecution. Hardly anywhere else would it be as simple to dispute wrong statements as in x-ray reports. In an effort to meet the demand of well-known authorities, that more physicians ought to be better able to compile expert reports, factually accurate and clearly formulated x-ray reporting can be a significant contribution.

15 Axial Computer Tomography in the Diagnosis of Skull-Brain Trauma

Axial computer tomography of the skull has added new dimensions to diagnostic traumatology. With it, the slightest differences in density within the cranial cavity can be demonstrated. These differences can be even more clearly visualized when contrast medium is administered intravenously.

Intracranial hemorrhages, which, with cerebral angiography, can only be indirectly inferred by the displacement of vessels or defined avascular areas, or which are not favorably located, can now be directly demonstrated. Acute traumatic hematomas have an essentially higher density than the surrounding brain tissue and, therefore, appear as white areas. The epidural and subdural location can frequently be distinguished by the different forms of the hematomas. Epidural hematomas are usually biconvex or planoconvex (Fig. 15.1); subdural hematomas are sickle-shaped.

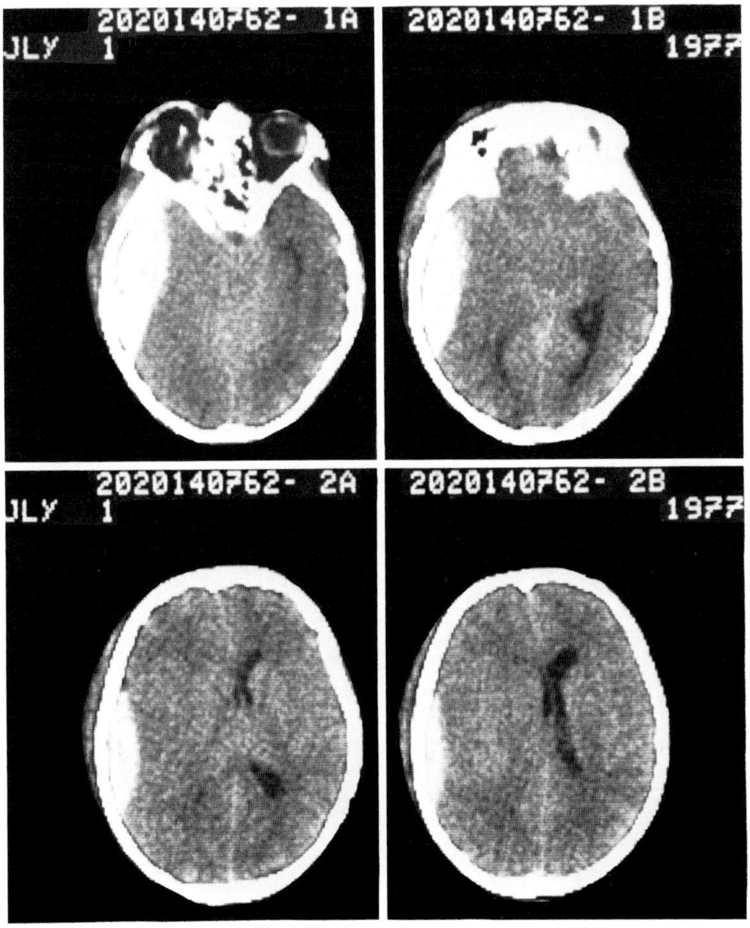

a b c d

Fig. 15.1a–d. Large epidural hematoma in left temporoparietal region, lateral displacement of ventricle system to the right, and subtotal compression of left lateral ventricle. Orbital hematoma on left and ethmoid hemorrhage.

The certainty of the subdural hematoma diagnosis is impaired by the fact that the structure, and therefore also the density, is changed by increasing liquefaction soon after the hematoma appears. At first the image is extremely dense, but then it becomes isodense and finally hypodense. In the isodense stage, the hematoma cannot be seen on the ct film. If unilateral space filling, is present it can only be indentified by the displacement of the lateral ventricle (Fig. 15.2).

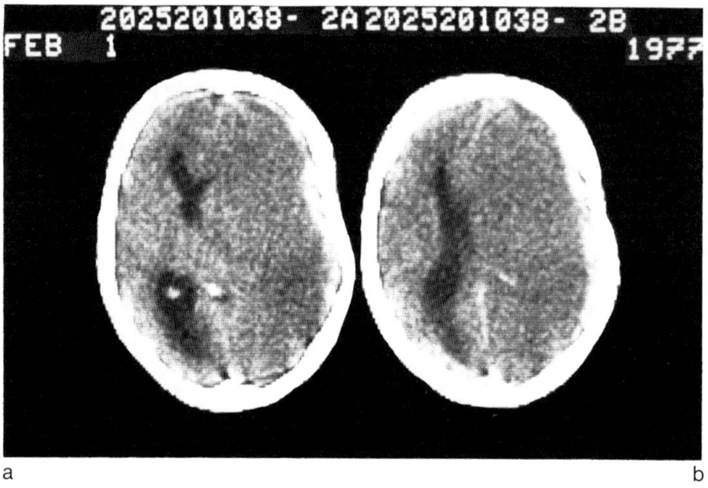

Fig. 15.2a and b. Very large isodense subdural hematoma in right parietal region with fresh narrow marginal hemorrhage. High-grade lateral displacement of ventricle system to the left and considerable compression of right lateral ventricle, particularly in the area of the cornu posterius ventriculi lateralis.

Bilateral subdural hematomas in the isodense stage with a centrally positioned ventricle system cannot be demonstrated and, for this reason, may lead to an incorrect diagnosis with fatal consequences. Older chronic subdural hematomas are usually imaged as clearly defined, sickle-shaped hypodense zones; the membrane of the hematoma sometimes appears as a marginal border of higher density (Fig. 15.3).

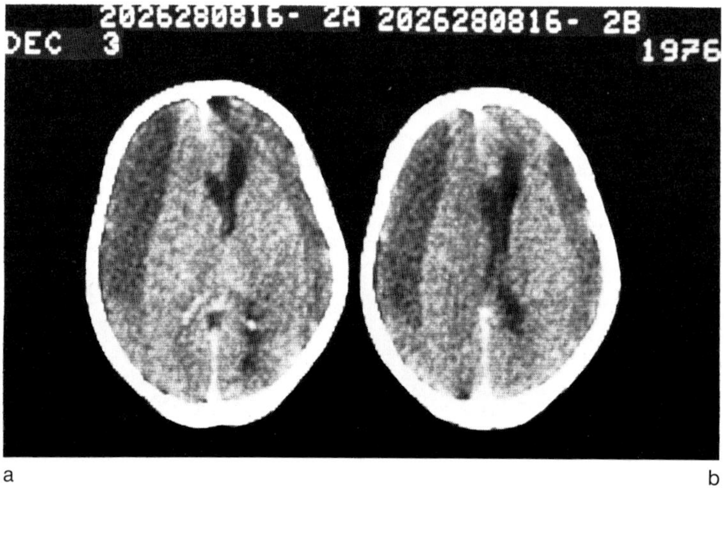

Fig. 15.3a and b. Older chronic subdural hematoma unilaterally in parietal region, left side considerably larger than right. Slight capsular density on left (after concentration of intravenously administered contrast medium), pronounced lateral displacement of ventricle system to the right.

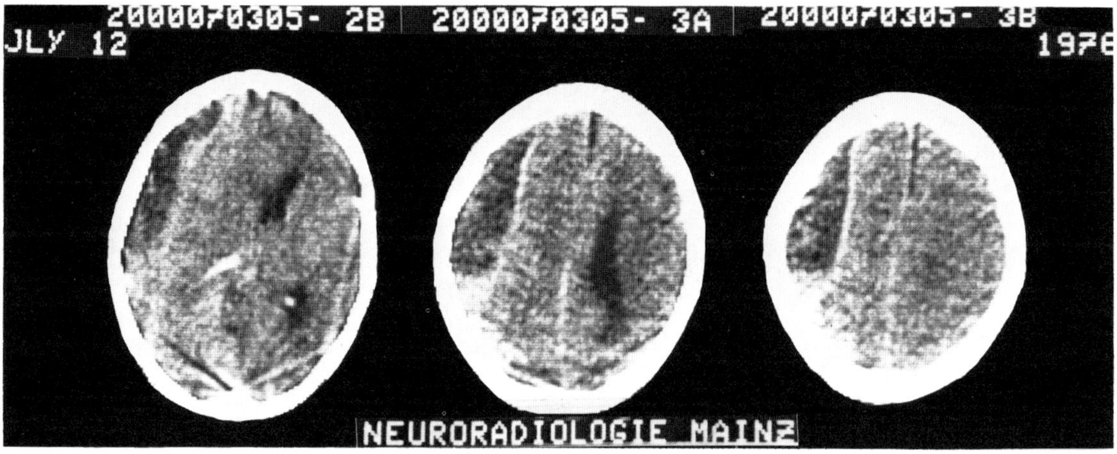

c d e

Fig. 15.3 c, d and e. Older post-traumatic chronic subdural hematoma in left parietal region with residual coagulum in dorsal part of encapsulated hemorrhage. Increased contrast medium at capsule, compression of left lateral ventricle.

The hygroma is the terminal state of an old subdural hemorrhage; the density corresponds to that of the cerebrospinal fluid spaces (Fig. 15.4).

Smaller traumatic intracerebral hemorrhages are usually located near the cortex. The ventricles are unchanged, or a local deformity is present (Fig. 15.5).

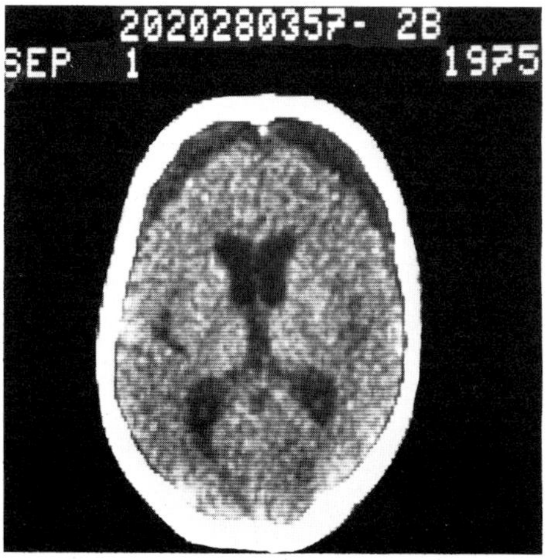

Fig. 15.4. Post-traumatic hygroma bilaterally in frontal region, sickle-shaped hypodense zone. Moderate post-traumatic hydrocephalus internus.

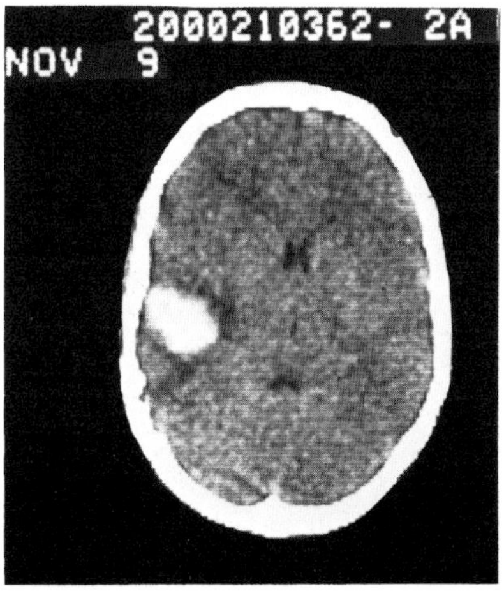

Fig. 15.5. Postcontusive intracerebral hematoma in left parietal region, marginal edema. Slight lateral displacement of ventricle system.

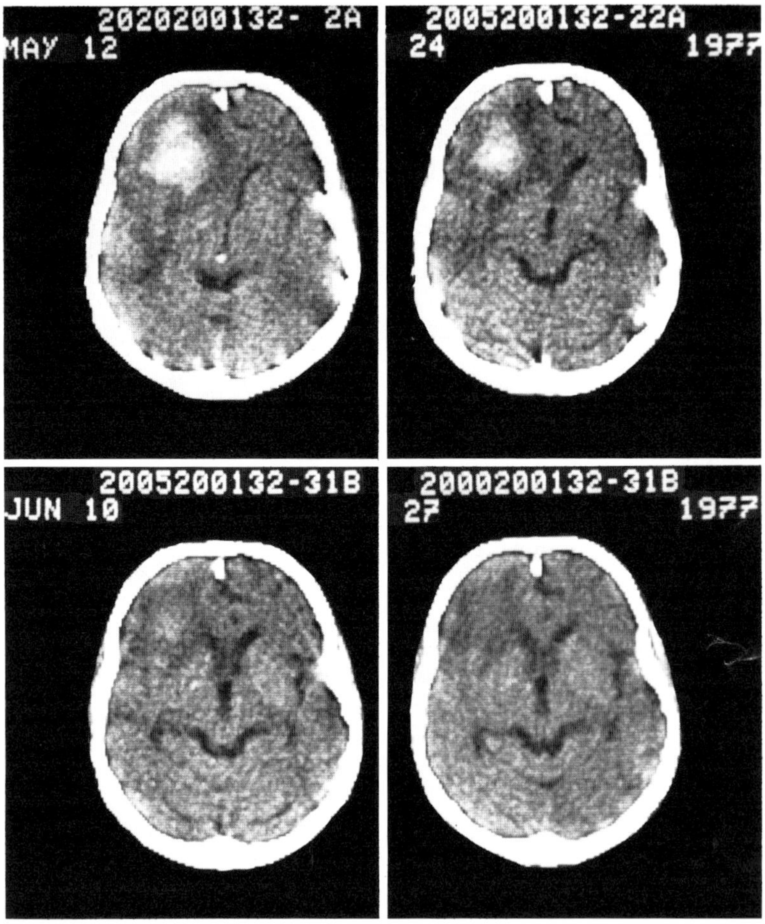

a b c d

Fig. 15.6a–d. a) Large intracerebral hematoma in left frontal region with indistinct limitation and hypodense marginal zone. Lateral displacement of ventricle system to the right and compression of left lateral ventricle. b–d) Gradual resorption of hematoma, regression of lateral displacement, terminal state with slight hypodense zone and enlargement of ventricle in the course of 8 weeks.

Large intracerebral hematomas develop which are imaged as indistinct zones of higher density with surrounding marginal edema (translucent zone). Figure 15.6 shows the course following such a hemorrhage with gradual resorption of the hematoma and the residual state with hypodense zone.

The important demonstration of the smallest hemorrhages in the brain stem, in the mesencephalon, and in the ventricle system (prognostically unfavorable) is now possible with computer tomography (Fig. 15.7).

Surgically approachable hematomas at the posterior cranial fossa which were difficult or impossible to demonstrate with angiography can now be identified.

Extracranial subgaleal hemorrhages (Fig. 15.8) and intracranial foreign bodies (e.g., bone fragments and metal, glass, or wood splinters) can be easily recognized with the help of computer tomography.

Mention should also be made of orbital diagnostics. Retrobulbar hemorrhages are almost always demonstrated as circumscribed dense areas or as a dense area which fills the whole retrobulbar space. Since the fatty tissue of the orbit absorbs little radiation, hemorrhages in all stages are particularly well imaged (s. Fig. 15.1a).

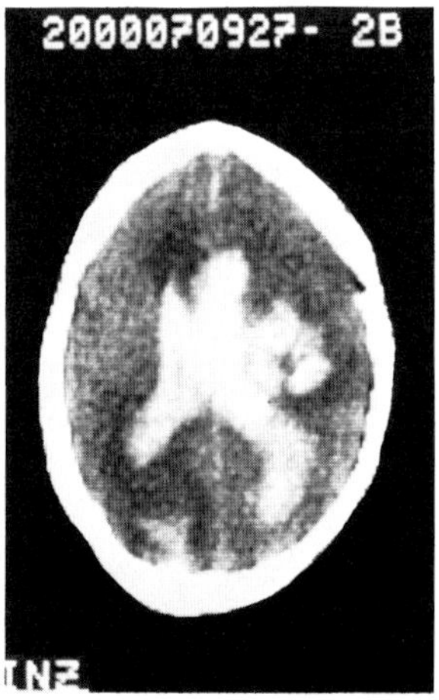

Fig. 15.7. Large postcontusive periventricular hemorrhage on right, invasion of right cella media ventriculi lateralis, almost total tamponade of both lateral ventricles.

Fractures of the vault of the cranium can only be recognized on the computer tomogram when the fracture line is wide enough and is perpendicular to the sectional plane, or when the fragments are displaced (e.g., depressed fracture).
Local post-traumatic cerebral edema with hemorrhage can be identified as an irregular zone of lower density. In the most favorable situation, the hematoma is replaced by the normal structural density of the brain after the edema has subsided, or a relatively sharply contrasted form of considerably lower density and/or a widening of the cerebral sulci can be seen with destruction of cerebral matter. General malignant cerebral edema usually begins hours after the traumatic event. It is characterized by the absence of the cerebral sulci, reduction in the size of the lateral ventricles, or total compression of the ventricles; a border of lower density can be seen around the lateral ventricle. Total compression of the lateral ventricle should be interpreted as a sign of extremely high cerebral compression; the patient seldom survives. With reversible edema, the hypodense marginal edge of the lateral ventricle slowly disappears over a period of weeks. The ventricles are considerably enlarged in the terminal state.
Computer tomography provides information for evaluating the consequences of a skull-brain injury which could not have been obtained earlier. This is particularly true when the whole course of a disease, from traumatic event to terminal state, has been recorded on films collected from repeated examinations. Circumscribed defects in the cerebral matter and general post-traumatic damage as extensive as hydrocephalus internus can, therefore, be identified as local zones of lower density (Fig. 15.9).

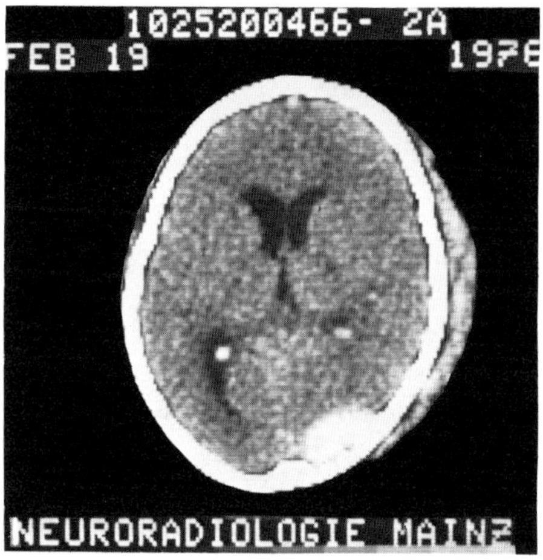

Fig. 15.8. Extensive hematoma of galea on right. Intracerebral hemorrhage in right occipital region from contusion, compression and frontal displacement of right cornu posterius ventriculi lateralis.

In spine-spinal cord trauma, axial computer tomography of the whole body has not yet been widely accepted. At this point we are not in a position to present a report of our experience. It is, however, already possible to identify epidural and subdural hemorrhages of the spinal canal as well as intramedullary hemorrhages.
The technical aspects of using computer tomography for diagnostic traumatology should be mentioned. Since the equipment sometimes requires a fairly long time to warm up (as much als 20 minutes), it must always be kept in operating order so that the examination be immediately performed in emergency cases. This presupposes that adequate personnel are available. In addition the present scanning time is so long that the patient must remain absolutely still; movement artefacts impair or even prevent an exact diagnosis.

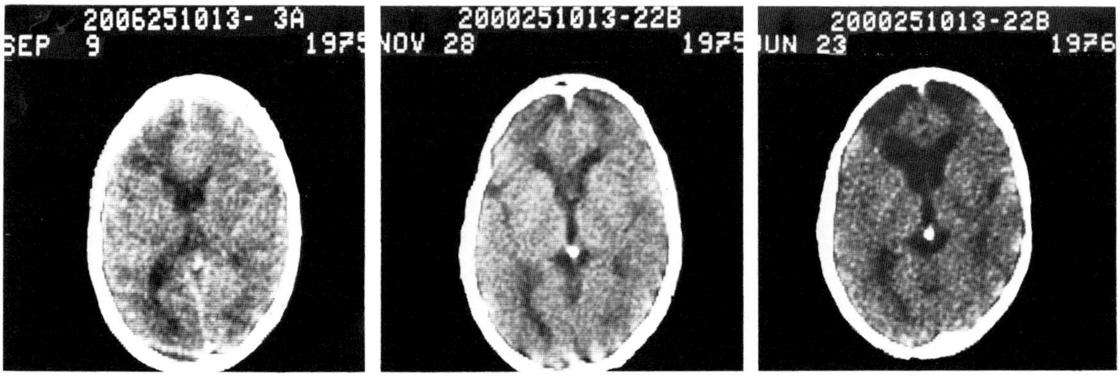

a b c

Fig. 15.9a–c. a) Shortly after severe skull-brain trauma. No hemorrhage, but postcontusive edema with translucent zone in left frontal region and to a lesser extent in right occipital region (contrecoup); b) Disappearance of edematous zones, gradual enlargement of ventricle; c) Terminal state 9 months later, bilateral defect of cerebral matter in frontopolar region, pronounced enlargement of cornu anterius medullae spinalis on left and of third ventricle.

References

General References

Athanasoulis, C. A., A. C. Waltman, S. T. Baum: Angiography of Trauma. *In* Cave, E., et al.: Trauma Management. Year Book Medical Publishers, Chicago 1974, pp. 197–212

Ballinger, W. F., R. B. Rutherford, G. D. Zuidema: The Management of Trauma. 2nd ed. W. B. Saunders Co., Philadelphia 1973

Büchner, H.: Radiometrie. Theorie und Praxis röntgenologischer Meßmethoden. Springer, Berlin 1963

Cave, E. F., J. F. Burke, R. J. Boyd: Trauma Management. Year Book Medical Publishers, Chicago 1974

Committee on Trauma, American College of Surgeons: Early Care of the Injured Patient. 2nd ed. W. B. Saunders Co., Philadelphia 1976

Ehalt, W.: Unfallchirurgie im Röntgenbilde. Maudrich, Wien 1952

Ehalt, W.: Unfallpraxis de Gruyter, Berlin 1968

Ell, P. J., J. Dash, J. Raymond: Bone scanning. A review on purpose and method. Skeletal Radiol. 1 (1976) 33–45

Feneis, H.: Anatomisches Bildwörterbuch. Thieme, Stuttgart 1970

Freedman, G. S.: Radionuclide imaging of the injured patient. Radiol. Clin. N. Amer. 11 (1973) 461–477

Fu, W. R.: Angiography of Trauma. Charles C. Thomas, Springfield, Ill. 1972

Grashey, R., R. Birkner: Atlas typischer Röntgenbilder vom normalen Menschen, 10th ed. Urban & Schwarzenberg, Munich 1964

Graul, E. H., J. Stockhausen: Strahlenschutzfibel. Deutscher Ärzteverlag, Köln 1968

Janker, R., Röntgenaufnahmetechnik, 7th ed. Parts 1 and 2. Barth, Munich 1966/1971

Köhler, A., E. A. Zimmer: Grenzen des Normalen und Anfänge des Pathologischen im Röntgenbilde des Skelettes. Thieme, Stuttgart 1967

Langenbach, H. J.: Röntgen-Einstelltechnik. Barth, Leipzig 1957

Littleton, J. T.: Transportation of the traumatized patient. Radiol. Clin. N. Amer. 11 (1973) 449–460

Lusted, L. B., Th. E. Keats: Atlas of Roentgenographic Measurement. Year Book Medical Publishers, Chicago 1967

Matsumoto, T.: Current Management of Trauma in Surgery and General Practice. Charles C. Thomas, Springfield Ill. 1975

Mayo, E. T.: Clinical Evaluation of the Critically injured. Charles C. Thomas, Springfield, Ill. 1975

Mittermaier, R.: Hals-Nasen-Ohren-Krankheiten im Röntgenbild. Thieme, Stuttgart 1969

Mohr, H.: Röntgenuntersuchung unfallverletzter Patienten.Radiologie 8 (1968) 239–241

Neiss, A.: Röntgenidentifikation. Thieme, Stuttgart 1968

Nelson, S. W.: Some important diagnostic and technical fundamentals in the radiology of trauma, with particular emphasis on skeletal trauma. Radiol. Clin. N. Amer. 4 (1966) 241–259

Otto, W. J.: Use and Abuse of X-ray in Trauma. *In* Cave, E., et al.: Trauma Management. Year Book Medical Publishers, Chicago 1974, pp. 191–196

Röntgenverordnung: Verordnung über den Schutz vor Schäden durch Röntgenstrahlen. Bundesgesetzblatt No. 18 (1973) Part I.

Schinz, H. R., W. E. Baensch, E. Friedl, E. Uehlinger: Lehrbuch der Röntgendiagnostik, Vols. I, II, Thieme, Stuttgart 1952

Schinz, H. R., W. E. Baensch, W. Frommhold, R. Glauner, E. Uehlinger, J. Wellauer: Lehrbuch der Röntgendiagnostik, Vol. III. Thieme, Stuttgart 1966

Schlosser V.: Traumatologie. Thieme, Stuttgart 1968

Schmidt, H., K.-H. Bauch, H.-G. Coerper: Erfahrungen mit einem neuen Transportsystem für Unfallverletzte. Der Krankenhausarzt 42 (1969) 252–254

Schoen, H.: Medizinische Röntgentechnik, Vol. I. Thieme, Stuttgart 1956

Schwartz, S. S. (ed.): Symposium on trauma. Radiol. Clin. N. Amer. 11 (1973) 3

Utz, D. C.: System for X-ray detection of foreign bodies at operation. Mayo Clin. Proc. 43 (1968) 368–372

Walt, J. A., R. F. Wilson: Management of Trauma. Pitfalls and Practice. Lea & Febiger, Philadelphia 1975

Zatzkin, H. R.: The Roentgen Diagnosis of Trauma. Year Book Medical Publishers, Chicago 1965

Chapters 1 to 3

Adams, A. E.: Einige diagnostische und therapeutische Probleme bei frischen Schädel-Hirn-Traumen. Dtsch. med. Wschr. 92 (1967) 1173

Alker, G. J., Y. S. Oh, E. V. Leslie, J. Lehotay, V. A. Panaro, E. G. Eschner: Postmortem radiology of head and neck injuries in fatal traffic accidents. Radiology 114 (1975) 611–617

Allen, W. E., E. L. Kier, S. L. G. Rothman: Pitfalls in the evaluation of skull trauma. Radiol. Clin. N. Amer. 11 (1973) 479–503

Archer, C. R., M. Sundaram: Uncommon sphenoidal fractures and their sequelae. Radiology 122 (1977) 157–161

Babcock, J. L.: Cervical spine injuries. Diagnosis and classification Arch. Surg. 111 (1976) 646

Baier, H.: Bedeutung der Tomographie in der Frakturdiagnostik der Stirnhöhlenhinterwand und der Siebbeinzellen. Fortschr. Röntgenstr. Beih. (1966) 158–160

Barnett, H. G., E. S. Connolly: Lumbosacral nerve root avulsion. Report of a case and review of the literature. J. Trauma 15 (1975) 532–535

Bell, R. S., J. W. Loop: The utility and futility of radiographic skull examination for trauma. New Engl. J. Med. 284 (1971) 236–239

Ben-Menachem, Y., J. H. Duke, B. L. Harberg, S. J. Hite: Preoperative angiography in vascular trauma. Report of four unusual cases. J. Trauma 15 (1975) 209–216

Bergeron, R. T., C. L. Rumbaugh: Non space-occupying sequelae of head trauma. Radiol. Clin. N. Amer. 12 (1974) 315–331

Betz, H., G. Groß, R. Schüttler: Raumfordernde traumatische Pneumatocele. Fortschr. Röntgenstr. 109 (1968) 803–805

Briggs, M.: Traumatic pneumocephalus. Brit. J. Surg. 61 (1974) 307–312
Brocher, J. E. W.: Die verkannten Wirbelsäulenverletzungen und Pseudofrakturen der Wirbelsäule. Thieme, Leipzig 1944
Brown, O. L., J. J. Longacre, G. A. De Steffano, R. W. Wood, J. B. Kahl: Roentgen manifestations of blow-out fracture of the orbit. Radiology 85 (1965) 908–913
Buetti-Bäuml, C.: Funktionelle Röntgendiagnostik der Halswirbelsäule. Regensburger Jahrbuch für Ärztliche Fortbildung, Vol. IV. (1955) 280–288
Carroll, T. B. Seat belt fractures. Radiology 91 (1968) 517–518
Chiroff, R. T., B. L. Sachs: Discontinuity of the spinous process on standard roentgenographs as an aid in the diagnosis of unstable fractures of the spine. J. Trauma 16 (1976) 313–316
Clementschitsch, F.: Die Röntgendarstellung des Gesichtsschädels. Urban & Schwarzenberg, Vienna 1951
Dart, C. H., H. E. Braitman: Traumatic rupture of thoracic aorta. Diagnosis and management. Arch Surg., 111 (1976) 697
Driesen, W.: Verletzungen des Hirnschädels. Fortschr. Röntgenstr. Beiheft (1966) 130–133
Dublin, A. B., B. N. French, J. M. Rennick: Computed tomography in head trauma. Radiology 122 (1977) 365–369
Etter, L. E.: Opacification studies of normal and abnormal paranasal sinuses. Amer. J. Roentgenol. 89 (1963) 1137–1146
Frey, K. W.: Die Tomographie in der Unfalldiagnostik des Mittelohrs. Fortschr. Röntgenstr. 103 (1965) 449–463
Friedenberg, M. J., P. Lake, S. Landau: Bilateral incomplete traumatic occlusion of internal carotid arteries. Amer. J. Roentgenol. 118 (1973) 546–549
Friedmann, G., R. A. Frowein: Röntgendiagnostik des akuten Schädelhirntraumas. Röntgenblätter 19 (1966a) 83–92
Friedmann, G., R. A. Frowein: Die Bedeutung der Schädelfrakturen für die klinische Behandlung. Fortschr. Röntgenstr. Beiheft (1966b) 170–171
Fueger, G. F., A. T. Milauskas, W. Britton: The roentgenologic evaluation of orbital blow-out injuries. Amer. J. Roentgenol. 97 (1966) 614–617
Funk, F. J., R. E. Wells: Injuries of the cervical spine in football. Clin. Orthop. 109 (1975) 50–58
Gehweiler, J. A., D. E. Duff, S. Martinez, M. D. Miller, W. M. Clark: Fractures of the atlas vertebra. Skeletal Radiol. 1 (1976) 97–102
Göhring, K., E. Weber: Das Röntgenübersichtsbild als Gradmesser für die Schwere des Schädel-Hirn-Traumas. Chir. Praxis 6 (1962) 415–428
Gould, H. R., C. O. Titus: Internal orbital fractures. The value of laminagraphy in diagnosis. Amer. J. Roentgenol. 97 (1966) 618–623
Han, S. Y., D. M. Witten, J. P. Mussleman: Jefferson fracture of the atlas. Report of six cases. J. Neurosurg. 44 (1976) 368–371
Hegenbarth, R., K. D. Ebel: Roentgen findings in fractures of the vertebral column in childhood. Examination of 35 patients and its results. Pediat. Radiol. 5 (1976) 34–39
Hemmer, R.: Über atypische posttraumatische epidurale Blutungen und die Ursachen ihrer Fehldeutung. Dtsch. med. Wschr. 90 (1965) 1945
Herrmann, H. D.: Das Schleudertrauma der Halswirbelsäule. Terminologie und Diagnose. Med. Welt 21 (1970) 1797–1800
Hinz, P., L. Tamska: Arteria vertebralis und Schleuderverletzung der Halswirbelsäule. Postmortale angiographische Untersuchungen an 31 Verkehrstoten. Arch. orthop. Unfall-Chir. 64 (1968) 268
Huber, P.: Zerebrale Angiographie beim frischen Schädel-Hirn-Trauma. Thieme, Stuttgart 1964
Huber, P.: Die zerebrale Angiographie-Indikationen, Gefahren, Aussagewert. Schweiz. med. Wschr. 99 (1969) 1398–1411
Huelke, D. F., H. Kaufer: Vertebral column injuries and seat belts. J. Trauma 15 (1975) 304–318
Jackson, W. D., L. L. Wilste, R. J. Ciarinione: Spondylolysis in the female gymnast. Clin. Orthop. 117 (1976) 68–73
Jacobs, B.: Cervical fractures and dislocations. Clin. Orthop. 109 (1975) 18–32
Jonasch, E.: Die isolierten Brüche der Wirbeldornfortsätze. Münch. med. Wschr. 109 (1967) 2001–2002
Käufer, C.: Die Bestimmung des Todes bei irreversiblem Verlust der Hirnfunktion. Fortschr. Med. 89 (1971) 651–654
Kewalramani, L. S., R. G. Taylor: Brachial plexus root avulsion. Role of myelography. J. Trauma 15 (1975) 603–608
Koneczny, O.: Auswertung und Dokumentation traumatischer Wirbelsäulenschäden. Hefte zur Unfallheilkunde 90 (1967) 33–72
Lang, E. K.: The role of arteriography in trauma. Radiol. Clin. N. Amer. 14 (1976) 353–370
Liliequist, B.: Roentgenologic appearances of traumatic lesions of middle meningeal artery. Report of two cases. Acta radiol. Diag. 6 (1967) 513–518
Lloyd, G. A. S.: Orbital Emphysema. Brit. J. Radiol. 39 (1966) 933–938
Lob, A.: Die Wirbelsäulenverletzungen und ihre Ausheilung. Thieme, Leipzig 1941
Lorenz, R.: Röntgenuntersuchungen der frischen Verletzung der Occipito-cervical-Gegend mit Berücksichtigung bereits vorhandener Schäden der Halswirbelsäule. Fortschr. Röntgenstr. Beiheft (1966) 160–161
Mayer, K.:Wertung und Behandlung des Schädelhirntraumas in der Praxis. Ärzteblatt Baden-Württemberg (1967) 16–21
McCoy, S. H., K. A. Johnson: Sagittal fracture of the cervical spine. J. Trauma 16 (1976) 310–312
Meinecke, F.-W.: Rückenmarkschäden bei Schleuderverletzungen der Halswirbelsäule. Dtsch. med. Wschr. 95 (1970) 1209–1212
Möller, W.-D., L. Stappenbeck: Die stereoskopische Schädelaufnahme. Med. Welt 23 (1972) 978–979
Müller, E.: Das Schleudertrauma der Halswirbelsäule und seine verschiedenen Folgen. Dtsch. med. Wschr. 91 (1966) 588–593
Naidich, J. B., T. P. Naidich, C. Garfein, A. L. Liebeskind, R. A. Hyman: The widened interspinous distance. A useful sign of anterior cervical dislocation in the frontal projection. Radiology 123 (1977) 113–116
Nelson, S. W., A. K. Freimanis: Angiographic features of convexity subdural hematomas with emphasis on the differential diagnosis between unilateral and bilateral hematomas. Amer. J. Roentgenol. 90 (1963) 445–461
Parvey, L. S., B. Gerald: Arteriographic diagnosis of brain death in children. Pediat. Radiol. 4 (1976) 79–82
Pay, N. T., A. E. George, M. V. Benjamin, T. Bergeron, J. P. Lin, I. I. Krichoff: Positive and negative contrast myelography in spinal trauma. Radiology 123 (1977) 103–111
Psenner, L.: Über Schädelveränderungen nach alten Traumen. Wien klin. Wschr. 80 (1968) 921–925
Pye, I. F., M. C. Hickey: Traumatic arachnoid diverticula. A report of two cases causing spinal cord compression. Brit. J. Radiol. 48 (1975) 889–893
Re, G.: L'indagine radioligica nella traumatologia maxillofacciale. Minerva stomat. 14 (1965) 595–609
Rehn, J.: Die Frakturen der Wirbelsäule, ihre Diagnostik und Beurteilung. Röntgenblätter 7 (1968) 318–328
Ricklin, P.: Der Straßenverkehrsunfall. Helv. chir. Acta. Suppl. 9 (1958)
Robinson, A. E., B. M. Meares, J. A. Goree: Traumatic sphenoid sinus effusion. Amer. J. Roentgenol. 101 (1967) 795–801
Roche, J.: Fractures of the temporal bone involving the ear. Austral. Radiol. 19 (1975) 317–325
Rothman, S. L. G., W. E. Allen, E. L. Kier: Stereo roentgenography in craniofacial injuries. A revival of fundamental ideas. Radiol. Clin. N. Amer. 11 (1973) 683–696
Russin, L. D., F. C. Guinto: Multidirectional tomography in cervical spine injury. J. Neurosurg. 45 (1976) 9–11
Saldeen, T.: Fatal neck injuries caused by use of diagonal safety belts. J. Trauma 7 (1967) 856–862
Schmorl, G., H. Junghanns: Die gesunde und die kranke Wirbelsäule in Rötgenbild und Klinik. Thieme, Stuttgart 1968
Schneider, R. C., K. E. Livingstone, A. J. E. Cave, D. Hamilton: Hangman's fracture of the spine. J. Neurosurg. 22 (1965) 141
Schoen, H.: Medizinische Röntgentechnik, Vol. I. Thieme, Stuttgart 1956
Schüle, H.: Röntgendiagnostik nach Kiefergelenktraumen. Beih. Deutscher Röntgenkongreß 1965, Part A. Thieme, Stuttgart (1966) 142–149
Schürmann K.: Sofortmaßnahmen bei Schädel-Hirn-Verletzungen. Fortschr. Med. 86 (1968) 297–300
Seeger, W.: Frontobasale Frakturen. Dtsch. med. Wschr. 92 (1967) 1009–1012
Seljeskog, E. L., S. N. Chou: Spectrum of Hangman's fracture. J. Neurosurg. 45 (1976) 3–8

Shapiro, R., A. S. Youngberg, S. L. G. Rothman: The differential diagnosis of traumatic lesions of the occipito-atlanto-axial segment. Radiol. Clin. N. Amer. 11 (1973) 505–526
Shrago, G. G.: Cervical spine injuries. Association with head trauma. A review of 50 patients. Amer. J. Roentgenol. 118 (1973) 670–673
Slepyan, D. H.: A case of orbital floor eruption. J. Trauma 16 (1976) 320–322
Smith, G. R., C. H. Northrop, J. W. Loop: Jumper's fractures. Patterns of thoracolumbar spine injuries associated with vertical plunges. A review of 38 cases. Radiology 122 (1977) 657–663
Sonnabend, E.: Traumatische Zahnschäden, Frakturen des Alveolarfortsatzes und des Unterkiefers. Fortschr. Röntgenstr. Beih. Deutscher Röntgenkongreß 1965, Part A. Thieme Stuttgart (1966) 149–155
Spenler, C. W., J. R. Benfield: Esophageal disruption from blunt and penetrating external trauma. Arch. Surg. 111 (1976) 663
Stewart, G. C., J. A. Gehweiler, R. H. Laib, S. Martinez: Horizontal fracture of the anterior arch of the atlas. Radiology 122 (1977) 349–352
Switzer, P., R. G. Pitman, J. P. Fleming: Pneumomediastinum associated with zygomaticomaxillary fracture. J. Can. Assoc. Radiol. 25 (1974) 316–318
Talim, S. T., F. E. Anita: A roentgenographic evaluation for implanted teeth. Surgery 21 (1966) 602–608
Tänzer, A.: Die Röntgendiagnostik der Impressionsfraktur des Orbitabodens (blow-out fracture). Fortschr. Röntgenstr. Beiheft Deutscher Röntgenkongreß 1965, Part A. Thieme Stuttgart (1966) 155–157
Tönnis, W., R. A. Frowein, K. H. Euler: Zur Erkennung der akuten traumatischen intrakraniellen Hämatome. Chirurg. 34 (1963) 145–151
Torklus, G., W. Gehle: Die obere Halswirbelsäule. Thieme, Stuttgart 1970
Trzebicki, J., M. Niewiadomska: Traumatische arteriovenöse Fistel der Arteria meningica media. Fortschr. Röntgenstr. 109 (1968) 104–105
Ueno, T., T. Oka, Y. Miyagawa, Y. Kobayashi: Clinical and experimental studies on the location and lines of mandibular fractures. Bulletin Tokyo med. dent. Univ. 4 (1957) 245–251
Vinik, M., F. P. Gargano: Orbital fractures. Amer. J. Roentgenol. 97 (1966) 607–613
Vogelsang, H.: Neuroradiologische Diagnostik bei Wirbelsäulenverletzungen. Dtsch. med. Wschr. 94 (1969) 723–725
Webber, R. L., J. Folio: Radiographic detectability of occipital and temporal-parietal fracture induced in cadaver heads. J. Trauma 16 (1976) 115–124
Weidenbach, W., F. Schmidberger, G. Weiß, B. Lex: Schwere Schädel-Hirn-Traumen. Fortschr. Med. 87 (1969) 673–676
Zatzkin, H. R.: The Roentgen Diagnosis of Trauma. Year Book Medical Publishers, Chicago 1965

Chapters 4 to 6

Arndt, J. H., A. D. Sears: Posterior dislocation of the shoulder. Amer. J. Roentgenol. 94 (1965) 639–645
Bernett, P.: Talusfrakturen. Fortschr. Med. 87 (1969) 647–652
Bernett, P., H. J. Wiendl: Hüftgelenk. Frakturen und Verrenkungsfrakturen. Fortschr. Med. 87 (1969) 365–369
Bernett, P., G. W. Prokscha, M. Stock: Mittelfußfrakturen. Fortschr. Med. 87 (1969) 1353–1355
Bernett, P., W. Hartl, F. Lechner, H. Scholze: Zur Behandlung der Schenkelhalsfrakturen. Fortschr. Med. 87 (1969) 370–373
Bernett, P., W. Hartl. P. Maurer, H. J. Wiendl: Zur Behandlung von Malleolarfrakturen. Fortsch. Med. 87 (1969) 551–555
Bernett, P., D. Mack, W. Rademacher, H. Wenzel: Die Behandlung der Unterarmschaftfrakturen. Fortschr. Med. 87 (1969) 1355–1357
Bernett, P., H. Scherer, H. Schmid, H. Scholze: Kniegelenksbrüche. Fortschr. Med. 87 (1969) 531–538
Bernett, P., P. Härtel, P. Maurer, W. Rademacher, H. Scholze: Bauchverletzungen. Fortschr. Med. 87 (1969) 662–667
Blom, J. M. H., S. P. Strijk: Lesions of the trochlea tali. Osteochondral fractures and osteochondritis dissecans of the trochlea tali. Radiol. Clin. Biol. (Basel) 44 (1975) 387–396
Das Sarkar, S.: Unstable hemipelvic fractures with internal rotation displacement. J. Trauma 16 (1976) 402–405
Debrunner, A. M.: Distale Radiusfrakturen. Schweiz. Med. Wschr. 97 (1967) 820–822
Epstein, H. C.: Posterior fracture-dislocations of the hip. Long-term follow up. J. Bone Jt. Surg. 56 A (1974) 1103–1127
Foster, S. C., R. R. Foster: Lisfranc's tarsometatarsal fracture-dislocation. Radiology 120 (1976) 79–83
Gilchrist, M. R., D. H. Peterson: Pelvic fracture and associated soft-tissue trauma. Radiology 88 (1967) 278–280
Gordon, S. L., E. J. Dunn, T. H. Malin: Lateral collateral ligament ankle injuries in young athletic individuals. J. Trauma 16 (1976) 225–231
Harris, N. H., R. O. Murray: Lesions of the symphysis in athletes. Brit. Med. J. 4 (1974) 211–214
Imatani, R. J.: Fractures of the scapula. A review of 53 fractures. J. Trauma 15 (1975) 473–478
Jacobs, B., P. A. Wade: Acromioclavicular-joint. J. Bone Jt. Surg. 48-A (1966) 475–486
Jonasch E.: Die traumatischen Knorpel-Knochenabsprengungen von der Kniescheibe und von den Oberschenkelknochen. Mschr. Unfallheilk. 65 (1962) 191–197
Jonasch E.: Erkennung und Beurteilung der Meniskusverletzung des Kniegelenkes durch das gewöhnliche Röntgenbild. Hefte zur Unfallheilkunde No. 90. Springer, Berlin 1967
Kolar, J., W. Penn: Progessive posttraumatic pelvic destruction. Radiol. Clin. Biol. (Basel) 42 (1973) 373–384
Kotzen, L. M.: Roentgen diagnosis of rotator cuff tear. Report of 48 surgically proven cases. Amer. J. Roentgenol. 112 (1971) 507–511
Küpfer, K.: Sogenannte Kontusionen und Distorsionen der Finger. Schweiz. Med. Wschr. 98 (1968) 1480
Mauermayer, W., G. Scharrer: Urologische Nebenverletzungen bei Beckenbrüchen. Fortschr. Med. 87 (1969) 668–671
Morehouse, D. D., K. J. MacKinnon: Urological injuries associated with pelvic fractures. J. Trauma 9 (1969) 479–496
Nettles, J. L.: Sternoclavicular dislocations. J. Trauma 8 (1968) 158
Newman, A.: The Supracondylar process and its fracture. Amer J. Roentgenol. 105 (1969) 844–849
O'Reilly, R. J., G. Blatt: Accidental high-pressure injection-gun injuries of the hand. The role of the emergency radiologic examination. J. Trauma 15 (1975) 24–31
Patscheider, H.: Über Anprallverletzungen der unteren Gliedmaßen bei Straßenverkehrsunfällen. Fortschr. Med. 85 (1967) 47–50
Ring, E. J., A. C. Waltman, C. Athanasoulis, J. C. Smith, Jr., S. Baum: Angiography in pelvic trauma. Surg. Gynecol. Obstet. 139 (1974) 375–380
Rogers, L. F., S. Jones, A. R. Davis, G. Dietz: "Clipping injury" fracture of the epiphysis in the adolescent football player. An occult lesion of the knee. Amer. J. Roentgenol. 121 (1974) 69–78
Schneider, R., J. J. Kaye, B. Ghelman: Adductor avulsive injuries near the symphisis pubis. Radiology 120 (1976) 567–569
Sinistrero, G., G. Toscano: Aspetti radiografici e clinici delle fratture del pisiforme. Minerva fisioter. (Torino) 10 (1965) 114–117
Smith, G. R., J. W. Loop: Radiologic classification of posterior dislocations of the hip. Refinements and pitfalls. Radiology 119 (1976) 569–574
Smith, K., Y. Ben-Menachem, J. H. Duke, G. L. Hill: The superior gluteal. An artery at risk in blunt pelvic trauma. J. Trauma 16 (1976) 273–279
Terry, D. W., J. E. Ramin: The navicular fat stripe. A useful roentgen feature for evaluating wrist trauma. Amer. J. Roentgenol. 25 (1975) 25–28
Thiele, K.: Schienbeinkopfbrüche. Bruchformen, Behandlung, Spätergebnisse bei 486 Fällen. Hefte zur Unfallheilkunde, No. 95. Springer, Berlin 1968
Torok, G.: Bilateral sacroiliac joint dislocation with intrapelvic intrusion of the intact lumbosacral spine and sacrum. J. Trauma 16 (1976) 930–934
Veihelmann, D., S. Weller: Die sogenannte zentrale Hüftgelenksluxation und ihre Behandlung. Dtsch. Med. Wschr. 94 (1969) 602–605
Wallner, H.: Das Beckentrauma aus geburtshilflicher Sicht. Fortschr. Med. 87 (1969) 671
Warrick, C. K.: Posterior dislocation of the shoulder joint. Brit. J. Radiol. 38 (1965) 758–761

Weber, B. G.: Malleolarfrakturen. Schweiz. Med. Wschr. 97 (1967) 790–792
Weller, S., E. Köhnlein: Die Traumatologie des Kniegelenkes. Thieme, Stuttgart 1962
Weston, W. J.: The soft tissue signs with rupture of the long head of biceps. Brit. J. Radiol. 42 (1969) 539–540
Wilson, D. W.: Functional capacity following fractures of the os calcis. Canad. med. Ass. J. 95 (1966) 908–911
Zatzkin, H. R.: The Roentgen Diagnosis of Trauma. Year Book Medical Publishers, Chicago 1965

Chapter 7

Barnes, G. R., J. L. Gwinn: Distal irregularities of femur simulating malignancy. Amer. J. Roentgenol. 122 (1974) 180–185
Cheli, C., C. A. Crivellaro, F. Bonadimani, A. Campanati: Fracture costali in pazienti affete da cancro mammario operate ed irradiate. Ann. Radiol. diagn. 41 (1968) 284–302
Delahaye, R. P., J. Jouffrey, H. Laurent, P. C. Loze: Les fractures de fatigue. J. Radiol. electrol. 47 (1966) 525–533
Devas, M. B.: Stress fractures in children. J. Bone Jt. Surg. 45 B (1963) 528
Drennan, D. B., J. S. Fahey, D. J. Maylahn: Fracture through large nonossifying fibromas. J. Bone Jt. Surg. 54 A (1972) 1794
Eichler, J.: Tumorähnliche Knochenveränderungen bei Hämophilie. Fortschr. Röntgenstr. 104 (1966) 103–107
Engh, C. A., R. A. Robinson, J. Milgram: Stress fractures in children. J. Trauma 10 (1970) 532
Fries, G.: Zur Röntgendiagnostik osteoradionekrotischer Hüftveränderung nach Röntgen-Radiumbestrahlung weiblicher Genitalkarzinome. Strahlentherapie 132 (1967) 113–127
Haller, T., S. Amit, D. Segal: Fatigue fractures of tibia and femoral shaft in soldiers. Clin. Orthop. 118 (1976) 35–43
Handelsman, J. E.: Spontaneous fractures in spina bifida. J. Bone Jt. Surg. 54 B (1972) 381
Hansen, S. T., T. K. F. Taylor, J. C. Honet, F. R. Lewis: Fracture-dislocations of the ankylosed thoracic spine in rheumatoid spondylitis. Ankylosing spondylitis, Marie-Strümpell disease. J. Trauma 7 (1967) 827
Jensen, T. M., W. L. Dillon, F. W. Reckling: Changing concepts in the management of pathological and impending pathological fractures. J. Trauma 16 (1976) 496–502
Korhonen, B. J.: Fractures in myelodysplasia. Clin. Orthop. 79 (1971) 145
Levin, C., E. M. Blazina, E. Levine: Fatigue fractures of the shaft of the femur: simulation of malignant tumor. Radiology 89 (1967) 883–885
Maeyama, J., S. Sato, S. Goto: Carcinomas metastatic to bone at the National Cancer Center Hospital in Japan. J. Jap. orthop. Ass. 40 (1966) 221–229
Marmor, L.: Stress fracture of the pubic ramus simulating a loose total hip replacement. Clin. Orthop. 121 (1976) 103–104
Martel, W., G. G. Bole: Pathologic fracture of the odontoid process in rheumatoid arthritis. Radiology 90 (1968) 948–952
Miller, H. E., H. J. Schneider, J. L. Bronson, D. McLain: A new consideration in athletic injuries. The classical ballet dancer. Clin. Orthop. 111 (1975) 181–191
North, K. A. K.: Multiple stress fractures simulating osteomalacia. Amer. J. Roentgenol. 97 (1966) 672–675
Ochsner, S. F.: Eosinophilic granuloma of bone; experience with 20 cases. Amer. J. Roentgenol. 97 (166) 719–726
Pogonowska, M. J., L. C. Collins, H. L. Dobson: Diabetic osteopathy. Radiology 89 (1967) 265–271
Robin, G. C.: Fractures in poliomyelitis in children. J. Bone Jt. Surg. 48 A (1966) 1048-1054
Schlosser, V.: Beitrag zur operativen Behandlung pathologischer Frakturen. Fortschr. Med. 86 (1968) 311
Wiltse, L. L., E. H. Widell, D. W. Jackson: Fatigue fracture. Basic lesion in isthmic spondylolisthesis. J. Bone Jt. Surg. 57 A (1975) 17–22

Chapter 8

Barrie, J., R. Sarrazin, M. Reichenecker: Eléments du diagnostic des ruptures traumatiques de l'oesophage (par traumatismes indirects). Ann. Chir. (Paris) 19 (1965) 510–514
Bennett, D. E., J. K. Chery: The natural history of traumatic aneurysms of the aorta. Surgery 61 (1967) 516–523
Benrey, J., E. C. Price, E. K. Massin, J. C. Bowers, D. A. Cooley: Coronary occlusion secondary to nonpenetrating chest trauma. Tex. Med. 71 (1975) 60–64
Christiansen, L. A., P. Stage, E. B. Brahe, S. Bertelsen: Rupture of the diaphragm. Thorax 29 (1974) 559–563
Crawford, W. O.: Pulmonary injury in thoracic and non-thoracic trauma. Radiol. Clin. N. Amer. 11 (1973) 527–541
Dart, C. H., H. E. Braitman: Traumatic rupture of thoracic aorta. Diagnosis and management. Arch. Surg. 111 (1976) 697
Eller, J. L., F. M. H. Ziter: Avulsion of the innominate artery from the aortic arch. An evaluation of roentgenographic findings. Radiology 94 (1970) 75–78
Fagan, C. J.: Traumatic lung cyst. Amer. J. Roentgenol. 97 (1966) 186–194
Fallazadeh, H., E. T. Mays: Disruption of the diaphragm by blunt trauma. New dimensions of diagnosis. Amer. Surg. 41 (1975) 337
Fishbone, G., D. I. Robbins, D. J. Osborn, V. Grnja: Trauma to the thoracic and great vessels. Radiol. Clin. N. Amer. 11 (1973) 543–554
Foley, W. D., R. R. Stewart: Angiographic findings in diaphragmatic rupture. Austral. Radiol. 20 (1976) 150–153
Freed, T. A., L. A. Bosher: Arteriographic demonstration of laceration of great vessels secondary to blunt chest trauma. Radiology 90 (1968) 88–89
Fu, W. R.: Angiography of Trauma. Charles C. Thomas, Springfield, Ill. 1972
Glaudemans, P. W.: Pulmonary hematoma caused by nonpenetrating chest injury. J. belge Radiol. 48 (1965) 730–742
Gremmel, G., H. Vieten: Stumpftraumatische Thoraxverletzungen. Röntgenblätter 19 (1966) 65–75
Grewe, H. E.: Der Chylothorax. Chir. Praxis 10 (1966) 103–110
Grill, W.: Die geschlossenen und offenen Verletzungen des Brustkorbs und der Brustorgane. Enke, Stuttgart 1966
Harlacher, A., H. Brebeck: Schwere Thoraxverletzungen und Grundzüge ihrer Behandlung. Fortschr. Med. 87 (1969) 1231–1235
Hensinger, R. N., H. A. Berkoff: Traumatic non-union of the sternum. Report of a case. J. Trauma 15 (1975) 159–162
Jimenez, J. P., R. G. Lester: Pulmonary complications following furniture polish ingestion. A report of 21 cases. Amer. J. Roentgenol. 98 (1966) 323–333
Johnson, J., G. W. Schwegman: Iatrogenic and spontaneous perforation of the esophagus. Amer. J. Gastroent. 47 (1967) 365–372
Jones, J. W., R. L. Hewitt, T. Drapanas: Cardiac contusion. Ann. Surg. 181 (1975) 567
Keller, J. W., C. V. Meckstroht, L. Sanzenbacher, W. G. Pace: Thoracic injuries due to blunt trauma. J. Trauma 7 (1967) 541–550
Kermond, A. J.: The dislocated heart. An unusual complication of major chest injury. Radiology 119 (1976) 56–60
Kessler, E., A. Stein: Diaphragmatic hernia as a long-term complication of stab wounds of the chest. Amer. J. Surg. 132 (1976) 34
Krauß, H.: Die Bronchusruptur. Dtsch. med. Wschr. 13 (1956) 429
Kümmerle, F.: Die stumpfen Bauchverletzungen. Ihre Erkennung und Behandlung. Enke, Stuttgart 1959
Kümmerle, F.: Beitrag zur traumatischen Ruptur der thorakalen Aorta. Hefte zur Unfallheilkunde, Heft 81 (1965) 21–24
Lorenz, D.: Verletzungen großer Körperhöhlen. Wehrmed. Mschr. 10 (1966) 286–295
Martin, W.: Die akute Barbiturat-Intoxikation. Fortschr. Med. 87 (1969) 1158–1160
McCune, R. P., C. P. Roda, C. Eckert: Rupture of the diaphragm caused by blunt trauma. J. Trauma 16 (1976) 531– 537
Muth, de W. E., A. E. Baue, J. A. Odom: Contusions of the heart. J. Trauma 7 (1967) 443–455
Noon, G. P., A. C. Beall Jr., M. E. De Bakey: Surgical management of penetrating esophageal injuries. J. Trauma 8 (1968) 458–464
Noon, G. P., D. Boulafendis, C. A. Beall: Rupture of the heart secondary to blunt trauma. J. Trauma 11 (1971) 122–128
Orringer, M. B., M. M. Kirsh, H. Sloan: Congenital and traumatic diaphragmatic hernias exclusive of the hiatus. Curr. Problems Surg. (Mar. 1975)
Panaro, V. A., E. S. Leslie: Spontaneous rupture of the esophagus. Radiology 84 (1965) 252–258
Pearce, W., E. Blair: Significance of the electrocardiogram in heart contusion due to blunt trauma. J. Trauma 16 (1976) 136–140

Pierce, G. E., J. A. Maxwell, M. D. Boggan: Special hazards of 1st rib fractures. J. Trauma 15 (1975) 264–267
Puijlaert, C. B. A. J.: Roentgen diagnosis of traumatic rupture of the aorta. Radiol. Clin. Biol. (Basel) 45 (1976) 217–235
Razemon, P., M. Ribet, C. Gauthier: Les hématomes pulmonaires. Ann. Chir. (Paris) 2 (1963) 78–87
Richardson, J. D., F. L. Grover, J. K. Trinkle: Early operative management of isolated sternal fractures. J. Trauma 15 (1975) 156–158
Rosenkranz, K. A.: Die traumatische Herzschädigung. Die Auswirkungen stumpfer Brustkorbtraumen auf das Herz. Experimentelle Grundlagen. Fortschr. Med. 87 (1969) 1181–1184
Klinische Beobachtungen. Fortschr. Med. 87 (1969) 1226–1230
Sanborn, J. C., R. Heitzman, B. Markarian: Traumatic rupture of the thoracic aorta. Radiology 95 (1970) 293–298
Sherborn, K. J.: Traumatic rupture of the thoracic aorta. The radiologist's responsibility. Austral. Radiol. 19 (1976) 164–171
Silbiger, M. L., L. N. Kushner: Tracheobronchial perforation: its diagnosis and treatment. Radiology 85 (1965) 242–246
Soulen, R. L., E. Freeman: Radiologic evaluation of traumatic head disease. Radiol. Clin. N. Amer. 9 (1971) 285–298
Spengler, C. W., J. R. Benfield: Esophageal disruption from blunt and penetrating external trauma. Arch. Surg. 111 (1976) 663
Steinberg, I., L. Miscall: Angiocardiographic findings in traumatic rupture of a bronchus. Amer. J. Roentgenol. 96 (1966) 962–966
Stevens, E., A. W. Templeton: Traumatic nonpenetrating lung contusion. Radiology 85 (1965) 247–252
Strug, B., G. P. Noon, A. C. Beall Jr.: Traumatic diaphragmatic hernia. Ann. Thorac Surg. 17 (1974) 444
Sturm, J. T., et al.: Hemopneumothorax following blunt trauma of the thorax. Surg. Gynecol. Obstet. 141 (1975) 539
Stutz. E., H. Vieten: Die Bronchographie. Thieme, Stuttgart 1955
Ting, Y. M.: Pulmonary parenchymal findings in blunt trauma to the chest. Amer. J. Roentgenol. 98 (1966) 343–349
Truckenbrodt, H., F. Gall: Zur Diagnose und Therapie der Bronchusruptur. Radiologe 8 (1968) 315–318
Tscherne, H., H. Schreyer, F. Magerl: Pulmonale und kardiale Röntgenbefunde bei traumatischer Fettembolie. Forstchr. Röntgenstr. 106 (1967) 703–710
Waridel, D., F. Saegesser: Les ruptures traumatiques fermées du diaphragme. Schweiz. med. Wschr. 99 (1969) 465–473
Wülfing, D.: Zur Problematik der Thoraxverletzung. Röntgenblätter 19 (1966) 75–83

Chapter 9

Aakhus, T., I. Enge: Angiography in traumatic rupture of the spleen. Brit. J. Radiol. 40 (1967) 855–861
Allison, R. C.: Urethrography in pelvic trauma. Urology 3 (1974) 453–455
Altemus, R., D. Charles, J. R. Stock: Hysterography used in the diagnosis of intrauterine trauma. Amer. J. Roentgenol. 104 (1968) 865
Aragon, G. E., B. Eiseman: Abdominal stab wounds. Evaluation of sinography. J. Trauma 16 (1976) 792–797
Bass, E. M., J. H. Crosier: Percutaneous control of post-traumatic hepatic hemorrhage by gelfoam embolization. J. Trauma 17 (1977) 61–63
Baudisch, E.: Angiographische Untersuchungen bei stumpfen Nierenverletzungen. Radiol. diagn. (Berl.) 5 (1964) 703–721
Baudisch, E., E. Hienzsch: Zur Indikationsstellung der Röntgenuntersuchung bei Nierenverletzungen. Urologe 4 (1965) 126–129
Bergmann, M.: Der Wert und die Indikation der Angiographie bei Nierenverletzungen. Verh. dtsch. Ges. Urol. (1965) 201
Bergqvist, D., H. Hedelin: Roll seat belt induced injury of the duodenum. J. Trauma 16 (1976) 390–394
Berk, R. N., J. M. Wholey: The application of splenic arteriography in the diagnosis of rupture of the spleen. Amer. J. Roentgenol. 104 (1968) 662
Berk, R. N., M. H. Wholey, R. Stockdale: The angiographic diagnosis of splenic and hepatic trauma. J. Can. Assoc. Radiol. 21 (1970) 230–234
Boijsen, E., M. P. Judkins, A. Simay: Angiographic diagnosis of hepatic rupture. Radiology 86 (1966) 66
Budin, E., G. Jacobson: Roentgenographic diagnosis of small amounts of intraperitoneal fluid. Amer. J. Roentgenol. 99 (1967) 62–70
Burell, M., R. Toffler, R. Lowman: Blunt trauma to the abdomen and gastrointestinal tract. Plain film and contrast study. Radiol. Clin. N. Amer. 11 (1973) 561–578
Buschmann, O., L. Kerk: Zur Röntgendiagnostik der Nierenverletzungen. Fortschr. Röntgenstr. 103 (1965) 683–689
Bussey, H. J., R. N. McGehee, K. R. T. Tyson: Isolated gastric rupture due to blunt trauma. J. Trauma 15 (1975) 190–191
Cimmino, C. V.: Ruptured spleen: some refinements in its roentgenologic diagnosis. Radiology 82 (1964) 57–62
Cornell, W. P., P. A. Ebert, G. D. Zuidema: X-ray diagnosis of penetrating wounds of the abdomen. J. surg. Res. 5 (1965) 142–145
Cornell, W. P., P. A. Ebert, L. J. Greenfield, G. D. Zuidema: A new nonoperative technique for the diagnosis of penetrating injuries to the abdomen. J. Trauma 7 (1967) 307–314
Depner, T. A., et al.: Post-traumatic renal artery stenosis. Cure of hypertension by late revascularization. Arch. Surg. 110 (1975) 1150
Elkin, M., M. H. Chien, G. R. DeParedes: Roentgenologic evaluation of renal trauma with emphasis on renal angiography. Amer. J. Roentgenol. 98 (1966) 1–26
Enge, I., O. Knutrud, T. Normann: Central rupture of the liver with traumatic haemobilia. Brit. J. Radiol. 41 (1968) 789–791
Evans, R. A., M. J. V. Smith: Violent injuries to the upper ureter. J. Trauma 16 (1976) 558–561
Farman, J., D. Stein, H. Krige: Duodenal haematomas. Clin. Radiol. (Edinb.) 17 (1966) 177–179
Freemann, L. M., C. J. Kay, C. H. Meng: The contribution of renal scanning in the evaluation of renal trauma. Radiology 86 (1966) 1021–1029
Fu, W. R.: Angiography of Trauma. Charles C. Thomas, Springfield, Ill. 1972
Guerrier, K., D. J. Albert, S. A. Mahoney, R. J. Izant, L. Persky: Delayed nephrectomy after trauma. J. Trauma 9 (1969) 465
Gumbert, J. L., P. M. Waitt, F. W. Taylor: Gunshot wounds of the abdomen: Evaluation of treatment. Surgery 59 (1966) 376–380
Hepp, J., J. Caroli, J. Moreaux, P. Opolon, H. Bismuth: Les hémobilies par lésion traumatique de l'artère hépatique dans les contusions de l'abdomen. Ann. Chir. (Paris) 20 (1966) 359–367
Hienzsch, E.: Die Verletzungen der Blase. Verh. dtsch. Ges. Urol. (1965) 159–169
Hodel, C.: Pathologische Leberruptur mit intraabdomineller Verblutung bei Leberkarzinom. Acta hepato-Splenologica 15 (1968) 252
Houston, H. E., J. H. Gilbaugh Jr., R. B. Wallace: Traumatic transection of horseshoe kidney. Mayo Clin. Proc. 43 (1968) 444–448
Kalish, M., et al.: Traumatic renal hemorrhage treatment by arterial embolization. J. Urol. 112 (1974) 138
Kaude, J.: Traumatic rupture of the abdominal wall with subcutaneous herniation of the transverse colon and perforation of small bowel. Brit. J. Radiol. 39 (1966) 950–951
Klieber, H.: Stumpfe Bauchverletzungen. Dissertation, Freiburg 1958
Kümmerle, F.: Die stumpfen Bauchverletzungen, ihre Erkennung und Behandlung. Enke, Stuttgart 1959
Lang, E. K.: Arteriography in the assessment of renal trauma.The impact of arteriographic diagnosis on preservation of renal function and parenchyma. J. Trauma 15 (1975) 553–556
Lorenz: D.: Verletzungen großer Körperhöhlen. Wehrmed. Mschr. 10 (1966) 286–295
Lundstrom, B.: Angiographic demonstration of rupture of the spleen. Acta Radiol. 10 (1970) 145–150
Mattox, K. L., R. Espada, A. C. Beall: Traumatic injury to the portal vein. Ann. Surg. 181 (1975) 519
McCort, J. J.: Radiographic Examination in Blunt Abdominal Trauma. Saunders, Philadelphia 1966
Morton, J. R., G. L. Jordan: Traumatic duodenal injuries. Review of 131 cases. J. Trauma 8 (1968) 127–139
Nelson, R. P., M. J. Sullivan, J. Richter, M. Russo: Complete avulsion of the renal pedicle with survival. Case reports and literature review. J. Trauma 16 (1976) 157–162
Nick, W. V., R. W. Zollinger, W. G. Pace: Retroperitoneal hemorrhage after blunt abdominal trauma. J. Trauma 7 (1967) 652

Osborn, D. J., M. G. Glickman, V. Grnja, G. Ramsby: The role of angiography in abdominal nonrenal trauma. Radiol. Clin. N. Amer. 11 (1973) 579–592

Popovsky, J., S. N. Wiener, P. A. Felder, A. Biramje, M. Reydman: Liver trauma. Conservative management and the liver scan. Arch. Surg. 227 (1974) 753–756

Rabinowitz, R., S. E. Price, M. M. Marshall, D. H. Barnhouse, S. H. Johnson: Isolated ureteral injury secondary to transperitoneal stab wound. J. Trauma 16 (1976) 164–168

Redman, H. C., S. R. Reuter, J. J. Bookstein: Angiography in abdominal trauma. Ann. Surg. 169 (1969) 57–66

Reiss, M. D.: Traumatic rupture of renal cyst into the calyceal system. Amer. J. Roentgenol. 100 (1967) 696–699

Richter, M. W., B. Lytton, D. Myerson, V. Grnja: Radiology of genitourinary trauma. Radiol. Clin. N. Amer. 11 (1973) 593–631

Richter, R. M.: Traumatic rupture of an exogastric leiomyosarcoma. Amer. J. Gastroent. 50 (1968) 144

Schorr, S., J. Danon: Rupture of the spleen: A new roentgen sign. Amer. J. Roentgenol. 99 (1967) 616–624

Scott, R., C. E. Carlton, M. Goldman: Penetrating injuries of the kidney: An analysis of 181 patients. J. Urol. (Baltimore) 101 (1969) 247

Shennan: J.: Seat-belt injuries of the left colon. Brit. J. Surg. 60 (1973) 673–675

Stables, D. P.: Unilateral absence of excretion at urography after abdominal trauma. Radiology 121 (1976) 609–615

Strum, J. T., J. F. Perry, S. C. Alexander: Renal artery and vein injuries following blunt trauma. Ann. Surg. 182 (1975) 696

Tomatis, L. A., F. A. Doornbos, J. A. Beard: Circumferential intimal tear of aorta with complete occlusion due to blunt trauma. J. Trauma 8 (1968) 1096–1101

Toxopeus, M. D., C. E. Lucas, K. L. Krabbenhoft: Roentgenographic diagnosis in blunt retroperitoneal duodenal rupture. Amer. J. Roentgenol. 115 (1972) 281–288

Unger, J. L., C. Bare, J. Haight: Traumatic bilateral renal artery thrombosis. J. Trauma 17 (1977) 64–68

Vielberg, H., E. Schnepper: Die Röntgendiagnostik stumpfer Bauchtraumen. Röntgenblätter 19 (1966) 405–424

Wanebo, H. J., T. K. Hunt, C. Mathewson: Rectal injuries. J. Trauma 9 (1969) 712

Weinstein, E. C., V. Pallais: Rupture of the pregnant uterus from blunt trauma. Report of a case. J. Trauma 8 (1968) 1111–1113

Westcott, J. L., J. R. V. Smith: Mesentery and colon injuries secondary to blunt trauma. Radiology 114 (1975) 597–600

Wilson, R. F., J. P. Tagett, J. P. Pucelik, J. A. Walt: Pancreatic trauma. J. Trauma 7 (1967) 643–651

Wolfel, D. A., B. G. Brogdon: Intrahepatic air. A sign of trauma. Radiology 91 (1968) 952–953

Yajko, R. D., F. Seydel, C. Trimble: Rupture of the stomach from blunt abdominal trauma. J. Trauma 15 (1975) 177–183

Chapter 10

Benedict, E. B.: An extraordinary foreign body in the esophagus. New. Engl. J. Med. 269 (1963) 146

Büchner, H.: Lokalisationsverfahren. *In:* Lehrbuch der Röntgendiagnostik, Vol. I. hrsg. *von H. R. Schinz, W. E. Baensch, W. Frommhold, R. Glauner, E. Uelinger, J. Wellauer.* Thieme, Stuttgart (1965) 166–188

Comberg, W.: Ein neues Verfahren zur Röntgenlokalisation am Augapfel. Albrecht v. Graefes Arch. klin. exp. Ophthal. 118 (1927) 175

Daum, R., K. Köhler: Verschluckte Fremdkörper im Kindesalter. Münch. med. Wschr. 108 (1966) 1261–1266

Dimond, F. C., N. M. Rich: M–16 Rifle wounds in Vietnam. J. Trauma 7 (1967) 619–625

Fink, D. W., F. M. Boyden: Gas in portal veins. A report of two cases due to ingestion of corrosive substances. Radiology 87 (1966) 741–743

Fischer, E.: Der Nachweis von Holz- und kleinen Glassplittern durch die Weichstrahlaufnahme. Fortschr. Röntgenstr. 118 (1973) 309

Freick, H. J., H. C. Crosta: Verschluß des Ductus, Choledochus durch eingewanderten Granatsplitter. Fortschr. Med. 87 (1969) 49–52

Führer, H.: Medizinische Toxikologie, Thieme, Leipzig 1947

Hill, M. C., W. B. Bieber, R. L. Koch, W. Coulson: Extraperitoneal perforations of the gastrointestinal tract. Amer. J. Roentgenol. 101 (1967) 315–321

Kainberger, F.: Die Beurteilung und das Verhalten nativ sichtbarer Fremdkörper im Gastrointestinaltrakt auf dem Röntgenbild. Wien, klin. Wschr. 80 (1968) 263–269

Kern, E., J. Klöß, A. Bremer: Verschluckte Fremdkörper und Bezoare im Gastrointestinaltrakt. Dtsch. med. Wschr. 89 (1964) 480–487

Letts, R. M., D. Miller: Gunshot wounds of the extremities in children. J. Trauma 16 (1976) 807–811

Maurer, R., H. Hoefer-Janker: Zur Differentialdiagnostik und Therapie intrathorakaler Fremdkörper. Dtsch. med. Wschr. 91 (1966) 2254–2258

Minnigerode, B.: Fremdkörper der tieferen Luft- und Speisewege. Dtsch. Ärztebl. 69 (1972) 1926–1929

Naumann, P.: Gesichtsverletzungen durch splitternde Windschutzscheiben. Dtsch. Ärztebl. 38 (1968) 2050–2052

Neiß, A. W.: Bei Verdacht auf Tötung durch Schuß sollte geröntgt werden. Fortschr. Röntgenstr. 109 (1968) 668–669

O'Reilly, R. J., C. Blatt: Accidental high pressure injection gun injuries of the hand. The role of the emergency radiologic examination. J. Trauma 15 (1975) 24–31

Park, W. H., W. E. DeMuth: Wounding capacity of rotary lawn mowers. J. Trauma 15 (1975) 36–38

Payne, R. F.: Foreign bodies in the frontal sinus. Br. J. Radiol. 40 (1967) 778–780

Rodriguez, M. A., M. R. Rodger: Right axillary artery bullet embolus following gunshot wound of the back. J. Trauma 15 (1975) 170–173

Shacklett, R. S., K. D. Dolan, E. F. Rose: A "piggy-back" bullet wound of the head. Amer. J. Roentgenol. 122 (1974) 576–579

Taxin, R. N., F. Feldman: The tumbling bullet sign in a post-traumatic bone cyst. Amer. J. Roentgenol. 123 (1975) 140–143

Thiel, R.: Röntgendiagnostik des Schädels bei Erkrankungen des Auges und seiner Nachbarorgane. Springer, Berlin (1932) 31, 68

Trede M., A. Encke: Iatrogene Fremdkörper im Herzen und in den großen Gefäßen. Thoraxchirurgie 18 (1970) 405–409

Valtonen, E. J.: Shellac and lipoid bezoars and other concretions of the stomach. Gastroenterologia 104 (1965) 309–320

Vogt, A.: Skelettfreie Röntgenaufnahme des vorderen Bulbusabschnittes. Schweiz. med. Wschr. 7 (1921) 145

Wadolowski, W.: Spontaner Abgang verschluckter Fremdkörper. Bruns' Beitr. klin. Chir. 210 (1965) 409–414

Wanebo, H. J., T. K. Hunt, C. Mathewson: Rectal injuries. J. Trauma 9 (1969) 712–722

Welin, S.: Fremdkörper der Speiseröhre. *In:* Lehrbuch der Röntgendiagnostik, hrsg. von *H. R. Schinz, W. E. Baensch, E. Friedl, E. Uehlinger:* Thieme, Stuttgart 1952

Wiesner, B., G. Laszig: Diagnostische Probleme der Fremdkörper im Tracheobronchialsystem. Z. ärztl. Fortbild. (Jena) 60 (1966) 79–82

Zatzkin, H. R.: The Roentgen Diagnosis of Trauma. Year Book Medical Publishers, Chicago 1965

Chapter 11

Becker, C. H., H. W. Becker: Nontraumatic percutaneous catheterization of blood vessels with guide wires. Acta Radiol. 7 (1968) 348–354

Bole, P. V., R. Munda, R. T. Purdy, A. Lande, R. Gomez, R. H. Clauss, K. K. Kazarian, W. L. Mersheimer: Traumatic pseudoaneurysms. A review of 32 cases. J. Trauma 16 (1976) 63–70

Bricker, D., G. L. Hallmann: Complete transection of the thoracic aorta: Management of a case associated with massive total body injury. J. Trauma 10 (1970) 420–426

Catalano, D.: Die Röntgendiagnostik der Aneurysmen der unteren Extremität. Radiographica (1965) 277–280

Creech, O., J. Gantt, H. Wren: Traumatic arteriovenous fistula at unusual sites. Ann. Surg. 161 (1965) 908–920

De Bakey, M. E., F. A. Simeone: Battle injuries of the arteries in World War II. Ann. Surg. 123 (1946) 534–579

Dost, K.: Der akute Arterienverschluß der Extremitäten. Med. Welt 22 (1969) 1275–1281

Fisher, G. W.: Acute arterial injuries treated by the United States Army medical service in Vietnam, 1965–1966. J. Trauma 7 (1967) 844–855
Fu, W. R.: Angiography of Trauma. Charles C. Thomas, Springfield, Ill. 1972
Gill, S. S., F. C. Eggleston, C. M. Singh, K. A. Abraham, S. Kumar, L. H. Lubo: Arterial injuries of the extremities. J. Trauma 16 (1976) 766–772
Girl, J.: Arteriography in arterial gunshot wounds. Acta radiol. Diagn. 11 (1971) 78, 84
Goerttler, U., V. Schlosser, J. Blümel: Der Beitrag der Angiographie zur Diagnostik und Therapie peripherer Arterienverletzungen. Bruns' Beitr. klin. Chir. 219 (1971) 129–137
Joffe, N.: Some sialographic findings in traumatic lesions of the parotid duct and gland. Amer. J. Roentgenol. 100 (1967) 656–663
Johnson, A. G., B. Lane, A. J. H. Rains, D. O'Connel, N. W. Ramsay: Large artery damage after X radiation. Brit. J. Radiol. 42 (1969) 937–939
Jimenez, J. P., A. J. Goree: Traumatic arteriovenous fistula of the superficial temporal artery; A report of a case. Amer. J. Roentgenol. 106 (1969) 279–281
Kelly, G. L., B. Eiseman: Civilian vascular injuries. J. Trauma 15 (1975) 507
Lipchik, E. O., J. A. DeWeese, S. M. Rogoff: Serial long-term phlebography after documented lower leg thrombosis. Radiology 120 (1976) 563–566
Love, L.: Arterial trauma. Seminars in Roentgenology 5 (1970) 267–283
Maurer, P., H. Scherer: Unfallbedingte Arterienverletzungen. Fortschr. Med. 87 (1969) 1317–1319
Piyachon, C., S. Arthachinta: Arteriography in trauma of the extremities. Amer. J. Roentgenol. 119 (1973) 580–585
Pochaczevsky, R., M. A. Mufti, J. N. LaGuerre, D. Bryk, E. G. Kassner, R. M. Richter, R. Levowitz: Arteriography of penetrating wounds of the extremities: Help or hindrance? J. Canad. Assoc. Radiol. 24 (1973) 354–361
Rich, N. M., C. W. Hughes, J. H. Baugh: Management of venous injuries. Ann. Surg. 171 (1970) 724–730
Rodriguez, M. A., M. R. Rodger: Right axillary artery bullet embolus following gunshot wound of the back. J. Trauma 15 (1975) 170–173
Smith, K., Y. Ben-Menachem, J. H. Duke, G. L. Hill: The superior gluteal. An artery at risk in blunt pelvic trauma. J. Trauma 16 (1976) 273–279
Staheli, L. T., L. R. Fry: Late popliteal false aneurysm complicating distal femoral fracture. J. Trauma 7 (1967) 322–326
Tice, D. A., R. H. Clauss, A. M. Keirle, G. E. Reed: Congenital arteriovenous fistulae of the extremities. Arch. Surg. 86 (1963) 460–465
Tomatis, L. A., F. A. Doornbos, J. A. Beard: Circumferential intimal tear of aorta with complete occlusion due to blunt trauma. J. Trauma 8 (1968) 1096–1101
Winegarner, F. G., A. G. Baker, J. F. Bascom, G. F. Jackson: Delayed vascular complications in Vietnam casualties. J. Trauma 10 (1970) 867–873

Chapter 12

Adams, J. E.:Bone injuries in very young athletes. Clin. Orthop. 58 (1968) 129–140
Adelson, L.: The battering child. J.A.M.A. 222 (1972) 159
Akbarnia, B., J. S. Torg, J. Kirkpatrick, S. Sussman: Manifestations of the battered-child syndrome. J. Bone Jt. Surg. 56 A (1974) 1159
Alexander, W. J., J. A. Kadish, J. S. Dunbar: Ingested foreign bodies in children. Prog. Pediatr. Radiol. 2 (1969) 256–285
Allen, M. L.: Air Force football injuries. J. A. M. A. 206 (1968) 1053–1058
Asch, M. J., A. G. Coran, P. W. Johnston: Gastric perforation secondary to blunt trauma in children. J. Trauma 15 (1975) 187–189
Audic, B., M. Maury: Secondary vertebral deformities in childhood and adolescence. Paraplegia 7 (1969) 10
Baker, D. H., W. E. Berdon: Special trauma problems in children. Radiol. Clin. N. Amer. 4 (1966) 289–305
Baker, D. H., W. E. Berdon, H. Grossman: Physical and chemical injuries to the respiratory tract. Progr. Pediatr. Radiol. 1 (1967) 326–345
Barnes, G. R., J. L. Gwinn: Distal irregularities of femur simulating malignancy. Amer. J. Roentgenol. 122 (1974) 180–185
Biemann othersen, H., F. T. Moore, E. T. Boles: Traumatic pancreatitis and pseudocyst in childhood. J. Trauma 8 (1968) 535–546
Bingas, B.:Die wachsende Schädelfraktur im Kindesalter. Berl. Med. 15 (1964) 317–319
Blount, W. T.: Fractures in Children. Williams & Wilkins, Baltimore, 1955
Borden, S.: Traumatic bowing of forearm in children. J. Bone Jt. Surg. 56 A (1974) 611–616
Boyd, H. B., J. C. Boals: The Monteggia lesion. A review of 159 cases. Clin. Orthop. 66 (1969) 94
Braunstein, P. W., et al.: Concealed hemorrhage due to pelvic fracture. J. Trauma 4 (1964) 832
Brogdon, B. G., N. E. Crow.: Little Leaguer's elbow. Amer. J. Roentgenol. 83 (1960) 671–675
Bryan, R. S.: Monteggia fracture of the forearm. J. Trauma 11 (1971) 992
Bufkin, W. J.: The avulsive cortical irregularity. Amer. J. Roentgenol. 112 (1971) 487–492
Burke, D. C.: Spinal cord trauma in children. Paraplegia 9 (1971) 1
Caffey, J.: Multiple fractures in the long bones of infants suffering from chronic subdural hematoma. Amer. J. Roentgenol. 56 (1946) 163
Cattell, H. S., D. L. Filtser: Pseudo-subluxation and other normal variations in the cervical spine in children. J. Bone Jt. Surg. 47 A (1965) 1295
Chasler, C.: The newborn skull. The diagnosis of fracture. Amer. J. Roentgenol. 100 (1967) 92–99
Christensen, J. B., K. O. Cho, J. P. Adams, L. Miller: A study of the interosseous distance between the radius and ulna during rotation of the forearm. J. Bone Jt. Surg. 46 B (1964) 778
Cooper, R. G.: Fractures in children. Fundamentals of management. J. Iowa Med. Soc. 54 (1964) 472
Dixon, G. L., Jr., N. F. Moon: Rotational supracondylar fractures of the proximal phalanx in children. Clin. Orthop. 83 (1972) 151
Dougall, A. J.: Severe fractures of the neck of the radius in children. J. Roy. Coll. Surg. Edinb. 14 (1969) 220
Dunbar, J. S., H. F. Owen, M. B. Nogrady, R. McLeese: Obscure tibial fracture of infants; the toddler's fracture. Canad. Ass. Radiol. 15 (1964) 136–144
Ekgengren, K., Söderlund: Radiological findings in traumatic lesions of the pancreas in childhood. Fortschr. Röntgenstr. 105 (1966) 908–909
Eraklis, A. J.: Abdominal injury related to the trauma of birth. Pediatrics 39 (1967) 421–424
Everett, W. G.: Traumatic lumbar hernia. Injury 4 (1973) 354
Fagon, C. J., L. E. Swischuk: Traumatic lung paramediastinal pneumatoceles. Radiology 120 (1976) 11–18
Fahey, J. J., E. T. O'Brien: Fracture-separation of the medial humeral condyle in a child confused with fracture of the medial epicondyle. J. Bone Jt. Surg. 53 A (1971) 1102
Felman, A. H., B. M. Rodgers, J. L. Talbert: Traumatic paramediastinal air cyst. A case report. Pediatr. Radiol. 4 (1976) 120–121
Fielding, J. W.: Radio-ulnar union following displacement of the proximal radial epiphysis J. Bone Jt. Surg. 46 A (1964) 1277
Franken, E. A.: Spinal cord injury in the newborn infant. Pediatr. Radiol. 3 (1975) 101–104
Gaul, R. W.: Recurrent traumatic dislocation of the hip in children. Clin. Orthop. 90 (1973) 107
Geiger, H., F. Schmid: Geburtstraumatisch bedingte Metaphysenverletzungen. Fortschr. Med. 8 (1967) 321–323
Genieser, N. B., M. H. Becker: Head trauma in children. Radiol. Clin. N. Amer. 12 (1974) 333–342
Gooding, C. A., M. E. Hurwitz: Avulsed vertebral rim apophysis in a child. Pediatr. Radiol. 2 (1974) 265–268
Gordon, S. L., E. J. Dunn, T. H. Malin: Lateral collateral ligament ankle injuries in young athletic individuals. J. Trauma 16 (1976) 225–231
Grantham, S. A., H. A. Kiernan: Displaced olecranon fracture in children. J. Trauma 15 (1975) 197–204
Griffiths, S. C.: Fracture of odontoid process in children. J. Pediatr. Surg. 7 (1972) 680

Gruenagel, H. H., H. Junkat: Unfälle im Kindesalter. Dtsch. med. Wschr. 92 (1967) 141–146
Hakstian, R. W.: Cold induced digital epiphyseal necrosis in childhood. Canad. J. Surg. 15 (1972) 168
Hardacre, J. A., S. H. Nahigian, A. I. Froimson, J. E. Brown: Fractures of the lateral condyle of the humerus in children. J. Bone Jt. Surg. 53 A (1971) 1083
Hartung, K: Kindesmißhandlung. Fortschr. Med. 85 (1967) 753–754
Harwood-Nash, D. C.: Cranio-cerebral trauma in children. Curr. Probl. Radiol. 3 (1973) 3
Harwood-Nash, D. C., E. B. Hendrick, A. R. Hudson: The significance of skull fractures in children. A study of 1187 patients. Radiology 101 (1971) 151
Hecker, W. C., R. Daum: Zur Wiederherstellungschirurgie unfallverletzter Kinder. Kapsel 24 (1969) 867
Hegenbarth, R., K. D. Ebel: Roentgen findings in fractures of the vertebral column in childhood. Examination of 35 patients and its results. Pediatr. Radiol. 5 (1976) 34–39
Hendrick, E. B., D. C. Harwood-Nash, A. R. Hudson: Head injuries in children. Clin. Neurosurg. 11 (1965) 46
Henriksen, B.: Supracondylar fractures of the humerus in children. Acta Chir. Scand. 369 (1966) 1
Henriksen, B.: Isolated fractures of the proximal end of the radius in children, Acta Orthop. Scand. 40 (1969) 246
Hofmann, S.: Die Fraktur des Condylus radialis humeri im Kindesalter. Pädiat. Fortbild. Prax. 5 (1966) 445–456
Hofmann, S., P. Petrausch: Die Perforation des Magen-Darm-Kanals im Säuglings- und Kleinkindesalter. Dtsch. med. Wschr. 93 (1968) 1503–1509
Huittinen, V. M.: Lumbosacral nerve injury in fracture of the pelvis. Acta Chir. Scand. (Suppl.) (1972) 429
Hunter, G. A.: Non-traumatic displacement of the atlanto-axial joint. J. Bone Jt. Surg. 50B (1968) 44
Hutchinson, R. J., M. B. Nogrady: Late sequelae of renal trauma in the pediatric age group. J. Canad. Assoc. Radiol. 24 (1973) 3–11
Ingram, A. J., B. Bachynski: Fractures of the hip in children. J. Bone Jt. Surg. 15 A (1953) 867
Izant, R. J., W. R. Drucker: Duodenal obstruction due to intramural hematoma in children. J. Trauma (Baltimore) 4 (1964) 797–813
Jennett, W. B.: Head injuries in children. Dev. Med. Child. Neurol. 14 (1972) 137
Jokl, P.: Athletic injuries. Radiol. Clin. N. Amer. 11 (1973) 657–664
Jones, E. R. W., M. Esah: Displaced fractures of the neck of the radius in children. J. Bone Jt. Surg. 53 B (1971) 429
Kaplan, S. S., F. W. Reckling: Fracture separation ot the lower humeral epiphysis with medial displacement. J. Bone Jt. Surg. 53 A (1971) 1105
Kay, S. P., J. E. Hall: Fracture of the femoral neck in children and its complications. Clin. Orthop. 80 (1971) 53
Kempe, C. H., F. N. Silverman: The battered-child syndrome. J.A.M.A. 181 (1962) 105
Kilfoyle, R. M.: Fractures of the medial condyle and epicondyle of the elbow in children. Clin. Orthop. 41 (1965) 43
Kilfoyle, R. M., J. I. Foley, P. L. Norton: Spine and pelvic deformity in childhood adolescent paraplegia. J. Bone Jt. Surg. 47 A (1965) 659
Kilman, J. W., E. Charnock: Thoracic trauma in infancy and childhood. J. Trauma 9 (1969) 863–873
Kogutt, M. S., L. E. Swischuk, C. J. Fagan: Patterns of injury and significance of uncommon fractures in the battered child syndrome. Amer. J. Roentgenol. 121 (1974) 143–149
Kolihova, E., D. Obenbergerova, B. Apetaurova: Total severance of renal pedicle caused by blunt trauma in children. Pediatr. Radiol. 1 (1973) 59–62
Krenz, J., J. D. G. Troup: The structure of the pars interarticularis of the lower lumbar vertebrae. J. Bone Jt. Surg. 55 B (1973) 735
Kuner, E., S. Weller, H. Thoma: Epiphysiolysis traumatica. Dtsch. med. Wschr. 93 (1968) 1423–1427
Lam, S. F.: Fractures of the neck of the femur in children. J. Bone Jt. Surg. 53 A (1971) 1165
de Lange, C.: Congenital hypertrophy of the muscles, extrapyramidal motor disturbances and mental deficiency. Amer. J. Dis. Child. 48 (1934) 243–268
Lauber, I.: Verschluckte Fremdkörper im Verdauungstrakt des Kindes. Med. Welt 44 (1967) 2621–2627
Letts, R. M., D. Miller: Gunshot wounds of the extremities in children. J. Trauma 16 (1976) 807–811
Mahboubi, S., H. J. Kaufmann: Intramural duodenal hematoma in children. The role of the radiologist in its conservative management. Gastrointest. Radiol. 1 (1976) 167–171
Mau, H.: Rezidivierende Hüftgelenksluxation nach leichterem Trauma und Spontanluxation bei mongoloiden Hüften. Arch. orthop. Unfall-Chir. 63 (1968) 176–186
Maurer, G., E. Hipp, P. Bernett: Wirbelfrakturen im Wachstumsalter. Fortschr. Med. 88 (1970) 633–636
McCue, F. X., R. Honner, M. C. Johnson, J. H. Gieck: Athletic injuries of the proximal interphalangeal joint requiring surgical treatment. J. Bone Jt. Surg. 52 A (1970) 937
Miller, W. E.: Fractures of the hip in children from birth to adolescence. Clin. Orthop. 92 (1973) 155
Mustarde, J. C.: Plastic Surgery in Infancy and Childhood. W. B. Saunders Co., Philadephia 1971
Nelson, S. W.: Some important diagnostic and technical fundamentals in the radiology of trauma, with particular emphasis on skeletal trauma. Radiol. Clin. N. Amer. 4 (1966) 241–259
Neuhauser, E. B. D., T. Griscom: Aspiration pneumonitis in children. Progr. Pediatr. Radiol. 1 (1967) 256–293
Parker, J. J., V. G. Mikity, G. Jacobson: Traumatic pneumoperitoneum in the newborn. Amer. J. Roentgenol. 95 (1965) 203–207
Pearson, D. E., R. J. Mann: Traumatic hip dislocation in children. Clin. Orthop. 92 (1973) 189
Pellerin, D., M. Fortier-Beaulieu, J. Gueguen: The fate of swallowed foreign bodies. Experience of 1250 instances of subdiaphragmatic foreign bodies in children. Progr. Pediatr. Radiol. 2 (1969) 286–302
Pia, H. W.: Zur Pathogenese und Frühbehandlung der wachsenden Schädelfraktur im Kindesalter. Dtsch. Z. Nervenheilk. 172 (1954) 1–11
Pollen, A. G.: Fractures and Dislocations in Children. Churchill Livingstone, Edinburgh 1973
Quinby, W. C.: Fractures of the pelvis and associated injuries in children. J. Pediatr. Surg. 1 (1966) 353
Rang, M.: Children's Fractures. J. B. Lippincott Co., Philadelphia 1974
Ratliff, A. H. C.: Traumatic separation of the upper femoral epiphysis in young children. J. Bone Jt. Surg. 50 B (1968) 757
Ratliff, A. H. C.: Complications after fractures of the femoral neck in children and their treatment. J. Bone Jt. Surg. 52 B (1970) 175
Rigault, P., F. Iselin, J. Moreau, J. Judet: Fractures du col du fémur chez l'enfant. Rev. Chir. orthop. 52 (1966) 325–336
Rogers, L. F., S. Jones, A. R. Davis, G. Dietz: "Clipping injury" fracture of the epiphysis in the adolescent football player. An occult lesion of the knee. Amer. J. Roentgenol. 121 (1974) 69–78
Rothman, L., J. S. Rose, D. W. Laster, R. Quencer, M. Tenner: The spectrum of growing skull fracture in children. Pediatrics 57 (1976) 26–31
Salter, R. B., C. Zaltz: Anatomic investigations of the mechanism of injury and pathologic anatomy of "pulled elbow" in young children. Clin. Orthop. 77 (1971) 141
Schneider, R., J. J. Kaye, B. Gheiman: Adductor avulsive injuries near the symphysis pubis. Radiology 120 (1976) 567–569
Sharrard, W. J. W.: Paediatric Orthopaedics and Fractures. Blackwell, Oxford 1971
Siffert, R. S.: Displacement of the distal humeral epiphysis in the newborn infant. J. Bone Jt. Surg. 45 A (1963) 165
Silverman, F. N.: Unrecognized trauma in infants, the battered child syndrome, and the syndrome of Ambroise Tardieu. Radiology 104 (1972) 337
Sinclair, M. C., T. C. Moore, M. J. Asch: Penetrating abdominal injuries in children and adolescents. Amer. Surg. 41 (1975) 342
Solomon, A., F. Rosen: The aspect of trauma in the bone changes of congenital lues. Pediatr. Radiol. 3 (1975) 176–178
Sorsdahl, O. A., J. W. Powell: Cavitary pulmonary lesions following nonpenetrating chest trauma in children. Amer. J. Roentgenol. 95 (1965) 118–124
Spackman, T. J.: Pediatric trauma. Medical abuse of infants. Radiol. Clin. N. Amer. 11 (1973) 633–656
Stein F., S. L. Grabias, P. A. Deffer: Nerve injuries complicating Monteggia injuries. J. Bone Jt. Surg. 53 A (1971) 1432–1436
Sterioff, S., R. J. Izant, L. Persky: Perineal injuries in children. J. Trauma 9 (1969) 56–61

Stern, E. W., R. W. Rand: Birth injuries to the cord. Amer. J. Obstet. Gynecol. 78 (1959) 498
Stockhausen, J.: Kindesmißhandlung und ärztliche Schweigepflicht. Dtsch. Ärztebl. 64 (1967) 837–838, 65 (1968) 541
Stucchi, C. A., R. Faggioni: Jeux interdits et lésions oculaires. Schweiz. med. Wschr. 99 (1969) 254–258
Swischuk, L. E.: Spine and spinal cord trauma in the battered child syndrome. Radiology 92 (1969) 733–738
Tachdjian, M. O.: Pediatric Orthopedics. W. B. Saunders Co., Philadelphia 1972
Theodorou, S. D.: Dislocation of the head of the radius associated with fracture of the upper end of the ulna in children. J. Bone Jt. Surg. 51 B (1969) 700
Tompkins, D. G.: Anterior Monteggia fracture. J. Bone Jt. Surg. 53 A (1971) 1109–1114
Truesdell, E. D.: Birth Fractures and Epiphyseal Displacements. Hoeber, New York 1917
Vassy, L. E., R. L. Klecker, E. Koch, T. S. Morse: Traumatic gastric perforation in children from blunt trauma. J. Trauma 15 (1975) 184–186
Wadsworth, T. G.: Injuries of the capitular (lateral humeral condylar) epiphysis. Clin. Orthop. 85 (1972) 127
Weiner, D. S., H. W. O'dell: Fractures of the hip in children. J. Trauma 9 (1969) 62–76
Willich, E.: Röntgendiagnostik der Schädelfrakturen im Kindesalter. Fortschr. Röntgenstr. 109 (1968) 653–661
Wilson, D. W.: Traumatic dislocation of the hip in children. J. Trauma 6 (1966) 739–743
Wiltse, L. L., E. H. Widell, D. W. Jackson: Fatigue fracture. Basic lesion in isthmic spondylolisthesis. J. Bone Jt. Surg. 57 A (1975) 17–22
Wortzman, G., F. P. Dewar: Rotary fixation of the atlanto-axial joint. Radiology 90 (1968) 479
Young, L. W., J. T. Adams: Roentgenographic findings in localized trauma to the pancreas in children. Amer. J. Roentgenol. 101 (1967) 639–648
Zelson, C., et al.: The incidence of skull fractures underlying cephalhematomas in newborn infants. Pediatrics 85 (1974) 371
Zolczer, L., Kazar G., J. Manninger, E. Nagy: Fracture of the femoral neck in adolescents. Injury 4 (1973) 41

Chapter 13

Allgöwer, M., G. Segmüller: Biomechanische Prinzipien bei der Metallverwendung am Knochen. *In:* Handbuch der Plastischen Chirurgie, Vol. I/16, *E. Gohrbandt, J. Gabka, A. Berndorfer* (eds); de Gruyter, Berlin 1965
Allgöwer, M., R. Ehrsam, R. Ganz, P. Matter, S. M. Perren: Klinische Erfahrungen mit der neuen Kompressionsplatte DCP. Acta orthop. scand., Suppl. 125, 1969
Beabout, J. W.: Radiology of total hip arthroplasty. Radiol. Clin. N. Amer. 12 (1975) 3–19
Brown, C. S., W. J. Knickerbocker: Radiologic studies in the investigations of the causes of total hip replacement failures. J. Canad. Assoc. Radiol. 24 (1973) 245–253
Charnley, J.: Fracture of femoral prostheses in total hip replacement. A clinical study. Clin. Orthop. 111 (1975) 105–120
Clarke, I. C., T. Gruen, M. Matos, H. C. Amstutz: Improved methods for quantitative radiographic evaluation with particular reference to total-hip arthroplasty. Clin. Orthop. 121 (1976) 83–91
Contzen, H., F. Straumann, E. Paschke: Grundlagen der Alloplastik mit Metallen und Kunststoffen. Thieme, Stuttgart 1967
Danis, R.: Théorie et pratique de l'ostéosynthèse. Masson, Paris 1949
Debrunner, A. M., O. Cech: Biomechanik der Osteosynthese pertrochanterer Frakturen. Z. Orthop. 106 (1969) 516
DeLee, J. G., J. Charnley: Radiological demarcation of cemented sockets in total hip replacement. Clin. Orthop. 121 (1976) 20–32
Dolinskas, C., R. E. Campbell, R. H. Rothman: The painful Charnley total hip replacement. Amer. J. Roentgenol. 121 (1974) 61–68
Frank, E., H. Zitter: Metallische Implantate in der Knochenchirurgie. Springer, Wien 1971
Freedman, M. T.: Radiologic aspects for femoral head replacements and cup mold arthroplasties. Radiol. Clin. N. Amer. 12 (1975) 45–56
Ganz, R., J. Brennwald, W. Hunter, S. M. Perren: The recovery of medullary circulation after osteotomy and internal fixation of the rabbit tibia. Europ. Surg. Res. 2 (1970) 106
Gilula, L. A., T. W. Staple: Miniature atlas of total hip prostheses. Radiol. Clin. N. Amer. 12 (1975) 21–44
Gilula, L. A., T. W. Staple: Radiology of recently developed total knee prostheses. Radiol. Clin. N. Amer. 12 (1975) 57–66
Herzog, K.: Nagelung der Tibiaschaftbrücke mit einem starren Nagel. Dtsch. Z. Chir. 276 (1953) 227
Kaushal, S. P., J. O. Galante, R. McKenna, F. Bachmann: Complications following total knee replacement. Clin. Orthop. 121 (1976) 181–187
Kuner, E. H., F. Weyand: Indikation zur operativen Behandlung kindlicher Frakturen. Act. traumatol. 2 (1971) 63
Kuner, E. H., F. Weyand, B. Domres: Zur Leistungsfähigkeit autologer Spongiosa bei der Behandlung knöcherner Defekte. Mschr. Unfallheilk. 75 (1972) 189
Küntscher, G.: Die Marknagelung von Knochenbrüchen. Arch. klin. Chir. 200 (1940) 443
Lane, W. A.: The Operative Treatment of Fractures, 2nd ed. Medical Publishing, London 1914
v. Lüdinghausen, M., P. Meister, J. Probst: Osteosynthese und Metallose. Med. Welt 21 (1970) 1913
Maatz, R.: Über die Formschlüssigkeit bei der Küntschernagelung. Zbl. Chir. 70 (1943) 1641
Marmor, L.: Stress fracture of the pubic ramus simulating a loose total replacement. Clin. Orthop. 121 (1976) 103–104
Müller, M. E.: Biomechanische Fehlleistungen. Langenbecks Arch. klin. Chir. 329 (1971) 1144
Müller, M. E., M. Allgöwer, H. Willenegger: Technik der operativen Frakturenbehandlung, Springer, Berlin 1963
Müller, M. E., M. Allgöwer, H. Willenegger: Manual der Osteosynthese. Springer, Berlin 1969
Mullins, M. F., R. N. Sutton, G. S. Lodwick: Complications of total hip replacement. A roentgen evaluation. Amer. J. Roentgenol. 121 (1974) 55–60
Pauweis, F.: Grundriß einer Biomechanik der Frakturheilung. Verh. dtsch. orthop. Ges. 34 (1940) 62
Perren, S. M., A. Huggler, M. Russenberger, F. Straumann, A. E. Müller, M. Allgöwer: A method of measuring the change in compresson applied to living cortical bone. Acta orthop. scand., Suppl. 125 (1969) 5
Rhinelander, F. W.: Some aspects of the microcirculation of healing bone. Clin. Orthop. 40 (1965) 12
Roberts, J. B.: Management of fractures and fracture complications of the femoral shaft using the ASIF compression plate. J. Trauma 17 (1977) 20–28
Salvati, E. A., V. Chuem Im, P. Aglietti, P. D. Wilson: Radiology of total hip replacements. Clin. Orthop. 121 (1976) 74–82
Schenk, R.: Personal communication, 1972
Schenk, R., H. Willenegger: Zum histologischen Bild der sogenannten Primärheilung der Knochenkompakta nach experimentellen Osteotomien am Hund. Experientia 19 (1963) 593
Scheuba, G.: Korrosionsgefahr bei der Osteosynthese subtrochanterer Oberschenkelfrakturen. Mschr. Unfallheilk. 72 (1969) 388
Schuster, J.: Entstehung von Metallbrüchen bei Osteosynthesen. Fortschr. Med. 90 (1972) 227
Spirig, B.: Die Diagnose der Achsenfehler der unteren Extremität. Z. Unfallmed. Berufskr. 59 (1966) 11
Weller, S., E. H. Kuner: Das Röntgenbild bei der Beurteilung der Knochenbruchheilung. Hippokrates 39 (1968) 98
Wieser, C.: Die primäre Knochenbruchheilung und ihre Störung im Röntgenbild. Langenbecks. Arch. klin. Chir. 308 (1964) 434
Wieser, C., M. Allgöwer: Die Beurteilung der Knochenheilung nach stabiler Osteosynthese im Röntgenbild. Radiol. clin. 31 (1962) 297
Willenegger, H., S. M. Perren, R. Schenk: Primäre und sekundäre Knochenbruchheilung. Chirurg. 42 (1971) 241

Chapter 14

Barber, J. W.: Delayed bone and joint changes following electrical injury. Radiology 99 (1971) 49–53
Becker, T.: Krebs und Unfall. Barth, München 1966
Betzler, H. J.: Weichteilsarkom und Trauma in der Unfallbegutachtung. Enke, Stuttgart 1964

Birzle, H., W. Vogel, C. Mittermayer, P. Ostendorf: Lungenveränderungen im traumatischen Schock. Radiologe 13 (1973) 192–195

Böhler, L.: The Treatment of Fractures. Grune & Stratton, New York 1958

Brinn, L. B., J. E. Moseley: Bone changes following electrical injury: case report and review of literature. Amer. J. Roentgenol. 97 (1966) 682–686

Brunner, A.: Röntgenkontrolle nach Thoraxoperationen: *In:* Lehrbuch der Röntgendiagnostik, Vol. III, *H. R. Schinz, W. E.* Baensch, E. Friedl, E. Uehlinger (eds.). Thieme, Stuttgart 1952 (p. 2549).

Bücheler, E., E. Raschke, R. Felix: Abszeß in der Bursa omentalis nach traumatischer Pankreasruptur. Fortschr. Röntgenstr. 107 (1967) 293–296

Burri, C.: Post Traumatic Osteomyelitis. H. Huber, Bern 1975

Dennis, D. L., C. G. Peterson, W. S. Fletcher: Candida septicemia in the severely traumatized patient. J. Trauma 8 (1968) 177–185

Ehalt, W.: Unfallchirurgie im Röntgenbilde. Maudrich, Wien 1952

Featherstone, D. F.: Sports Injuries, Their Prevention and Treatment. John Wright & Sons, Ltd. Bristol 1957

Feldman, F., K. Ellis, W. M. Green: Fat embolism syndrome. Radiology 114 (1975) 535–542

Geiser, M.: Die radiologische Beurteilung der Frakturheilung nach Fixation von Schaftfrakturen mit metallischen Implantaten. Radiol. clin. biol. 36 (1967) 65–81

Gondos, D.: Tennis elbow. A re-evaluation. Amer. J. Roentgenol. 79 (1958) 684

Grauberger, W., H. Scherer, W. Theisinger: Meniskusverletzungen. Diagnostische Leistungsfähigkeit der Arthrographie. Fortschr. Med. 87 (1969) 1350–1352

Groh, H.: Überlastungsschäden am Bewegungsapparat beim Sport. Hippokrates 40 (1969) 870–873

Gumbert, J. L., P. M. Waitt, F. W. Taylor: Gunshot wounds of the abdomen: evaluation of the treatment. Surgery (St. Louis) 59 (1966) 376–380

Günther, E., R. Hymmen: Unfallbegutachtung. de Gruyter, Berlin 1968

Gurdjian, E. S., L. M. Patrick: Protection of the head and neck in sports. J.A.M.A. 182 (1962) 509

Heberer, G., H. J. Castrup: Die Ösophago-Trachealfistel nach stumpfem Thoraxtrauma. Thoraxchirurgie 12 (1965) 384–393

Hipp, E., G. Thiemel: Zur Diagnose und Differentialdiagnose der aseptischen Epiphysennekrose, der Osteochondrosis dissecans und der Chondromatose am Ellenbogen. Fortschr. Med. 86 (1968) 6–10

Hupe, K.: Fettembolie. Fortschr. Med. 85 (1967) 663–666

Jonasch, E.: Erkennung und Beurteilung der Meniskusverletzung des Kniegelenkes durch das gewöhnliche Röntgenbild. Hefte z. Unfallheilkunde, No. 90, Berlin 1967

Kouba, R.: Preßluftschäden bei Steinarbeitern. Ergebnisse der Röntgenkontrolle nach vier Jahren. Zbl. Arbeitsmed. 17 (1967) 67–73

Lorenz, D.: Verletzungen großer Körperhöhlen. Wehrmed. Mschr. 10 (1966) 286–295

Marx, H. H.: Gutachten-Fibel. Thieme, Stuttgart 1967

McLaughlin, H. L.: Trauma. W. B. Saunders Co., Philadelphia 1959

Mills, M.: Pulmonary effects of nonthoracic trauma – The clinical syndrome. J. Trauma 8 (1968) 651

Mittermayer, C., W. Vogel, H. Burchardi, H. Birzle, K. Wiemers, W. Sandritter: Pulmonale Mikrothrombosierung als Ursache der respiratorischen Insuffizienz bei Verbrauchskoagulopathie (Schocklunge). Dtsch. med. Wschr. 95 (1970) 1999–2002

Morton, J. R., G. L. Jordan: Traumatic duodenal injuries J. Trauma 8 (1968) 127–139

Nietlispach, L.: Besonderheiten beim stumpfen Bauchtrauma. Gastroenterologia 103 (1965) 209–219

Peiper, H.-J., K. H. Wellmer: Zur Wertigkeit bei der Versorgung von Kombinationsverletzungen. Chirurg 38 (1967) 448–454

Psenner, L.: Über Schädelveränderungen nach alten Traumen. Wien. klin. Wschr. 80 (1968) 921–925

Rauber, A.: Ein wenig bekanntes Röntgensymptom bei älteren Meniskusaffektionen. Z. Unfallmed. Berufskr. 37 (1944) 168–172

Rosenkranz, K. A.: Die traumatische Herzschädigung. Fortschr. Med. 87 (1969) 1437–1440

Russe, O.: Die Entwicklung eines interventrikulären Shunts als Spätkomplikation einer Herzverletzung. Wien. klin. Wschr. 80 (1968) 517–520

Salter, R. B.: Textbook of Disorders and Injuries of the Musculoskeletal System. Williams & Wilkins, Baltimore 1970

Schinz, H. R.: Zirkulatorische Knochenveränderungen. *In:* Lehrbuch der Röntgendiagnostik, 5th ed. Vol. I, *H. R. Schinz, W. E. Friedl, E. Uehlinger* (eds.). Thieme, Stuttgart 1952 (p. 222)

Schlosser, V.: Traumatologie. Thieme, Stuttgart 1968

Schlosser, V., K. Körner: Die Pseudarthrosen langer Röhrenknochen im Lichte moderner Behandlungsverfahren. Fortschr. Med. 85 (1967) 239–242

Schmidt, H. D., K. Spohn, M. Auerbach: Zur Klinik der Pankreaspseudozysten. Fortschr. Med. 88 (1970) 461–465

Scholler, K. L., W. Vogel, K. Wiemers, H. Burchardi, J. Groh-Bruch: Die Langzeitbeatmung in der Behandlung von Thoraxverletzten. Dtsch. med. Wschr. 93 (1968) 747–753

Schulte-Brinkmann, W.: Zur Röntgendiagnostik der Milzzysten. Dtsch. med. Wschr. 93 (1968)

Schuster, J.: Gefahren bei Osteosynthesen. Fortschr. Med. 88 (1970) 580–582

Stutz, E.: Beitrag zum Problem Krebs und Trauma. Strahlentherapie 95 (1954) 416–423

Tauber, R., H. Kübler, H. Pelzl: Richtlinien zur Frakturbehandlung. Fortschr. Med. 88 (1970) 603–604, 606–609, 648–651

Theisinger, W., P. Bernett: Sportverletzungen. Fortschr. Med. 88 (1970) 62–66

Thorndike, A.: Athletic Injuries, Prevention, Diagnosis and Treatment. 4th ed. Lea & Febiger, Philadelphia 1956

Vogel, W.: Die Bedeutung der disseminierten intravasalen Gerinnung in der terminalen Lungenstrombahn für die postoperative und posttraumatische respiratorische Insuffizienz. Habilitationsschrift, Freiburg 1972

Webb, W. R.: Pulmonary complications of non-thoracic trauma: summary of the national research council conference. J. Trauma 9 (1969) 700–711

Wegener, K., H. Wesch, H. Kampmann: Retikuloendotheliales System und Thorotrastose nach diagnostischer Angiographie. Dtsch. med. Wschr. 96 (1971) 1977–1981

Weller, S., E. Kuner: Das Röntgenbild bei der Beurteilung der Knochenbruchheilung. Hippokrates (1968) 98–101

Wenz, W.: Thorotrast-Tumoren. Experimentelle Untersuchungen zum Dosis-Wirkungsproblem. Fortschr. Med. 83 (1965) 423–426

Wilhelm, K., F. L. Ruéff, R. Bedacht, M. Wilhelm: Die Frakturheilung im Röntgenbild bei operativen und konservativen Behandlungsmethoden. Radiologe 9 (1969) 209–214

Wilson, R. F., J. P. Tagett, J. P. Pucelik, A. J. Walt: Pancreatic trauma. J. Trauma 7 (1967) 643–651

Wissinger, H. A., E, J. McClain, J. H. Boyes: Turret exostosis. Ossifying hematoma of the phalanges. J. Bone Jt. Surg. 48 (1966) 105–110

Index

G

H